Clinical Use of Drugs in Patients with Kidney and Liver Disease

Edited by

ROBERT J. ANDERSON, M.D.

Associate Professor of Medicine,
Division of Renal Diseases,
University of Colorado School of Medicine,
Denver, Colorado

ROBERT W. SCHRIER, M.D.

Professor and Chairman,
Department of Medicine,
University of Colorado School of Medicine,
Denver, Colorado

Drug Reference Tables edited by

JOHN G. GAMBERTOGLIO, Pharm. D.

Assistant Clinical Professor of Pharmacy,
University of California, San Francisco

1981 W. B. SAUNDERS COMPANY/Philadelphia/London/Toronto/Sydney

W. B. Saunders Company: West Washington Square
Philadelphia, PA 19105

1 St. Anne's Road
Eastbourne, East Sussex BN21 3UN, England

1 Goldthorne Avenue
Toronto, Ontario M8Z 5T9, Canada

9 Waltham Street
Artarmon, N.S.W. 2064, Australia

Library of Congress Cataloging in Publication Data

Main entry under title:

Clinical use of drugs in patients with kidney and liver disease.

1. Drugs—Side effects. 2. Kidneys—Diseases—Complications and sequelae. 3. Liver—Diseases—Complications and sequelae. I. Anderson, Robert James, 1943– II. Schrier, Robert W. III. Gambertoglio, John G. [DNLM: 1. Drug therapy—Adverse effects. 2. Kidney diseases—Complications. 3. Kidney diseases—Drug therapy. 4. Liver diseases—Complications. 5. Liver diseases—Drug therapy. WJ 300 C641]

RM302.5.C56 616.6′1 80–54856

ISBN 0–7216–1239–3 AACR2

Clinical Use of Drugs in Patients with Kidney and Liver Disease ISBN 0-7216-1239-3

Last digit is the print number: 9 8 7 6 5 4 3 2 1

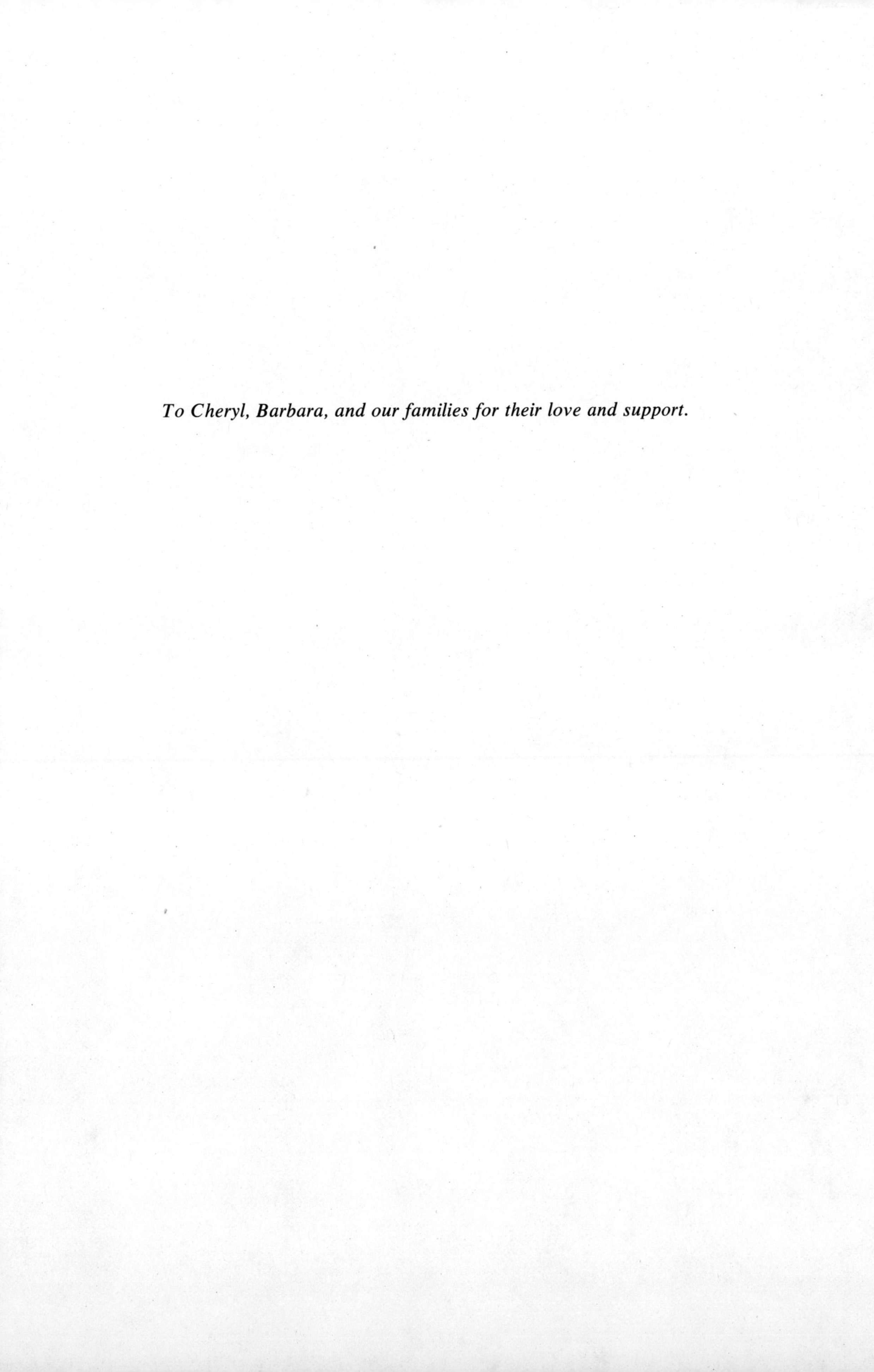

To Cheryl, Barbara, and our families for their love and support.

Contributors

Melton B. Affrime, Pharm.D.

Assistant Professor of Medicine and Pharmacology, Likoff Cardiovascular Institute of Hahnemann Medical College and Hospital, Philadelphia, Pennsylvania.

Analgesics, Sedatives, and Sedative Hypnotics; Cardiac Glycosides and Anti-Arrhythmic Drugs

Robert J. Anderson, M.D.

Associate Professor of Medicine, Division of Renal Diseases, University of Colorado Health Sciences Center, Denver, Colorado.

Mechanisms of Adverse Drug Reactions; Drug-Induced Chronic Renal Failure

William M. Bennett, M.D.

Professor of Medicine and Head, Division of Nephrology, University of Oregon Health Sciences Center, Portland, Oregon. Attending Physician, University Hospital; Head, Dialysis Unit, Portland Veterans Administration Hospital, Portland, Oregon.

Altering Drug Dose in Patients with Diseases of the Kidney and Liver

Pravit Cadnapaphornchai, M.D.

Associate Professor of Internal Medicine, Wayne State University School of Medicine, Detroit, Michigan. Chief of Nephrology, Detroit Receiving Hospital, Detroit, Michigan.

Drug-Induced Fluid and Electrolyte Disorders

Jack W. Coburn, M.D.

Professor of Medicine, UCLA School of Medicine, Los Angeles, California. Director of Training in Nephrology, Veterans Administration Wadsworth Medical Center, Los Angeles, California.

Drug-Induced Immunologic-Renal Disease

Robert E. Cronin, M.D.

Assistant Professor of Medicine, University of Texas Southwestern Medical School, Dallas, Texas. Staff Physician, Dallas Veterans Administration Hospital, Dallas, Texas.

Antimicrobial Agent Nephrotoxicity

Antoine M. De Torrenté, M.D.

Privat-Docent, University of Geneva Medical School, Geneva, Switzerland. Associate Chief of Medicine, Hôpital Communal, La Chaux-de-Fonds, Switzerland.

Drug-Induced Chronic Renal Failure

LAWRENCE E. FEINBERG, M.D.

Assistant Professor of Medicine, University of Colorado Health Sciences Center, Denver, Colorado. Attending Physician, University of Colorado Medical Center, Denver, Colorado.

Drug-Induced Hepatitis

CURT R. FREED, M.D.

Associate Professor of Medicine and Pharmacology, University of Colorado Health Sciences Center, Denver, Colorado. Attending Physician, Denver General Hospital and Veterans Administration Hospital, Denver, Colorado.

Clinical Pharmacology for the Clinician

JOSEPH GAL, Ph.D.

Assistant Professor of Pharmacology, University of Colorado Health Sciences Center, Denver, Colorado.

Clinical Use of Drug Assays

JOHN G. GAMBERTOGLIO, Pharm.D.

Assistant Clinical Professor of Pharmacy, University of California, San Francisco, School of Medicine. Attending Clinical Pharmacist, Kidney Transplant Service, University of California Hospital, San Francisco, California.

Neuropsychiatric Drug Use; Drug Reference Tables

SERAFINO GARELLA, M.D.

Associate Professor of Medicine, Brown University Program in Medicine, Providence, Rhode Island. Director, Division of Renal Diseases, Rhode Island Hospital, Providence, Rhode Island.

Use of Dialysis and Hemoperfusion in Drug Overdose

JOHN G. GERBER, M.D.

Assistant Professor of Medicine and Pharmacology, University of Colorado Health Sciences Center, Denver, Colorado. Attending Clinical Pharmacologist, Colorado General Hospital, Denver, Colorado.

Antihypertensive Agents and Diuretics

L. MICHAEL GLODE, M.D.

Assistant Professor of Medicine, University of Colorado Health Sciences Center, Denver, Colorado.

Cytotoxic and Immunosuppressive Drugs

WILLIAM L. HENRICH, M.D.

Assistant Professor of Internal Medicine, University of Texas Southwestern Medical School, Dallas, Texas. Chief, Home Dialysis Service, Dallas Veterans Administration Hospital, Dallas, Texas.

Nephrotoxicity of Heavy Metals, Organic Solvents, Radiographic Contrast Agents, and Prostaglandin Inhibitors

DAVID W. KNUTSON, M.D.

Associate Professor of Medicine, University of Rochester School of Medicine and Dentistry, Rochester, New York. Director, Nephrology Laboratory Research, Strong Memorial Hospital, Rochester, New York.

Drug-Induced Immunologic-Renal Disease

ROGER M. LAUER, M.D.

Lecturer, Department of Psychiatry, University of California, San Francisco, School of Medicine, San Francisco, California.

Neuropsychiatric Drug Use

JOEL S. LEVINE, M.D.

Assistant Professor of Medicine, Division of Gastroenterology, University of Colorado Health Sciences Center, Denver, Colorado.

Drug-Induced Cholestasis

JONATHAN A. LORCH, M.D.

Assistant Professor of Clinical Medicine, Columbia University College of Physicians and Surgeons, New York, New York. Attending Physician, Division of Nephrology, St. Luke's-Roosevelt Hospital Center, New York, New York.

Use of Dialysis and Hemoperfusion in Drug Overdose

DAVID T. LOWENTHAL, M.D.

Professor of Medicine and Pharmacology, and Director, Division of Clinical Pharmacology, Likoff Cardiovascular Institute of Hahnemann Medical College and Hospital, Philadelphia, Pennsylvania.

Analgesics, Sedatives, and Sedative Hypnotics; Cardiac Glycosides and Anti-Arrhythmic Drugs

DAVID M. MELIKIAN, Pharm.D.

Assistant Professor of Clinical Pharmacology, University of Colorado Health Sciences Center, Denver, Colorado. Assistant Director of Clinical Programs, University of Colorado Medical Center, Denver, Colorado.

Treatment of Infectious Complications

ALAN S. NIES, M.D.

Professor of Medicine and Pharmacology, University of Colorado Health Sciences Center, Denver, Colorado. Attending Physician, University of Colorado Medical Center, Denver, Colorado.

Clinical Use of Drug Assays

RASHMI V. PATWARDHAN, M.D.

Assistant Professor of Medicine, Vanderbilt University School of Medicine, Nashville, Tennessee. Attending Physician—Gastroenterology, Vanderbilt University Medical Center and Veterans Administration Hospital, Nashville, Tennessee.

Drug Use in Patients with Liver Disease

STEVEN SCHENKER, M.D.

Professor of Medicine and Biochemistry, and Director of Gastroenterology, Vanderbilt University School of Medicine. Attending Physician, Veterans Administration Hospital, Nashville, Tennessee

Drug Use in Patients with Liver Disease

ROBERT W. SCHRIER, M.D.

Professor and Chairman, Department of Medicine, University of Colorado Health Sciences Center, Denver, Colorado. Staff Physician, University of Colorado Medical Center, Denver, Colorado.

Mechanisms of Adverse Drug Reactions

JAMES C. STEIGERWALD, M.D.

Associate Professor of Medicine, University of Colorado Health Sciences Center, Denver, Colorado. Attending Physician, University of Colorado Medical Center, Denver, Colorado.

Treatment of Musculoskeletal Disorders

SAADI TAHER, M.D.

Associate Professor of Internal Medicine, Wayne State University School of Medicine, Detroit, Michigan. Attending Nephrologist, Hutzel Hospital, Detroit, Michigan.

Drug-Induced Fluid and Electrolyte Disorders

Preface

Patients with diseases of the kidney and liver are susceptible to multiple medical problems, not only hypertension and heart disease but also a variety of other afflictions, and are therefore the potential recipients of numerous pharmacologic agents. In a recent survey of 1023 patients on chronic maintenance hemodialysis, we found that the mean number of prescribed drugs per patient was 7.7. Moreover, 24 per cent of all patients were receiving 10 or more medications.

Most drugs in common use are excreted at least partly by the kidney. Many are metabolized in part by the liver. For patients in whom function of either organ is impaired, the administration of drugs must be modified appropriately if the therapy is not to prove worse than the disease. The combination of drug administration and impaired function of the kidneys or liver may lead to significant drug accumulation and potential toxicity. Surveillance studies and clinical observations confirm that the presence of kidney and liver disease leads to a high frequency of adverse drug reactions. Careful selection and appropriate dosage modifications are necessary when administering drugs to patients with kidney and liver diseases.

This book has been developed to provide the clinician with information needed to insure safe, efficacious drug therapy in such patients. To this end, the book can be broadly divided into four sections. The first four chapters deal with basic pharmacologic principles necessary for understanding the methods of altering drug dosage in patients with kidney and liver diseases. Chapters 5 through 12 deal with drug-induced disorders of the kidneys and liver. Chapters 13 through 20 discuss use of specific pharmacologic agents for patients with kidney and liver disease in numerous clinical settings. Finally, the last section of the book provides an appendix of tabular data on the pharmacologic properties and effects of kidney and liver disease on the disposition of several commonly used drugs.

We would like to acknowledge the superb administrative and secretarial support of Loretta Durkin who contributed in so many ways during the course of the writing and publication of this book.

In closing, our hope is that *Clinical Use of Drugs in Kidney and Liver Disease* may assist physicians in their goal of enhancing patients' health by the knowledgeable and judicious use of the many effective but potentially toxic drugs.

Robert J. Anderson, M.D.
Robert W. Schrier, M.D.

Contents

Chapter 1

Clinical Pharmacology for the Clinician

by

Curt R. Freed

Liver and kidney disease complicate the task of prescribing drugs and evaluating therapeutic response. Because the liver and the kidneys are the organs responsible for biotransformation and elimination of most drugs, any reduction in their functional status may prolong the action of a drug and may, therefore, require the physician to reduce maintenance doses. The high metabolic activity of the liver and the kidneys and the concentrating ability of the nephron add a second complication. During drug metabolism and elimination, toxic quantities of parent drug or metabolites may accumulate and cause organ damage. A third kind of problem is caused by systemic effects of organ disease. Both liver and kidney disease can alter the distribution and protein binding of drugs in the body. Renal disease, for example, is accompanied by increased circulating organic acids that can displace phenytoin (Dilantin) from plasma proteins and change the therapeutic plasma drug level.

Plasma drug levels have been shown to correlate with clinical effects for many drugs and have made therapeutics easier, especially for the patient with liver or kidney disease who has impaired drug elimination. Plasma drug levels are discussed in Chapter 4. The empiric nature of the "therapeutic range," however, must be stressed. Definite guidelines for therapeutic blood levels in patients with organ failure are not available for many drugs, since variability in clinical response is large in this population. Still, plasma levels are established in renal disease for some drugs, such as phenytoin and digoxin. Nevertheless, changing the dose of a drug because of reduced metabolism by the liver or diminished elimination by the kidney is an imperfect science. Even for a well-studied example like digoxin in the patient with renal failure, guidelines for changing dose are approximate. The best and easiest technique is simply to decrease the maintenance dose by half for the patient with moderate to severe renal impairment and then use plasma level measurements to regulate dose more precisely. Similarly, patients with cardiac or liver disease have a reduction in hepatic clearance of lidocaine. The severity of the reduction is impossible to gauge clinically and must be assessed by plasma drug level measurement.

Pharmacokinetics is the formal science that describes how loading and maintenance doses can be predicted from plasma drug concentrations. The concepts of volume of distribution, rate of metabolism, drug clearance, and drug half-life are basic for understanding pharmacokinetics and will be explained for both the normal patient and the patient with kidney or liver disease to show how organ pathology changes drug requirements. The overlying theme of the pharmacokinetics discussion is that there are two goals for drug dosing. The first is to achieve a therapeutic blood level with a loading dose and the second is to sustain that amount of drug with a maintenance dose. While liver and kidney failure may occasionally change the body load of drug necessary to get a clinical effect, disease in these organs most often slows drug elimination. Because maintenance doses simply replace the drug lost during metabolism and excretion, reduced elimination of drug means lowered maintenance doses. The use of diazepam (Valium) in patients with cirrhosis illustrates this point. Very large doses of drug may be needed to blunt ethanol withdrawal, but once the desired therapeutic effect is reached, maintenance doses may not be needed at all because drug elimination is so impaired in the cirrhotic liver.[1] The physician who prescribes a high maintenance dose of diazepam will unwittingly overdose the cirrhotic patient.

DRUG ABSORPTION AND BIOAVAILABILITY

The speed and intensity of a drug effect depend on the route of administration. Drugs given by intravenous bolus usually have immediate effects, while subcutaneous depot preparations, such as testosterone in oil or phenothiazines in wax, offer drug effects for days or weeks. Oral and intramuscular administration offer an intermediate onset of action. The primary advantage of intramuscular dosing is that the drug bypasses the gut and liver so that bioavailability may be improved. However, for some drugs, such as phenytoin and chlordiazepoxide, the intramuscular route is less effective than the oral route because the drugs are insoluble at tissue pH and form a dense precipitate in the muscle. Because chlordiazepoxide absorption from the site may be erratic and incomplete, the intramuscular route should not be used.[2]

Sometimes local application of drug is appropriate and effective. The best examples are inhaled bronchodilators, poorly absorbed antibiotics like neomycin for gut sterilization, and drugs used in ophthalmology. While efforts have been made to infuse cancer chemotherapeutic drugs selectively into arteries leading to solid tumors, most drug targeting has been of limited success.

Drugs can be systemically administered by routes as diverse as sublingual, rectal, and dermal. The problem with each of these routes is that the practical absorptive surface area is small. Only potent, lipid-soluble drugs, such as nitroglycerin, are suitable for direct absorption from the mouth. For nitroglycerin, this route is nearly equivalent to intravenous dosing, since the drug rapidly crosses the oral epithelium and also bypasses the liver where much of the drug would otherwise be destroyed. It is for this reason that sublingual nitroglycerin is more predictable and more potent than nitrate preparations that are swallowed. The skin can absorb a number of drugs although the diffusion barrier across keratin is much greater than across the oral mucosa. While the skin offers a potentially large surface area, in practical terms it is limited because of uncertainty about rate and extent of drug absorption. Nitroglycerin in the form of nitrol paste can be successfully administered through the skin. More often the skin may be an undesired absorptive surface. Gamma benzene hexachloride (Kwell) treatment for scabies can lead to some systemic absorption; convulsions and aplastic anemia have been reported from its use.[3] Rectal administration is not usually desirable. While some drugs, such as prochlorperazine (Compazine), given for vomiting are effective by the rectal route, others, such as theophylline, are erratically absorbed.[4]

The oral route is generally effective and safe for most drugs. Since normal nutrition requires absorption of ionic as well as lipid-soluble foods, most drugs find an absorption site during intestinal transit. Obviously, a drug like ethanol, which is miscible but also highly lipid soluble, can be absorbed from any part of the gastrointestinal tract so that drug absorption is rapid and complete. Phenytoin is insoluble in the acid pH of the stomach but has limited solubility in the more alkaline pH of the small intestine so that absorption begins there. Because some drug must be absorbed before additional drug can dissolve, absorption is slow and takes place over 6 to 8 hours. In patients with normal gastrointestinal motility 80 per cent of a dose is eventually absorbed. If motility is increased during an episode of gastroenteritis, phenytoin absorption may fall and plasma drug levels can drop to the subtherapeutic range. Convulsions may occur. Ethanol and phenytoin represent extremes of oral absorption; most drugs are absorbed with peak levels in less than 2 hours and total absorption is usually greater than 80 per cent.

An important constraint on effective oral absorption is the chemical stability of the drug being administered. Penicillin G is unstable in the acid pH of the stomach and will be hydrolyzed. A semisynthetic preparation such as penicillin V-K is resistant to acid hydrolysis and so is popular as an oral penicillin. Because

TABLE 1–1. DRUGS WITH EXTENSIVE FIRST-PASS METABOLISM

Drugs	Useful Orally	Comments
Amitriptyline	++++	Active metabolite
L-Dopa	++++	Can block catabolism with carbidopa
Isoproterenol	0	
Lidocaine	0	> 90% metabolism; toxic metabolite
Meperidine	++	Toxic metabolite
Metoprolol	++++	
Morphine	0	
Organic nitrates	+	Nearly complete catabolism
Propranolol	++++	

about 30 per cent of penicillin G is absorbed, an oral dose three times larger than that of penicillin V-K can still be effective, and economy could dictate such use of a cheaper though less stable drug.

A major problem with oral administration of drugs is metabolism occurring in the gastrointestinal mucosa and in the liver. This so-called "first-pass effect" results from the fact that all orally absorbed drug must enter the liver via the portal vein before reaching the systemic circulation. For drugs like morphine or lidocaine, metabolism is so complete that these drugs are ineffective orally. For propranolol and some orally administered analgesics, first-pass metabolism varies from 50 to 90 per cent of the administered dose. Increasing the dose of propranolol can overcome these losses. First-pass metabolism is the reason that propranolol must be given in doses of 160 mg/day orally, while intravenous infusions can be as low as 40 mg/day.[5]

Patients with cirrhosis have reduced first-pass metabolism because of shunting of portal blood around the remaining functional hepatocytes. While this shunt predisposes to hepatic coma, it offers some interesting pharmacologic phenomena. Lidocaine can be an effective oral drug in the cirrhotic patient because some drug escapes metabolism. Similarly, propranolol can appear to be a more potent drug in these patients because of less first-pass metabolism. Table 1–1 shows a list of drugs with substantial first pass metabolism whose oral potency could be affected in the patient with cirrhosis.[6]

Bioavailability is the overall fraction of orally administered drug that reaches the circulation. It is defined by comparison of blood levels achieved after similar oral and intravenous doses. The details of this comparison are presented in the pharmacokinetics section. As suggested by the preceding paragraphs, bioavailability is reduced by first-pass metabolism and chemical instability. Bioavailability is also affected by tablet composition, including such simple variables as pill compression. Manufacturers have become more aware of potential problems in formulation and generally conduct tests of bioavailability in quality control operations. More difficult to control are drug interactions in the gut. Milk or other sources of divalent cations, such as antacids, can lead to drug malabsorption. This is of particular importance in patients with renal disease who often receive phosphate-binding antacids and in patients with liver disease who receive antacids as prophylaxis for gastrointestinal hemorrhage. Similarly, foods interfere with drug absorption, probably by a combination of chelation, increased enzyme activity, and competition for uptake sites. Most drugs are absorbed best in an empty stomach. Table 1–2 lists a number of drugs that may have pharmacologic activity altered by antacids.[7]

TABLE 1–2. DRUGS INTERACTING WITH ANTACIDS

Drug	Mechanism
Digoxin	Bioavailability ↓ 25%
Iron	↓ Absorption
Salicylate	↑ Renal excretion ↓ Plasma levels 30–70%
Tetracycline	Chelation reduces absorption 80%
Other antimicrobial agents (ampicillin, isoniazid, sulfonamides)	Unknown

Neomycin is an example of a nephrotoxic drug that is clinically useful as a result of poor bioavailability. Because this drug is poorly absorbed when taken orally, drug action is restricted to the gastrointestinal tract and systemic toxicity is avoided. Reduction in gut flora can be achieved for treatment of hepatic coma. Toxic systemic levels do not occur in patients with normal renal function because the drug is cleared as rapidly as it is absorbed. Unfortunately, the patient with renal failure is unable to excrete the drug as rapidly as it is absorbed so that significant blood and tissue levels are reached and the patient is likely to suffer further renal damage from this potent nephrotoxin. The drug should, therefore, be used with caution in patients with renal insufficiency.

DRUG METABOLISM AND ELIMINATION

Most of the problems with drug administration in organ failure are caused by a reduction in the capacity to metabolize and eliminate drugs. Many drugs are sufficiently polar so that they can be eliminated unchanged by glomerular filtration. Digoxin is an example of a drug that is eliminated by the kidney at a rate nearly equal to that of creatinine clearance. Other drugs like penicillin have tubular secretion as their primary mode of elimination. This process is so rapid that probenecid is a useful adjunct for slowing secretion and thereby maintaining high plasma penicillin levels. Many drugs are lipid soluble. Although they are filtered by the glomerulus, these compounds easily cross the renal tubular epithelium by passive diffusion and are not excreted. These drugs must be made more polar by metabolism before urinary excretion can take place. While the kidney has some metabolic capacity, the liver is the most common site of drug metabolism. The chemical changes produced are generally those that increase the polarity of the drug. A compound with a benzene ring may be oxidized to a phenol, which may be made even more polar by conjugation with sulfate or glucuronide. These chemical modifications most often result in inactivation of the drug, and because the more polar metabolite can be excreted in the bile or eliminated by glomerular filtration, the metabolite will usually have a shorter half-life than the parent drug.

Sometimes drug metabolism will convert the parent drug to another active form. The antidepressant amitriptyline (Elavil) is metabolized by loss of a methyl group to nortriptyline. Both drugs are active and each happens to be independently marketed. The patient taking amitriptyline is, therefore, receiving two drugs that are in approximately equal concentration in the plasma during chronic treatment.[8] The nortriptyline-treated patient has only a single active compound in his body. The antiarrhythmic agent procainamide is metabolized to *N*-acetylprocainamide which has some antiarrhythmic activity. Because the parent drug appears to be responsible for the lupus syndrome seen with procainamide, the acetylated metabolite has been evaluated as a potentially better and less toxic antiarrhythmic agent. Unfortunately, these studies have shown that it does not have the same efficacy as procainamide for all patients.[9] The anticonvulsant methsuximide is so rapidly and extensively metabolized to *n*-desmethylmethsuximide that only the plasma level of the metabolite appears to correlate with clinical effect.[10] Primidone (Mysoline) is an anticonvulsant that is metabolized to two active metabolites, one of which is phenobarbital. Studies vary in their estimate of the relative importance of the parent drug and metabolites, but plasma phenobarbital levels derived from primidone may reach therapeutic concentrations equivalent to phenobarbital administration alone.[11]

In patients with liver or kidney disease, the complex relationships between parent drug and metabolites may be changed. In renal failure, the procainamide metabolite *N*-acetylprocainamide can accumulate to toxic levels.[12] In hepatic failure, chlordiazepoxide and diazepam metabolism is slowed; therefore, the parent drug will persist. Each drug is also converted to an active metabolite that has a prolonged half-life.[13] The difficulty in estimating additive pharmacologic effects in such a setting suggests that these drugs should not be used in patients with liver disease. Oxazepam (Serax), a benzodiazepine that can be directly excreted by the kidney, is a preferable substitute. Drugs that form active metabolites will be discussed in Chapter 3.

PHARMACOKINETICS

PLASMA DRUG LEVELS

Plasma drug level measurements have made it easier to treat many diseases and can be critically important for gauging drug dose in patients with liver or kidney diseases. Plasma drug levels are discussed in detail in Chapter 4. Traditionally, physicians used standard doses of drugs, estimated clinical responses, and then gave more drug if the response seemed inadequate or decreased the dosage if a toxic response developed. This approach is still a useful one for some conditions like atrial fibrillation. Digoxin doses can be given until ventricular response slows. For most conditions, however, there is no immediately measurable clinical effect. For example, in epilepsy, seizures may be infrequent. Optimizing drug dosing could take months or years. In fact, the therapeutic plasma level of phenytoin was established only after 3 years of experimental observation of a group of clinic patients in Sweden.[14] Another problem with clinical assessment is that drugs may cause the condition they are being used to control. Antiarrhythmic drugs, such as lidocaine, can occasionally induce ventricular arrhythmias as a manifestation of toxicity. Additional drug in that setting can be catastrophic. Aminoglycoside antibiotics can lead to nephrotoxicity in some patients, even at therapeutic concentrations, but the risk is increased with higher doses or in renal failure.[15] While all patients should have renal status assessed during treatment, aminoglycoside blood levels have been important in preventing blood level–related ototoxic reactions. Before theophylline blood level measurements became available, some physicians increased the dose until the patient became nauseated. Unfortunately, seizures and death sometimes occurred first; thus, this dangerous practice should not be used.

Not all drug treatments need plasma drug level measurements. If a drug is not toxic, then large excess doses can be given. An example is penicillin. Because the drug is inexpensive and high doses can be given safely to most patients, doses can be given that are known to produce many times the bactericidal concentrations in blood. Plasma drug concentrations are relatively unimportant. In general, plasma drug measurements are important for drugs in which therapeutic effects are closely followed by toxic effects.

Nevertheless, even though a drug has a narrow therapeutic range, plasma levels may not be helpful. A study must have been performed in a large group of patients to show good correlation between blood level and clinical response. Recent criticism of digoxin blood levels has been based on the observation that some patients show signs of drug toxicity even in the therapeutic range of 1.0 to 2.0 ng/ml, while others require levels above 2.0 ng/ml to control ventricular response to atrial fibrillation.[16] Since individual patients may not obey the population estimates, the therapeutic window should be viewed as a probability scale. At the lower end of the therapeutic range, the drug may produce a clinical effect. At the high end and beyond, therapeutic effect may be more likely, but the risk of toxicity is also increased. Plasma drug levels should be seen in the context of the total clinical picture; a level that is "therapeutic" neither guarantees clinical benefit nor excludes toxicity.

Digoxin treatment of heart failure illustrates another shortcoming of therapeutics. About 50 per cent of patients taking digoxin chronically for congestive heart failure can have the drug discontinued without clinical deterioration, while others may develop heart failure without change in plasma drug level.[17] These facts demonstrate that chronic digoxin therapy may be unnecessary in some patients and that others develop resistance to its inotropic effect. The blood level in these patients is meaningless, since the drug itself is without efficacy.

VOLUME OF DISTRIBUTION

The most basic relationship in pharmacokinetics is that between the dose of drug given and the blood level that results. The goal in giving a drug is to reach and then sustain a therapeutic plasma drug level. A loading dose is one that immediately produces a plasma level in the therapeutic range. Because a dose of drug is in milligrams and plasma concentration can be expressed in milligrams per liter, a constant with the units of liters has been created to make it possible to equate dose to plasma concentration. This constant is defined as the apparent volume of distribution. In equation form:

$$\frac{\text{Dose}}{V_d} = C_p \text{ or } V_d = \frac{\text{Dose}}{C_p} \text{ or Dose} = C_p \cdot V_d \quad (1)$$

Where dose is in milligrams, V_d is the volume of distribution in liters and C_p is the plasma concentration in milligrams per liter. Every drug has its own volume of distribution that has been experimentally determined by giving a known intravenous dose of drug to a large population of people and measuring the resulting plasma levels. Because renal disease, heart failure, and cirrhosis can alter the distribution characteristics of drugs, patients with these diseases may have different volumes of distribution from those determined in subjects without organ disease. Volumes of distribution, therapeutic levels, and loading doses for selected drugs in normal patients and patients with renal and hepatic disease can be found in the Appendix.

Two examples will illustrate how different the volume of distribution can be for different drugs. An ethanol dose of 40 gm to a 70-kg man will produce a blood level of 100 mg/dl or 1000 mg/L. The volume of distribution can be calculated from equation (1).

$$\text{Dose} = 40 \text{ gm}$$

$$C_p = 1000 \text{ mg/L} = 1 \text{ gm/L}$$

$$V_d = \frac{\text{Dose}}{C_p} = \frac{40 \text{ gm}}{1 \text{ gm/L}}$$

$$V_d = 40 \text{ L}$$

Since the patient weighs 70 kg, the volume of distribution can also be expressed in relation to weight.

$$V_d = \frac{40 \text{ L}}{70 \text{ kg}} = 0.6 \text{ L/kg}$$

For most individuals, the volume of distribution of ethanol will be 0.6 L/kg times body weight. While it is tempting to say that this volume of distribution represents total body water, it need not be true that ethanol distributes into body water. The only meaning of the volume of distribution is that it establishes the relation between a dose of drug and a measured plasma concentration. Digoxin demonstrates the abstract nature of the volume of distribution. A dose of 0.5 mg will produce a plasma drug level of 1 ng/ml or 1 μg/L in a 70-kg man. Using equation (1):

$$\text{Dose} = 0.5 \text{ mg} = 500 \text{ } \mu\text{g}$$

$$C_p = 1 \text{ } \mu\text{g/L}$$

$$V_d = \frac{500 \text{ } \mu\text{g}}{1 \text{ } \mu\text{g/L}}$$

$$V_d = 500 \text{ L}$$

The surprising observation that a 70-kg man can have an apparent volume of distribution of 500 L for digoxin shows that the volume of distribution is not related to any real volume. What such a large volume does mean is that the plasma level is very low, which implies that the drug must be present in some tissue at a much higher concentration than in the blood. Although plasma concentrations of digoxin are low, they still correlate with drug concentration at the site of action as shown by the clinical response.

The most important use of the volume of distribution is to predict a loading dose of a drug. An example will demonstrate this point. Since the volume of distribution of digoxin is 500 L for a 70-kg man, it is 7 L/kg. To reach a digoxin level of 1 μg/L in a 50-kg woman the required dose can be calculated.

$$V_d = (7 \text{ L/kg}) \cdot (50 \text{ kg}) = 350 \text{ L}$$

$$\text{desired } C_p = 1 \text{ ng/ml} = 1 \text{ } \mu\text{g/L}$$

using equation (1),

$$\text{Dose} = (1 \text{ } \mu\text{g/L}) \cdot (350 \text{ L})$$

$$\text{Dose} = 350 \text{ } \mu\text{g} = 0.35 \text{ mg}$$

This dose is smaller than that for the 70-kg man simply in relation to the difference in body weight.

Phenytoin is a second example of a drug often given by loading dose. To stop convulsions, a blood level of 10 to 20 mg/L is required. The volume of distribution for phenytoin is 0.6 L/kg. For a 70-kg man the dose to achieve a level of 10 mg/L can be estimated.

$$V_d = (0.6 \text{ L/kg}) \cdot (70 \text{ kg}) = 42 \text{ L}$$

$$\text{desired } C_p = 10 \text{ mg/L}$$

$$\text{Dose} = (10 \text{ mg/L}) \cdot (42 \text{ L})$$

$$\text{Dose} = 420 \text{ mg}$$

A commonly used intravenous loading dose is 500 mg. This will produce a level of approximately 12 mg/L in a 70-kg man. Some clinicians use a dose of 1000 mg of phenytoin. This doubling of dose will double the plasma concentration to 24 mg/L and produce a level somewhat above the accepted therapeutic range. The best approach for using loading doses is to give a dose that will produce a plasma concentration in the lower end of the therapeutic range; if it is ineffective, then a second dose can be given to reach the high end of the therapeutic range. For phenytoin, an initial dose of 500 mg should be given. If seizures stop, then only maintenance doses need to be given thereafter. If seizures persist, a second 500-mg dose will raise the plasma concentration to 24 mg/L. No further phenytoin doses are likely to be of benefit until 12 to 24 hours have elapsed and significant drug elimination has occurred.

The plasma concentrations mentioned in these examples are those achieved after the drug has an opportunity to distribute and before drug elimination has taken place. Loading doses can be given by any effective route but are most often given intravenously. Rapid intravenous doses can be dangerous because of transiently high plasma drug levels. A loading dose of 500 mg of phenytoin should be given no faster than 50 mg per minute.

The volume of distribution can also be used to estimate how much drug is in the body. In overdoses, a blood level can be determined and then multiplied by the volume of distribution to get an estimate of how much drug was taken. Aspirin is an example.

$$\text{Measured } C_p = 1500 \text{ mg/L} = 1.5 \text{ gm/L}$$

$$V_d = 40 \text{ L}$$

$$\text{Dose} = (40 \text{ L}) \cdot (1.5 \text{ gm/L})$$

$$\text{Dose} = 60 \text{ gm}$$

$$\text{Tablet size } 325 \text{ mg}$$

$$\text{Dose} = 185 \text{ tablets}$$

This technique can be helpful for providing an objective correlate to the drug dose stated in the patient history.

DRUG ELIMINATION HALF-LIFE

Once a loading dose has been administered, a maintenance dose must be given to replace drug lost by metabolism and renal excretion. Even without a loading dose, drug will accumulate over time so that the maintenance dose will ultimately determine the long-term plasma drug level. It is the maintenance dose that most often requires adjustment in patients with kidney or liver disease.

As mentioned before, some drugs require metabolism, while others can be directly excreted by the kidney. Despite this difference, most drugs are eliminated in direct proportion to the concentration of the drug in the plasma; the higher the plasma concentration, the larger the absolute amount of drug eliminated. This fortunate fact simplifies dosing. It is the reason that doubling drug dose will lead to exact doubling of the steady-state plasma concentration.

Drugs that are eliminated in direct proportion to their concentration in plasma are said to obey first-order kinetics; that is, the drugs are removed in proportion to the plasma concentration raised to the first power. Figure 1–1 shows how the plasma concentration falls with time after a single intravenous dose of a drug with first-order elimination. The curve has two parts. The first part, termed the distribution phase, or the *α phase*, has a rapid fall that

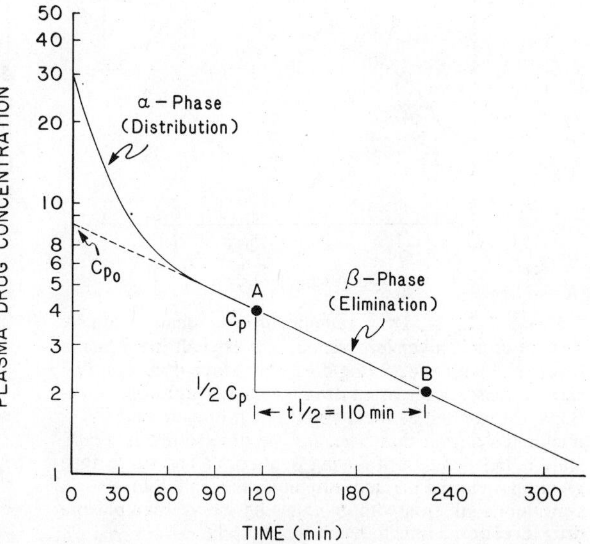

Figure 1–1. Plasma drug concentrations after an intravenous bolus of drug. Plasma concentrations fall rapidly as the drug moves into its volume of distribution (α-phase) and then more slowly as the drug is eliminated from the body (β-phase). C_{p_0} is the plasma concentration that would have been present if the drug immediately passed into the volume of distribution. The log-linear fall of the plasma concentration during the elimination phase shows that this drug obeys first order kinetics.

represents the drug moving into its volume of distribution. The second part, the elimination phase, or the *β phase*, has an exponential shape. From this second phase the half-life can be calculated. The half-life is the time that it takes for the blood level to fall to half of some previous level regardless of the absolute magnitude of the previous level. Half of the drug is eliminated from the body in one half-life, independent of how much drug is present.

The most profound effect of the half-life is on drug accumulation. Figure 1–2 shows the plasma concentrations that result from multiple intravenous doses. The same dose given every half-life will eventually lead to plateau levels that have a peak value twice as high as the first dose produced and a trough value equal to the level the first dose produced. The plateau is reached after about five half-lives. Nothing in the dosing regimen affects the time taken to reach these steady-state levels; an infusion that gives an equivalent dose per half-life will reach the same average level as multiple boluses and the steady-state level will also be reached in five half-lives. Of course, there are no peaks and troughs with an infusion. Drugs have widely variable half-lives depending on the site of drug elimination and on the volume of distribution of the drug. The half-lives of most drugs in normal patients and in patients with hepatic failure and renal failure are given in the Appendix.

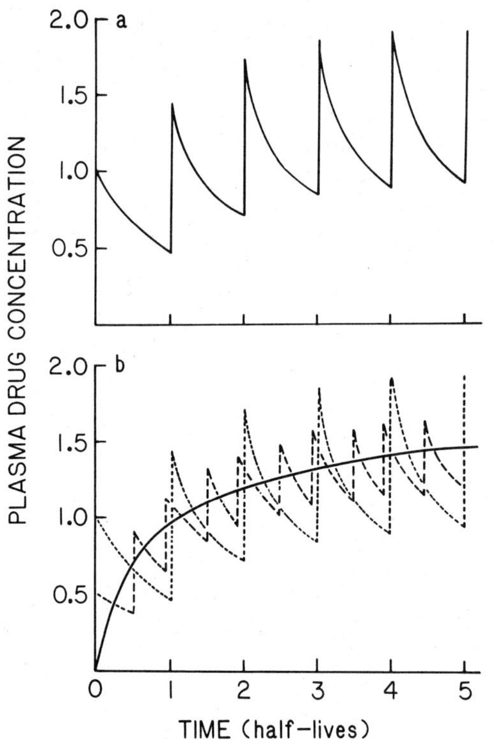

Figure 1–2. *A*, Drug accumulation to steady state. A dose of drug is given intravenously every half-life. Plasma levels rise with succeeding doses but since drug removal rate increases with rising drug levels, plateau concentrations are reached as the amount given in each half-life is eliminated during that time. *B*, The time to reach steady state is independent of dosing frequency. The same dose given in *a* can be divided into multiple small boluses or a continuous infusion without changing the average plasma drug level or the time to reach steady state.

Lidocaine illustrates a number of pharmacokinetic principles discussed thus far. Because it is given for rapid control of arrhythmias, the first dose is usually an intravenous bolus. For a 70 kg-man, a commonly chosen first dose is 100 mg. This dose is often effective at stopping ventricular ectopy. Frequently, however, arrhythmias may recur in 15 to 20 minutes, even if a lidocaine infusion has been started. The reason for this is shown in Figure 1–3. The bolus of 100 mg produces an initial blood level in the therapeutic range of 2 to 4 mg/L and stops the arrhythmia. If the initial bolus is pushed too rapidly (in less than 1 minute), then a transient level of 10 mg/L or more can be reached and convulsions may occur. As the drug distributes from the plasma into the full volume of distribution, the initial level falls rapidly and a subtherapeutic plasma concentration results. An infusion started at the same time as the bolus will not produce a therapeutic plasma level until many hours have passed. Because the half-life of lidocaine is about 1.5 hours in patients without heart failure or liver disease, steady-state concentrations will not be reached for over 7 hours.

The problem with this dosing regimen is that 100 mg of lidocaine is not an adequate loading dose for most patients. The volume of distribution of lidocaine is 1.7 L/kg. Using equation (1), the concentration of lidocaine after the distribution phase can be calculated.

$$\text{Dose} = 100 \text{ mg}$$
$$V_d = 1.7 \text{ L/kg} \times 70 \text{ kg} = 120 \text{ L}$$
$$C_p = \frac{100 \text{ mg}}{120 \text{ L}} \simeq 0.83 \text{ mg/L}$$

The level of 0.83 mg/L is subtherapeutic. This problem can be solved by giving a second 100-mg bolus after the first dose has been distributed. The second bolus will raise the level from 0.83 to 1.7 mg/L when it distributes. A third bolus of 100 mg would insure a plasma

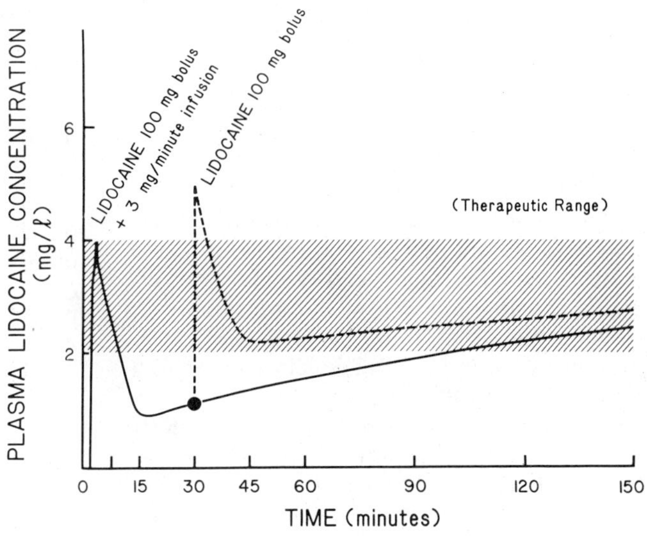

Figure 1–3. Lidocaine bolus and infusion to 70 kg patient. At time 0 a 100 mg intravenous bolus and a 3 mg/minute infusion of lidocaine is given. Because of subtherapeutic plasma levels at 15 minutes, an additional 100 mg intravenous bolus is administered.

concentration in the therapeutic range — 2.5 mg/L — but this subsequent bolus is also more likely to produce a transient toxic level, since it is added to the existing plasma concentration. Some physicians, therefore, prefer giving incremental doses of 50 mg after the two 100-mg boluses have been administered.[18]

Once the loading dose has been given, a maintenance dose must be determined. Because lidocaine has a relatively short half-life of 90 minutes, it is convenient to give the drug by infusion rather than by intermittent boluses. Recommended infusion rates for lidocaine are 2 to 4 mg/min for patients without heart failure or hepatic disease. A conceptual rationale for this dose comes from considering the total amount of drug in the body when a therapeutic steady-state level of 3 mg/L is reached.

$$C_p = 3 \text{ mg/L}$$

$$V_d = 120 \text{ L}$$

$$\text{Drug in the body} = (3 \text{ mg/L}) \cdot (120 \text{ L})$$

$$\text{Drug in the body} = 360 \text{ mg}$$

Since in every half-life, half of the body load must be replaced, the following calculation can be made:

$$\text{Dose each half-life} = \frac{\text{Drug in the body}}{2} = \frac{360 \text{ mg}}{2} = 180 \text{ mg}$$

Because lidocaine $t_{\frac{1}{2}} = 90$ minutes

$$\frac{180 \text{ mg}}{90 \text{ min}} = 2 \text{ mg/min}$$

This infusion rate is actually a somewhat low estimate for maintaining a level of 3 mg/L. The reason is that more than half of the body load of drug is lost in one half-life because the level is not permitted to undergo exponential decay during an infusion. In the following section of drug clearance a more exact estimate is made. Intuitively, however, it is useful to look at maintenance drug dosing as replacing a part of total body drug.

DRUG CLEARANCE

Whether drug is eliminated by the liver or the kidney, the concept of clearance is useful. In analogy with creatinine clearance, drug clearance is defined as a certain volume of blood completely cleared of drug in a unit time. It is especially useful for calculating steady-state infusion doses. Because lidocaine is cleared rapidly by the liver at a rate nearly equal to liver blood flow or 900 ml/min in an adult, the drug must be given in relatively high doses. The infusion dose to maintain a steady-state level is simply the dose needed to replace the drug in the blood that is being cleared. Since in this example the desired blood level is 3 mg/L, 3 mg of drug must be given each time 1 L of blood is cleared of drug.

Infusion dose = (clearance) · (C_p)

Clearance = 900 ml/min = 0.9 L/min

Dose = (0.9 L/min) · (3.0 mg/L)

Dose = 2.7 mg/min

In heart failure and hepatic cirrhosis clearance can fall to 500 ml/min or less. In cirrhosis, the reduced hepatic mass can receive an effective flow that is also low. In both situations, lidocaine infusions must be less; only measurement of plasma drug levels can predict reliably the appropriate dose.

Lidocaine dosing in heart failure has another complication. The volume of distribution of the drug is reduced so that both the loading dose and the maintenance dose must be decreased. As little as 100 mg is adequate to reach a therapeutic blood level of 2 mg/L, indicating a volume of distribution of 50 L instead of 120 L. Caution must be used for both loading and maintenance doses.

Clearance, half-life, and volume of distribution can be related by introducing the concept of the first order rate constant of elimination, k_e. Because most drugs are eliminated at a rate directly proportional to the plasma concentration C_p, a rate constant can be defined.

Rate of fall of plasma concentration = $-k_e \cdot C_p$

Expressed in integral calculus terms:

$$\frac{dC_p}{dt} = -k_e \cdot C_p$$

Rearranging:

$$\frac{dC_p}{C_p} = -k_e dt$$

Integrating:

$$\ln\left(\frac{C_p}{C_{p_0}}\right) = -k_e \cdot t$$

And

$$C_p = C_{p_0} e^{-k_e t} \qquad (2)$$

This is the expression that governs the exponential decay of blood levels after a single intravenous dose. Even though the concept of half-life is very familiar in science, the half-life is a less fundamental relationship than the rate constant and is in fact derived from this equation. After one half-life, the plasma concentration will fall to half of some previous value. Thus, after one half-life, $C_p = 1/2\ C_{p_0}$. After substitution into equation (2) and taking the natural logarithm of both sides, the half-life or $t_{\frac{1}{2}}$ can be expressed as $t_{\frac{1}{2}} = 0.693/k_e$. This derivation shows that the commonly used term half-life comes directly from the less familiar first-order rate constant, k_e. The first-order rate constant is a percentage. Using lidocaine as an example:

$$t_{\frac{1}{2}} = 1.5 \text{ hours}$$

$$k_e = \frac{0.693}{t_{\frac{1}{2}}}$$

$$k_e = \frac{0.693}{1.5 \text{ hr}}$$

$$k_e = 0.46 \text{ hr}^{-1}$$

The first-order rate constant of 0.46 hr^{-1} indicates that 46 per cent per hour of a lidocaine infusion dose will be eliminated. Expressed in clearance terms, 46 per cent of the volume of distribution will be cleared every hour. Calculating clearance this way:

$$k_e = 0.46 \text{ hr}^{-1}$$

$$V_d = 120 \text{ L}$$

$$\text{Clearance} = (0.46 \text{ hr}^{-1}) \cdot (120 \text{ L})$$

$$= 55 \text{ L/hr}$$

$$= 920 \text{ ml/min}$$

This value is nearly the same as the 900 ml/min estimate of drug clearance based on hepatic blood flow even though this calculation has used the abstract volume of distribution and the first-order rate constant for the calculation. In the same way, infusion rates at steady state can be estimated using the first-order rate constant. Since the amount of drug in the body is being held constant by the infusion and is being eliminated at a fractional rate indicated by the first-order rate constant, the replacement infusion will be predicted by the following calculations. From equation (1):

Drug in the body = $C_p \cdot V_d$

= (3 mg/L) · (120 L)

= 360 mg

First-order rate constant

$k_e = 0.46\ hr^{-1}$

$$\begin{aligned}\text{Rate of drug infusion} = \text{Rate of drug elimination} &= k_e \cdot C_p \cdot V_d \\ &= (0.46\ \text{hr}^{-1}) \cdot (360\ \text{mg}) \\ &= 166\ \text{mg/hr} \\ &= 2.8\ \text{mg/min}\end{aligned}$$

Not surprisingly, this infusion rate is the same as that estimated by knowing the clearance and the desired steady-state plasma level. Elimination rate constants for commonly utilized drugs can be found in Chapter 2.

SATURATION KINETICS

A few drugs are given in doses that nearly saturate the hepatic enzymes that metabolize the drug. Aspirin, phenytoin, and alcohol are the most common examples. Maintenance doses of these drugs are difficult to establish because there is no simple relationship between the dose of drug and the steady-state plasma concentration. Doubling dose will more than double the plasma concentration. If the dose exceeds the maximum rate of hepatic metabolism, the patient will become progressively toxic as the blood level increases without any upper limit. The equation for steady-state levels for this class of drug is adapted from Michaelis-Menten enzyme kinetics.

$$C_{p_{ss}} = \frac{(k_m) \cdot (\text{dose/time})}{V_{max} - (\text{dose/time})} \qquad (3)$$

Where $C_{p_{ss}}$ is the steady-state plasma drug concentration, k_m is the plasma concentration at which the enzymes are half-saturated, and V_{max} is the maximum rate of metabolism of the drug. For phenytoin, a daily dose of 300 mg may lead to therapeutic blood levels of 10 to 20 mg/L in many patients. However, if the blood level is subtherapeutic at 7 mg/L in an individual patient, an increase of only 100 mg may increase the steady-state level to 15 mg/L as the dose more closely approaches the maximum rate of metabolism. A typical value for k_m is 8 mg/L so that most patients are well beyond the half-saturation point of their liver enzyme capacity when they are in the therapeutic range of 10 to 20 mg/L. The concept of half-life is meaningless for phenytoin, since the liver cannot increase the amount of drug eliminated as the dose is increased. The time required to reach a new steady-state level is also unpredictable. Drug may accumulate gradually for days to weeks after a change in dose.

For patients with liver disease, the maximum rate of metabolism, V_{max}, may be reduced in proportion to the reduction in liver mass. No estimate can be made for adjusting dose except by following plasma levels after a conventional loading dose.

There is a technique for adjusting phenytoin dosage to a new therapeutic level that does not require weeks of monitoring. If the patient taking 300 mg/day has a subtherapeutic level of 7 mg/L, the level can be brought to 15 mg/L by a single incremental dose. A new maintenance dose can be chosen and started immediately. If plasma levels continue to rise, then the new dose is high; if plasma drug levels fall from 15 mg/L, the new dose is low. For a 70-kg man the calculations are:

Increase C_p from 7 to 15 mg/L:
Dose = (8 mg/L) (0.6 L/kg) · (70 kg)
Dose = 336 mg

This single extra dose will be given in addition to an increased maintenance dose of 400 mg/day. Plasma levels are measured 1 day and 5 days after the additional loading dose and the new, higher daily dose.

Observations: Day 1 level = 15 mg/L
Day 5 level = 19 mg/L

Conclusion: Too much drug is being given

Analysis of drug accumulation:
19 − 15 = 4 mg/L
= (4 mg/L) (0.6 L/kg) (70 kg)
= 168 mg in 4 days
= 42 mg/day

The drug is accumulating at 42 mg/day. Reducing dose from 400 mg to 360 mg/day (or for simpler dosing, 350 mg) should lead to constant levels of 15 mg/L. In exactly the same way, falling blood levels will indicate underdosing and the appropriate increment in dose can be calculated.

When hepatic disease reduces the maximum rate of metabolism, drugs that are eliminated by saturable enzyme systems are more difficult to regulate than drugs removed by first order processes. If a drug obeying first order kinetics is eliminated by the kidney at a rate equal to creatinine clearance and creatinine clearance is reduced by 50 per cent, then the half-life will be doubled. The doubling of half-life will eventually lead to a doubling of the steady-state plasma concentration. By contrast, reductions in maximum rate of metabolism caused by loss of hepatic parenchyma are much more ominous. For many patients, the maximum daily rate of metabolism of phenytoin is 600 mg. If a patient with liver disease has a 50 per cent reduction in V_{max} to 300 mg, any dose more than 300 mg of phenytoin per day will lead to an infinite steady-state blood level. Drug toxicity will be certain if dosing is maintained. Fortunately, even in severe hepatic disease, most drugs maintain first-order metabolism and saturation kinetics do not apply.

Aspirin is a complex drug because it is eliminated by the liver with saturation kinetics and is also partly cleared by the kidney with first-order kinetics. In the liver, maximal rates of metabolism are approximately 100 mg/hr. This means that about 2400 mg/day of aspirin can be metabolized. This amount corresponds to 7 tablets/day. Additional aspirin is excreted by the kidneys with a half-life of about 40 hours at urine pH 5.0. If patients consume more than 7 tablets per day, renal elimination will control drug accumulation. Because of the long half-life of urinary elimination, aspirin can accumulate for over 1 week before a steady-state level is reached. Insidious chronic salicylate poisoning has been increasingly recognized as a cause of chronic metabolic acidosis.[19] The patient with rheumatoid arthritis taking high-dose aspirin must be followed with serum electrolyte and salicylate measurements to avoid drug intoxication.

AREA UNDER THE CURVE – BIOAVAILABILITY

The plasma concentration–time curve provides a simple way to compute the effective oral absorption of a drug. Using integral calculus and a simple first-order kinetic decay model (excluding the distribution phase), it is possible to show that the area under the plasma concentration–time curve is directly related to the dose of drug given. The ratio of the area under the curve achieved by an oral dose to the area produced by an identical intravenous dose will give the fraction of the oral dose that has been absorbed.

PROTEIN BINDING

Plasma proteins are a common binding site for drugs. Warfarin is an acidic drug tightly bound to albumin. Because such a large fraction of the total body load of drug is in the plasma, the volume of distribution is small, as low as 10 L in a 70-kg man. Because only the free drug is active, the presence of a high concentration of bound drug is not usually a concern. However, if the patient also takes another acidic drug, such as aspirin, serious problems can result. The aspirin can displace warfarin from albumin-binding sites and expose the liver to much higher anticoagulant concentrations. Although metabolism of warfarin will eventually restore the free drug level to its previous steady-state value, the surge of released drug may cause severe depletion of clotting factors and subsequent bleeding. Other acidic drugs given in gram quantities, such as sulfa antibiotics and phenylbutazone, will have the same displacing effect on bound warfarin.

Aspirin illustrates another feature of protein binding. At low doses, aspirin is extensively bound to albumin and, therefore, has an apparent volume of distribution of 15 L in a 70-kg man.[20] As dose is increased, the protein sites are saturated so that relatively more drug distributes to tissue. In an army experiment in the 1950's, volunteers were given 20 gm of aspirin and blood levels were measured.[21] These values indicate that the volume of distribution is about 40 L at this dose. Measurement of free drug not bound to plasma protein, however, would show a comparable volume of distribution at either dose.

Changes in protein binding can alter the interpretation of plasma drug measurements and will be discussed in detail in Chapter 4. Phenytoin binding has been studied in patients with normal renal function and in patients with renal failure. Ordinarily, 90 per cent of plasma phenytoin is bound to protein. In renal disease, a low-molecular-weight compound accumulates and displaces some phenytoin, reducing bound phenytoin by up to 50 per cent.[22] Figure 1–4 shows the correlation between the

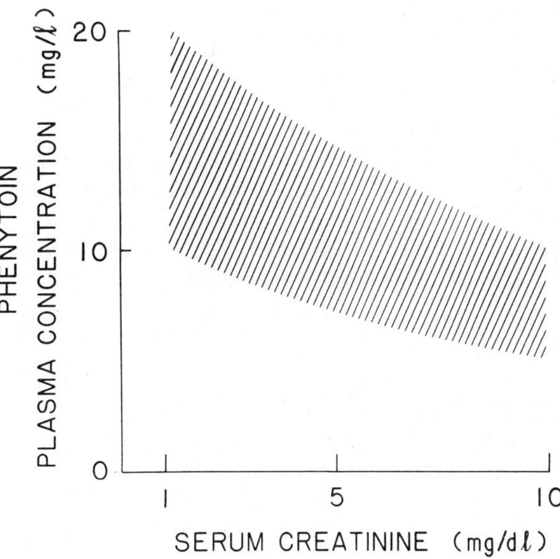

Figure 1–4. Renal failure changes therapeutic plasma concentrations of phenytoin. Since the amount of protein-bound phenytoin is reduced in renal failure and the plasma assay measures both bound and free drug, therapeutic plasma concentrations decline with rising creatinine despite the fact that free drug concentrations remain constant.

fraction of phenytoin bound and the serum creatinine level.

Because free drug levels of phenytoin are unchanged in renal failure, the ratio of free to total drug increases. Since the conventional plasma drug measurement includes both bound and free drug, the total drug level will be lower in patients with renal failure. The therapeutic window will be reduced from normal values of 10 to 20 mg/L to 5 to 10 mg/L. Free drug remains 1 to 2 mg/L. The physician must recognize that the therapeutic window is redefined for this patient group. Since phenytoin tissue distribution and metabolism are usually normal in patients with renal failure, standard doses can be given despite the fact that the plasma levels will reach only 5 to 10 mg/L. If necessary, free drug levels can be determined. While free drug levels can be measured from blood by equilibrium dialysis techniques, free levels can be more easily obtained by assaying saliva. Because saliva is a protein-free plasma filtrate, it is a convenient medium for confirming that unbound plasma phenytoin levels are therapeutic.[23]

The effect of protein binding can be very important when a drug is more than 90 per cent bound (Table 1–3). While acidic drugs like warfarin and phenytoin bind to albumin, basic drugs such as lidocaine have been shown to bind to the plasma protein α_1-acid glycoprotein. The importance of this protein is that its concentration may increase in diseases such as congestive heart failure or myocardial infarction. The increase will lead to more drug in plasma and a reduction in the apparent volume of distribution. These changes in binding protein may be a partial explanation for the problems with lidocaine administration in patients with heart disease.[24]

TABLE 1–3. DRUGS HIGHLY BOUND TO PROTEIN (> 90%)

Acidic Drugs (Albumin)	Basic Drugs (Albumin and α_1-Acid Glycoprotein)
Aspirin	Chlordiazepoxide
Diazoxide	Chlorpromazine
Furosemide	Diazepam
Indomethacin	Diphenhydramine
Penicillin	Lidocaine
Phenylbutazone	Propranolol
Phenytoin	Quinacrine
Probenecid	Quinidine
Sulfinpyrazone	Quinine
Sulfonamides	Tricyclic antidepressants
Tolbutamide	
Warfarin	

DRUG SELECTION

The basic goals in treating patients with renal or hepatic failure are to use the fewest drugs possible and then to select those with the best understood pharmacokinetics. Preferably, drugs can be chosen that are excreted without requiring the diseased organ. Since quinidine is primarily metabolized in the liver, patients with cirrhosis could be treated with disopyramide, which is excreted by the kidneys. The spectrum of antiarrhythmic activity is similar for the two drugs. Because digitoxin is eliminated by the liver and digoxin by both the kidneys and liver, some physicians have proposed using digitoxin instead of digoxin in renal failure.[25] Because most physicians do not ordinarily use digitoxin and because the dose adjustment for digoxin is easily made for the patient with renal disease, there is probably no need to resort to digitoxin. Table 1–4 lists some alternate drug choices for patients with either liver or kidney disease. Unfortunately, pharmacokinetic data in hepatic and renal disease are available for only a few drugs. In the absence of specific information, the physician should use drugs with which he is most familiar and ones for which plasma drug level measurements are available. Therapeutic levels may be redefined for some drugs as they have been for phenytoin in renal failure, but until specific studies are performed for each drug, the accepted therapeutic range is the only available guideline. Methods of altering drug dosages in patients with renal and liver disease are discussed in Chapter 2.

The risk of drug toxicity cannot be eliminated; it can only be controlled by techniques such as drug level monitoring. For the patient with hepatic or renal failure, skillful clinical judgment remains the critical element for synthesizing laboratory measurements and patient response.

TABLE 1–4. DRUG ALTERNATIVES IN HEPATIC OR RENAL FAILURE

Drug	*Alternative*
RENAL	
Acetazolamide	Furosemide
Acetohexamide	Insulin
Aminoglycosides	Other antibiotic or ↓ dose
Aspirin	Acetaminophen
Cephaloridine	Cephalothin
Chlorothiazide	Furosemide
Chlorpropamide	Insulin
cis-Platinum	↓ dose
Cycloserine	Other antitubercular
Decamethonium	Suxamethonium
Ethacrynic acid	Furosemide
Gallamine	Suxamethonium or *d*-Tubocurare
Lithium	Other antipsychotic or careful plasma monitoring
Meperidine	Morphine
Methotrexate	↓ dose
Methoxyflurane	Halothane
Nitrofurantoin	Other antibiotic
Organic mercurials	Furosemide
Phenformin	Insulin
Phenylbutazone	Indomethacin
Probenecid	Allopurinol
Procainamide	Quinidine, lidocaine
Spironolactone	Furosemide
Streptozocin	Other antineoplastic
Sulfinpyrazone	Allopurinol
Tetracyclines	Doxycycline
Tolbutamide	Insulin
Triamterene	Furosemide
HEPATIC	
Drug	*Alternative*
Chloramphenicol	Other antibiotic
Chlordiazepoxide	Oxazepam
Cytosine arabinoside	Other antineoplastic or ↓ dose
Diazepam	Oxazepam
5-Fluorouracil	Other antineoplastic or ↓ dose
Halothane	Other anesthetic
Lidocaine	Disopyramide or ↓ dose
6-Mercaptopurine	Other antineoplastic or ↓ dose
Methotrexate	Other antineoplastic or ↓ dose
Quinidine	Disopyramide
Rifampicin	Other antitubercular
6-Thioguanine	Other antineoplastic or ↓ dose
Vitamin D	25-Hydroxy vitamin D

REFERENCES

1. Klotz U, Avant GR, Hoyumpa A, Schenker S, Wilkinson GR: The effects of age and liver disease on the disposition and elimination of diazepam in adult man. J. Clin. Invest. *55*:347–359, 1975.
2. Greenblatt DJ, Koch-Weser J: Intramuscular injection of drugs. N. Engl. J. Med., *295*:542–546, 1976.
3. Kastrup EK, Boyd JR: Facts and Comparisons. St. Louis: Facts and Comparisons Inc., 1979, p. 1478.
4. Ogilvie RE: Clinical pharmacokinetics of theophylline. Clin. Pharmacokinet., *3*:267–293, 1978.
5. Chidsey CA, Morselli P, Bianchetti G, Morganti A, Leonetti G, Zanchetti A: Studies of the absorption and removal of propranolol in hypertensive patients during therapy. Circulation *52*:313–318, 1975.
6. Blaschke TF: Hepatic first pass metabolism in liver disease. Clin. Pharmacokinet. *4*:423–432, 1979.
7. Hurwitz A: Antacid therapy and drug kinetics. Clin. Pharmacokinet. *2*:269–280, 1977.
8. Kupfer DJ, Hanin, I, Spiker DG, Graw T, Coble P: Amitriptyline plasma levels and clinical response in primary depression. Clin. Pharm. Ther. *22*:904–911, 1977.
9. Kluger J, Drayer D, Reidenberg M, Ellis G, Lloyd V, Tyberg T, Hayes J: The clinical pharmacology and antiarrhythmic efficacy of acetylprocainamide in patients with arrhythmias. Amer. J. Cardiol. *45*:1250–1257, 1980.
10. Strong JM, Abe T, Gibbs EL, Atkinson AJ: Plasma levels of methsuximide and N-desmethylmethsuximide during methsuximide therapy. Neurology *24*:250–255, 1974.
11. Penry JK, Newmark ME: The use of antiepileptic drugs. Ann. Int. Med. *9*:207–218, 1979.
12. Karlsson E: Clinical pharmacokinetics of procainamide. Clin. Pharmacokinet. *3*:97–107, 1978.

13. Andreasen PB, Hendel J, Greisen G, Hvidberg EF: Pharmacokinetics of diazepam in disordered liver function. Eur. J. Clin. Pharm. *10*:115–120, 1976.
14. Lund L: Anticonvulsant effect of diphenylhydantoin relative to plasma levels. A prospective three year study in ambulatory patients with generalized epileptic seizures. Arch. Neurol. *31*:289–294, 1974.
15. Appel GB, New HC: The nephrotoxicity of antimicrobial agents. N. Engl. J. Med. *296*:663–670, 722–728, 784–787, 1977.
16. Ingelfinger JA, Goldman P: The serum digitalis concentration — Does it diagnose digitalis toxicity? N. Engl. J. Med. *294*:867–870, 1976.
17. Johnston GD, McDevitt DG: Is maintenance digoxin necessary in patient with sinus rhythm? Lancet *1*:567–570, 1979.
18. Greenblatt DJ, Bolognini V, Koch-Weser, J, Harmatz, JS: Pharmacokinetic approach to the clinical use of lidocaine intravenously. J.A.M.A. *236*:273–277, 1976.
19. Anderson RJ, Potts DE, Gabow, PA, Rumack BH, Schrier, RW: Unrecognized adult salicylate intoxication. Ann. Int. Med. *85*:745–748, 1976.
20. Levy G, Tsuchiya T: Salicylate accumulation kinetics in man. N. Engl. J. Med. *287*:430–432, 1972.
21. Swintosky JV: Illustrations and pharmaceutical interpretations of first order drug elimination rate from the bloodstream. J. Am. Pharm. Assn., *45*:395–400, 1956.
22. Reidenberg MM, Affrime M: Influence of disease in binding of drugs to plasma proteins. Ann. N.Y. Acad. Sci. *226*:115–126, 1973.
23. Bochner F, Hooper WD, Sutherland JM, Eadie MI, Tyrer JH: Diphenylhydantoin concentrations in saliva. Arch. Neurol. *31*:57–59, 1974.
24. Piafsky KM: Disease induced changes in the plasma binding of basic drugs. Clin. Pharmacokinet. *5*:246–262, 1980.
25. Perrier D, Mayersohn M, Marcus FI: Clinical pharmacokinetics of digitoxin. Clin. Pharmacokinet. *2*:292–311, 1977.

Chapter 2

Altering Drug Dose in Patients with Diseases of the Kidney and Liver

by

William M. Bennett

Drug prescribing in patients with renal or liver dysfunction often involves adjustment of usual dosage regimens in order to avoid drug accumulation and, thus, adverse effects. For practical purposes, it is essential that the physician consider all the factors at play in the individual patient and not rely on a fixed drug regimen or formula.[1] This is particularly true in clinical situations involving multiple drugs and complicated pathophysiologic disturbances. For example, it is now widely recognized that the altered physiology of renal failure may affect hepatic capacity to metabolize and biotransform drugs. Likewise, hepatic failure is often associated with diminished renal function. To the clinician treating such patients, these factors and other variables that affect drug action, such as changes in the volume of distribution, binding to plasma proteins, irregular absorption, intercurrent drug removal with dialysis, and drug interactions, often appear overwhelming. However, drug prescribing in these disease states follows some general principles that will be reviewed in this chapter. It is obvious that the best guide to appropriate therapy is a thorough knowledge of a drug's pharmacokinetic parameters, a careful analysis of the factors at play in any individual patient, and, when indicated, plasma drug level analysis (see Chap. 4).

This chapter will attempt to provide the framework for a practical approach to the individual patient. In patients with renal failure, drugs usually eliminated by the kidneys require the most modification. The level of renal function should be determined as the basis for dosage modification. To insure efficacy, the initial loading dose should be near normal. Maintenance doses can be adjusted by lengthening the interval between doses or by reducing the size of individual doses. Tables, nomograms, elimination rate constants, or plasma half-life can serve as an approximation for these adjustments if the limitations of these methods are kept in mind. Whenever possible, serum levels can be used to guide therapy for drugs with narrow therapeutic toxic ratios. Since decreased binding to plasma proteins in uremia can result in toxic concentrations of free drug despite normal blood levels, special care should be taken in interpretation of drug blood levels, and careful clinical evaluation of the patient is needed. Hemodialysis and peritoneal dialysis may remove enough drug to require supplemental doses. The clinician caring for patients with renal disease is best advised to become familiar with the clinical pharmacology of the drugs most frequently required by this challenging group of patients.

The best approach to drug therapy in individual patients with liver disease is less clear. This is largely due to a lack of readily obtainable hepatic functional parameters that correlate well with alterations in hepatic drug metabolism. For an individual patient, the alert clinician often can anticipate situations in which drugs may produce adverse reactions. A knowledge of drugs that undergo extensive hepatic metabolism or first-pass extraction is useful. These drugs are likely to demonstrate high plasma levels in patients with significant liver disease. In addition, consideration of possible diminished drug protein binding, for example, owing to hypoalbuminemia, and decreased liver blood flow producing decreased delivery of drug to site of metabolism, should serve to warn the physician of the need to reduce dosage. As in patients with renal failure, properly interpreted blood level measurements are often valuable adjuncts.

LABORATORY ASSESSMENT OF RENAL AND LIVER FUNCTION

RENAL FUNCTION

Most dosage adjustments in patients with renal failure depend on a knowledge of renal function. Since the serum half-life of drugs predominantly excreted by the kidney is inversely proportional to glomerular filtration rate (GFR), assessment of GFR is necessary for current dosage determinations. Little information is available correlating pharmacokinetics of drugs eliminated by the kidney with other parameters of renal function, such as urine concentrating ability or renal blood flow. For clinical purposes, serum creatinine or endogenous creatinine clearance are the most practical indices of glomerular filtration rate.

When renal function is not changing, the serum creatinine level is determined by rate of production and endogenous clearançe. During abrupt changes in renal function, as in patients with acute renal failure, the serum value is also affected by changes in the apparent volume of distribution. The chief disadvantage of endogenous creatinine clearance is the requirement for carefully timed urine collections. Cockroft and Gault have developed a useful formula for estimating creatinine clearance from serum creatinine without the need for urine collection.[2] These workers utilize the fact that creatinine excretion is proportional to body mass and inversely proportional to age. In this formula:

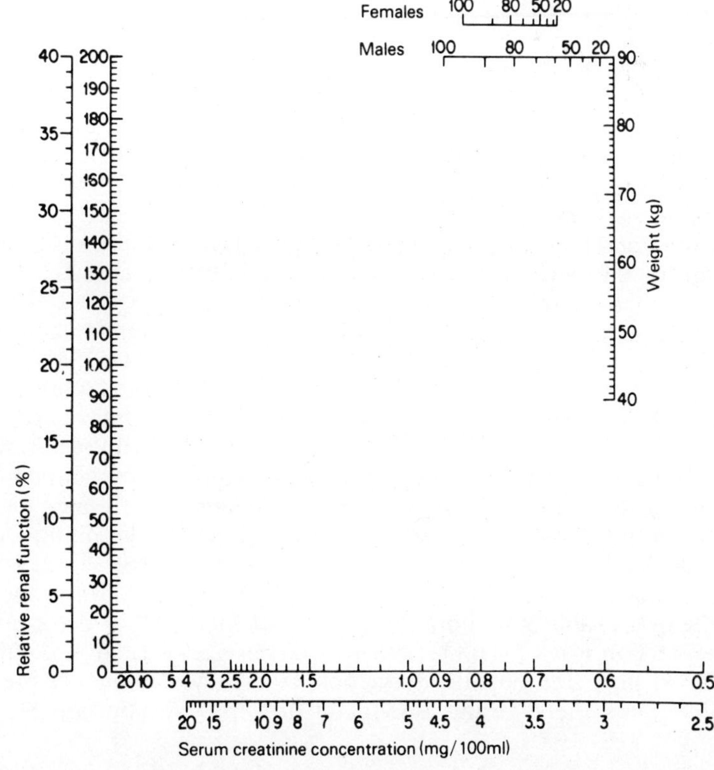

Figure 2–1. Nomogram for determining relative renal function from serum creatinine concentrations in adults. (From Bjornsson TD: Clin. Pharmacokinet. *4*:200–222, 1979, with permission.) To use, define a point where lines perpendicular to patient's age and sex cross. Draw a line from that point through the origin. For any serum creatinine, the per cent of renal function can be read on the ordinate using the outer scales for serum creatinine higher than 2.5 mg/dl.

Creatinine clearance =

$$\frac{(140 - \text{age})\ (\text{body weight in kg})}{72 \times \text{serum creatinine in mg/dl}}$$

The value calculated should be reduced 10 to 15 per cent in women.[2] The formula may overestimate the creatinine clearance in pregnancy and, possibly, in patients with ascites or edema.[3]

Bjornsson has derived a useful nomogram for the same purpose (Fig. 2–1). Relative renal function in units of per cent of normal function can be read directly.[4] This value can then be used in conjunction with the nomograms for dosage modification described later in this chapter. The Siersbaek-Nielsen nomogram is equally useful in estimating creatinine clearance from the serum creatinine value.[5]

If the relationship between serum creatinine and endogenous creatinine clearance is established for any individual patient, the serum value can usually be safely used to infer renal function. However, it may be incorrect to anticipate normal renal function from "normal" serum creatinine values, particularly if the patient is wasted or elderly. In these situations, presumption of normal renal function can result in serious overdoses with drugs that have narrow therapeutic:toxic ratios, such as aminoglycoside antibiotics and digitalis glycosides. Diet, corticosteroid therapy, and state of catabolism are extrarenal factors that influence the blood urea nitrogen, making it an unsuitable parameter on which to base dosage adjustments in renal failure. In patients with acute renal failure or with changing renal function, creatinine clearance and serum creatinine may become inaccurate until steady-state conditions are reached. To modify dosage in this situation, a measured creatinine clearance using a midpoint serum creatinine provides a reasonable estimate.

LIVER FUNCTION

A number of factors are involved in determining the rate of hepatic drug metabolism and elimination.[6-12] Several drugs, such as indocyanine green and bromsulphalein are efficiently extracted on a single pass through the liver (Table 2–1). For these drugs with high extraction rates (> 0.6), both rate of hepatic blood flow and hepatic extraction efficiency determine the rate and amount of drug processed by the liver.[6-8] Hepatic extraction is determined by hepatocyte mass and function. In patients with liver disease, hepatic blood flow can be increased (viral hepatitis), normal (early cirrhosis), and decreased (moderate cirrhosis, alcoholic hepatitis). In general, all forms of liver disease are associated with some reduction in hepatocyte function. Hepatic mass varies depending on the type and duration of liver disease. To date, no consistent clinical or readily available laboratory parameters provide a means to assess accurately liver blood flow, function, and mass. Thus, prediction of the degree of altered drug pharmacokinetics is often difficult in the individual patient with liver disease.

TABLE 2–1. DRUGS BELIEVED TO HAVE HIGH HEPATIC FIRST-PASS METABOLISM

Acetylsalicylic acid	Nitroglycerin
Alprenolol	Nortriptyline
Chlorpromazine	Paracetamol
Isoproterenol	Pentazocine
Lidocaine	Prazosin
Methylphenidate	Propoxyphene
Metoprolol	Propranolol
Meperidine	Salicylamide
Morphine	

Disease processes that affect the liver may decrease hepatic drug metabolism and increase systemic availability of orally administered drugs. For most orally administered drugs, absorption occurs across gastrointestinal epithelium that is drained by the portal vein. For oral drugs efficiently extracted by the liver, the drug is often metabolized before it can exert its effect. These drugs are often called "first-pass" drugs and are depicted in Table 2–1.[9, 12, 13] Not only hepatocyte dysfunction but also intra- and extrahepatic portosystemic shunts occur in patients with liver disease and markedly increase the oral bioavailability of these first-pass drugs.[9, 12, 13] Thus, extra caution should be utilized when administering these high hepatic clearance compounds to patients with liver disease.

Biliary excretion is an important route for elimination of many parent drugs and drug metabolites (Table 2–2). Chemical structure, polarity, and molecular weight are all factors that determine a drug's excretion into bile.[14] Chemical structure exerts a profound effect on biliary excretion. For example, in the rat substitution of simple chemical groups (such as

TABLE 2–2. DRUGS CONCENTRATED IN BILE (Bile/plasma ratio > 1)

Acebutolol	Doxycycline
Ampicillin	5-Fluorocytosine
Carbenoxolone	Indomethacin
Cephamandole	Metronidazole
Chloramphenicol	Pivampicillin
Chlortetracycline	Practolol
Clindamycin	Sex steroids
Demethylchlortetracycline	Spironolactone
Digoxin	Terbutaline
Doxorubicin	Vincristine

the hydroxyl groups) has a major influence on whether or not a drug is eliminated in bile.[14]

Most drugs excreted in human bile are either ionized or highly polar. A drug excreted into bile crosses two cell membranes. First, it must be taken up by the hepatocyte and subsequently transported across the canalicular membrane into bile. At least three active transport systems exist for the excretion of organic compounds into the bile of rats: one for organic acids, one for organic bases, and another for neutral organic compounds. Some evidence suggests a similar system exists in humans.[14] It is generally assumed that drugs are transported across both the sinusoidal and canalicular membranes of the hepatocyte by carrier-mediated transport systems. However, organic acids may be transferred from plasma to liver cells by binding to a binding protein (ligandin), which binds organic anions and is localized in cell cytosol.

The third feature of a drug important in determining biliary excretion is molecular weight. In rats, compounds with molecular weights above 325 are excreted into bile, while substances with lower molecular weights are not. In humans, there is also a tendency for high-molecular-weight substances to be excreted in the bile. However, many exceptions exist.

A drug excreted in the bile may be reabsorbed from the gastrointestinal tract and undergo enterohepatic circulation. Moreover, a drug conjugate excreted in bile may be hydrolyzed by gastrointestinal bacteria, liberating free drug. Thus, enterohepatic circulation may prolong the pharmacologic effect of drugs and their metabolites. However, in humans, this pathway appears to be of minor quantitative importance.

Cholestatic liver disease (Chap. 10) would be anticipated to result in impaired elimination of drugs normally excreted in large amounts in bile (Table 2–2). Thus, under these circumstances, empiric reduction in dosage may be indicated.

Taken together, it is apparent that a large number of variables affect hepatic metabolism and elimination of drugs. These variables include rate of hepatic blood flow, the presence of portosystemic shunts, hepatocellular mass and function, and bile flow. Some reported disease processes (e.g., severe alcoholic hepatitis) may affect all of these parameters. Alternatively, some liver processes (e.g., moderate hepatic cirrhosis) may affect drug metabolism to a variable extent in any group of patients, making generalizations regarding dosage modification difficult. Unlike renal disease, there is no clinically available test that uniformly correlates with hepatic drug clearance to guide dosage modifications.

An excellent example of the difficulties encountered in administering drugs to patients with liver disease has recently been published by Pirttiaho and co-workers.[15] They observed that alcoholics with normal liver function tests and histology had an increased rate of drug elimination associated with an increased cytochrome P-450 system in liver tissue. Induced induction of hepatic drug-metabolizing enzymes by chronic alcoholic ingestion can lead to reduced half-lives for such drugs as phenobarbital and phenytoin. Alcoholics with only fatty liver changes did not demonstrate abnormalities in either drug clearance or liver cytochrome P-450. In contrast, both alcoholic hepatitis and alcohol-associated cirrhosis had significantly reduced cytochrome P-450 content and prolonged drug clearance. Poor correlation between conventional liver function tests and drug elimination was noted. Thus, in all patients with known liver disease, the prescribing physician must exercise extreme caution when using drugs that require hepatic metabolism or biotransformation for elimination from the body. For several drugs, including propranolol, amylobarbital, phenylbutazone, and phenobarbital, the largest decreases in systemic clearance were found in patients with low serum albumin and prolonged prothrombin time.[6,16]

In summary, there are no readily available laboratory or clinical parameters that provide a practical guide to assist in drug dosage alterations in patients with liver disease. In general, acute hepatitis and cholestatic jaundice affect drug metabolism less than moderate or severe hepatic parenchymal processes. Patients with liver disease and associated hypoalbuminemia, prolonged prothrombin time, and clinical evidence of portal hypertension are most likely to have the greatest changes in drug metabolism. In these patients, the drugs listed in Tables 2–1 and 2–2 should be utilized with a great deal of caution.

IMPORTANCE OF A LOADING DOSE

For intermittent therapy in patients with renal disease, it is most often necessary to prescribe an initial dose larger than the usual maintenance dose. After the first dose, the blood level of a drug will reach a steady state in an interval equal to four to five elimination half-lives. If the half-life is prolonged because of impaired renal drug excretion and a loading dose is not given, a delay in reaching therapeutically effective concentrations may result. The loading dose is particularly important in clinical situations requiring prompt pharmacologic action, such as antiarrhythmic, antibiotic, or cardiac glycoside treatment. Figure 2–1 shows the influence of the loading dose on the achievement of desired blood levels.

It is difficult to assess precisely how much of the usual loading dose should be given to patients with renal failure. If other pharmacokinetic parameters, such as protein binding and apparent volume of distribution, are unaltered, the loading dose may be kept exactly the same as in patients without renal failure. This seems to be true for aminoglycoside antibiotics. However, the binding of digoxin to myocardial receptors is reduced in uremia, resulting in a decrease in the apparent volume of distribution. In this setting, most authors recommend only one-half to two thirds of the usual digitalizing dose.[17]

For clinical practice, the principle to be emphasized is that a loading or increased initial dose is required for drugs in which the half-life is prolonged by renal failure. If the desired drug concentration at steady state and the apparent volume of distribution are known, the loading dose can be calculated as:

$$D_L = AVD \times C_{SS}$$

where D_L equals the loading dose, AVD is the apparent volume of distribution, and C_{SS} is the desired concentration at steady state. For example, the AVD of gentamicin (in liters) is 25 per cent of body weight (in kilograms) and is approximately 17.5 L in a 70-kg individual. A desired steady-state concentration (C_{ss}) of gentamicin is 6 μg/dl. Thus, the loading dose would be:

$$\begin{aligned} D_L &= (17.5 \text{ L})\ (6 \text{ mg/l}) \\ &= 105 \text{ mg or } 1.5 \text{ mg/kg} \end{aligned}$$

The loading dose can also be estimated at approximately twice the dose given during each half-life to maintain a steady state; i.e., twice the maintenance dose. The calculations assume that the total drug administered enters the bloodstream. For orally administered drugs, variable amounts remain unabsorbed or undergo first-pass hepatic inactivation.

At the present time, there is no general rule about initial drug doses in patients with liver diseases. Drugs that undergo liver biotransformation to inactive metabolites or orally administered compounds that undergo extensive hepatic first-pass metabolism should be given cautiously with frequent observation of the patient.[8]

METHODS OF ALTERING MAINTENANCE DOSES IN RENAL FAILURE

Modification of drug dosage regimen in renal disease is usually only necessary when creatinine clearance is less than 30 to 40 ml/min. This is particularly true for drugs such as cephalosporin antibiotics in which adverse effects are minor despite high blood levels. Conversely, no general formula or rule will completely prevent adverse reactions for drugs such as cardiac glycosides or aminoglycoside antibiotics that have low safety margins and that almost entirely depend on renal excretion for elimination. In these latter circumstances, the clinician must be constantly vigilant, especially when serum concentrations cannot be monitored.

Drugs are ideally prescribed to maintain a desired concentration in the blood or at tissue receptors without toxic accumulation. Two general strategies can be adopted. The first employs a reduction in the size of each dose without changing the usual dosage interval. The second method increases the interval between doses, but keeps the size of each dose the same as would be employed in patients without renal failure. As an example, if a drug is excreted entirely unchanged by the kidney, the dosage interval must be doubled or the dosage size reduced by one-half if renal function is decreased to 50 per cent of that of normal. The best approach for any individual drug is determined by the drug's pharmacokinetics, the clinical situation, and, to some extent, physician preference.

EXTENSION OF DOSAGE INTERVALS

The method is most useful in situations where drugs with long serum half-lives are to be prescribed. If the usual dosage interval is the same or less than the serum half-life, this method will avoid unsafe drug accumulation. The new dosing interval for drugs excreted entirely by the kidney can be calculated by the formula: Dosing interval in renal failure = dose interval normal × (present creatinine clearance/normal creatinine clearance). When the drug in question has some elimination pathway other than renal excretion of unchanged drug, the formula becomes:

$$\text{Dose interval in renal failure} = \text{normal dose interval} \times \frac{1}{\text{f (patient's creat. clearance/normal creat. clearance} - 1)} + 1$$

where f = the fraction of drug normally eliminated unchanged by the kidney. For example, if a drug that is normally excreted 60 per cent unchanged by the kidney and usually is given every 6 hours to a patient with a creatinine clearance of 10 ml/min, the interval modification calculation would be:

$$\text{Dose interval} = 6\text{ hr} \times \frac{1}{0.6 \times (0.1/1)} + 1$$

$$= 6\text{ hr} \times \frac{1}{0.46} = 13\text{ hr}$$

The method of interval lengthening will result in intermittency of therapeutic concentrations with relatively wide swings from peak to trough serum levels. For drugs with a narrow therapeutic range, toxic or nontherapeutic levels may result.

REDUCTION OF DOSAGE SIZE

The amount of drug given can be reduced using dosage intervals that do not change from normal individuals. This reduces the differences between maximum and minimum plasma concentrations in patients with renal failure. This may be an advantage for drugs in which it is desirable to maintain a reasonably constant steady-state level, such as antibiotics with short serum half-lives and some antiarrhythmic drugs. However, if the extent of renal dysfunction is underestimated or if toxicity is dependent on a certain level of drug available for tissue transport, the risk of an adverse reaction might be increased. There is some experimental evidence that nephrotoxic potential is increased by frequent doses in aminoglycoside nephrotoxicity.[18] The general formula to find the correct dose in renal failure is: Dose size in renal failure = normal dose × (normal creatinine clearance/patient's creatinine clearance). This assumes that the drug is excreted unchanged by the kidney exclusively. If some portion of the drug is eliminated by hepatic biotransformation, the formula becomes:

$$\text{Dose size in renal failure} = \text{normal dose} \times \text{f}\,\frac{\text{(normal creat. clearance/patient's creat. clearance} - 1)}{1} + 1$$

where f = the fraction of drug normally eliminated unchanged by the kidney. In practice, a combination of the dosage reduction and interval extension is frequently used.

DOSAGE NOMOGRAMS

Total body drug clearance is equal to the sum of renal clearance plus nonrenal clearance. Drugs tend to cluster into one of three groups: those with exclusive renal clearance, those with predominant nonrenal clearance, and those with a combination of renal and nonrenal clearance. A graphic representation of these types of body elimination is shown in Figure 2–2. The slope of the line relating total plasma clearance to creatinine clearance represents the elimination rate constant for that drug in units of fraction per hour or day (Fig. 2–3). The intercept on the ordinate represents clearance by such nonrenal means as hepatic metabolism. A nomogram can be constructed that allows a graphic estimate of plasma clearance in renal failure. The nomogram is based on changes in the plasma fraction (relative to subjects with normal renal function) as a linear function of creatinine clearance. By connect-

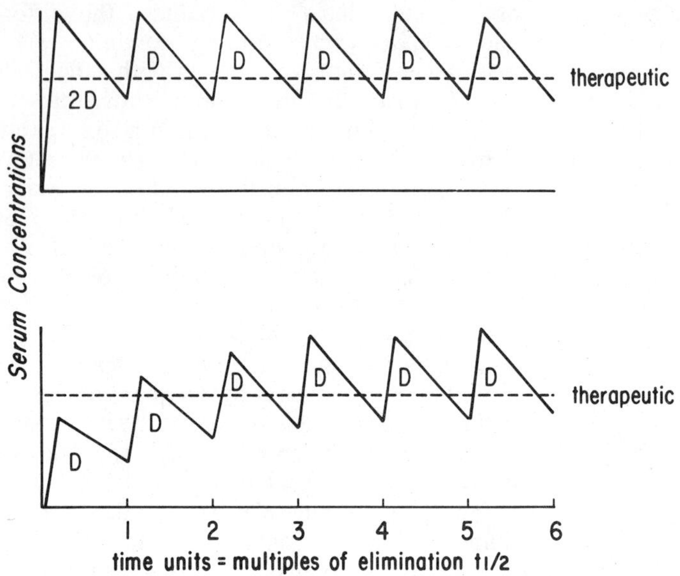

Figure 2–2. Influence of a loading dose on blood level of a theoretical drug. Bottom panel – maintenance dose D given at interval equal to elimination half-life. Top panel – loading dose equal to twice maintenance dose (2D) followed by usual maintenance therapy. Note the prompt appearance of therapeutic blood levels.

ing the intercept on the ordinate (the dose fraction in anuric patients) with the right upper corner of the nomogram, a dosing line for a specific drug can be drawn. Dettli has published elimination rate fractions for anuric patients.[19] The point of intersection between the patient's creatinine clearance and the dosing line will read that patient's plasma clearance fraction. Using this fraction, the clinician can multiply the usual dose to obtain the proper maintenance dose, or divide into the usual interval to calculate the correct dosage interval for renal failure. Alternately, the amount of drug usually given over any dosing interval in normal subjects can be multiplied by the proper plasma clearance fraction to obtain a modified rate of administration for renal failure.

Figure 2–4 represents an example of such a nomogram adapted to antibiotic therapy by Aronoff and Luft[20] from a more inclusive nomogram of Bryan and Stone.[21] The maintenance dose is defined by the product of the dose in patients with normal renal function

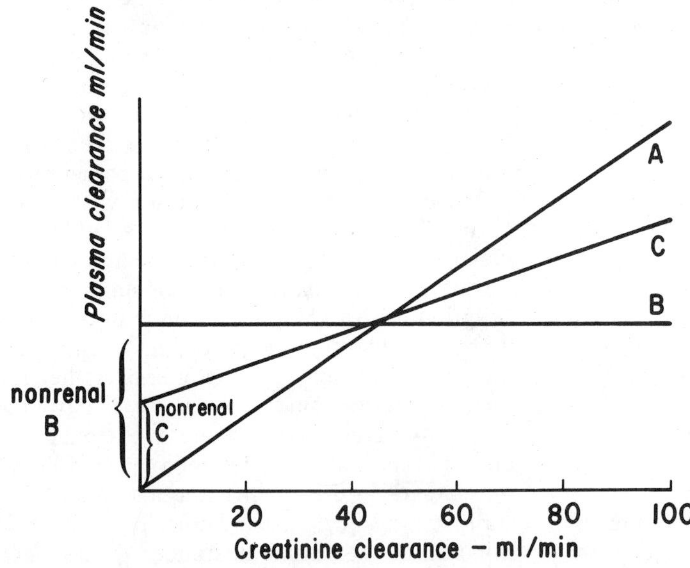

Figure 2–3. Total plasma clearance versus creatinine clearance for three prototype drugs exhibiting renal (drug A), nonrenal (drug B), or combination (drug C) elimination. The intercept on the ordinate represents nonrenal clearance. Nonrenal clearance of A = 0.

times the dose fraction read off the nomogram. As an example, to prescribe gentamicin for a 70-kg patient with a creatinine clearance of 40 ml/min, an initial loading dose similar to the usual loading dose is given (1.5 mg/kg). Reading from Figure 2–4, the dosing line A intersects with the patient's creatinine clearance at a dose fraction of 0.42. Thus, we can multiply the normal maintenance dose of 1 mg/kg (70 mg) by 0.42 to get a new dose of 29 mg every 8 hours. Alternatively, the usual dosage interval of 8 hours can be divided by the dose fraction 0.42 to obtain the correct dosage interval of 19 hours for this degree of renal failure. Finally, the rate of administration, 70 mg/8 hr or 8.8 mg/hr, can be multiplied by 0.42 to get a new rate of 3.7 mg/hr.

Tozer has developed a different type of nomogram (shown in Fig. 2–5) that is applicable to all drugs, provided the fraction of the drug normally eliminated unchanged in the urine is known.[22] The intersection of the lines representing the fraction of drug excretion unchanged and the fraction of normal kidney function provides a Q value, indicating the extent of the increase in drug half-life in the body. Using the Q value, the dose size or interval may be adjusted.

In using these nomograms, the simplifying

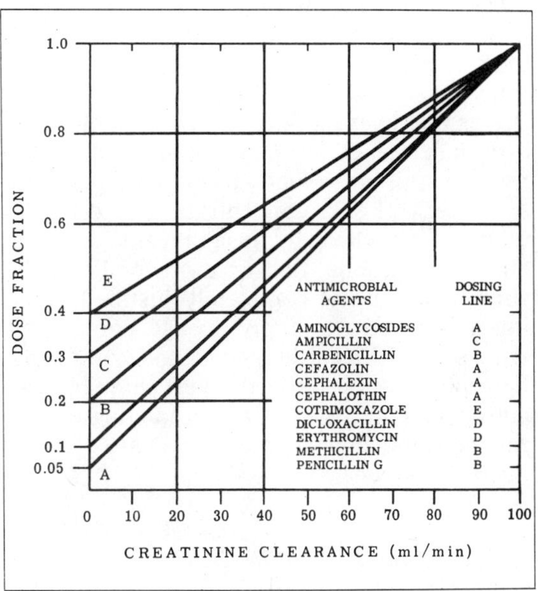

Figure 2–4. Dose fraction as a function of creatinine clearance. Lines A through E are dosing lines appropriate for different antibiotics based on the dose fraction for anephric patients. (Data from Aronoff GR and Luft FG: Antimicrobial therapy in patients with impaired renal function. Dialysis Transpl. *8*:14–77, 1979; Bryan CS and Stone WJ: Antimicrobial dosage in renal failure: A unifying nomogram. Clin. Nephrol. *7*:81–84, 1977, with permission.)

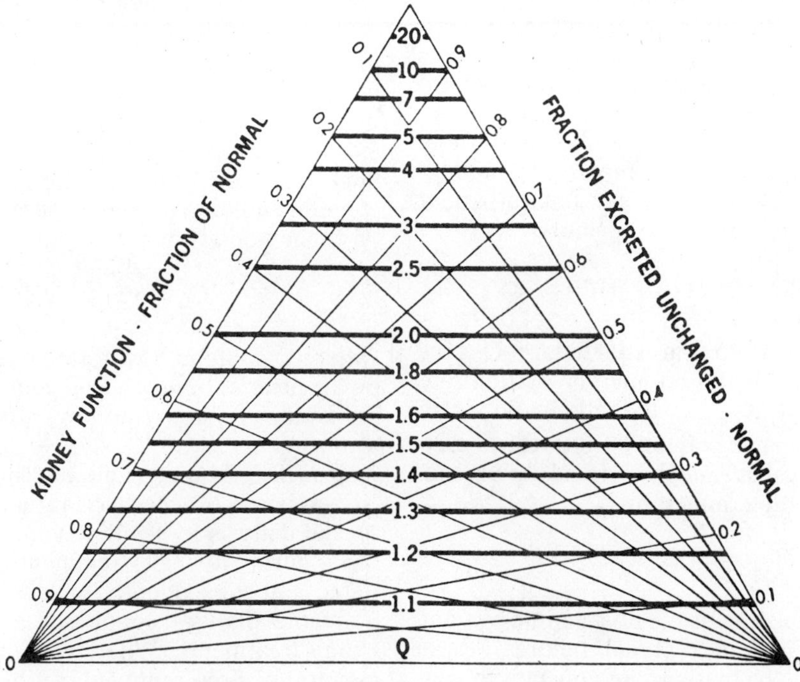

Figure 2–5. Dosage adjustment nomogram based on fraction of drug excreted unchanged in the urine. Q-value indicates the extent of increase in drug half-life due to renal failure. (From Tozer TN: Nomogram for modification of dosage regimens in patients with chronic renal function impairment. J. Pharmacokinet. Biopharm. *2*:13–28, 1974, with permission.)

assumptions and limitations that are implicit need to be kept in mind. First, renal function must remain constant and factors other than renal function that affect drug pharmacokinetics cannot change. Second, it is assumed that drug metabolites are pharmacologically inactive. Lastly, individual variations in response to a given plasma concentration of drug are taken to be clinically insignificant. In most clinical situations, one or more of these assumptions are not completely justified, making it necessary to apply dosage nomograms with sound clinical judgment and careful patient observation. Indeed, even with sophisticated computer models for predicting dosage regimens the clinician must be aware of unexpected reactions.

ELIMINATION RATE CONSTANT AND PLASMA HALF-LIFE

Dettli has published equations describing the rate of drug elimination as a linear function of glomerular filtration rate.[19] The proportionality factor relating renal drug elimination to the level of renal function plus the rate constant for extrarenal elimination equals the overall elimination rate constant, K_e. It is assumed that a first-order, one-compartment model describes with sufficient accuracy the elimination of the drugs in question. Experimentally derived elimination rate constants for normal and anuric patients are available[23] and these constants for some of the more commonly utilized agents are shown in Table 2–3. If these constants are known, the maintenance dose for an anuric renal failure patient can be calculated from the formula

$$D_{RF} = D\ (K_{e_{RF}}/K_e)$$

where D_{RF} is the dose in renal failure, D is the usual dose, K_e is the normal elimination rate constant, and $K_{e_{RF}}$ is the elimination rate constant in anuric patients. Likewise, a new dosage interval in anephric renal failure patients can be determined by

$$T_{RF} = T\ (K_e/K_{e_{RF}}$$

where T equals the usage dosage interval and T_{RF} is the interval in renal failure. As an example, the elimination rate constant of gentamicin in normal subjects is 0.30 hr^{-1} and in anephric patients 0.01 hr^{-1}. The usual dose is 1 mg/kg every 8 hours (0.33 day). The new interval for gentamicin in an anephric patient not undergoing dialysis would be

$$0.33\ (0.03/0.03) = 9.9 \text{ days}$$

Since $K_e = 0.693/t_{\frac{1}{2}}$, the elimination rate constant can be used to calculate the plasma half-life for the degree of renal failure present. For practical purposes, the half-life is defined as the time required for the serum drug concentration to decline by 50 per cent. Half-lives for various drugs in patients with normal renal function and renal failure are given in the Appendix and several standard sources.[24, 25] If the ratio of normal half-life to the half-life in renal failure is divided by the usual dosing interval, the dosing interval for renal failure can be estimated. Likewise, if the ratio of the normal half-life in renal failure is multiplied by the usual dose, the new reduced maintenance dose is obtained.

ADJUSTMENT OF DOSAGE FOR DIALYSIS

Gibson and Nelson have reviewed the variables that influence drug removal during clinical hemodialysis.[26] The increase in plasma drug clearance that may occur with dialysis is described by the equation

$$C_p = C_R + C_{NR} + C_D$$

where C_p is the plasma clearance, C_R is the renal clearance, C_{NR} is the nonrenal clearance, and C_D is the drug dialyzer clearance. The general equation used to describe drug removal by hemodialysis is

$$C_D = Q\ (A-V)/A$$

where Q is blood flow through the dialyzer, A is the arterial (inflow) drug concentration, and V is the venous (outflow) drug concentration.

If a drug is dialyzable and maintenance of serum levels is necessary, replacement of projected dialysis losses is required. Recovery of drug during a single treatment can be quantitated and subsequently replaced. This is best if stable dialysis conditions are present for many treatments. When the C_D is known, the amount of drug removed can be estimated by the equation: predicted removal − plasma clearance × dialysis time × midpoint arterial

TABLE 2–3. ELIMINATION RATE CONSTANTS OF COMMONLY USED DRUGS

Drug	Normal K/hr	Anephric K(K/Hr)
Penicillins		
Amoxicillin	0.70	0.10
Ampicillin	0.70	0.10
Carbenicillin	0.60	0.05
Cloxacillin	1.40	0.35
Methicillin	1.40	0.17
Nafcillin	1.20	0.48
Oxacillin	1.40	0.35
Penicillin G	1.40	0.05
Ticarcillin	0.60	0.06
Cephalosporins		
Cephacetrile	0.70	0.03
Cephalexin	1.00	0.03
Cephaloridine	0.50	0.03
Cephalothin	1.40	0.04
Cefazolin	0.40	0.04
Aminoglycosides		
Amikacin	0.40	0.04
Gentamicin	0.30	0.01
Kanamycin	0.40	0.01
Streptomycin	0.27	0.01
Tobramycin	0.36	0.01
Antituberculotic-Antifungal Agents		
Amphotericin B	0.04	0.02
Ethambutol	0.58	0.09
Fluorocytosine	0.24	0.01
Isoniazid (fast acetylators)	0.60	0.20
(slow acetylators)	0.20	0.08
Rifampin	0.25	0.25
Tetracyclines		
Chlortetracycline	0.10	0.10
Doxycycline	0.03	0.03
Minocycline	0.05	0.03
Oxytetracycline	0.08	0.02
Tetracycline	0.08	0.01
Miscellaneous Antimicrobials		
Chloramphenicol	0.30	0.20
Clindamycin	0.47	0.10
Colistimethate	0.20	0.04
Erythromycin	0.50	0.14
Lincomycin	0.15	0.06
Polymyxin B	0.16	0.02
Sulfadiazine	0.08	0.03
Sulfamethoxazole	0.70	0.70
Trimethoprim	0.60	0.02
Vancomycin	0.12	0.003
Antiarrhythmic-Antihypertensive Agents		
Alpha-methyldopa	0.17	0.03
Lidocaine	0.40	0.36
Procainamide	0.22	0.01
Propranolol	0.20	0.16
Quinidine	0.07	0.06
Cardiac Glycosides		
Digitoxin	0.004	0.003
Digoxin	0.017	0.006

concentration. Since changes in protein binding, patient variables and dialyzer factors make precise clinical adjustments difficult, it is best to check drug levels prior to the next scheduled dose. Serum concentrations measured immediately postdialysis can underestimate total body burden, since equilibration from extravascular sites may take place over several hours following dialysis. Supplemental doses are generally given at the conclusion of dialysis in order to maintain total body drug concentrations. If no specific data are available concerning clearance of a dialyzable drug, it is best to administer a full maintenance dose.

Consideration should also be given to common therapeutic agents lost during peritoneal dialysis. The large peritoneal surface area and longer duration of treatment may result in removal of larger solutes than during hemodialysis. To prevent marked fluctuations in serum concentrations, drug can be added to peritoneal dialysate at concentrations equal to the desired serum level. Table 2–4 lists drugs that undergo enough clearance during routine dialysis to require dosage supplementation.

MODIFYING FACTORS FOR GENERAL FORMULAS

Patients with renal failure often demonstrate alterations in pharmacokinetic parameters that do not have a precise correlation with the conventional clinical measure of renal function, i.e., the creatinine clearance. Changes in the volume of drug distribution and gastrointestinal absorption or drug-protein binding induced by uremia may alter serum half-life. The extent of these alterations may be difficult to predict for any individual patient making fixed dosing formulas subject to error, even for drugs whose elimination depends entirely on renal mechanisms. For drugs whose pharmacokinetics are more complex or in cases in which renal failure alters hepatic drug metabolism, the clinician must depend more heavily on careful observation of the patient for drug toxicity and serum drug levels if available.

If data on prescribing a specific drug in renal failure are available from the literature in a well-designed study, these recommendations should be used as initial dosing guidelines in preference to any general formulas. Several tables compiling data on commonly used drugs are available.[24,25] In this regard, the Appendix also provides a valuable source of information. It should be recognized that the data base on which recommendations for drug prescribing in renal failure depend is often lacking or conflicting. Furthermore, few studies have been reported that compare the predictions of kinetic models or the suggestions from dosage tables to data obtained in clinical practice. Losses of drug during clinical dialysis further complicate the situation, since wide individual variability exists.

TABLE 2–4. COMMON DRUGS REQUIRING SUPPLEMENTAL DOSAGE AFTER HEMODIALYSIS AND PERITONEAL DIALYSIS

Hemodialysis	
Antibiotics	
Aminoglycosides	amikacin, gentamicin, kanamycin, tobramycin, streptomycin
Cephalosporins	cephalothin, cephalexin, cephapirin, cephazolin
Penicillins	amoxicillin, ampicillin, carbenicillin, penicillin G
Others	sulfonamides, trimethoprim-sulfamethoxazole
Antituberculous	ethambutol, isoniazid
Antifungal	5-fluorocytosine
Analgesics	acetylsalicylic acid
Cardiovascular	procainamide, quinidine
Immunosuppressive-antineoplastic	azathioprine, cyclophosphamide, methotrexate
Miscellaneous	long-acting barbiturates, lithium, phenytoin
Peritoneal Dialysis	
Antibiotics	
Aminoglycosides	amikacin, gentamicin, kanamycin, tobramycin, streptomycin
Cephalosporins	cephalexin, cephalothin, cephradine
Penicillins	ticarcillin
Others	sulfonamides, trimethoprim-sulfamethoxazole
Antituberculous	ethambutol
Antifungal	5-fluorocytosine
Analgesics	acetylsalicylic acid
Cardiovascular	procainamide
Miscellaneous	phenytoin

DRUG PRESCRIBING IN LIVER DISEASE

There are few general rules to aid the clinician in prescribing for patients with liver disease. This is due to variable extents of liver involvement by disease processes and lack of clinical measures of hepatic drug metabolism or clearance. The hepatic clearance of a drug is equal to the product of hepatic blood flow and the extraction ratio. Unfortunately, the extraction ratio is not constant for any particular drug and depends on hepatic blood flow, intrinsic hepatic drug removal capacity, and drug binding to plasma proteins.[7] In addition, certain drugs induce microsomal enzymes that may increase their own or other drugs' hepatic removal. Thus, unlike the situation with renal failure, the prolongation of drug half-life by decreased hepatic function is less certain, particularly since volume of distribution may also change. The situation may be more predictable when drugs are given parenterally. During oral administration, the liver may be variably involved in presystemic drug removal. Drugs that undergo substantial hepatic first-pass metabolism may exhibit large increases in bioavailability and should be used with caution in liver disease.[9, 12]

In any situation in which liver hemodynamics are likely to be compromised, such as congestive heart failure or shock, the removal of drugs normally exhibiting high liver clearance may be reduced (Table 2–1). Drugs in this category, such as lidocaine, should be administered with caution starting with lower doses. With intrinsic liver disease, there may be associated hepatic circulatory abnormalities, such as reduced total blood flow, intrahepatic shunting, or extrahepatic shunting of blood.[6]

Nies has proposed a classification of drugs based on their intrinsic hepatic clearance.[7] If a drug is more than 70 per cent extracted by the liver and, thus, possesses an intrinsic clearance greater than hepatic blood flow, it is a high-clearance drug. Disposition from the body of such drugs is dependent on hepatic blood flow and less so on liver enzyme metabolizing capacity. Low-clearance drugs are those in which liver extraction less than 20 per cent of liver blood flow and removal is determined by hepatic metabolic enzyme capability.[7]

Since liver function and hepatic blood flow must decrease to a considerable extent before plasma levels rise, only drugs with a low therapeutic index are likely to cause problems. The only real guidelines a clinician can use are related to assessment of the likely degree of hepatic perfusion and a knowledge of individual drug pharmacology.

Certain drugs or their metabolites have major excretion in bile. Cholestatic liver disease may impair drug excretion and increase the risk of toxicity. For example, digoxin and spironolactone excretion in bile may be impaired in liver disease.[14]

Liver disease may also cause impaired drug binding to plasma proteins, either because of decreased albumin concentration or qualitative changes in drug-binding properties of the proteins.[8] With high-clearance drugs, such as propranolol, a decrease in plasma protein binding will not change clearance, since their rate of metabolism is dependent on hepatic blood flow. Decreased binding might prolong half-life if the volume of distribution increases.

Other drugs normally exhibit high binding to plasma proteins and dependence on a fixed liver enzyme capacity for metabolism. Liver diseases, by decreased protein binding, may cause increased availability of free drug for metabolic conversion, lowering total drug concentrations; warfarin, tolbutamide, and phenytoin are drugs that exhibit this phenomenon. However, if liver disease leads to both decreased drug-protein binding and a reduc-

TABLE 2–5. DRUGS WITH POTENTIAL FOR ADVERSE REACTIONS IN LIVER DISEASE[8, 24, 26, 27]

Analgesics	acetylsalicylic acid, acetaminophen
Antiarrhythmics	lidocaine, verapamil
Antidepressants	imipramine, nortriptyline
Beta-adrenergic Blocking Drugs	alprenolol, labetalol, metoprolol, oxyprenolol, propranolol
Cardiovascular Drugs or Antihypertensives	digoxin, prazosin, spironolactone, nitroglycerin
Opiates	meperidine, morphine, naloxone, pentazocine, propoxyphene
Miscellaneous	chlorpromazine, antineoplastic drugs, diazepam, tolbutamine, warfarin, phenytoin, phenylbutazone

tion of intrinsic drug clearance, as in acute hepatitis, free drug levels will rise, often leading to adverse reactions. If protein binding of a drug is normally less than 30 per cent, liver disease will usually cause problems only if intrinsic metabolic capacity is decreased.[8]

Table 2–5 categorizes some drugs that have been studied in relation to liver disease. Physicians who prescribe these drugs in liver disease should be alert for the necessity to reduce dose or increase dosing interval to avoid excessive accumulation and toxicity.

USE OF SERUM LEVELS TO MONITOR THERAPY

Even in normal individuals there is marked difference in therapeutic response to a given dose of a drug. To avoid serious over- or underdosage, serum drug concentrations can be used as guides to safety and efficacy[27] (see Chap. 4). Usual therapeutic ranges are being increasingly defined as methodology for measuring various drugs in biologic fluids becomes widely available. Interpretation of drug levels must take into account the complex relationships between the dose prescribed and pharmacologic or therapeutic effects. Most drugs exert pharmacologic actions after free drug combines with a receptor located at the site of action. Most analytic methods currently used for measuring drug levels give a total concentration, including both free drug and any fraction bound to plasma proteins. Thus, the relationship between drug effects and plasma drug concentration may change if protein binding is affected by liver or kidney disease. Both the serum albumin concentration and the ability of serum proteins to bind drug may be decreased in liver disease.[8] The same is true for patients with renal disease who may have nephrotic syndrome, renal failure, or both.[28-30] With some agents, a normal or even low total drug concentration may be associated with serious adverse reactions if the unbound concentration is increased. Decreased protein binding does not inevitably lead to enhanced pharmacologic activity. With phenytoin, elimination is enhanced when binding is reduced because of increased availability of free drug for metabolic conversion.[30]

Serum or plasma levels can be understood fully only if the elapsed time from the last dose and the elimination half-life in that particular patient are known. To obtain the best estimate of the peak blood concentration, samples should be obtained 1 to 2 hours after an oral dose and 30 minutes to 1 hour following parenteral dosing. A minimum of trough concentration is obtained just prior to the next dose. For drugs with half-lives longer than the usual dosing interval, such as digoxin, timing following maintenance doses is less critical. This presumes, of course, that a steady state has been reached during chronic dosing and the dose has not been recently changed.

Clinical judgment is still required even when serum levels are known. Cardiac glycoside toxicity, for example, may occur with "therapeutic" or even low serum levels if hypokalemia or metabolic alkalosis is present. Thus, the patient's physiologic and biochemical milieu must be carefully considered when evaluating serum levels in pathologic states of liver or kidney disease. It is also helpful to know the reproducibility of drug assays in the laboratory available to the physician and any possible interference by other drugs in the test results. Desirable levels for individual drugs are available in this book (see Appendix).

CONCLUSIONS

This chapter has summarized the practical aspects of drug prescribing for patients with renal and liver disease. In renal failure, determination of glomerular filtration rate by endogenous creatinine clearance provides the best basis for adjustment of drug dosage. Unfortunately, there is no liver function test that correlates well enough with hepatic drug metabolism to provide a similar framework in hepatic disease. Thus, the use of serum drug concentrations to monitor therapy is encouraged in severe liver failure whenever possible.

In renal disease, various formulas, nomograms, or tables are available as guides to dosage. However, any fixed approach to the complex patient should be tempered with sound clinical judgment and knowledge of side effects of the drug being used. This is of even greater importance in hepatic disease in which general information is less readily available.

REFERENCES

1. Bennett WM: Drug prescribing in renal failure. Drugs *17*:111–123, 1979.
2. Cockroft DW, Gault MH: Prediction of creatinine clearance from serum creatinine. Nephron *16*:31–41, 1976.
3. Parker RA, Bennett WM, Porter GA: Clinical estimation of creatinine clearance without urine collection. Dialysis Transpl. *9*:257, 1980.
4. Bjornsson TD: Use of serum creatinine concentrations to determine renal function. Clin. Pharmacokinet. *4*:200–222, 1979.
5. Siersbaek-Nielsen K, Hansen JM, Kampmann J, et al.: Rapid evaluation of creatinine clearance. Lancet *1*:1133–1134, 1971.
6. Wilkinson GR, Schenker S: Drug disposition and liver disease. Drug Metab. Rev. *4*:139–175, 1975.
7. Nies AS, Shand DG, Wilkinson GR: Altered hepatic blood flow and drug disposition. Clin. Pharmacokinet. *1*:135–155, 1976.
8. Blaschke TF: Protein binding and kinetics of drugs in liver diseases. Clin. Pharmacokinet. *2*:32–44, 1977.
9. Blaschke TF, Rubin PC: Hepatic first-pass metabolism in liver disease. Clin. Pharmacokinet. *4*:423–432, 1979.
10. Wood AJ, Villeneuve JP, Branch RA, Rogers LW, Skind DG: Intact hepatocyte theory of impaired drug metabolism in experimental cirrhosis in the rat. Gastroenterology *76*:1358–1362, 1979.
11. Shand DG: Hepatic circulation and drug disposition in cirrhosis. Gastroenterology *77*:184–186, 1979.
12. Neal EA, Meffin DJ, Gregory PB, Blaschke TF: Enhanced bioavailability and decreased clearance of analgesics in patients with cirrhosis. Gastroenterology *77*:96–102, 1979.
13. George CF: Drug kinetics and hepatic blood flow. Clin. Pharmacokinet. *4*:433–448, 1979.
14. Rollins DE, Klaassen CD: Biliary excretion of drugs in man. Clin. Pharmacokinet. *4*:368–379, 1979.
15. Pirttiaho HI, Sotaniemi EA, Ahlqvist J, Pitkanen U, Pelkonen RO: Liver size and indices of drug metabolism in alcoholics. Europ. J. Clin. Pharmacol. *13*:61–67, 1978.
16. Branch RA, Shand DG: Propranolol disposition in chronic liver disease: A physiological approach. Clin. Pharmacokinet. *1*:264–279, 1976.
17. Fabre J, Balant L: Renal failure, drug pharmacokinetics and drug action. Clin. Pharmacokinet. *1*:99–120, 1976.
18. Bennett WM, Plamp CE, Gilbert DN, et al.: The influence of dosage regimen on experimental gentamicin nephrotoxicity: dissociation of peak serum levels from renal failure. J. Infect. Dis. *140*:576–580, 1979.
19. Dettli L: Drug dosage in renal disease. Clin. Pharmacokinet. *1*:126–134, 1976.
20. Aronoff GR, Luft FG: Antimicrobial therapy in patients with impaired renal function. Dialysis Transpl. *8*:14–77, 1979.
21. Bryan CS, Stone WJ: Antimicrobial dosage in renal failure: A unifying nomogram. Clin. Nephrol. *7*:81–84, 1977.
22. Tozer TN: Nomogram for modification of dosage regimens in patients with chronic renal function impairment. J. Pharmacokinet. Biopharm. *2*:13–28, 1974.
23. Dettli L: Individualization of drug dosage in patients with renal disease. Med. Clin. N. Am. *58*:977–985, 1974.
24. Bennett WM, Muther RS, Parker RA, et al.: Drug therapy in renal failure: Dosing guidelines for adults. Ann. Intern. Med. *93*:62–89; 286–325, 1980.
25. Cutler RE, Krichman KH, Blair AD: Pharmacology of drugs in renal failure. *In* Current Nephrology (H Gonick, ed.) Boston: Houghton Mifflin Co., 1979, pp. 397–435.
26. Gibson TP, Nelson HA: Drug kinetics and artificial kidneys. Clin. Pharmacokinet. *2*:403–416, 1977.
27. Koch-Weser J: Drug therapy: serum drug concentrations as therapeutic guides. N. Engl. J. Med. *287*:227–231, 1972.
28. Gugler R, Shoeman DW, Huffman DH, et al.: Pharmacokinetics of drugs in patients with the nephrotic syndrome. J. Clin. Invest. *55*:1182–1189, 1975.
29. Reidenberg MM: The binding of drugs to plasma proteins and the interpretation of measurements of plasma concentrations of drugs in patients with poor renal function. Am. J. Med. *62*:466–468, 1977.
30. Odar-Cederlof I, Borga O: Kinetics of diphenylhydantoin in uremic patients: consequences of decreased plasma protein binding. Eur. J. Clin. Pharmacol. *7*:31–37, 1974.

Chapter 3

Mechanisms of Adverse Drug Reactions

by

Robert J. Anderson
and Robert W. Schrier

ADVERSE REACTIONS TO ESTABLISHED DRUGS

Adverse effects resulting from use of prescribed as well as "over-the-counter" pharmacologic agents are a major problem of contemporary medicine. As illustrated in Table 3–1, several studies published during the past two decades found that adverse reactions to pharmacologic agents occurred in 1 to 30 per cent of hospitalized patients.[1-12] A number of factors, including ambiguities in the definition of adverse drug reactions, variability in patient populations studied, difficulties in establishing a clear cause-effect relationship, and frequent lack of control populations, suggest that the data in Table 3–1 be interpreted cautiously.[13, 14] Nevertheless, conservative estimates of drug-induced adverse effects from long-term prospective studies carried out in several countries (United States, Canada, Israel, Scotland, Italy, Germany, and New Zealand) suggest that approximately 5 per cent of hospitalized patients will develop a per cent of hospitalized patients will develop a significant adverse drug reaction.[15] Moreover, a review of more than 16,000 hospital admissions documents that 2 to 4 per cent of admissions to medical services were directly related to adverse drug effects (Table 3–2).[12, 16-19] Taken together, it is clear that the widespread use of established pharmacologic agents car-

TABLE 3–1. ADVERSE DRUG REACTIONS OCCURRING IN HOSPITALIZED PATIENTS

Study	Duration of Surveillance (months)	Number of Patients Evaluated	Frequency of Adverse Drug Reactions
Schimmel, 1964[1]	8	1,014	10%
MacDonald and MacKay, 1964[2]	12	9,557	1%
Seidl et al., 1964, 1966[3, 4]	3	714	13.6%
Smith et al., 1966[5]	12	900	10.8%
Ogilvie and Ruedy, 1967[6]	12	731	18%
Hoddinott et al., 1967[7]	2	104	15%
Reidenberg, 1968[8]	24	86,100	0.9%
Simmons et al., 1968[9]	3	219	12.3%
Hurwitz and Wade, 1969[10]	12	1,160	10.2%
Wang and Terry, 1971[11]	12	8,291	1.5%
Grey et al., 1973[12]	2	170	30%

TABLE 3–2. ADVERSE DRUG REACTIONS CAUSING HOSPITAL ADMISSIONS

Study	Duration of Surveillance (months)	Number of Admissions Evaluated	Per Cent Admissions Due To Adverse Drug Reactions
Hurwitz, 1969[16]	12	1,268	2.9
Gray et al., 1973[12]	2	170	1.7
Miller, 1974[17]	34	7,017	3.7
Caranasas, 1974[18]	36	6,063	2.9
Levy et al., 1979[19]	84	2,499	4.1

ries with it a substantial potential for drug-related adverse effects.

ADVERSE REACTIONS TO NEWLY MARKETED DRUGS

It is important for the practitioner to acknowledge that previously unrecognized adverse effects of new drugs are often observed only after drug marketing. Current practices of drug evaluation in the United States are divided into three phases. Phase one involves studies of drug pharmacology and toxicity carried out in animals and in tissue specimens. Phase two consists of acute and chronic toxicity studies carried out in generally healthy human volunteers. Phase three studies involve clinical trials carried out in selected human populations. The two major objectives of these three phases of premarketing drug testing are evaluation of effectiveness and assessment of risk. Evaluation of effectiveness, since it often involves quantitative assessment of well-defined results in a selected population (for example, lowering of blood pressure in patients with hypertension), is relatively easy. In contrast, risks are an open-ended issue, often without advanced knowledge of a specified end point. Although hematologic, renal, and hepatic function tests are usually carried out in premarketing drug testing, there can be no guarantee that the clinical and laboratory observations will detect all adverse effects. Moreover, since phase two and three trials are carried out on relatively small numbers of patients (approximately 500 to 3000), adverse drug reactions that are infrequently encountered (e.g., 1 in 1000) may not be detected prior to drug marketing.[20, 21] Furthermore, very few patients in phase three studies undergo prolonged (> 6 to 12 months) therapy.[20, 21] Thus, adverse effects that are dependent on chronic drug exposure may go undetected. In addition, many patients particularly susceptible to adverse drug reactions, such as patients with kidney and liver disease, are not included in phase three studies. These factors, when combined with the present lack of a structured system of postmarketing drug surveillance in the United States,[21] demand that new drugs be used with special caution. Numerous deaths due to fulminant hepatic failure following the new uricosuric-diuretic agent ticrynafen (discussed in detail in Chap. 10) illustrates this point.

In view of the potential for substantial morbidity from use of established and new drugs, avoidance of adverse drug reactions becomes an important issue. This chapter will review several "risk factors" that may predispose to adverse drug effects. Particular emphasis will be placed on the mechanisms whereby the presence of renal and hepatic disease increases the likelihood of adverse drug effects. Based on a knowledge of epidemiologic factors associated with adverse drug reactions and the mechanisms involved in some of these reactions, practical guidelines helpful in avoidance of adverse drug effects will become apparent.

FACTORS PREDISPOSING TO ADVERSE DRUG REACTIONS

TYPES OF ADVERSE DRUG REACTIONS

As utilized in this and subsequent chapters, an adverse drug effect is defined as any unintended response to a drug that is noxious and occurs with doses conventionally utilized for prophylaxis, diagnosis, or therapy.[22] This definition has recently been expanded to exclude failure to accomplish the intended effect of the drug.[13] Of note, this definition excludes adverse effects resulting from intentional drug overdose.

EXAGGERATION OF DESIRED PHARMACOLOGIC RESPONSE

Adverse drug reactions can be divided into four major categories. One adverse pharmacologic reaction is a noxious, undesired extension of the known effects of a drug. An example of this form of reaction is prolonged sedation following a standard dose of a sedative-hypnotic agent administered to a patient with advanced hepatic cirrhosis. In general, such pharmacologic reactions comprise 30 to 70 per cent of all adverse drug reactions and are thus among the most common adverse drug effects currently recognized.[1, 6, 10, 12] This type of adverse drug reaction is particularly common in patients with kidney and liver disease in whom drug biotransformation and elimination are often impaired.

IMMUNOLOGIC REACTIONS

Another form of adverse drug reaction can be broadly classified as "immunologic"-mediated reactions and account for 10 to 40 per cent of adverse drug effects.[1, 6, 10, 12] Increasing knowledge has expanded this form of drug reaction from anaphylactic reactions and hypersensitivity skin rashes to a broad spectrum of disease states. Briefly, immunologic reactions to drugs can be mediated either by humoral mechanisms, which include direct cellular toxicity as well as cell damage due to immune complex deposition, or by cellular immune mechanisms. For a review of the multiple mechanisms and resultant end-organ effects of drug-induced immunologic diseases of the kidney and liver, see Chapters 7 and 11. There is no evidence that either kidney or liver disease predisposes to immunologic adverse drug reactions. However, a drug-induced immunologic disorder may be either more severe or more prolonged in the presence of renal and hepatic disease that diminishes elimination and thereby lengthens the half-life of the offending drug.

TOXIC DRUG REACTIONS

An additional 10 to 40 per cent of adverse drug reactions can be termed toxic reactions on the basis of drug-induced cellular-organ toxicity not explicable on an immunologic basis.[1, 6, 10, 12] These reactions were formerly called idiosyncratic reactions. The oto- and nephrotoxicity observed following aminoglycoside antimicrobial agents are examples of this form of adverse drug reaction. Some toxic reactions exhibit a clear-cut direct relationship between drug dosage and likelihood of toxicity. There is debate as to whether or not renal and hepatic disease predispose to toxic adverse drug reactions (see Chaps. 5 and 10). Inasmuch as some toxic drug reactions may be dose dependent, the combination of administration of standard doses of agents normally eliminated by the kidney and liver to patients with diseases of these organ systems may predispose to some toxic reactions.

METABOLIC LOADS

A smaller number of adverse reactions to pharmacologic agents are due to "metabolic loads" concomitantly administered with drugs. These loads are discussed in detail in Chapter 9. Because of already precarious fluid and electrolyte balance occurring in patients with renal and hepatic disease, these disease states predispose to this form of adverse drug reaction.

DRUG-RELATED FACTORS PREDISPOSING TO ADVERSE DRUG REACTIONS

Both drug-related and patient-related factors play important roles in the development of adverse drug reactions (Table 3–3). Drug-related factors can usually be directly controlled by the clinician. Thus, consideration of these factors is an important starting point for

TABLE 3–3. PREDISPOSING FACTORS IN ADVERSE DRUG REACTIONS

- I. Drug-related Factors
  - Type of drug administered
  - Dosage of drug administered
  - Number of drugs administered
- II. Patient-related Factors
  - Presence of renal, hepatic, and cardiac disease
  - Age
  - Compliance
  - Previous adverse drug reaction
  - Genetic influences
  - Sex
  - Miscellaneous (diet, smoking, body habitus, environmental exposures)

avoidance of adverse drug reactions. The most important drug-related factor affecting development of drug reactions is the therapeutic index of the administered drug. Adverse drug reactions are most often encountered following large doses of drugs with narrow therapeutic indices. Examples of such agents include immunosuppressive-antineoplastic agents, to which adverse reactions will be observed in up to 75 per cent of cases.[15] Other types of therapeutic agents with narrow therapeutic indices and therefore relatively high rates of adverse drug reactions (10 to 30 per cent) include anticoagulants and cardiovascular agents, such as digitalis preparations, antiarrhythmics, antihypertensive agents, and diuretics. The importance of choosing the lowest effective dosage of the least toxic available therapeutic agent has been demonstrated in a recent study. In this surveillance study, 4.1 per cent of 2499 patients admitted to a general medical ward were hospitalized because of an adverse drug reaction.[19] Life-threatening or fatal reactions were encountered in 15 per cent of those admitted for an adverse reaction. Most important, 27 per cent of these adverse drug admissions could have been avoided by a more careful choice and dosage of drug.[19]

Another drug-related factor important in the frequency of adverse drug reactions is the number of concomitantly administered drugs. A relationship between the number of drugs and the frequency of adverse reactions was first emphasized by Smith and associates.[5] In these studies, a logarithmic association between number of drugs and adverse reactions occurring in hospitalized patients was present. Thus, with less than five drugs, the adverse drug reaction rate was 4.2 per cent, which increased to 24 to 45 per cent when the number of drugs exceeded 10. A direct relationship between number of administered drugs and frequency of adverse reactions has been subsequently confirmed by several investigators.[10, 12, 23]

Several factors underlie the association of adverse drug reactions and number of drugs. The additive effects of individual drug reactions increase the overall adverse reaction rate. Patients treated with large numbers of drugs often have serious underlying disease, including impaired function of kidneys and liver leading to diminished drug biotransformation and elimination. Pharmacologic factors can also contribute to the relationship between number of drugs and likelihood of adverse effects.[24] Drugs can interact by altering metabolism of other drugs via inhibition or induction of hepatic microsomal enzymes, by altering binding of other drugs to plasma proteins or tissue receptor sites, by delaying or enhancing the excretion of other drugs, and by facilitating or impairing the absorption of other agents. Since patients with kidney and liver disease have a number of medical problems (e.g., infections, hypertension, fluid and electrolyte disturbances), they are often treated with several pharmacologic agents. For example, in a recent survey, we have found that more than 25 per cent of patients treated in chronic maintenance dialysis facilities are treated with more than 10 drugs (Unpublished data). The relationship between number of drugs and frequency of adverse reactions demands that the clinician make every effort to maintain the number of drugs at a minimum.

PATIENT-RELATED FACTORS PREDISPOSING TO ADVERSE DRUG REACTIONS

Although the clinician is less able to manipulate patient-related factors of potential importance in the frequency of adverse drug reactions, a knowledge of these factors may lead to more enlightened drug prescribing.

PRESENCE OF RENAL DISEASE

The presence of renal disease has been clearly demonstrated to enhance the frequency of adverse drug reactions. Smith and associates found that the incidence of adverse drug reactions was 9 per cent when the blood urea nitrogen was less than 20 mg/dl, and this rate increased to 24 per cent once the blood urea nitrogen exceeded 40 mg/dl.[5] Similar results have been observed in other surveillance studies, in which patients with high blood urea nitrogen values had increased rates of adverse drug reactions.[12, 19] In another surveillance study, Jick found that even slight increases in admission values for blood urea nitrogen significantly increased the rate of adverse reactions to ampicillin, tetracycline, chloral hydrate, flurazepam, chlorpromazine, spironolactone, hydrochlorothiazide, digoxin, procainamide, methyldopa, and Maalox.[15] In a series of patients with renal failure admitted with signs and symptoms of neurologic disease, adverse central nervous system effects of drugs were the most common identifiable etiologic factor.[25] Thus, taken together, there can be no doubt that renal failure leads to an increased frequency of adverse drug effects.

PRESENCE OF LIVER DISEASE

Although it is widely held that liver disease predisposes to adverse drug reactions,[26-28] there is little epidemiologic evidence directly related to this issue.[5, 10] However, much circumstantial evidence supports the view that advanced liver disease predisposes to adverse drug reactions. As discussed in detail in Chapter 12, numerous drugs, including aminophylline, amobarbital, carbenicillin, chlordiazepoxide, diazepam, hexobarbital, lidocaine, meperidine, meprobamate, pentobarbital, phenobarbital, phenylbutazone, and rifampicin, have increased bioavailability, decreased plasma clearance, and prolonged half-lives in patients with advanced hepatic disease. In a prospective analysis of the causes of 100 consecutive episodes of hepatic coma, Fessel and Conn found that 43 per cent were directly related to drugs.[29]

Patients with advanced hepatic disease have been demonstrated to have diminished tolerance to morphine,[30] hexobarbital,[31] thiopental,[32] and chlorpromazine.[33] High rates of occurrence of adverse reactions to potent diuretic agents have also been found in patients with advanced hepatic disease.[34] Taken together, several studies support an effect of severe hepatic disease to predispose to adverse drug reactions.

Some evidence suggests that impaired cardiac output also results in impaired drug disposition.[35] Thus, the elimination of lidocaine, indocyanine green, canrenone, aprindine, prazosin, and procainamide appears to be diminished in cardiac failure.[35] The effects of cardiac failure on drug disposition, however, have not been dissociated from concomitant decreases in hepatic blood flow and renal function.

ADVANCED AGE

An additional patient-related factor postulated to be of importance in rate of adverse drug reactions is patient age.[36-38] In two studies of adverse drug reactions in hospitalized patients, a significant relationship between advancing age (especially age over 60 years) and drug reactions was found.[3, 23] However, other studies have not found age to be an important factor in predisposing to adverse drug effects.[5, 6, 12, 19] There are several reasons why increasing age may, in some cases, predispose to drug reactions. Elderly patients tend to be treated with more drugs than younger patients.[36] Moreover, the aging process may alter drug distribution, metabolism, and elimination.[37, 38] For example, a decrease in total body water occurs with increasing age; therefore, increased levels of drugs distributed in body water may occur.[39] Increasing age from 25 to 80 years is associated with a decline in plasma albumin from 4 to 3.8 gm/dl.[40] The diminished albumin concentration with age may influence drug protein binding and distribution. Advancing age from 20 to 25 as compared to 75 to 80 years is also associated with a 35 to 40 per cent reduction in hepatic blood flow and glomerular filtration rate.[41, 42] Both of these factors would be expected to significantly diminish drug elimination. In this regard, increasing age is associated with diminished hepatic clearance of antipyrine, a drug dependent on hepatocellular function for metabolism.[43] Finally, the elderly have been demonstrated to have diminished tolerance to such drugs as digoxin, flurazepam, and morphine.[44-46] Thus, there are several reasons to exert caution in the use of pharmacologic agents in the elderly.

GENETIC INFLUENCES

Important genetic influences have recently been recognized to be responsible for some of the large (three- to fortyfold) interindividual variations in drug disposition.[50, 51] Thus, the large variations in drug disposition between individuals disappears in monozygotic (identical) twins, but persists in dizygotic (nonidentical) twins.[50, 51] Genetically controlled differences in drug disposition among normal subjects are due primarily to differences in hepatic drug metabolism rather than drug absorption, distribution, or excretion.[50, 51] Several additional poorly defined factors, such as smoking, dietary intake, body habitus, and exposure to a variety of chemicals, toxins, and other environmental factors, have been postulated to be important in determining the disposition of drugs.[50, 52] The mechanism(s) whereby these factors alter drug disposition and the effect of these factors to predispose to adverse drug reactions remain to be elucidated.

COMPLIANCE

Compliance is another patient-related problem that potentially plays a role in adverse drug reactions. Although most noncompliance involves omission of prescribed drugs, other compliance problems, such as taking drugs not currently prescribed and utilizing prescribed drugs inappropriately, comprise up to 30 to 40 per cent of compliance problems.[47] The potential role for medication noncompliance in adverse drug reactions demands careful education programs by the clinician. In some difficult cases, reinforcement of medication instructions by a relative, friend, or other household member, as well as use of a medication calendar may provide some help.[48, 49]

PREVIOUS ADVERSE DRUG REACTION AND FEMALE SEX

Two additional patient-related factors — a history of previous adverse drug reaction and female sex — have been associated with increased likelihood of development of adverse drug effects. A history of previous adverse drug effect, regardless of the type of prior adverse effect, results in a twofold increase in the chance of a new adverse drug effect.[5, 19, 23] Thus, cautious use of pharmacologic agents in patients with a convincing history of a previous significant adverse drug reaction appears warranted. The frequency of adverse drug reactions in females has been consistently higher than in males in a number of reports.[5, 12, 19, 23] The mechanism(s) underlying this sex-related effect remains to be elucidated.

MECHANISMS WHEREBY KIDNEY AND LIVER DISEASES PREDISPOSE TO ADVERSE DRUG REACTIONS

DIMINISHED DRUG METABOLISM

Pharmacologic mechanisms that may be involved in the high frequency of adverse drug reactions in patients with hepatic and renal diseases are depicted in Table 3–4. Many

TABLE 3–4. MECHANISMS OF ADVERSE DRUG REACTIONS IN PATIENTS WITH KIDNEY AND LIVER DISEASE

I. Increased Drug Levels
   - Decreased drug metabolism
   - Decreased elimination of parent drug
   - Decreased elimination of active metabolite

II. Increased Drug Sensitivity
   - Decreased drug-protein binding
   - Target organ alterations

III. Administration of Metabolic Loads

drugs undergo metabolism or biotransformation before elimination (Chap. 1).[53] These processes occur predominantly in the liver and result in the formation of water-soluble metabolites that are more readily excreted. The major pathway of drug metabolism occurs in two phases. The first phase is drug oxidation, followed by a second phase of glucuronide, glycine, or sulfate conjugation reactions. Drugs can also undergo reduction and hydrolysis reactions during the first phase and methylation and acetylation during the second phase, although these reactions are less common. Obviously, advanced liver disease will substantially affect metabolism of a number of drugs, and may lead to diminished drug clearance and prolonged drug half-life. It has also become increasingly apparent in recent years that renal failure *per se* can lead to abnormalities in the hepatic metabolism of some drugs.[53] For example, recent experimental studies demonstrate that renal insufficiency in the rat results in a decrease in the specific activity of the hepatic mixed function oxidation system.[54, 55] In contrast, in uremic patients, oxidation reactions are generally normal or rapid; although quinidine, which is metabolized by oxidative processes, is delayed.[53] Other first-step drug metabolism pathways, such as reduction and hydrolysis reactions, are often impaired in the uremic state.[53] Moreover, second phase reactions, such as conjugation and acetylation, are also impaired in uremia.[53] In this regard, uremic animal studies have found abnormalities in activities of enzymes that modulate these reactions.[56] However, the exact mechanisms whereby the uremic state results in alterations in hepatic enzyme systems modulating drug biotransformation remains to be elucidated. Thus, both advanced hepatic and renal disease may result in high blood drug levels by impaired drug metabolism.

DIMINISHED DRUG ELIMINATION

The kidneys and the biliary tract serve as major sites of drug elimination. The rates of renal elimination of drugs are based on both extrarenal and renal considerations. Among the extrarenal considerations are (1) percentage of protein binding of the drug (protein-bound drugs are not filtered at the glomerulus); (2) apparent volume of distribution (AVD) of the drug (drugs with large AVD values are not as readily available for renal removal in a specified time period as compared with drugs with small AVD values); and (3) the rate of metabolism of the drug (rapid metabolism precludes significant renal excretion of unchanged drug). Among the renal considerations are (1) renal blood flow (delivery of drug to the kidney); (2) glomerular filtration rate (entry of drug into tubule fluid); and (3) tubule transport of the drug, including both secretion and reabsorption (entry into and removal of drug from tubule fluid). Drugs that are predominantly eliminated unchanged by the kidneys are listed in Table 3–5.

Many drugs undergo significant tubule reabsorption.[57] Several processes, including simple passive diffusion, govern tubule reabsorption of drugs. Passive diffusion often proceeds rapidly because readily diffusable forms of drugs become significantly concentrated in tubule fluid, thereby creating large concentration gradients for reabsorption. Drugs can also be reabsorbed by active transport processes. This mode of drug transport has not been studied extensively. However, chlormerodrin[57,58] and oxypurinol[59] may undergo active reabsorption. Finally, it should be noted that therapeutic agents such as fluoride, bromide, and lithium are reabsorbed actively in the proximal tubule. Maneuvers that decrease proximal tubule reabsorption, such as saline infusion, increase the renal clearance of fluoride, bromide, and lithium. Conversely, volume depletion and sodium restriction enhance tubule reabsorption of these ions and may lead to toxic plasma levels.

Nonionic back-diffusion is another means whereby various drugs can be reabsorbed by the renal tubules. Since numerous drugs are either weak acids or weak bases (Table 3–6), they exist in a mixture of ionic and nonionic forms, depending on the pK_a of the drug and the pH of the urine. For example, weak acids (low pK_a) will be in a nonionized form in acid urine. Since the nonionized form of the drug is more easily reabsorbed than the ionized form, an elevated tubule fluid pH will retard absorption and enhance renal excretion of weak acids. The enhancement of renal excretion of drugs through alterations in urine pH can optimally be achieved under the following conditions: (1) if the pK_a of the drug is in the range of achievable urine pH (5 to 8), (2) if the glomerular filtration rate is normal, and (3) if there is a relatively low rate of hepatic drug metabolism. From a practical standpoint, forced alkaline diuresis has resulted in clinically efficacious enhanced excretion of weak acids such as salicylate[60] and phenobarbital[61] and forced acid diuresis has increased excretion of the weak base amphetamine.[62]

A number of weakly acidic or weakly basic drugs are known to be secreted into the urine by tubule transport mechanisms.[37,63] Some commonly encountered drugs that undergo

TABLE 3–5. DRUGS WITH RENAL EXCRETION AS THE MAJOR PATHWAY OF ELIMINATION

Ampicillin	Kanamycin
Carbenicillin	Methotrexate
Cephalexin	Methyldopa
Cephalothin	Neomycin
Cephazolin	Procainamide
Colistin	Streptomycin
Cycloserine	Sulfinpyrazone
Digoxin	Tetracycline
Ethambutol	Tobramycin
5-Fluorocytosine	Vancomycin
Gentamicin	

TABLE 3–6. WEAK ACIDS AND WEAK BASES THAT MAY BE REABSORBED BY NONIONIC BACK DIFFUSION

Weak Acids	Weak Bases
Acetazolamide	Amphetamines
Cephaloridine	Chloroquine
Ethacrynic acid	Dopamine
Furosemide	Meperidine
Hydrochlorothiazide	Morphine
Methotrexate	Neostigmine
Mersalyl	Quinine
Penicillin	Quinidine
Phenobarbital	Thiamine
Phenylbutazone	Tricyclic drugs
Probenecid	Trimethoprim
Sulfonamides	
Salicylic acid	

TABLE 3–7. DRUGS THAT UNDERGO TUBULAR SECRETION

Carbenicillin	Methotrexate
Cephalosporins	Penicillin G
Chlorothiazide	Probenecid
Ethacrynic acid	Procainamide
Fluorouracil	Pyrazinamide
Furosemide	Sulfonamides
Guanethidine	Triamterene

tubule secretion are listed in Table 3–7. In general, there appear to be separate pathways for the secretion of weak organic acids and bases.[64, 65] Although competitive inhibition of secretion of one organic acid by another may occur, no effect of an organic base on the acid transport system has been observed. It is important to emphasize that drug metabolites, as well as the parent drug, may be secreted by the renal tubule.

It is also important to note that several drugs are metabolized to pharmacologically active metabolites. These pharmacologically active metabolites are in turn excreted by the kidneys (Table 3–8).[66] Thus, renal retention of the parent drug as well as pharmacologically active metabolites may predispose to drug toxicity in the uremic state.

With regard to elimination of drug via the biliary tract, factors governing drug excretion by this route are less well defined.[67] Drugs highly concentrated in bile are listed in Chapter 2. A drug excreted into bile must cross the hepatocyte cell membrane and the sinusoidal cell membrane. At least three active transport systems exist for organic compound excretion in the rat — one for organic acids, one for organic bases, and one for neutral compounds.[68] At least two factors are important in determining biliary drug transport and excretion. The first is molecular weight. In contrast to elimination by the kidneys, in which substances with molecular weights less than 300 daltons are readily filtered (provided they are not extensively protein bound), only higher (>325 daltons) molecular weight substances are readily excreted into bile.[67] In addition to molecular weight, drug polarity appears to be important in biliary drug excretion, since most drugs excreted into bile are highly polar.[67] Although the effects of cholestatic liver disease on drug elimination have not been extensively studied, cholestasis results in diminished biliary recovery of some drugs known to be excreted in bile, including cardiac glycosides and spironolactone.[67] Moreover, impaired hepatocellular function *per se* may increase drug half-life and diminish drug clearance, either by decreasing drug uptake into hepatocytes or by decreasing drug metabolism by the hepatocyte. Thus, in the presence of significant liver disease, accumulation of drugs may occur that are normally excreted into the bile in substantial quantity or metabolized by the liver.

INCREASED DRUG SENSITIVITY

Some patients with kidney and liver disease exhibit increased drug sensitivity that does not appear explicable on the basis of accumulation of parent drug or active metabolites. For example, patients with both renal and hepatic disease are inordinately sensitive to centrally active sedative hypnotic agents[30-33, 69] (Chap. 14). One of the mechanisms postulated to be responsible for this heightened drug sensitivi-

TABLE 3–8. DRUGS THAT FORM ACTIVE METABOLITES

Drug	Metabolite	Used in Renal Failure
Acetohexamide	Hydroxyhexamide	No
Allopurinol	Oxypurinol	↓ dose
Azathioprine	6-Mercaptopurine	Yes
Chlordiazepoxide	Oxazepam	Yes
Diazepam	Oxazepam	Yes
Meperidine	Normeperidine	No
Methsuximide	*N*-Desmethylmethsuximide	Yes
Primidone	Phenobarbital	Yes
Procainamide	*N*-Acetylprocainamide	↓ dose
Propranolol	4-Hydroxypropranolol	Yes
Propoxyphene	Norpropoxyphene	No

ty is diminished protein binding of drugs.[53] Once in the circulation, the intensity of drug effect is generally related to the concentration of unbound drug in plasma water, since only the "free" (nonprotein bound) portion of a drug is capable of diffusing into the cell and inducing a pharmacologic effect. Most analytical methods of estimating the plasma concentration of a drug measure both the "free" and "protein-bound" fractions. Thus, as discussed in Chapter 4, a good relationship between the intensity of drug effect and the plasma concentration of a drug will exist only if drug-protein binding is constant. Renal failure and liver disease induce alterations in the protein binding of several drugs, as shown in Table 3–9.[53, 70] It is of interest to note that the majority of drugs that exhibit decreased protein binding in renal failure are acidic drugs. In fact, only one acidic drug studied to date —indomethacin — has demonstrated normal protein-binding characteristics in uremia. By contrast, most basic drugs, including dapsone, desmethylimipramine, *d*-tubocurarine, propranolol, quinidine, and trimethoprim, exhibit normal protein-binding characteristics in uremia.

The reasons for the impaired protein binding of drugs in uremia and liver disease have not been elucidated. However, some of the decreased protein binding of drugs can be related to the hypoalbuminemia that may accompany these disorders. In addition, several lines of evidence suggest that "competitive displacers" may be present in uremia. Thus (1) renal failure is associated with accumulation of a number of acidic metabolites, and protein binding of acidic drugs is predominantly affected by renal failure; (2) charcoal treatment of serum of patients with renal failure may restore the protein-binding characteristics of several drugs;[71, 72] (3) *in vitro* dialysis increases protein binding of drugs in some, but not all, patients with renal failure;[73, 74] (4) adding normal plasma proteins to an ultrafiltrate of plasma from patients with renal failure may decrease drug binding;[75] and (5) more recently, strong evidence supporting an "inhibitor" of drug–plasma protein binding in uremia has been found.[76] In these studies, a nonionic polystyrene-divinylbenzene copolymer resin was used to treat acidified uremic plasma. This resin resulted in a marked improvement in binding of phenytoin to plasma proteins. Moreover, an alcohol eluate of the resin produced a substance which, when reconstituted with normal plasma, caused a dose-dependent decrease in phenytoin and tryptophan protein binding. This inhibitor was water soluble, heat stable, and dialyzable across plasma membranes. Alternatively, it has been suggested that the uremic state may result in either biochemical or ultrastructural abnormalities that alter normal drug-binding sites on albumin.[74, 77] In this regard, the amino acid composition of albumin from uremic patients differs from that found in normal subjects[77] and isoelectric focusing techniques demonstrate abnormalities of the B band of albumin from uremic patients that correlate with decreased protein binding of drugs.[77]

The clinical significance of alterations in drug-protein binding are difficult to predict. On one hand, the increased amount of "free" drug would be anticipated to lead to a more intense pharmacologic effect. Conversely, impaired binding may lead to more rapid total body clearance, since many drug elimination processes proceed at rates proportional to the "free" level of the drug. In studies performed in hypoalbuminemic patients with normal renal and hepatic function, the anticipated increased per cent of "free" (unbound) drugs was present.[78] However, this increased per cent of free drug was balanced by an increased volume of distribution of the drugs studied and increased total body clearance rates so that the absolute plasma concentrations of "free"

TABLE 3–9. DRUGS WITH DECREASED PROTEIN BINDING IN RENAL AND HEPATIC FAILURE

Renal Failure	Hepatic Disease
Barbiturates	Amylbarbitone
Benzylpenicillin	Diazepam
Clofibrate	Morphine
Congo red	Phenylbutazone
Diazepam	Phenytoin
Diazoxide	Propranolol
Dicloxacillin	Quinidine
Digitoxin	Thiopentone
Furosemide	Tolbutamide
Metolazone	
Morphine	
Papaverine	
Phenylbutazone	
Phenytoin	
Salicylate	
Sulfonamides	
Thyroxine	
Triamterene	
Tryptophane	
Warfarin	

drug were equivalent.[78,79] Although these experimental observations suggest that diminished drug-protein binding has little clinical consequence, a number of clinical studies demonstrate an increased rate of adverse drug reactions in the setting of diminished protein binding of drugs and/or hypoalbuminemia. Thus, hypoalbuminemia has been demonstrated to increase the frequency of adverse effects of phenytoin, prednisone, and benzodiazepines.[80-82] Taken together, it is important to recognize that renal and hepatic disease may be associated with increased amounts of "free" drug and enhanced pharmacologic effect at normal plasma concentrations.

Another mechanism potentially responsible for the increased drug sensitivity of patients with kidney and liver disease is the presence of underlying disease in the target organs of administered pharmacologic agents. With regard to target organ alterations in uremia predisposing to drug toxicity, a practical example is the susceptibility of the uremic patient to the effects of central nervous system depressants, such as sedative hypnotic drugs.[69] The effect of uremia *per se* on the central nervous system may be to potentiate the effects of these drugs. Alternatively, the uremic state may be associated with alterations in the blood-brain barrier that allow for excessive brain concentrations of these drugs. In a similar manner, uremia-induced alterations in gastrointestinal mucosa and platelet function may predispose the uremic patient to the gastrointestinal irritant effect of a number of drugs and may increase the hemorrhagic tendency of uremic patients following administration of drugs with platelet-inhibiting properties (e.g., carbenicillin).[83] Finally, it should be kept in mind that administration of multiple drugs may result in substantial metabolic loads (Chap. 9). These metabolic loads may have catastrophic effects when administered to patients whose fluid and electrolyte status is already precarious.

GUIDELINES FOR USE OF DRUGS IN PATIENTS WITH KIDNEY AND LIVER DISEASE

In consideration of the above-mentioned mechanisms of enhanced drug toxicity in renal and hepatic disease, several simple guidelines will serve to lessen adverse drug reactions in these conditions.

1. Do not use drugs in patients with renal and hepatic failure unless specific indications exist.
2. Review medication lists frequently and avoid the use of multiple pharmacologic agents.
3. Be familiar with the pharmacologic and potential toxic effects of all drugs used in patients with renal and hepatic failure.
4. Base dosage modifications for drugs on an accurate, timed measurement of creatinine clearance as an index of renal function rather than on the serum creatinine level alone.
5. When possible, modify drug dosage and dosage regimens by using drug dosage schedules previously evaluated in patients with renal and liver failure.
6. Supplement the dosage regimen with clinical monitoring of the pharmacologic effect, as well as with monitoring of drug level (when available).

REFERENCES

1. Schimmel EM: The hazards of hospitalization. Ann. Intern. Med. *60*:100–110, 1964.
2. MacDonald MG, MacKay BC: Adverse drug reactions — experience of Mary Fletcher Hospital during 1962. J.A.M.A. *190*:1071–1074, 1964.
3. Seidl LG, Thorton GF, Cluff LE: Epidemiological studies of adverse drug reactions. Am. J. Public Health *55*:1170–1175, 1964.
4. Seidl LG, Thorton GF, Smith JW, Cluff LE: Studies on the epidemiology of adverse drug reactions. III. Reactions in patients on a general medical service. Bull. Johns Hopkins Hospital *119*:299–315, 1966.
5. Smith JW, Seidl LG, Cluff LE: Studies on the epidemiology of adverse drug reactions. V. Clinical factors influencing susceptibility. Ann. Intern. Med. *65*:629–640, 1966.
6. Ogilvie RI, Ruedy J: Adverse drug reactions during hospitalization. Canad. Med. Assoc. J. *97*:1450–1457, 1967.
7. Hoddinott BC, Gowdey CW, Coulter WK, Parker JM: Drug reactions and errors in administration on a medical ward. Canad. Med. Assoc. J. *97*:1101–1106, 1967.
8. Reidenberg M: Registry of adverse drug reactions. J.A.M.A. *203*:31–37, 1968.
9. Simmons M, Parker JM, Gowdey CW, Coulter WK: Adverse drug reactions during hospitalization. Canad. Med. Assoc. J. *98*:175, 1968.
10. Hurwitz N, Wade OL: Intensive hospital monitoring of adverse reactions to drugs. Brit. Med. J. *1*:531–536, 1969.
11. Wang, RI, Terry IC: Adverse drug reactions in a Veterans Administration Hospital. J. Clin. Pharmacol. *11*:14–18, 1971.
12. Gray RK, Adams LL, Fallon HJ: Short term intense surveillance of adverse drug reactions. J. Clin. Pharmacol. *13*:61–67, 1973.

13. Karch FE, Lasagna L: Adverse drug reactions. A critical review. J.A.M.A.*234*:1236–1244, 1975.
14. Koch-Weser J, Sellers EM, Zacest R: The ambiguity of adverse drug reactions. Eur. J. Clin. Pharmacol. *11*:75–78, 1977.
15. Jick H: Adverse drug effects in relation to renal function. Am. J. Med. *62*:514–518, 1977.
16. Hurwitz N: Admissions to hospital due to drugs. Brit. Med. J. *1*:539–540, 1969.
17. Miller RR: Hospital admissions due to adverse drug reactions. Arch. Intern. Med. *134*:219–223, 1974.
18. Caranasas GJ, Stewart RB, Cluff LE: Drug-induced illness leading to hospitalization. J.A.M.A. *228*:713–717, 1974.
19. Levy M, Lipshitz M, Eliakin M: Hospital admissions due to adverse drug reactions. Am. J. Med. Sci. *277*:49–56, 1979.
20. Temple RJ, Jones JK, Crout JR: Adverse effects of newly marketed drugs. N. Engl. J. Med. *300*:1046–1047, 1979.
21. Stone D, Shapiro S, Miettinen OS, Finkle WD, Statley PD: Drug evaluation after marketing. Ann. Intern. Med. *90*:259–261, 1979.
22. World Health Organization: International drug monitoring — the role of the hospital. Drug Intelligence Clin. Pharmacol. *4*:101, 1970.
23. Hurwitz N: Predisposing factors in adverse reactions to drugs. Brit. Med. J. *1*:536–539, 1969.
24. Adverse interactions of drugs. Med. Let. *21*:5–19, 1979.
25. Richet G, Fabre J, de Freudenreich J, Podevin R: La tolérance médicamenteuse des uremiques. Presse Med. *74*:2339, 1966.
26. Block M: Liver disease and drug therapy. Med. Clin. North Am. *58*:1051–1057, 1974.
27. Najanjo CA, Busto U, Mardones R: Adverse drug reactions in liver cirrhosis. Eur. J. Clin. Pharmacol. *13*:429–434, 1978.
28. Klotz U: Influence of liver disease on the elimination of drug. Eur. J. Drug Metab. Pharmacokinet. *1*:129–140, 1976.
29. Fessel JM, Conn HO: An analysis of the cause and prevention of hepatic coma. Gastroenterology *62*:191, 1972.
30. Laidlow J, Road AE, Sherlock S: Morphine tolerance in hepatic cirrhosis. Gastroenterology *40*:389–396, 1961.
31. Richter E, Zilly W, Brachtel D, Becker S: Zur Frage der Barbiturattoleranze bei Patienten mit akuter Hepatitis. Dtsch. Med. Wchenschr. *97*:254–255, 1972.
32. Shideman FE, Kelly AR, Lee LE, Lowell VF, Adams BJ: The role of the liver in the detoxication of thiopental (pentothal) by man. Anesthesiology *10*:421–428, 1949.
33. Read AE, Laidlow J, McCarthy CF: Effects of chlorpromazine in patients with hepatic disease. Brit. Med. J. *3*:497–499, 1969.
34. Naranjo CA, Pontigo E, Valdenegro C, Gonzalez G, Ruiz I, Busto U: Furosemide-induced adverse reactions in cirrhosis of the liver. Clin. Pharmacol. Ther. *25*:154–160, 1979.
35. Williams RL, Benet LZ: Drug pharmacokinetics in cardiac and hepatic disease. Ann. Rev. Pharmacol. Toxicol. *20*:389–413, 1980.
36. Smith CR: Use of drugs in the aged. Johns Hopkins Med. J. *145*:61–64, 1979.
37. Schumukker DL: Age related changes in drug disposition. Pharmacol. Rev. *30*:445–456, 1978.
38. Gillette JR: Biotransformation of drugs during aging. Fed. Proc. *38*:1900–1909, 1979.
39. Novak LP: Aging, total body potassium, fat-free mass and cell mass in males and females between ages 18 and 85 years. J. Gerontol. *27*:438–443, 1972.
40. Misra DP, Loudon JM, Staddon GE: Albumin metabolism in elderly patients. J. Gerontol. *30*:304–306, 1975.
41. Bender AD: The effect of increasing age on the distribution of peripheral blood flow in man. J. Am. Geriatric Soc. *13*:192–198, 1965.
42. Rowe JW: The effect of age on creatinine clearance in man: a cross-section and longitudinal study. J. Gerontol. *31*:155–163, 1976.
43. Vestal RE, Norris AH, Tobin JD, Cohen BH, Shock NW, Andres R: Antipyrine metabolism in man: influence in age, alcohol, caffeine, and smoking. Clin. Pharmacol. Ther. *18*:425–432, 1975.
44. Greenblatt DJ, Allen MD, Shader RI: Toxicity of high-dose flurazepam in the elderly. Clin. Pharmacol. Ther. *21*:355–361, 1976.
45. Bellville JW, Forrest WH, Miller E, Brown BW: Influence of age on pain relief from analgesics. J.A.M.A. *217*:1835–1841, 1971.
46. Cusack B: Pharmacokinetics of digoxin in the elderly. Brit. J. Clin. Pharmacol. *6*:439–440, 1978.
47. Schwartz D: Medication errors made by elderly chronically ill patients. Am. J. Public Health *52*:2018–2029, 1962.
48. Levine DM, Green LW, Deeds SG, Chwalow J, Russell RP, Finlay J: Health education for hypertensive patients. J.A.M.A. *241*:1700–1708, 1979.
49. Wadless I, Davie JW: Can drug compliance in the elderly be improved? Brit. Med. J. *1*:359–361, 1977.
50. Vesell ES: Why are toxic reactions to drugs so often undetected initially? N. Engl. J. Med. *302*:1027–1029, 1980.
51. Vesell ES: Advances in pharmacogenetics. Prog. Med. Genet. *9*:291–367, 1973.
52. Vestal RE, Wood AJ, Branch RA, Shond DG, Wilkinson GR: Effects of age and cigarette smoking on propranolol disposition. Clin. Pharmacol. Ther. *26*:8–15, 1979.
53. Reidenberg, MM, Drayer DE: Drug therapy in renal failure. Ann. Rev. Pharmacol. Toxicol. *20*:45–54, 1980.
54. Leber HW, Schutterle E: Oxidative drug metabolism in liver microsomes from uremic rats. Kidney Int. *2*:152–158, 1972.
55. Dundee JW, Annis D: Barbiturate narcosis in uremia. Brit. J. Anesth. *27*:114–123, 1955.
56. Leber HW: Drug metabolism in uremia. Proc. 13th Congress European Dialysis Transplant Assoc., Hamburg, Germany, 1976, p. 617.
57. Cafruny EJ: Renal tubular handling of drugs. Am. J. Med. *62*:490–496, 1977.
58. Cafruny EJ: Reabsorptive transport of drugs. *In* Renal Pharmacology (JW Fisher, ed.). New York: Appleton-Century-Crofts, 1971, pp. 1–20.
59. Elion GB, Yu TF, Gutman AB, Hitchings GF: Renal clearance of oxypurinol, the chief metabolite of allopurinol. Am. J. Med. *45*:69–77, 1968.
60. Anderson RJ, Potts DE, Gabow PA, Rumack GH, Schrier RW: Unrecognized adult salicylate intoxication. Ann. Intern. Med. *85*:745–748, 1976.
61. Bloomer HA: A critical evaluation of diuresis in the treatment of barbiturate intoxication. J. Lab. Clin. Med. *67*:898–905, 1966.

62. Gary NE, Saidi P: Methamphetamine intoxication. A speedy new treatment. Am. J. Med. *64*:537–540, 1978.
63. Weiner IM: Transport of weak acids and bases. *In* Handbook of Physiology, Section 8: Renal Physiology (J Orloff and RW Berliner, eds.). Washington, D.C.: Am. Physiol. Soc. 1973, pp. 521–554.
64. Depopoulos A: A definition of substrate specificity in renal transport of organic anions. J. Theor. Biol. *8*:163–192, 1965.
65. Peters L: Renal tubular excretion of organic bases. Pharmacol. Rev. *12*:1–35, 1960.
66. Drayer DE: Active drug metabolites and renal failure. Am. J. Med. *62*:486–489, 1977.
67. Rollins DE, Klaassen CD: Biliary excretion of drugs in man. Clin. Pharmacokinet. *4*:368:379, 1979.
68. Klaassen CD: Biliary excretion. *In* Handbook of Physiology: Reaction to Environmental Agents (HC Lea, ed.): Washington, D.C.: Am. Physiol. Soc., 1977, pp. 537-553.
69. Taclob L, Needle M: Drug-induced encephalopathy in patients on maintenance hemodialysis. Lancet *2*:704–705, 1976.
70. Blaschke TF: Protein binding and kinetics of drugs of liver diseases. Clin. Pharmacokinet. *2*:32–44, 1977.
71. Sjoholm I, Kober A, Odar-Cederlof I, Borga A: Protein-binding of drugs in uremic and normal serum. The role of endogenous binding inhibitors. Biochem. Pharmacol. *25*:1205–1213, 1976.
72. Dromgoole SH: The effect of hemodialysis on the binding capacity of albumin. Clin. Chim. Acta *46*:469–472, 1973.
73. Reidenberg MM, Odar-Cederlof I, VonBahr C, Borga ML, Sjoqvist F: Protein binding of diphenylhydantoin and desmethylimipramine in plasma from patients with poor renal function. N. Engl. J. Med. *285*:264–267, 1971.
74. Shoeman DW, Azarnoff DL: The alterations of plasma proteins in uremia as reflected in their ability to bind digitoxin and diphenylhydantoin. Pharmacology *7*:169–177, 1972.
75. Tilstone WJ, Dargie H, Dargie EN, Morgan HG, Kennedy AC: Pharmacokinetics of metolazone in normal subjects and in patients with cardiac or renal failure. Clin. Pharmacol. Ther. *16*:322–329, 1974.
76. Depner TA, Gulyassy PF: Plasma protein binding in uremia: extraction and characterization of an inhibitor. Kidney Int. *18*:86–94, 1980.
77. Boobis SW: Alteration in plasma albumin in relation to decreased drug binding in uremia. Clin. Pharmacol. Ther. *22*:147–153, 1977.
78. Gugler R, Shoeman DW, Huffman DH, Cohlmia JB, Azarnoff DL: Pharmacokinetics of drugs in patients with the nephrotic syndrome. J. Clin. Invest. *55*:1182–1189, 1975.
79. Gibaldi M: Drug distribution in renal failure. Am. J. Med. *62*:471–474, 1977.
80. Boston Collaborative Drug Surveillance Program. Diphenylhydantoin side effects and serum albumin levels. Clin. Pharmacol. Ther. *14*:529–532, 1973.
81. Lewis GP, Juskow WJ, Burke CW, Graves L: Prednisone side-effects and serum protein levels. Lancet *2*:778–780, 1971.
82. Greenblatt DJ, Koch-Weser J: Clinical toxicity of chlordiazepoxide and diazepam in relation to serum albumin concentration. Eur. J. Clin. Pharmacol. *7*:259–262, 1974.
83. Brown CH, Natelson EA, Bradshaw MW, Williams TW, Alfrey CP: The hemostatic defect produced by carbenicillin. N. Engl. J. Med. *291*:265–270, 1974.

Chapter 4

Clinical Use of Drug Assays

by

Alan S. Nies and Joseph Gal

Rational therapeutics mandates that physicians individualize drug therapy for their patients. The average dose for a given therapeutic effect is the correct dose for the average patient. However, since most patients are not average, the average dose will be ineffective in some patients and toxic in others. Individualization of drug dosages can be accomplished only if the physician has well-defined therapeutic end points. Using these end points, the physician can adjust the dose to produce the desired result. Adjustment of dose is best accomplished when the therapeutic end point is an easily quantifiable effect of the drug. Thus, antihypertensive drugs can be given in a dose sufficient to lower blood pressure; oral anticoagulant drug doses can be increased until the prothrombin time is prolonged to the desired end point; and insulin dose in the diabetic patient can be adjusted until the blood sugar is decreased toward the normal range. With these drugs, it is not surprising to see a severalfold variation in the doses required to achieve the desired clinical effect, and since the effect is easily quantified, the use of an "average" dose is unnecessary.

For some drugs, however, the clinical effects are not easily measurable, either because there is no quantitative measurement of the effect, or the disease for which the drug is being given has sufficient variability in its expression so that the therapist may not be certain that a desired effect is being achieved at all times. Thus, in the treatment of diseases such as epilepsy or sporadic cardiac arrhythmias, drug dosage adjustments are difficult to make with precision. If an epileptic patient without treatment has one seizure a month, proper dosages for adequate control will be difficult to determine in a short period of time, and dosage adjustment based purely on clinical response may not give optimum management. Similarly, a patient with occasional ventricular arrhythmias may have an episode of sudden death as the first manifestation of inadequate drug dosage. Nonetheless, many patients will be placed on an average dose of an antiseizure or antiarrhythmic drug, and this dose may be continued in spite of an inadequate clinical response. Instead of adjusting the dose, the physician may label the drug a failure if the desired effect is not seen or if toxicity occurs at the average dose, and rather than adjusting doses in such a case, other drugs may be prescribed. In a review of phenytoin doses prescribed for seizures in 200 adult, ambulatory patients, Koch-Weser[1] found that 92 per cent of the patients received the "average" 300 mg dose, whereas in a similar review of 200 patients receiving warfarin, the doses varied widely from less than 2 mg/day to more than 11 mg/day with no dose being used in more than 20 per cent of patients (Fig. 4–1). This study illustrates that physicians are willing to individualize doses of drugs for which the therapeutic effects can be quantified, as is the case for warfarin, but frequently use an average dose for other drugs, such as phenytoin, for which quantitative effects cannot be determined.

In order to individualize doses for those drugs that do not have quantifiable clinical effects, physicians may use the emergence of drug toxicity as the therapeutic end point and

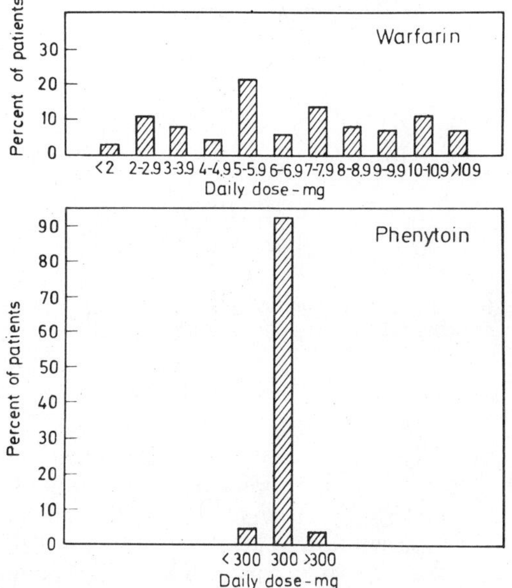

Figure 4–1. Distribution of doses of warfarin (*top*) and phenytoin (*bottom*) during chronic therapy in 200 ambulatory patients at the Massachusetts General Hospital. (Reproduced with permission from Koch-Weser, J.: The serum level approach to individualization of drug dosage. Eur. J. Clin. Pharmacol. 9:1–8, 1975.)

then decrease the dose somewhat. William Withering in 1785[2] suggested the use of digitalis toxicity as an end point to ascertain that sufficient glycoside had been given to produce an effect. Obviously, the use of drug toxicity as the therapeutic end point for dose adjustment entails considerable risk to the patient, especially for those drugs where serious toxicity can be the first sign of drug effect.

In recent years, it has become apparent that the concentration of a drug in plasma can be correlated with clinical efficacy in groups of patients where quantifiable end points in the individual patient are difficult to discern. For such drugs, monitoring of the drug concentration in plasma can be helpful for individualizing doses. Thus, in the study by Koch-Weser cited previously,[1] less than 30 per cent of patients given the average phenytoin dose of 300 mg/day achieved serum concentrations of the drug that have been found to be effective for optimal antiseizure activity, whereas 57 per cent had concentrations below and 16 per cent concentrations above the optimal range (Fig. 4–2). These data indicate that individualization of dosages is no less important for phenytoin than for warfarin, although it is less frequently done.

THE USE OF PLASMA LEVELS FOR INDIVIDUALIZATION OF DOSES

The basic tenet underlying the use of plasma levels to guide therapy is that drug present in the plasma is in dynamic equilibrium with drug at the site of action, and, therefore, alterations of the drug concentration in the plasma will reflect alterations in drug at the site of action with consequent alterations in effect (Fig. 4–3).

The sources of variation in response to a

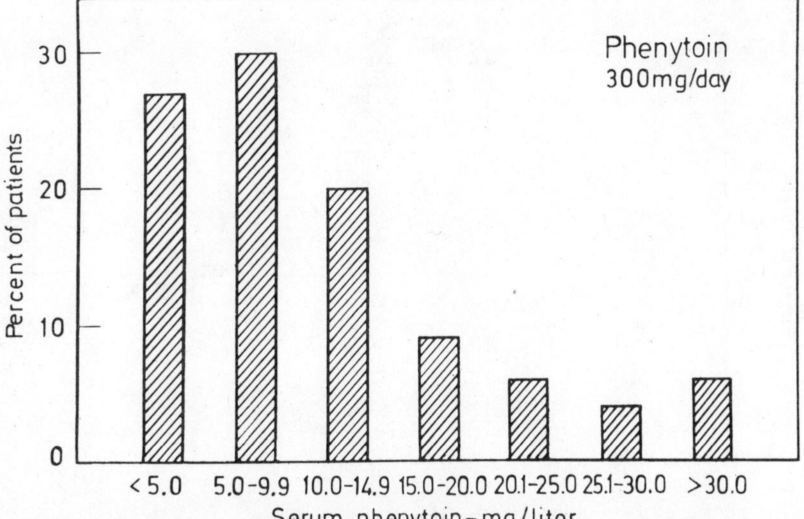

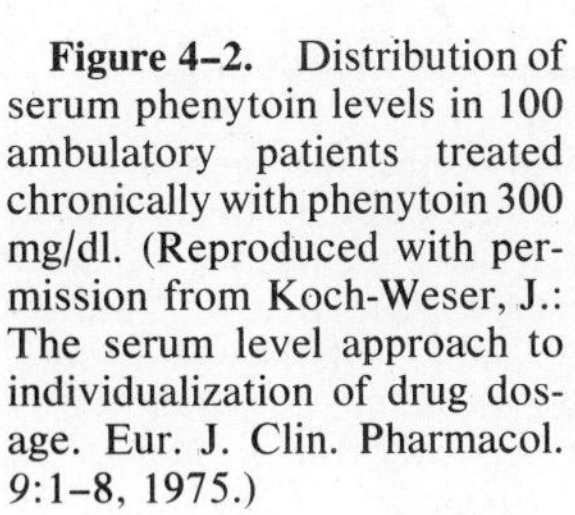
Figure 4–2. Distribution of serum phenytoin levels in 100 ambulatory patients treated chronically with phenytoin 300 mg/dl. (Reproduced with permission from Koch-Weser, J.: The serum level approach to individualization of drug dosage. Eur. J. Clin. Pharmacol. 9:1–8, 1975.)

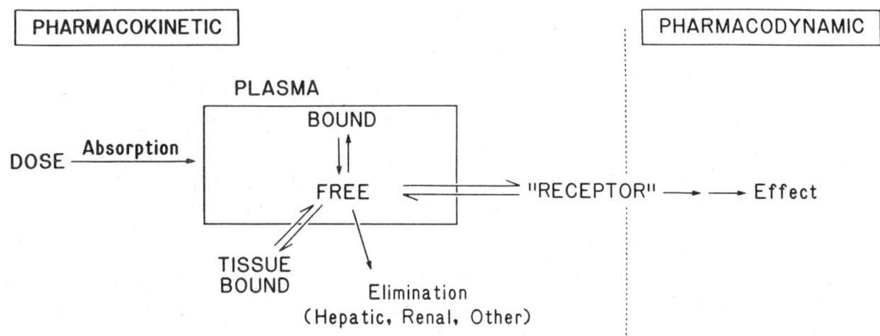

Figure 4–3. This diagram illustrates the variables controlling the effects of a given dose of drug. On the left-hand side of the figure are the pharmacokinetic variables and on the right-hand side, the pharmacodynamic variables.

given dose of drug can be divided into pharmacokinetic and pharmacodynamic factors. Those factors that result in variable plasma levels after a given dose are the pharmacokinetic factors, whereas those that account for the variable response to a given plasma level are the pharmacodynamic factors. If the pharmacodynamic factors are so large as to account for most of the variability in response to a drug, then plasma concentrations will not be a useful guide to therapy. Fortunately, however, the pharmacokinetic factors are the major source of variability for most drugs, and this variability can be minimized with the use of plasma level monitoring.

The range of drug concentrations required for optimum therapeutic effects with minimal toxicity is termed the "therapeutic window" (Fig. 4–4). This window must be determined empirically for each drug in a group of patients undergoing careful monitoring for therapeutic and undesirable effects. The width of the therapeutic window, i.e., the steepness of the concentration-effect curve, is an index of the pharmacodynamic variability between patients, whereas the separation between the therapeutic and toxic concentration-effect curves is an index of the toxicity of the drug, frequently called the "therapeutic index" (toxic dose/therapeutic dose). With all drugs there is more or less overlap between the toxic and therapeutic concentration-effect curves. The plasma level cannot, therefore, be an infallible guide to safe, effective therapy, since it cannot remove the pharmacodynamic variability between patients. However, plasma level monitoring does allow adjustment for the pharmacokinetic variability between patients,

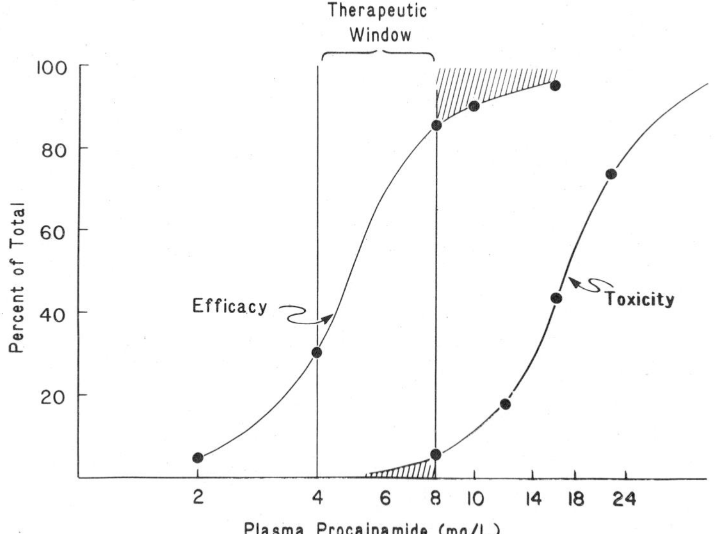

Figure 4–4. Plasma procainamide concentration in a group of patients is plotted against the per cent of patients achieving a desired effect or toxicity. The "therapeutic window" is indicated. Note the overlap of the efficacy and toxicity curves. (Reproduced with permission from Koch-Weser, J.: Clinical application of the pharmacokinetics of procainamide. Cardiovasc. Clin., *6* (Suppl. II):63–75, 1974.)

and for most drugs the correlation between plasma levels and effects is better than the correlation between dose and effect.[3]

SOURCES OF PHARMACOKINETIC VARIABILITY

There are a large number of reasons why patients achieve different drug concentrations in plasma when given the same dose. These pharmacokinetic variables are diagrammed in Figure 4–3 and are discussed in detail in Chapter 1. The important factors critical to interpretation of the plasma levels will be reiterated here.

DOSE ADMINISTERED

Clearly, a major determinant of the plasma level is the dose of drug prescribed; this is the one variable controlled by the physician. However, the amount of drug prescribed and the amount of drug absorbed are not necessarily the same thing. One of the common reasons for lack of efficacy of a drug is lack of patient compliance, but noncompliance with a therapeutic regimen is frequently difficult to detect. If plasma levels for a drug in a particular patient have been established for a given dose during supervised drug administration, then a change in the plasma level during the outpatient visits is most likely due to lack of compliance.

ABSORPTION

For drugs given parenterally, absorption is not usually a problem, although some drugs, such as phenytoin, are poorly absorbed from intramuscular sites. Absorption can be a considerable problem for some orally administered drugs. The amount of orally ingested drug reaching the systemic circulation is termed "bioavailability." The Food and Drug Administration in the United States has the responsibility to assure that the bioavailability of different marketed formulations of the same drug are equivalent. Until recently, different brands of the same drug (digoxin, phenytoin, corticosteroids, spironolactone, and others) did not have identical bioavailability with the consequence that a change in plasma level could occur even without a change in dose ingested if the patient received a formulation from a different manufacturer. Although such differences between brands of drugs should no longer exist, according to the Food and Drug Administration, the clinician should be aware of the potential for problems in this area.

Diseases and other drugs may alter the rate or extent of drug absorption from the gastrointestinal tract. For drugs given chronically, the rate of absorption is of little importance relative to the completeness of absorption. In fact, for sustained effects a slower rate of absorption is sometimes desirable. If the completeness of absorption is decreased, however, the plasma levels will fall.

One other factor influencing the bioavailability of drugs is the amount of drug removed by the liver prior to reaching the systemic circulation. This "presystemic" or "first-pass" elimination may be large (50 to 80 per cent for propranolol) and is a source of variation between patients. If there is shunting of blood from the mesenteric veins to the systemic circulation, as occurs with liver disease and portal hypertension, the first-pass elimination may be very small, leading to unexpectedly high plasma levels after a given dose of drugs, such as propranolol, that normally undergo extensive first-pass elimination.

DISTRIBUTION

Once the drug is absorbed into the systemic circulation, the concentration of drug in the plasma is determined by its distribution within the body. For most drugs, only a fraction of the drug in the body is contained in the blood (see Chap. 1). Disease and other drugs can alter the distribution of drugs in the body. Congestive heart failure alters the distribution of several drugs (lidocaine, quinidine, procainamide) so that higher plasma levels result from any given dose. However, the relationship between plasma drug concentration and effect does not seem to be altered by heart failure.[4]

Changes in binding of drug to plasma proteins can alter the distribution of the drug as well as the interpretation of the plasma concentration. If drug is less well bound to plasma proteins, more drug will be able to leave the circulation to be bound to tissue sites, and this will decrease the total drug concentration (bound plus free) in plasma. However, since it is the free concentration of drug in the plasma that is in equilibrium with drug at the site of action, the interpretation of the total drug concentration as reported from the laboratory will be altered by changes in protein binding. This problem will be discussed later in the section on "Pitfalls in Interpretation of Blood Concentrations."

DRUG ELIMINATION

Drug elimination is a large source of variability between patients, and the drug levels can be used to correct for this variability. In particular, diseases of the liver and kidney will alter the elimination of many drugs, allowing an increase in drug concentrations for any given dose. In patients with renal disease, a first approximation of adjustment in dosage for renally cleared drugs can be made by knowing the creatinine clearance. However, accurate adjustments of dosage can be made only with the feedback supplied by a plasma level determination.

Unfortunately, in liver disease, there is no quantitative estimate of liver function that allows one to make drug dosage adjustments for drugs that are metabolized. Therefore, plasma drug concentrations are critical for proper therapy in patients with liver disease who are receiving potentially toxic drugs for serious illnesses.

CLINICAL APPLICATION OF PLASMA LEVEL DATA

The drugs for which plasma levels have been correlated with the therapeutic and toxic responses are listed in Table 4–1. When using the table, the clinician needs to keep in mind the meaning of the therapeutic window (Fig. 4–2). The data are collected in groups of patients and not in an individual patient.[14] Most patients will have a response within the therapeutic range, but a few may have beneficial effects of a drug in a concentration below this range, and a few may require concentrations higher than this range. Toxicity begins to occur at the upper part of the therapeutic range in some patients, but the incidence of side effects increases sharply as the therapeutic range is exceeded. Thus, the ranges are guidelines and must be interpreted as a part of the data to guide clinical decisions and are not meant to supplant clinical judgment. A number of clinical features may require that a dose be increased even though the established therapeutic range is exceeded in an individual patient. Providing the clinician is aware of the risks and monitors the patient closely for adverse effects, individual patients may obtain benefit from such an increase in drug concentrations.

TABLE 4–1. THERAPEUTIC RANGES FOR DRUGS

Drugs	Therapeutic Range
Cardiovascular Drugs	
Digoxin	0.8–2.0 μg/L
Digitoxin	10–25 μg/L
Disopyramide	2–7 mg/L
Lidocaine	1.5–5.0 mg/L
Procainamide	4–8 mg/L
Quinidine	2–6 mg/L
Theophylline	8–20 mg/L
Antiepileptic Drugs	
Carbamazepine	2–6 mg/L
Ethosuximide	40–80 mg/L
Phenobarbital	15–30 mg/L
Primidone*	6–12 mg/L
Phenytoin	10–20 mg/L
*Antibiotics***	
Carbenicillin	100–300 mg/L
Gentamicin	4–12 mg/L
Penicillin G	1–25 mg/L
Others	
Salicylate	200–300 mg/L
Nortriptyline	50–150 μg/L
Lithium	0.5–1.5 mEq/L

*Metabolized to phenobarbital, which should also be measured.

**Actual concentration required related to minimal inhibitory concentration of the infecting organism. This list is not meant to be comprehensive.

The data in Table 4–1 can be most useful for drugs that have serious toxicities and, in particular, if the drugs are being used prophylactically (e.g., to prevent a seizure or an arrhythmia). Plasma levels will also be of use when there is disease of the organs of elimination or when drugs are being given that might interact with each other. Finally, the plasma levels can be of value in adjusting dose if there is a lack of efficacy or if drug toxicity occurs on the initial dose chosen.

PITFALLS IN INTERPRETATION OF PLASMA LEVELS

Several potential problems exist in interpretation of drug concentrations that must be recognized so that improper decisions can be avoided.

TIMING OF SAMPLES

The most common problem is obtaining the drug level at the wrong time after a dose. If blood is drawn shortly after an intravenous dose of drug, the plasma drug concentration may be very high and not reflect drug present at the site of action. The best time to obtain a plasma level for most drugs is either during steady-state infusions (e.g., with lidocaine) or just prior to a dose. This latter time of sampling will give the minimum or trough level and will determine whether the concentration is always above a minimum therapeutic concentration. If a peak level is desired, blood should be drawn 1 to 2 hours after an oral dose.[6]

ACTIVE METABOLITES

Some drugs form metabolites that also possess activity. For such drugs, the value of knowing only the concentration of the parent drug is limited to situations where the quantitative importance of any active metabolite is small. In conditions where the active metabolite accumulates, the metabolite must be measured along with the parent drug for proper interpretation. Drugs with active metabolites are discussed in Chapter 3.

ALTERED BINDING TO PLASMA PROTEINS

Many drugs are highly bound to plasma proteins (Fig. 4–3). For routine drug assays, the total (bound plus free) concentration of drug in plasma is determined. If the binding is constant, then the total concentration is an accurate index of the free drug concentration that is in equilibrium with tissues, including the site of action in the target tissues. If binding to plasma protein is altered by a disease or other drugs, then the meaning of a total drug concentration will be altered. Both liver and kidney diseases can alter protein binding of drugs, either by an alteration of the quantity of protein in plasma (decreased albumin in nephrotic syndrome and cirrhosis) or by competitive binding with endogenous compounds that accumulate in uremia.[7] If doubt exists as to the interpretation of a total blood concentration, the laboratory should have the expertise and facilities to evaluate the free drug levels. Drugs with altered protein binding in renal failure are discussed in Chapters 1 and 3.

PHARMACODYNAMIC VARIABLES

The relationship between plasma levels of a drug and the observed response can be altered by a number of factors. Tolerance developing during chronic therapy with some drugs may have a pharmacokinetic or pharmacodynamic basis. If tolerance is due to altered kinetics, the plasma level–effect relationship will not be altered. Pharmacodynamic tolerance, on the other hand, is defined as a decreasing effect for a given plasma concentration. The sedation seen during phenobarbital therapy decreases with time, and patients on long-term phenobarbital therapy may tolerate higher plasma concentrations than do patients beginning on the drug. The basis for tolerance may be at the receptor level, as has been described for beta-adrenergic agonists, or beyond. The exact mechanisms for the development of pharmacodynamic tolerance are, in general, unknown.

Tissue responsiveness to a drug also may be altered by a variety of physiologic and pharmacologic variables. Thus, the cardiac responses to a given concentration of digoxin may be altered by changes in serum potassium, calcium, and magnesium concentrations. Concomitant administration of other drugs may also alter the observed plasma level–effect relationship. Therefore, the plasma levels of a drug must never be viewed out of the context of other clinical data.

EXAMPLES OF THE USE OF DRUG CONCENTRATIONS

The subsequent section illustrates several points in the use of drug levels; it is not meant to review all drugs for which plasma level monitoring is justified (Table 4–1).

ANTIARRHYTHMIC DRUGS

Regulation of the dose of the antiarrhythmic drugs is usually accomplished by using plasma levels as a guide. Many arrhythmias have a sporadic occurrence so that judgment of efficacy is difficult, and failure of adequate prophylaxis in a patient with lethal arrhythmias cannot be tolerated. In addition, drug toxicity can be serious and may be attributed to the underlying disease rather than the therapeutic agent. Finally, patients with heart disease frequently have liver, kidney, and circulatory abnormalities that can alter the pharmacokinetics, requiring dosage adjustment. Plasma level measurement is the only practical guide to the proper dose in these situations.

Procainamide. The relationship of plasma levels to efficacy and toxicity for procainamide has been established by Koch-Weser as 4 to 8 mg/L.[5] Reference to Figure 4–4 indicates that some patients will achieve therapeutic effects at concentrations as low as 2 mg/L, and that toxicity begins to appear at the upper part of the therapeutic range in some patients. It is also apparent that some patients may require concentrations of procainamide in excess of the established range to achieve arrhythmia control and the risk of serious toxicity is not great until the concentration exceeds 12 to 16 mg/L. Since the data in Figure 4–4 have been compiled, it has been found that procainamide is metabolized to *N*-acetylprocainamide, an active, antiarrhythmic metabolite, which is entirely excreted in the urine. In patients with normal renal function, the contribution of the active metabolite to the efficacy and toxicity of procainamide is probably relatively small. However, with renal dysfunction, procainamide levels will rise for any given dose and *N*-acetylprocainamide will accumulate to levels severalfold higher than the parent drug.[8] For proper interpretation, especially in patients with renal dysfunction, analysis of parent drug and active metabolite should be done.

Lidocaine. Although not used frequently, lidocaine plasma levels can be of value in patients with heart failure and liver dysfunction in which the elimination of the drug is impaired and the distribution of the drug may be altered.[9] Patients who develop signs of lidocaine toxicity on the standard infusion rates should have a lidocaine level determined as a guide to further therapy with the drug. Ideally, the turn-around time for a lidocaine level should be about 1 hour. Frequently, the drug is said to be inefficacious or not tolerated because of too low or too high concentrations, whereas it may provide satisfactory effects if the proper dose is administered.

DIGOXIN

The use of digoxin plasma levels to guide therapy has been the topic of some controversy.[10] The major difficulty in the interpretation of plasma levels of digoxin is when they are in the range of 1 to 3 μg/L. In this range there is considerable overlap between the toxic and effective plasma level–response curves. In the interpretation of the plasma digoxin concentration, clinical judgment must be used. Digoxin concentration measurements are most helpful in patients who have an inadequate response to a given dose and those with renal disease in which drug elimination is decreased.

Recently, an unexpected, potentially serious drug interaction between digoxin and quinidine has been reported. When quinidine is added to a digoxin regimen, the plasma digoxin concentrations increase and toxicity may occur.[11] The pharmacokinetic basis for this interaction is apparently a decrease in both the apparent volume of distribution and the renal clearance of the drug. The interaction had not been suspected clinically because digoxin toxicity can mimic the underlying disease and is, therefore, easily overlooked in patients who have underlying arrhythmias. By monitoring blood levels, not only was the interaction detected, but quinidine and digoxin can now be used more safely in combination by adjusting the digoxin dose.

PHENYTOIN

It has been established that optimal seizure control occurs with phenytoin concentrations of 10 to 20 mg/L.[12] However, as was pointed out earlier, many patients receive a standard 300 mg/day dose without regard to the plasma levels (Figs. 4–1 and 4–2). For proper dosage adjustment, plasma levels of phenytoin are mandatory. Unlike most drugs, phenytoin does not obey "first-order" or "linear" kinetics, in which the plasma levels and dose are related in a linear way; e.g., if the dose is doubled, the plasma concentration is doubled. With phenytoin, a change in dose will give a proportionately greater change in plasma concentrations. This behavior may be due to saturation of the enzymes responsible for phenytoin metabolism or it may be due to inhibition of phenytoin metabolism by a metabolite. Some patients can go from a subtherapeutic to a toxic plasma concentration with a dosage change of 100 mg/day. Since patients differ in their ability to eliminate phenytoin, the blood concentration of the drug is the only practical way to adjust the dose.

Phenytoin also illustrates the potential problem of altered protein binding affecting the interpretation of plasma levels. Phenytoin is about 90 per cent bound to plasma albumin. Patients with renal disease have a decrease in the amount of phenytoin bound to as low as 70 per cent.[7] Since the free drug is the species available for metabolism, distribution, and action, the total plasma concentration will be lower for any given effect of the drug if the binding is 70 per cent versus the normal 90 per cent. The therapeutic range of total phenytoin concentrations with 90 per cent protein binding is 10 to 20 mg/L, which is equivalent to a free drug concentration range of 1 to 2 mg/L. If a patient has only 70 per cent phenytoin bound to plasma proteins, this free drug concentration range of 1 to 2 mg/L will be achieved at a total concentration of only 3.3 to 6.7 mg/L. Therefore, in order to interpret the total concentration of phenytoin in a patient with renal disease, the drug binding to plasma must be determined — a test that may not be available in some laboratories. Certainly, the dose of phenytoin should not be increased to achieve a total concentration of 10 to 20 mg/L in patients with uremia, inasmuch as toxicity will be the likely result.

DRUG ASSAY METHODOLOGY

The availability of assays suitable for therapeutic monitoring of drug concentrations in plasma is due in large measure to the recent advances in instrumentation technology and in the analytical chemistry of drugs. The earliest techniques for the quantitation of drugs in biological media were based on visible and ultraviolet spectrophotometry. The introduction of chromatographic methods, starting with gas-liquid chromatography (GLC) in the late 1960's, into drug analysis represented a major breakthrough. During the early 1970's high-performance liquid chromatography (HPLC) was introduced, and the use of this technique in therapeutic drug monitoring is undergoing a rapid increase. Among the nonchromatographic techniques, a variety of immunoassay methods are becoming increasingly popular in clinical drug analysis laboratories.

GAS-LIQUID CHROMATOGRAPHY (GLC)

Chromatographic systems are used in drug analysis to separate and quantitatively detect drugs present in a highly complex biologic medium. To achieve separation of the components of a mixture, the chromatographic system uses two components, a stationary phase and a mobile phase. In GLC, the stationary phase is a high-molecular-weight liquid polymer coated on particles of inert solid support. The stationary phase is contained in a column, usually made of glass. The mobile phase is a gas, most often nitrogen or helium, forced into the column at one end and exiting at the other. The system is kept at a sufficiently elevated temperature that the components of the mixture containing the drug are volatilized upon entering the GLC column. The components are then carried by the gas through the bed of stationary phase. The individual substances will travel along the column at different rates owing to their differing affinities for the stationary phase. The separated components emerging at the end of the column are detected by the detector. The flame-ionization detector (FID) is widely used and responds to most organic molecules. The electron-capture detector (ECD) and the nitrogen-phosphorus detector (NPD) are more selective and usually more sensitive than the FID. The ECD responds to "electron-capturing" groups, e.g., halogen-containing, while the NPD is highly selective for organic compounds containing nitrogen or phosphorus. Details of the GLC system have been well described.[13]

GLC assays generally require extraction of the drug from the aqueous biologic medium with an organic solvent. To correct for losses during extraction and other sample manipulations, an internal standard (i.s.) is commonly used in GLC (and other chromatographic) assays. The i.s., ideally a compound closely related chemically to the drug to be analyzed, is added to the specimen prior to extraction. Using the i.s., the concentration of the drug in the specimen is obtained by comparing the drug: i.s. peak-height ratio to a similar ratio derived from a known standard sample, or to a calibration curve.

Chemical derivatization is frequently used in GLC. Derivatization can improve the chromatographic behavior of the drug and/or the response of the detector to the drug. A variety of derivatizing agents are available.[14]

HIGH-PERFORMANCE LIQUID CHROMATOGRAPHY (HPLC)

Of the several types of HPLC techniques available,[15] the "reversed-phase" method is the most widely used for drug assays. The stationary phase in this type of HPLC is nonpolar, e.g., long-chain hydrocarbon chemically bonded to silica, and the mobile phase is polar, generally a mixture of water and a water-miscible organic solvent. The mobile phase is pumped through the column at high pressure, typically several thousand psi. The nature of reversed-phase HPLC is such that the less polar (more lipophilic) a drug is, the more affinity it will have for the nonpolar stationary phase, and, as a result, the longer it will take to travel through the column.

Detection of the components in HPLC drug assays is usually by ultraviolet (UV) absorbance, although the use of fluorescence detectors is increasing. Fixed-wavelength and variable-wavelength UV detectors are available; one advantage of the latter is the considerable specificity achievable by the judicious selection of the wavelength monitored.

Since the reversed-phase system is compatible with aqueous solutions, drug assays are often carried out by simple deproteinization of the specimen and injection of the resulting sample into the HPLC. While this procedure is attractive in its simplicity and rapidity, its disadvantage is that no purification prior to chromatography is achieved (other than removal of proteins). As a result, interference with the analysis of a drug may occur from other drugs or from substances present in the specimen normally or as a result of a disease state. Extraction of the drug to be analyzed from the plasma prior to HPLC is required in such cases.

Chemical derivatization may also be used in HPLC assays.[14] Typically, derivatives with enhanced UV absorption or fluorescence are prepared to increase the sensitivity of the assay.

The use of HPLC in drug assay laboratories has increased rapidly during the past 5 years owing to the simplicity, rapidity, high specificity, and sensitivity often achievable with this technique. Furthermore, many compounds not analyzable with GLC because of their thermal lability and/or low volatility are readily amenable to HPLC analysis.

SPECTROPHOTOMETRY

Many of the earlier UV and visible absorption spectrophotometric and spectrophotofluorometric drug assays have been replaced by more modern, chromatography-based assays. Nevertheless, nonchromatographic spectrophotometric methods continue to be used in the analysis of some drugs. The basis of the technique is measuring the absorption of light by a drug at a wavelength of high absorption by the drug. A variety of modifications of this procedure are often used to increase the specificity. Thus, the absorbance *difference* between two wavelengths may be measured; the absorbance at different pH levels can be measured in the case of drugs where the absorbance is significantly pH-dependent; the drug may be subjected to a chemical reaction resulting in a better absorbing molecule. Despite such refinements, however, these assays may still suffer from lack of specificity. For example, methadone and diphenhydramine can interfere with the determination of phenytoin based on oxidation to benzophenone,[16] since these drugs are also oxidized to benzophenone.

Some drugs possess the property of fluorescence where light is absorbed by the molecule with a maximum at one wavelength and is emitted at another. Since these wavelengths are characteristic of the chemical structure of the drug, interference from other drugs and natural substances can be minimized. Metabolites of the drug to be measured, however, can interfere unless they can be separated from the parent drug. The determination of quinidine by fluorescence, for example, involves separation of the parent drug from its metabolites by solvent extraction, and is a sensitive and specific procedure.[17]

It is clear that spectrophotometric methods are potentially subject to more interference than chromatography-based techniques. Nevertheless, if these dangers are appreciated and if appropriate measures are taken to minimize the interference, spectrophotometric drug assays can be useful.

IMMUNOLOGIC ASSAYS

Of the several different types of immunologic assays for drugs,[18] radioimmunoassay (RIA) is the most frequently used.

In this procedure, a radioactively labeled analog of the drug and antibody to the drug are added to the unknown specimen. The drug and its radiolabeled analog compete for binding to the antibody. After equilibration, the bound drug and bound radiolabeled drug are separated from the free (unbound) fraction, using one of the several methods available, and the bound or unbound radioactivity is counted. The amount of radioactive drug bound is dependent on the amount of unlabeled drug in the sample. By comparing the amount of bound radioactivity in the unknown specimen to a calibration curve obtained from a series of standards containing known varying amounts of the drug, the concentration of the drug in the unknown specimen can be determined. While RIAs for a large number of drugs have been described,[18] commercial kits are available for only a relatively few. The advantage of the kits is that they include the radiolabeled analog, the antiserum, and the appropriate series of standards. Most RIA drug assays use ^{125}I or ^{3}H (tritium) as the radioactive label. Tritium has a longer half-life and is safer than ^{125}I, but the latter is more convenient and less expensive to count. RIAs have several advantages: no extraction or cleanup is required; microsamples, typically 50 μl or less, are used; and the procedure is highly sensitive. On the other hand, RIAs are costly. Moreover, the specificity of the antibody may not be sufficiently high to avoid cross reaction with metabolites of the drug or with other drugs of closely related chemical structure. A highly successful use of RIA is in the therapeutic monitoring of digoxin. The therapeutic serum concentration of this drug is in the low ng/ml range, and its chemical structure is such that other analytical techniques currently available are not readily applicable to its routine determination. With commercial RIA procedures, however, serum digoxin concentrations as low as 0.5 ng/ml are readily measured.

Another immunoassay useful in drug analysis is the homogeneous enzyme immunoassay (a commercially available form is the EMIT system). The basic principle in this technique is the same as in RIA, i.e., the competition between the drug to be measured and its "labeled" analog for binding sites on the antibody. In the homogeneous enzyme assay, however, the "labeled" drug is the drug covalently bound to an enzyme (EMIT uses glucose-6-phosphate dehydrogenase). The catalytic activity of the enzyme is lost when the drug-enzyme complex binds to the antibody. In the assay procedure, the catalytic activity of the enzyme is measured and related to the amount of drug present in the specimen. Since the antibody-bound enzyme is catalytically inactive, determination of the enzymatic activity directly provides a measure of the amount of unbound "labeled" drug. Therefore, separation of the bound from the unbound fraction is unnecessary, a major advantage of the technique. In the EMIT procedure, the enzyme-catalyzed conversion of NAD to NADH is measured spectrophotometrically. EMIT is currently available for several antiepileptic drugs, digoxin, several antiarrhythmic agents, theophylline, methotrexate, and gentamicin. A disadvantage of the EMIT system is the high cost of the reagents.

Another variant of the immunoassay principle is the fluorescence immunoassay (FIA). In this technique, the unbound labeled drug fluoresces, while the antibody-bound labeled drug does not. The amount of fluorescence is measured with a fluorometer and is related to the concentration of the drug in the sample.

Immunoassays are sensitive and often use equipment already available in clinical laboratories, e.g., spectrophotometers and radioactivity counters. On the other hand, immunoassays can be costly, and specificity is sometimes less than desired. Finally, immunoassays are by nature unsuited to the simultaneous analysis of several drugs and metabolites. Chromatographic procedures, on the other hand, do have this capability.

OTHER ASSAY METHODS

Several other techniques have been used in drug assays. Thin-layer chromatography (TLC) is primarily useful in drug screening and is of limited value in quantitative drug analysis. Combined gas chromatography–mass spectrometry (GC–MS) is a highly sensitive and specific technique eminently suitable for drug assays. Owing to the high cost and complexity of the equipment involved, however, GC–MS has not gained routine use in clinical drug assay laboratories. Enzyme inhibition and microbiologic assays have also been used. The latter are being rapidly replaced by immunoassays and HPLC methods in the determination of antibiotics.

MEASUREMENT OF FREE DRUG CONCENTRATION

Routine drug assays using methods described previously generally provide the *total* drug concentration and do not distinguish between free and protein-bound drug. This is because the process of sample preparation or analysis abolishes protein binding. Solvent extractions, for example, denature the proteins and, thus, eliminate protein binding. In immunoassays, the antibodies have a sufficient affinity for the drug to remove it from plasma proteins, and, once again, only the total drug concentration is obtained. The free drug concentration can be obtained by ultrafiltration or dialysis of the plasma prior to analysis.[19] The protein binding of several basic drugs has been shown to be significantly inhibited by a plasticizer compound present in plasma when blood is collected in Vacutainer tubes.[20]

QUALITY CONTROL

Recent survey programs have demonstrated that there is a considerable interlaboratory variation in drug assays, and that, indeed, the interlaboratory variation for drug assays is greater than that seen in most other areas of the clinical laboratory. It is clear that a vigorous quality control program is indispensable in a drug assay laboratory. Quality control in such laboratories may be divided into two parts: routine sample controls and external quality control programs. The former are used to assure reliability in the daily routine analyses performed by the laboratory. Several different systems are in use. One system[21] uses two controls. One of these controls contains the drug at a known concentration and is run along with each batch of patient samples. If the value found for this control falls outside a specified range, the patient values must not be reported, and corrective action must be taken. The other of the two controls contains the drug at a concentration unknown to the analyst. Determined values of this control sample are recorded and collected for long-term analysis of assay performance. A different system is used in our laboratory: each batch of patient samples includes two control samples of known concentration, which on analysis must give values within the specified acceptable range. Whichever routine sample control system is used, however, the control samples must be of good quality and accuracy. Control samples may be prepared in the laboratory or purchased from external suppliers. The latter source appears more suitable, since it provides an independent check. For many drugs, however, no commercial controls are available, and when controls are commercially available, they may be rather expensive.

The second part of the overall quality control program involves participation in external proficiency testing and surveys. Several agencies, e.g., the College of American Pathologists, the American Association of Clinical Chemists, and the Center for Disease Control, offer proficiency testing programs in therapeutic drug monitoring. Participation in these provides the laboratory director with important information indicative of the quality and reliability of the laboratory.

CONCLUSIONS

Monitoring of the plasma concentration of drugs has been shown to be of use for a limited number of drugs. The procedure will not be of clinical use for those drugs (such as antihypertensive agents) with an effect that is easily measured and quantified, although plasma concentrations may have research value for such drugs to dissect pharmacokinetic from pharmacodynamic variables in responsiveness. Plasma level monitoring has no value for those drugs that produce effects that are irreversible and persist beyond elimination of the drug, such as the effect of aspirin to inhibit platelet function when one aspirin has an effect for over a week. Finally, plasma level monitoring has little practical importance when the drugs being used have a large therapeutic index and are used to treat illnesses that are mild and not life-threatening. Thus, the use of diazepam to treat anxiety is unlikely to be aided by monitoring the plasma concentration of diazepam.

Conversely, therapeutic plasma level monitoring will be most valuable for drugs with low therapeutic indices that are used to treat serious and life-threatening illnesses, in which the effects of the drug are not easily quantified, and the manifestation of the illness may be sporadic. Blood level monitoring is especially helpful in dosage adjustment in patients with circulatory, renal, and/or hepatic diseases that alter the drug's pharmacokinetics. In addition, drugs, like phenytoin, that have nonlinear pharmacokinetics cannot be adequately used without knowledge of the concentration in plasma. Finally, monitoring the drug concentration is one of the best ways to check for patient compliance to a therapeutic regimen. Whenever available, plasma concentration of drugs must be used to augment and complement clinical judgment. There are valid, justifiable reasons to use drug doses that produce levels below or above the therapeutic window in individual patients. One must never make the mistake of treating the laboratory data rather than the patient.

REFERENCES

1. Koch-Weser J: The serum level approach to individualization of drug dosage. Eur. J. Clin. Pharmacol. *9*:1–8, 1975.
2. Withering W: An Account of the Foxglove and Some of Its Medicinal Uses: With Practical Remarks on Dropsy and Other Diseases. London; C. G. J. and J. Robinson, 1785.
3. Koch-Weser J: Serum concentrations as therapeutic guides. N. Engl. J. Med. *287*:227–231, 1972.
4. Benowitz NL, Meister W: Pharmacokinetics in patients with cardiac failure. Clin. Pharmacokinet. *1*:389–405, 1975.
5. Koch-Weser J: Clinical application of the pharmacokinetics of procainamide. Cardiovas. Clin. 6(Suppl. II):63–75, 1974.
6. Richens A, Warrington S: When should plasma drug levels be monitored? Drugs *17*:488–500, 1979.
7. Reidenberg M: The binding of drugs to plasma proteins and the interpretation of measurements of plasma concentrations of drugs in patients with poor renal function. Am. J. Med. *62*:466–470, 1977.
8. Drayer DE, Lowenthal DT, Woosley RL, et al.: Accumulation of N-acetylprocainamide, an active metabolite of procainamide, in patients with poor renal function. Clin. Pharmacol. Ther. *22*:63–69, 1977.
9. Thomson PD, Melmon KL, Richardson JA, et al.: Lidocaine pharmacokinetics in advanced heart failure, liver disease, and renal failure in humans. Ann. Intern. Med. *78*:499–508, 1973.
10. Lasagna L: How useful are serum digitalis measurements. N. Engl. J. Med. *294*:898–899, 1976.
11. Bigger JT Jr: The quinidine-digoxin interaction. What do we know about it? N. Engl. J. Med. *301*:779–781, 1979.
12. Atkinson AJ Jr: Individualization of anticonvulsant therapy. Med. Clin. North Am. *58*:1037–1049, 1974.
13. Perry ES, Weissberger A (eds.): Organic Chemistry. New York: Intersciences, 1968.
14. Blau K, King G (eds.): Handbook of Derivatives for Chromatography. London: Heyden and Sons Ltd., 1978.
15. Johnson EL, Stevenson R: Basic Liquid Chromatography. Palo Alto, Calif.: Varian Assoc., 1978.
16. Dill WA, Chucot L, Chang T, et al.: Simplified benzophenone procedure for determination of diphenylhydantoin in plasma. Clin. Chem. *17*:1200–1201, 1971.
17. Huffman DH, Higmite CE: Serum quinidine concentrations: Comparison of fluorescence, gas-chromatographic, and gas-chromatographic/mass spectrometric methods. Clin. Chem. *22*:810–812, 1976.
18. Butler VP Jr: The immunological assay of drugs. Pharmacol. Rev. *29*:103–186, 1977.
19. Kutt H: Evaluation of unusual antiepileptic drug concentrations. *In* Antiepileptic Drugs: Quantitative Analysis and Interpretation (Pippenger CE, Penry JK, Kutt H, eds.): New York: Raven Press, 1978, pp. 312–313.
20. Borgå O, Piafsky KM, Nilsen OG: Plasma protein binding of basic drugs. I. Selective displacement from alpha 1-acid glycoprotein by tris (2-butoxyethyl) phosphate. Clin. Pharmacol. Ther. *22*:539–544, 1977.
21. Kalman SM, Clark DR: Drug Assay. New York: Masson Publ. U.S.A. Inc., 1979, p. 116.

Chapter 5

Antimicrobial Agent Nephrotoxicity

by

Robert E. Cronin

Antimicrobial agents frequently induce renal dysfunction. For example, in one prospective study, approximately 20 per cent of all cases of acute renal failure were due to antimicrobial agents.[1] Moreover, antibiotics cause a spectrum of injuries to the kidneys, only some of which can be classified as acute renal failure (Table 5–1). This chapter will deal primarily with those antibiotic reactions best described as acute renal failure due to direct tubular injury. These adverse reactions are characterized by a fall in glomerular filtration rate with histologic injury confined mainly to the proximal tubular epithelium. Drug-induced acute renal failure mediated by immunologic mechanisms will be discussed in Chapter 7.

In Table 5–2 are listed the antibiotics that cause acute renal failure. Before discussing these individual agents, several general comments are appropriate. A characteristic shared by most nephrotoxic antibiotics is that their elimination is primarily by renal excretion. Also, these agents are felt to be more likely to cause clinically recognizable renal damage in the presence of underlying renal impairment. However, there is some question as to whether this represents a real or an apparent increase in the risk of developing nephrotoxicity. For example, using the common clinical measurement of worsening renal function (a rise in serum creatinine), considerable renal damage (25 to 50 per cent loss in glomerular filtration rate) is required in a normal individual before an easily detectable change in serum creatinine is seen, whereas a detectable rise in serum creatinine occurs with less diminution in filtration rate in patients with preexisting renal disease. Figure 5–1 depicts the effect of a nephrotoxic antibiotic on measured renal function in two hypothetical patients. Prior to antibiotic therapy, patient 1 had normal renal function (serum creatinine of 1 mg/dl and

TABLE 5–1. SPECTRUM OF ANTIBIOTIC-INDUCED RENAL INJURY

Acute renal failure ("acute tubular necrosis")
Acute glomerulonephritis (hypersensitivity glomerular reaction; see Chap. 7)
Interstitial nephritis (hypersensitivity interstitial reaction; see Chap. 7)
Renal tubular acidosis (see Chap. 9)
Hypokalemic alkalosis (see Chap. 9)
Nephrogenic diabetes insipidus (see Chap. 9)
Tubular obstruction

TABLE 5–2. ANTIBIOTICS CAUSING ACUTE RENAL FAILURE

Aminoglycosides
Polymyxins
Cephalosporins
Vancomycin
Tetracyclines
Co-trimoxazole
Pentamidine

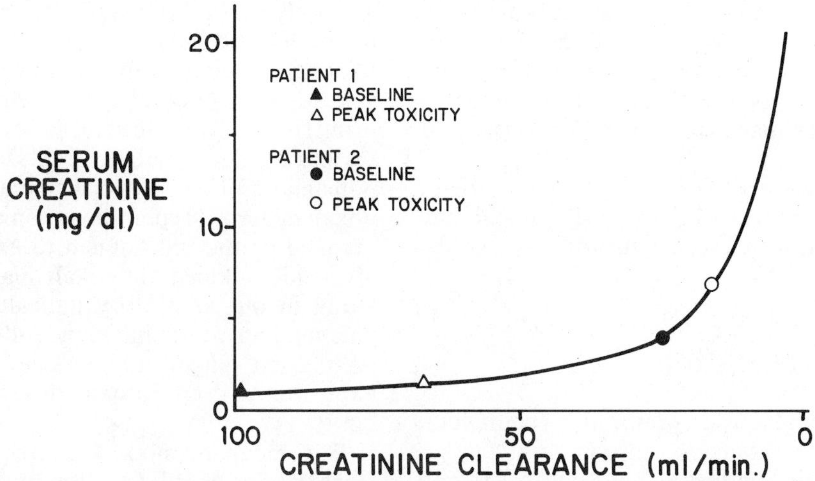

Figure 5–1. Comparative effect of a nephrotoxic antibiotic on serum creatinine and creatinine clearance in two hypothetical patients. While the absolute rise in serum creatinine for Patient 1 is smaller than for Patient 2, Patient 1 had greater nephrotoxicity when changes in the glomerular filtration rate are compared.

creatinine clearance of 100 ml/min). Patient 2 had chronic renal insufficiency (baseline serum creatinine of 4 mg/dl and a creatinine clearance of 25 ml/min). Following exposure to the antibiotic, both developed nephrotoxicity that resulted in a similar percentage reduction in creatinine clearance of 33 per cent. Patient 2, however, appeared to suffer greater renal injury, since the absolute rise in serum creatinine was 4 to 6 mg/dl, 2 mg/dl as compared to 1.0 to 1.5 mg/dl in patient 1. The latter might have even been overlooked as a variation in the laboratory determination. However, in an absolute sense, patient 1 lost more filtration capacity (100 to 67 ml/min or 33 ml/min) than patient 2 (25 to 17 ml/min or 8 ml/min).

These examples highlight several points that should be remembered when dealing with nephrotoxic drugs: (1) Reliance on the serum creatinine as a measure of nephrotoxicity may be misleading, since in patients with a low starting serum creatinine, a major loss of renal function may occur before a clinically apparent rise in serum creatinine is noted. (2) The assumption that such agents are more nephrotoxic in individuals with renal insufficiency may not be valid. Rather, because of the relationships depicted in Figure 5–1, it may be easier to appreciate nephrotoxicity in patients with lower filtration rates prior to drug administration. (3) A small rise in serum creatinine in a patient with normal renal function may represent greater renal injury than a larger rise in serum creatinine in a patient with impaired renal function.

As more experience accumulates with antibiotics, our interpretation of what constitutes nephrotoxicity has changed. The aminoglycosides are now recognized to cause significantly more nephrotoxicity than originally estimated. Moreover, with the aminoglycosides, the nephrotoxic reaction may not become clinically apparent until after the drug has been discontinued.[2] Careful scrutiny of patients receiving potentially nephrotoxic antibiotics has identified another important relationship. Although nephrotoxic drugs may have widely differing chemical structures and modes of action, when the kidney is exposed to two or more of them at the same time, the nephrotoxic effect of each is additive or potentiated.

A great deal of confusion exists regarding the role of monitoring antibiotic blood levels and the relationship of this to the prevention of nephrotoxicity. It is a common teaching that careful dosing of potentially nephrotoxic antibiotics based on the level of renal function will prevent nephrotoxicity. However, nephrotoxicity may occur in the presence of carefully prescribed doses and therapeutic blood levels. Clearly, other factors also must be involved in determining nephrotoxicity. Several published articles have outlined nomograms and formulas for proper dosing of antimicrobial agents, especially the aminoglycosides, in patients with impaired renal function.[3,4] However, even careful dosing of aminoglycosides supplemented with measurement of antibiotic blood levels still results in nephrotoxicity in as many as 15 per cent of treated patients.[5]

The following sections will discuss some of these problems as well as the clinical and laboratory features of nephrotoxicity for the specific antibiotics outlined in Table 5–2.

AMINOGLYCOSIDES

The aminoglycoside antibiotics (neomycin, kanamycin, gentamicin, tobramycin, amikacin, sisomicin, netilmicin, and streptomycin) are bactericidal agents that have nephrotoxicity as their major adverse effect. In bacteria, the aminoglycosides penetrate the cell wall and cytoplasmic membrane and act on the bacterial ribosomes, causing misreading of the genetic code. The resulting faulty proteins lead to death of the microorganism. The polycationic nature of the molecules is responsible for their poor oral absorption, poor penetration into the cerebrospinal fluid, and rapid renal excretion. Studies to be described later suggest that this polycationic charge also may be important in nephrotoxicity.

The reported incidence of nephrotoxicity with these drugs is increasing. In 1969, the reported incidence of gentamicin nephrotoxicity was 2 to 3 per cent,[6] while in 1979 an incidence ranging between 16 and 25 per cent was reported.[5,7] The reason for this increase is probably multifactorial but certainly includes an increase in the recommended dosage and more rigorous criteria for detecting toxicity. Longer courses of therapy, a more resistant spectrum of gram-negative organisms, and expanding indications for use of these drugs also play a part in the increased incidence of nephrotoxicity.

The clinical hallmark of aminoglycoside nephrotoxicity is nonoliguric acute renal failure. The clinical course is often milder than that of oliguric acute renal failure. Also, the onset of renal failure is usually slower and the daily rises in serum creatinine tend to be somewhat lower than observed in acute renal failure from other causes. Recovery from aminoglycoside nephrotoxicity is usually a slow process and may require more than a month. In some patients, particularly those with renal impairment prior to receiving the aminoglycoside, recovery to baseline renal function may be incomplete. In addition to nonoliguric acute renal failure, aminoglycoside administration can cause enzymuria, proteinuria, aminoaciduria, glucosuria, and a variety of electrolyte disorders, including hypomagnesemia,[8,9] hypocalcemia,[9,10] and hypokalemia.[8-10] Hyperaldosteronism has been invoked as the mechanism to explain aminoglycoside-induced hypokalemia.[8] A canine study in our laboratory indicates that hypokalemia can occur independently of an effect on plasma magnesium or calcium following exposure to nephrotoxic doses of gentamicin.[11]

The mechanism(s) whereby aminoglycosides impair renal function is not precisely known, but considerable investigative work on this topic has been undertaken during the past 10 years. Because of their highly basic charge, the aminoglycosides penetrate cells poorly. Nevertheless, in order to impair bacterial growth and presumably to damage kidney cells, at least a small fraction of administered aminoglycoside must gain access to the cell interior. While serum protein binding of aminoglycosides is minor and the renal clearance of gentamicin is very close to that of inulin, indicating little secretion or reabsorption, a small fraction of filtered gentamicin is known to gain access to proximal tubular cells. Of all the tissues in the body, those of the renal cortex stand alone in their ability to concentrate aminoglycosides many times over plasma. The relatively non-nephrotoxic streptomycin is the only exception to this rule. The proximal but not distal renal tubular cells concentrate aminoglycosides[12] and are the cells that demonstrate significant injury in experimental nephrotoxicity in the rat.[13] Morphologic changes in proximal tubular cells can be detected within hours of drug administration.[14] Gentamicin gains access to proximal tubular cytoplasm by a process of pinocytosis occurring at the brush border on the luminal surface of the cell.[14] However, studies of renal cortical tissue slices (in which gentamicin presumably cannot gain access to the tubule from the luminal side) also demonstrate significant tissue uptake of gentamicin,[15,16] suggesting the possibility of some uptake at the basolateral (contraluminal) surface as well. However, transtubular secretion of gentamicin could not be demonstrated by microperfusion of peritubular capillaries with ^{3}H-gentamicin,[12] supporting the idea that glomerular filtration is the only important route of aminoglycoside elimination.

Once inside the cell, gentamicin binds to subcellular organelles or is taken into lysozymes.[17] Kunin has demonstrated that the aminoglycosides (e.g., neomycin, streptomycin, kanamycin, and gentamicin) bind to cellular homogenates, especially of the liver and kidneys. The cellular fraction with greatest binding of aminoglycosides is that containing the bulk of microsomes and lysozymes. Binding of these agents to tissue homogenates occurs in proportion to the number of charged radicals (free amino groups) present on the molecule. Interestingly, there also is a direct relationship between number of charged radicals and nephrotoxicity. Several studies point to this tissue accumulation of aminoglycoside as being an important factor in the generation of nephrotoxicity. Luft and Kleit[18] measured the concentrations of gentamicin, tobramycin, kanamycin, and streptomycin in rat renal tissue after a single subcutaneous injection and found that gentamicin, tobramycin, and kanamycin accumulated to high levels in renal cortex, but streptomycin, clinically the least nephrotoxic, disappeared rapidly. The half-life of gentamicin in renal tissue is 109 hours and, once concentrated in renal tissues, may take several months to be excreted.[18] The method of administration of aminoglycosides has a marked effect on renal cortical uptake. Multiple injections cause greater tissue accumulation and nephrotoxicity than the same total dose on a weight basis given as a single bolus.[19]

While intracellular concentration of aminoglycosides correlates roughly with nephrotoxicity, other factors also appear to be involved. Gilbert et al.[20] noted that administration of gentamicin to rats for 6 weeks led to renal failure followed by recovery in spite of continued administration of the drug. Although recovery of renal function occurred, the renal cortical concentration of gentamicin remained high. This study suggests that the regenerating or immature proximal tubular cells are resistant to the nephrotoxic effect of these antibiotics; however, the mechanism of this protective effect remains to be clarified.

A preliminary study by Weinberg et al.[21] using isolated renal mitochondria demonstrated that all of the clinically used aminoglycosides (neomycin, gentamicin, tobramycin, kanamycin, and streptomycin) caused a significant reduction in renal oxidative phosphorylation and nephrotoxicity. The toxic component of the molecule appeared to be the polycationic charge, since polycationic dextran caused similar mitochondrial changes and nephrotoxicity. In additional studies on the pathogenesis of aminoglycoside nephrotoxicity, Bennett et al.[22] utilized rat studies to demonstrate that organic acid transport (PAH) is stimulated prior to development of overt renal failure. They postulated that early stimulation of PAH uptake may represent changes in membrane permeability.

In addition to tubular changes induced by gentamicin, at least one glomerular defect has been reported. Baylis et al.[23] demonstrated in the rat that gentamicin caused a marked decline in the glomerular capillary ultrafiltration coefficient (kf) at a time when both whole kidney glomerular filtration rate and single nephron glomerular filtration rate had fallen by 30 to 50 per cent. In this micropuncture study, neither tubular obstruction nor renal ischemia appeared to be involved in the reduction of glomerular filtration rate.

Several risk factors have been identified that appear to enhance the likelihood of developing aminoglycoside nephrotoxicity. The combination of an aminoglycoside with a known nephrotoxin, such as amphotericin,[24] *cis*-platinum,[25] and possibly x-ray contrast material,[26] leads to enhanced nephrotoxicity. In experimental animals, the combination of gentamicin plus methoxyflurane[27] also leads to worse renal damage than when either drug is used alone. The combined use of aminoglycosides with cephalosporin antibiotics appears to enhance the risk of nephrotoxicity. Initial reports on this question were retrospective and most, but not all, indicated greater toxicity when the two agents were combined.[28, 29] Adding to the confusion were several animal studies showing that the addition of a cephalosporin to an aminoglycoside actually resulted in decreased nephrotoxicity.[30, 31] However, three prospective studies done in the past few years clearly demonstrate that the combination of an aminoglycoside and a cephalosporin results in nephrotoxicity in approximately 20 per cent of cases, whereas the combination of an aminoglycoside and a penicillin derivative leads to nephrotoxicity in approximately 6 per cent of cases.[32-34] The reason for this enhanced nephrotoxicity is not precisely known, but cephalosporins also concentrate, at least transiently, in renal proximal tubular cells. Since a penicillin and an aminoglycoside generally provide comparable antibacterial efficacy, it seems prudent to avoid the combination of an aminoglycoside and a cephalosporin. Advancing age, volume depletion, and prior renal insufficiency reportedly enhance the likelihood of aminoglycoside nephrotoxicity, but as outlined previously, additional data on this latter relationship are needed.[35]

The specific aminoglycoside preparation utilized might also be an important factor in the frequency of nephropathy. As noted previously, both laboratory and clinical studies have demonstrated a direct relationship between the number of free amino groups on the drug and nephrotoxicity. In a prospective clinic study reported in 1977,[36] nephrotoxicity developed in 26 per cent of 72 patients given gentamicin and 12 per cent of 74 patients receiving tobramycin ($p < 0.25$). However, ototoxicity developed in 10 to 11 per cent of patients receiving both drugs. In spite of potent nephrotoxicity of the aminoglycosides, there is no substitute for these valuable drugs in the face of serious gram-negative infections. How can they be used safely? The nomograms and formulas designed to estimate the aminoglycoside dosage in patients with renal failure[2,3] may be helpful in planning the initial dose of drug (see Chap. 2). For accurate determination of subsequent doses, peak levels (drawn 1 hour post injection) and trough levels (drawn immediately before the next calculated doses) should be used in calculating subsequent therapy. These measurements will allow assurance of adequate but not excessive blood bactericidal levels to be achieved. In addition, peak and trough levels have been proposed as indicators of aminoglycoside nephrotoxicity; however, there is little evidence to support the belief that the blood level of these agents is an important risk factor for or indicator of nephrotoxicity. Bennett et al.[19] have shown in the rat that a single large dose of gentamicin producing a high peak blood level was less nephrotoxic than the same amount given in divided doses in which the resulting peak blood levels were much lower. A rising trough level, rather than indicating impending nephrotoxicity, represents drug retention owing to already reduced glomerular filtration rate.

In attempting to minimize clinical nephrotoxicity, several points should be emphasized. (1) Aminoglycoside nephrotoxicity relates to the dose and duration of drug administration. Thus, nephrotoxicity will be more likely to occur when large doses are given over prolonged periods, or when "normal" doses are given to individuals with renal impairment and, thus, have diminished capacity to excrete aminoglycoside antibiotics. Rather than be guided by rigid protocols regarding duration of therapy, the goal of treatment should be the shortest course of therapy compatible with clinical cure. When an aminoglycoside is begun to treat an infection subsequently proven to be due to aerobic gram-negative bacilli, it is appropriate to change therapy to a less toxic agent, such as ampicillin or a cephalosporin, provided the microorganism is susceptible. Such a change in therapy is recommended even if the patient is responding satisfactorily during the initial aminoglycoside therapy. (2) Since aminoglycoside nephrotoxicity is dose-duration dependent and since the renal cortical half-life of these drugs is long, administration of repetitive courses of these agents should be avoided if possible. (3) Empiric aminoglycoside therapy in a patient with presumed sepsis or other serious infection must be reevaluated when culture results are available. A "clinical response" in the absence of positive cultures is not usually sufficient justification for completing a full course of an empirically started aminoglycoside. (4) Aminoglycosides are best viewed as nephrotoxins for all patients who receive them. In most patients, nephrotoxicity is subclinical and beyond detection with the usual tests of renal function. Nevertheless, serial monitoring of renal function (serum creatinine three times per week) should be carried out in patients receiving aminoglycosides. (5) Concomitant administration of other potent nephrotoxins (cephalosporins, potent diuretics, radiographic contrast agents, amphotericin, and *cis*-platinum) should be avoided. (6) Attempts should be made to maintain optimal extracellular fluid volume and renal perfusion during aminoglycoside therapy. (7) Dosage estimates should be based on the best index of renal function available. A steady-state serum creatinine often will suffice. In elderly patients or patients with diminished renal function, however, a creatinine clearance is preferable. (8) Assessment of plasma drug levels is often of help, particularly when inadequate clinical response or impaired renal function is present.

POLYMYXINS

Colistin (sodium colistimethate, polymyxin E) is a cyclic polypeptide that differs from polymyxin B only by the absence of a single amino acid. Initial reports suggested that colistin was less nephrotoxic than polymyxin B, but the drugs were not administered at equivalent doses. When given in doses that result in blood concentrations of equal antibacterial effectiveness, the toxicity of colistin and polymyxin B was found to be similar.[37] The present discussion describing clinical and experimental toxicity can be equally applied to either agent. A prospective study of 288 patients who received colistin indicated adverse renal reactions in 20 per cent.[38] In a manner similar to the aminoglycoside antibiotics, renal function may continue to deteriorate for a week or more following cessation of therapy before improvement occurs.

The polymyxins are largely excreted by the kidneys; thus, the half-life in the blood is a function of the glomerular filtration rate. Like the aminoglycoside antibiotics, decreased renal function interferes with the excretion of the polymyxins and demands a reduction in dosage. Whether the presence of prior renal insufficiency *per se* enhances the likelihood of nephrotoxicity is not clear. One author suggests that preexisting renal disease is important in nephrotoxicity only to the extent that decreased renal function interferes with the excretion of the polymyxins and demands a reduction in dosage.[38] The combination of colistin with a cephalosporin antibiotic appears to enhance the risk of nephrotoxicity.[38, 39] Surprisingly, the combination of a polymyxin and an aminoglycoside does not further increase the risk of nephrotoxicity.

Healthy volunteers have been found to have a fall in creatinine clearance and a rise in serum creatinine after receiving colistin.[40] Generally, the damage is reversible after cessation of therapy, but in some cases, renal function may be permanently impaired. In experimental animals, parenteral administration of polymyxin caused a fall in glomerular filtration rate and histologic evidence of tubular injury.[41] Pathologic studies of human kidneys have demonstrated acute tubular necrosis.[42, 43] Colistin and polymyxin B nephrotoxicity may be associated with proteinuria, increased cellular elements, and cylindruria on urinalysis.[44]

The mechanism of the nephrotoxicity of these drugs is not well described, but several observations suggest that they affect the kidneys in a manner similar to the aminoglycoside antibiotics. Kunin and Bugg[45] have shown that polymyxins bind to cell membranes of liver, kidneys, muscle, lungs, and brain in a biologically inactive state. This tissue-bound drug is detectable in tissue long after disappearance from the blood and tends to accumulate with repeated administration. Kunin[17] demonstrated that the binding of antibiotics to specific tissue sites can be linked closely with the number of free amino groups. Colistin, polymyxin B, and the aminoglycoside antibiotics contain from three to six free amino radicals, which appears to be the reason why these drugs bind avidly to tissue, particularly in the kidneys. This electrostatic binding to tissue is likely to be a factor in both the biologic and the nephrotoxic effect of these agents. In the case of the polymyxins, biologic activity depends on their binding to polyphosphate groups of phospholipids in the bacterial cell membrane.[46] While the binding of aminoglycosides to renal tissues appears to be quite distinct from that observed with the polymyxins, the overall effect on renal function and clinical patterns of nephrotoxicity seems to be similar. Both classes of antibiotics may cause nonoliguric acute renal failure,[39] enhanced toxicity with concomitant cephalosporin administration,[34, 38, 39] a variety of serum electrolyte and mineral disturbances,[8-16, 47] and a protracted time for recovery following withdrawal of the drug.

In summary, colistin and polymyxin B are agents closely related in structure, antibacterial spectrum, and toxicity. While side-by-side comparisons of nephrotoxicity with the aminoglycoside antibiotics are not available, treatment with the polymyxin class of drugs appears to carry substantially greater risk for renal damage than comparable doses of the currently used group of aminoglycosides.

CEPHALOSPORINS

The cephalosporin antibiotics are generally regarded as having a low potential for nephrotoxicity. The major exception to this rule has been cephaloridine, which clearly causes acute renal failure, especially in the presence of underlying renal impairment.[48-50] Isolated reports have implicated cephalothin in causing acute renal failure.[51, 52] Many of these cases, however, are suggestive of an acute hypersensitivity reaction.

Renal clearance of the cephalosporins is rapid and they are excreted both by glomerular filtration and, with the exception of cephaloridine, by tubular secretion.[53] Most of an administered dose is recovered in the urine within 24 hours. The serum half-life of most cephalosporins is between 30 and 60 minutes. Cefazolin, cephaloridine, and cefamandole have longer half-lives (1½ to 2 hours). Protein binding is relatively high with cefazolin and cephalothin, but insignificant with cephaloridine.

The mechanism of nephrotoxicity of these antibiotics, particularly cephaloridine, has been studied in considerable depth. Tune and associates[54-56] have offered persuasive evidence indicating that high intracellular concentrations of cephaloridine are the ultimate reasons for nephrotoxicity. All the cephalosporins are transported via the organic anion secretory pathway of the kidney. However, in the case of cephaloridine, there is little or no excretion into the urine[57, 58] and high levels accumulate in renal cortical tissue.[59] The toxic effect of cephaloridine on renal function can be prevented by probenecid and other organic anions that inhibit tubular uptake of cephaloridine.[54, 57, 60] When the PAH (para-aminohippuric acid) transport system is immature, the kidney is less at risk for toxicity. Tune[56] reported that the renal cortical–to–serum cephaloridine concentration ratio was lower in newborn rabbits. Wold et al.[61] demonstrated that the development of susceptibility to cephaloridine nephrotoxicity paralleled the maturation of the renal anionic transport system in newborn rabbits. After entry into the proximal tubule, subsequent movement across the luminal cell membrane into tubular fluid is restricted.[56] Thus, the cortical–to–serum cephaloridine concentration ratio in the rabbit is twofold greater than that for PAH.[55, 57] Cefazolin, which is much less nephrotoxic compared to cephaloridine in experimental animals, shares with cephaloridine the association between transport and toxicity.[62] However, while there is a diffusion block for cephaloridine to move across the luminal border into the urine, cefazolin is secreted into the urine at a rate three to four times its estimated filtration rate.[63]

While the isolated use of cephalosporins other than cephaloridine has been incriminated occasionally in causing acute renal failure in humans, many of the reported cases have occurred when cephalosporins have been used in conjunction with aminoglycosides.[28, 29, 64] In these cases, it seems likely that the effect of the cephalosporin was to potentiate the nephrotoxicity of the aminoglycoside. Since both classes of drugs may concentrate to high levels in proximal tubular cells, it seems likely that tissue accumulation and concentration by the proximal tubular cells is an important factor in nephrotoxicity for both of these antibiotic groups.

In summary, nephrotoxicity is an uncommon event following administration of cephalosporin antibiotics alone. Cephaloridine is by far the most nephrotoxic drug in this class and the mechanism of toxicity appears to depend on the accumulation of high concentrations of the drug in proximal tubular cells. Accumulation occurs via the organic anion transport pathway. When cephalosporins are combined with aminoglycosides, the nephrotoxicity of the latter is enhanced.

VANCOMYCIN

Vancomycin was introduced into clinical use for staphylococcal infections in 1958, but in a few years was overshadowed by the appearance of the less toxic synthetic penicillins. While vancomycin was a very effective drug against penicillinase-producing staphylococci, initial use was associated with a high incidence of thrombophlebitis, fever, chills, rash, and, occasionally, nephrotoxicity.[65] Improvements in manufacturing techniques have eliminated many of the problems.[66] Vancomycin-associated hearing loss is the most serious adverse effect and has been reported only in patients with renal insufficiency and serum vancomycin levels exceeding 80 to 100 μg/ml.[67]

In recent years, vancomycin has become popular once again. It may be a very suitable agent in the following conditions: infections due to methicillin-resistant staphylococci; bacterial endocarditis in patients allergic to penicillin; staphylococcal enterocolitis; staphylococcal infections, particularly those in arteriovenous fistulas and shunts in patients undergoing hemodialysis; infections caused by penicillin-resistant diphtheroids; and prophylaxis of bacterial endocarditis in patients with prosthetic valves and penicillin allergy.[68]

In normal individuals, vancomycin is not detectable in the serum after oral administration; thus, parenteral administration is mandatory. The serum half-life of intravenously administered drug is 6 hours in patients with normal renal function. Vancomycin is excreted primarily by the kidneys in its unchanged active form.[69] Conversely, in the presence of severely reduced or absent renal function, excretion is greatly delayed and serum levels remain high for long periods. This property has been exploited in anatomically or functionally anephric patients on chronic dialysis therapy in whom staphylococcal shunt infections[70] or a staphylococcal peritonitis[71] can be treated successfully with a 1 gm dose given every 7 to 10 days.

A reversible impairment in renal function with vancomycin therapy was reported during the early experience with this drug,[72] but there is no uniformity on this question in the literature. In 1978, Hook and Johnson[65] reported on their 9-year experience using vancomycin therapy in the therapy of bacterial endocarditis. In the 15 patients reported, an average dose of 2 gm/day was administered over a 2 to 10-week period (average 5 weeks) with no evidence of nephrotoxicity, as estimated from changes in serum creatinine or urea nitrogen. In some cases, other antibiotics were also administered, but streptomycin was the only other potentially nephrotoxic agent. In another series, 33 cases of staphylococcal septicemia were treated without nephrotoxicity.[66] In cases of enterococcal endocarditis in which penicillin allergy exists, a vancomycin-gentamicin combination has been suggested as an alternative form of therapy to penicillin-streptomycin.[69] Although there are few data regarding renal toxicity with vancomycin-gentamicin in combination, the addition of a drug with low nephrotoxic potential (vancomycin) to one with a high risk of nephrotoxicity would be expected to enhance the toxicity of the latter.

In summary, the clinical use of vancomycin is undergoing a revival. It is a very useful drug for staphylococcal infections in patients unable to tolerate penicillins. Nephrotoxicity from the use of this agent is possible, but the frequency of its occurrence appears to be low and considerably less than that seen with the aminoglycoside antibiotics. However, this difference may depend as much on variables in the patient population likely to receive the two drugs (age, level of renal function, underlying disease) as on actual differences in toxicity between the two drugs.

TETRACYCLINES

Tetracyclines are broad-spectrum antibiotics that are partially metabolized by the liver and concentrated in the bile. Excretion from the body occurs primarily by urinary elimination of intact drug and metabolites with a small proportion excreted in the feces. However, in the case of doxycycline, the fecal route predominates. Protein binding varies from 35 per cent for oxytetracycline to 93 per cent for doxycycline.[73] As would be expected of a drug that depends primarily on the kidneys for elimination, in chronic renal failure, high tetracycline blood levels will result if the dose is not reduced.[74]

Azotemia is a well-described complication of tetracycline administration in normal individuals and in patients with chronic renal failure.[75] A disproportionate increase in blood urea nitrogen to creatinine ratio is often observed and is felt to be due to the antianabolic effect of tetracycline. Doxycycline, however, appears to have little antianabolic effect. In some cases, however, particularly in patients with underlying renal disease, doxycycline causes striking elevations in blood urea nitrogen. Both blood urea nitrogen and plasma creatinine concentration have been reported to increase during demeclocycline administration; until recently, this effect was thought to be due to either hypovolemia induced by polyuria or the antianabolic effects of tetracyclines.[76-78] However, Carrilho et al.[79] administered demeclocycline to three patients with cirrhosis, ascites, and hyponatremia to study the abnormal water retention associated with liver disease. An increase in blood urea nitrogen and serum creatinine was noted, as well as a 60 per cent reduction in inulin clearance. The abnormalities in renal function reversed with drug withdrawal. Carefully recorded weights did not change during drug administration, ruling out volume depletion as the cause of the fall in glomerular filtration rate. The mechanism of this demeclocycline effect on the glomerular filtration rate is unknown, but it appears to occur only in situations in which baseline renal function is already compromised (e.g., cirrhosis with ascites) and correlates with high plasma demeclocycline levels. In normal subjects receiving demeclocycline at doses of 600 to 1200 mg/day for 3 days to 6 weeks, impairment of inulin and para-aminohippurate clearance has not been observed.[80, 81] In cirrhotic patients, the complete recovery of baseline renal function occurs on withdrawal of the drug.[80] A parallel to this effect is the recently reported reversible reduction in glomerular filtration rate and renal blood flow in a patient with congestive heart failure[82] following administration of the prostaglandin inhibitor indomethacin. The reduction in glomerular filtration rate and renal blood flow in these patients may occur by unmasking of renal vasoconstriction when the vasodilating effect of renal prostaglandins is abolished by inhibition of cyclooxygenase with indomethacin. There is no direct evidence for a vascular site of action of demeclocyline, but a direct effect of demeclocycline at the tubular level is possible. The possibility of a direct effect on subcellular organelles is suggested by the observation that tetracyclines are concentrated in mammalian mitochondria.[83]

In addition to the effect on glomerular filtration rate, demeclocycline has been incriminated in another nephrotoxic reaction. Singer and Rotenberg[80] demonstrated renal concentrating defects in eight of 24 patients treated with demeclocycline for acne. The defect appeared to result from impaired generation of cyclic AMP (adenosine monophosphate), the secondary messenger for the action of vasopressin. This adverse effect of demeclocycline on urinary concentration has been used to advantage in the treatment of the syndrome of inappropriate antidiuretic hormone secretion.[84]

Degradation products of outdated tetracyclines may cause proximal tubular injury characterized by proteinuria, aminoaciduria, glucosuria, and phosphaturia.[85] Elimination of citric acid in the tetracycline capsules has eliminated this problem.[44]

In summary, the nephrotoxic potential of the tetracycline antibiotics is relatively low, but they should not be used in the presence of renal insufficiency or renal failure. While demeclocycline may be helpful in some cases of chronic syndrome of inappropriate antidiuretic hormone release, it should not be used to treat hyponatremic states resulting from hepatic dysfunction, since a serious reduction in glomerular filtration rate is likely to occur.

CO-TRIMOXAZOLE

Co-trimoxazole (trimethoprim-sulfamethoxazole) was introduced in 1968 and is widely used for the treatment of urinary tract infections and several other disorders. Reports of renal impairment following administration can be found,[86, 89] but the type of renal injury is difficult to classify. In almost all cases, patients who developed renal deterioration had underlying renal impairment as indicated by an elevated serum creatinine at the start of therapy. Renal deterioration tends to be characterized by a nonoliguric state.[86] Most authors feel that the sulfa component of this drug is the toxic moiety. Acetylated conjugated derivatives of sulfamethoxazole accumulate when renal function is impaired.

However, in spite of these case reports, when a large group (649) of hospitalized patients receiving co-trimoxazole was prospectively evaluated for toxic reactions, no evidence of renal injury was noted.[88] Even in high-risk cancer patients, chemoprophylaxis with co-trimoxazole prevented *Pneumocystis carinii* pneumonia, but was not associated with any renal injury.[89]

In summary, acute renal failure may occur with this agent, but the incidence appears to be low. When an acute reduction in renal function occurs with co-trimoxazole in the presence of a skin rash, acute interstitial nephritis rather than acute renal failure should be considered. A renal biopsy may be helpful to resolve these cases. The drug should be used with caution in patients with renal insufficiency.

PENTAMIDINE

Pentamidine has been in use as a therapeutic agent for 40 years, primarily to treat tropical diseases such as trypanosomiasis and leishmaniasis. In more recent years, it has been used effectively to treat *Pneumocystis carinii* pneumonia.[90] Pentamidine is a very toxic drug and almost half of the patients receiving it experience some side effects.[90-92] Azotemia, hypoglycemia, and changes in liver function are the major adverse effects. As with the other agents discussed in this chapter, adverse renal reactions tend to occur when pentamidine is administered with other nephrotoxic drugs.

In summary, the use of pentamidine carries a high risk of renal toxicity. The effective use in recent years of a less toxic antibiotic combination, trimethoprim and sulfamethoxazole (co-trimoxazole), for the treatment[92, 93] and prophylaxis[89] of this disease has relegated pentamidine to a second-line status.

REFERENCES

1. Anderson RJ, Linas SL, Berns AS, et al.: Nonoliguric acute renal failure: a prospective study. N. Engl. J. Med. *296*:1134–1138, 1977.
2. Gary NE, Buzzeo L, Salaki J, et al.: Gentamicin-associated acute renal failure. Arch. Intern. Med. *136*:1101–1104, 1976.
3. McHenry MC, Gavran TL, Gifford RW Jr, et al.: Gentamicin dosages for renal insufficiency: adjustments based on endogenous creatinine clearance and serum creatinine concentration. Ann. Intern. Med. *74*:192–197, 1971.
4. Hull JH, Sarubbi FA Jr: Gentamicin serum concentrations: pharmacokinetic predictions. Ann. Intern. Med. *85*:183–189, 1976.
5. Smith CR, Maxwell RR, Edwards CQ, et al.: Nephrotoxicity induced by gentamicin and amikacin. Johns Hopkins Med. J. *142*:85–90, 1978.
6. Falco FG, Smith HM, Arcieri GM: Nephrotoxicity of aminoglycosides and gentamicin. J. Infect. Dis. *9*:406–409, 1969.
7. Maki DG, Agger WA, Craig WA: Comparative clinical study of sisomicin and gentamicin. (Abstract.) Clin. Res. *26*:156A, 1978.
8. Holmes AM, Hesling CM, Wilson TM: Drug-induced secondary hyperaldosteronism in patients with pulmonary tuberculosis. Q. J. Med. *39*:299–314, 1970.
9. Patel R, Savage A: Symptomatic hypomagnesemia associated with gentamicin therapy. Nephron *23*:50–52, 1979.
10. Bar RS, Wilson HE, Mazzaferri EL: Hypomagnesemic hypocalcemia secondary to renal magnesium wasting: a possible consequence of high dose gentamicin therapy. Ann. Intern. Med. *82*:646–649, 1975.
11. Cronin RE, Bulger RE, Southern P, et al.: Natural history of aminoglycoside nephrotoxicity in the dog. J. Lab. Clin. Med. *95*:463–474, 1980.
12. Pastoriza-Munoz E, Bowman RL, Kaloyanides GJ: Renal tubular transport of gentamicin in the rat. Kidney Int. *16*:440–450, 1979.
13. Kosek, JC, Mazze RI, Cousin MJ: Nephrotoxicity of gentamicin. Lab. Invest. *30*:48–57, 1974.
14. Silverblatt FJ, Kuehn C: Autoradiography of gentamicin uptake by the rat proximal tubule cell. Kidney Int. *15*:335–345, 1979.
15. Bennett WM, Plamp CE, Parker RA, et al.: Renal transport of organic acids and bases in aminoglycoside nephrotoxicity. Antimicrob. Agents Chemother. *16*:231–233, 1979.
16. Kluwe WM, Hook JB: Analysis of gentamicin uptake by rat renal cortical slices. Toxicol. Appl. Pharmacol. *45*:513–539, 1978.
17. Kunin CM: Binding of antibiotics to tissue homogenates. J. Infect. Dis. *121*:55–64, 1970.
18. Luft FC, Kleit SA: Renal parenchymal accumulation of aminoglycoside antibiotics in rats. J. Infect. Dis. *130*:656–659, 1974.
19. Bennett WM, Plamp C, Gilbert DN, et al.: The effects of dosage regimen on experimental gentamicin nephrotoxicity: dissociation of peak serum levels from renal failure. J. Infect. Dis. *140*:567–580, 1979.
20. Gilbert DN, Houghton DC, Bennett WM, et al.: Reversibility of gentamicin nephrotoxicity in rats: recovery during continuous drug administration. Proc. Soc. Exp. Biol. Med. *160*:99–103, 1979.
21. Weinberg JM, Simmons CF, Humes HD: The molecular basis for aminoglycoside and diethylaminoethyl dextran nephrotoxicity. (Abstract.) Kidney Int. *16*:778A, 1979.
22. Bennett WM, Plamp CE, Parker RA, et al.: Alterations in organic ion transport induced by gentamicin nephrotoxicity in the rat. J. Lab. Clin. Med. *95*:32–39, 1980.
23. Baylis C, Helmut R, Rennke R, et al.: Mechanisms of the defect in glomerular ultrafiltration associated with gentamicin administration. Kidney Int. *12*:344–348, 1977.
24. Churchill DN, Seely J: Nephrotoxicity associated with combined gentamicin-amphotericin B therapy. Nephron *19*:176–181, 1977.
25. Dentino ME, Luft FC, Yum MN, et al.: Long term effect of cis-diamminedichloride platinum (CDDP) on renal function and structure in man. Cancer *41*:1274–1281, 1978.
26. Barshay ME, Kaye JH, Goldman R, et al.: Acute renal failure in diabetic patients after intravenous infusion pyelography. Clin. Nephrol. *1*:35–39, 1973.
27. Barr GA, Mazze RI, Cousins MJ, et al.: An animal model for combined methoxyflurane and gentamicin nephrotoxicity. Br. J. Anesth. *45*:306–311, 1973.
28. Kleinknecht D, Ganeval D, Droz D: Acute renal failure after high doses of gentamicin and cephalothin. Lancet *1*:1129, 1973.
29. Plager JE: Association of renal injury with combined cephalothin-gentamicin therapy among patients severely ill with malignant disease. Cancer *37*:1937–1943, 1976.
30. Luft FC, Patel V, Yum MN, et al.: Nephrotoxicity of cephalothin-gentamicin combinations in rats. Antimicrob. Agents Chemother. *9*:831–839, 1976.
31. Dellinger P, Murphy T, Pinn V, et al.: The protective effect of cephalothin against gentamicin induced nephrotoxicity in rats. Antimicrob. Agents Chemother. *9*:172–178, 1976.
32. Klastersky, J, Hensgens C, Debusscher L: Empiric therapy for cancer patients: comparative study of ticarcillin-tobramycin, ticarcillin-cephalothin, and cephalothin-tobramycin. Antimicrob. Agents Chemother. *7*:640–645, 1975.
33. EORTC International Antimicrobial Therapy Project Group: Three antibiotic regimens in the treatment of infections in febrile granulocytopenic patients with cancer. J. Infect. Dis. *137*:14–29, 1978.
34. Wade JC, Smith CR, Petty BG, et al.: Cephalothin plus an aminoglycoside is more nephrotoxic than methicillin plus an aminoglycoside. Lancet *2*:604–606, 1978.
35. Lane AZ, Wright GE, Blair DC: Ototoxicity and nephrotoxicity of amikacin. Am. J. Med. *62*:911–913, 1977.
36. Smith CR, Lipsky JJ, Laskin GL, et al.: Double-blind comparison of the nephrotoxicity and auditory toxicity of gentamicin and tobramycin. N. Engl. J. Med. *302*:1106–1108, 1980.
37. Nord MN, Hoeprich PD: Polymyxin B and colistin, a critical comparison. N. Engl. J. Med. *270*:1030–1035, 1964.
38. Eaton AE: Adverse effects of sodium colistimethate. Ann. Intern. Med. *72*:857–868, 1970.

39. Adler S, Sigel DP: Nonoliguric renal failure secondary to sodium colistimethate: a report of four cases. Am. J. Med. Sci. *261*:109–114, 1971.
40. Brumfitt W, Black M, Williams JD: Colistin in *Pseudomonas pyocyanea* infections and its effects on renal function. Br. J. Urol. *38*:495–500, 1966.
41. Vinnicombe J, Stamey TA: The relative nephrotoxicities of polymyxin B sulfate, sodium sulfomethyl-polymyxin B, sodium sulfomethyl-colistin (colymycin), and neomycin sulfate. Invest. Urol. *6*:505–519, 1969.
42. Ryan KJ, Schainuck LI, Hickman RO, et al.: Colistimethate toxicity: report of a fatal case in a previously healthy child. J.A.M.A. *207*:2099–2101, 1969.
43. Randall RE Jr, Bridi GS, Setter JH, et al.: Recovery from colistimethate nephrotoxicity. Ann. Intern. Med. *73*:491–492, 1970.
44. Appel GB, Neu HC: The nephrotoxicity of antimicrobial agents. N. Engl. J. Med. *296*:722–728, 1977.
45. Kunin CM, Bugg A: Binding of polymyxin antibiotics to tissue: the major determinant of distribution and persistence in the body. J. Infect. Dis. *124*:394–400, 1971.
46. Newton BA: The properties and mode of action of the polymyxins. Bacteriol. Rev. *20*:14–27, 1956.
47. Rodriguez V, Green S, Bodey GP: Serum electrolyte abnormalities associated with the administration of polymyxin B in febrile leukemic patients. Clin. Pharmacol. Ther. *11*:106–111, 1970.
48. Mandell GL: Cephaloridine. Ann. Intern. Med. *79*:561–565, 1973.
49. Kleinknecht D, Jungers P, Fillastre JP: Nephrotoxicity of cephaloridine. Ann. Intern. Med. *80*:421–422, 1974.
50. Rosenthal T, Boichis H: Nephrotoxicity of cephaloridine. Br. J. Med. *4*:115, 1971.
51. Engle JE, Drago J, Carlin B, et al.: Reversible acute renal failure after cephalothin. Ann. Intern. Med. *83*:232–233, 1975.
52. Burton JR, Litchenstein NS, Colvin RB, et al.: Acute renal failure during cephalothin therapy. J.A.M.A. *229*:679–682, 1974.
53. Thompson RL: The cephalosporins. Mayo Clin. Proc. *52*:625–630, 1977.
54. Tune BM: Effect of organic acid transport inhibitors on renal cortical uptake and proximal tubular toxicity of cephaloridine. J. Pharm. Exp. Ther. *181*:250–256, 1972.
55. Tune BM, Fernholt M: Relationship between cephaloridine and p-aminohippurate transport in the kidney. Am. J. Physiol. *225*:1114–1117, 1973.
56. Tune BM: Relationship between the transport and toxicity of cephalosporins in the kidney. J. Infect. Dis. *132*:189–194, 1975.
57. Child KJ, Dodds MG: Nephron transport and renal tubular effects of cephaloridine in animals. Br. J. Pharmacol. Chemother. *30*:354–370, 1967.
58. Tuano SB, Brodie JL, Kirby WM: Cephaloridine versus cephalothin: relation of the kidney to blood level differences after parenteral administration. Antimicrob. Agents Chemother. *6*:101–106, 1966.
59. Tune BM, Fernhold M, Schwartz A: Mechanism of cephaloridine transport in the kidney. J. Pharmacol. Exp. Ther. *191*:311–317, 1974.
60. Fleming PC, Jaffe D: The nephrotoxic effects of cephaloridine. Postgrad. Med. J. *43*(Suppl.):89–90, 1967.
61. Wold JS, Joost RR, Owen NV: Nephrotoxicity of cephaloridine in newborn rabbits: role of the renal anionic transport system. J. Pharmacol. Exp. Ther. *210*:778–785, 1977.
62. Silverblatt F, Harrison WO, Turck M: Nephrotoxicity of cephalosporin antibiotics in experimental animals. J. Infect. Dis. *128*(Suppl.):S367–S372, 1973.
63. Kirby WMM, Regamey C: Pharmacokinetics of cefazolin compared with four other cephalosporins. J. Infect. Dis. *128*(Suppl.):S341–S346, 1973.
64. Cabanilles F, Burgos RC, Rodriguez RC, et al.: Nephrotoxicity of combined cephalothin-gentamicin regimen. Arch. Intern. Med. *135*:850–852, 1975.
65. Hook EW, Johnson WD: Vanocomycin therapy of bacterial endocarditis. Am. J. Med. *65*:411–415, 1978.
66. Kirby WMM, Perry DM, Lane JL: Present status of vancomycin therapy of staphylococcal and streptococcal infections. Antibiot. Ann. 1958–59, p. 580, 1959.
67. Riley HD: Vancomycin and novobicin. Med. Clin. North Am. *54*:1277–1289, 1970.
68. Cook FV, Farrar WE: Vancomycin revisited. Ann. Intern. Med. *88*:813–818, 1978.
69. Geraci JE: Vancomycin. Mayo Clin. Proc. *52*:631–634, 1977.
70. Barcenas CG, Fuller TJ, Elms J, et al.: Staphylococcal sepsis in patients on chronic hemodialysis regimens. Arch. Intern. Med. *136*:1131–1134, 1976.
71. Ayus JC, Eneas JF, Tong TG, et al.: Peritoneal clearance and total body elimination of vancomycin during chronic intermittent peritoneal dialysis. Clin. Nephrol. *11*:129–132, 1979.
72. Waisbren BA, Kleinerman L, Skemp J, et al.: Comparative clinical effectiveness and toxicity of vancomycin, ristocetin and kanamycin. Arch. Intern. Med. *106*:179–193, 1960.
73. Anderson RJ, Gambertoglio JG, Schrier RW (eds.): Clinical Use of Drugs in Renal Failure. Springfield, Ill., Charles C Thomas, 1976.
74. Fabre J, DeFreudenreich J, Duchert A, et al.: Influence of renal insufficiency on the excretion of chloroquine, phenobarbital, phenothiazines and methacycline. Helv. Med. Acta *33*:307–316, 1967.
75. Wilson WR: Tetracyclines, chloramphenicol, erythromycin, and clindamycin. Mayo Clin. Proc. *52*:635–640, 1977.
76. Roth H, Becker KL, Shalhoub RJ, et al.: Nephrotoxicity of demethylchlortetracycline hydrochloride. A prospective study. Arch. Intern. Med. *120*: 433–435, 1967.
77. Cherril DA, Stote RM, Birge JR, et al.: Demeclocycline treatment in the syndrome of inappropriate antidiuretic hormone secretion. Ann. Intern. Med. *83*:654–656, 1975.
78. Shils ME: Renal disease and the metabolic effects of tetracycline. Ann. Intern. Med. *58*:389–408, 1963.
79. Carrilho F, Bosch J, Arroyo V, et al.: Renal failure associated with demeclocycline in cirrhosis. Ann. Intern. Med. *87*:195–197, 1977.
80. Singer I, Rotenberg D: Demeclocycline-induced nephrogenic diabetes insipidus. In-vivo and in-

vitro studies. Ann. Intern. Med. *79*:679–683, 1973.

81. Wilson DM, Perry HO, Sams WM Jr, et al.: Selective inhibition of human distal tubular function by demeclocycline. Curr. Ther. Res. *15*:734–740, 1973.
82. Walshe JJ, Venuto RC: Acute oliguric renal failure induced by indomethacin: possible mechanism. Ann. Intern. Med. *91*:47–49, 1979.
83. Dubuy HG, Showacre JL: Selective localization of tetracycline in mitochondria of living cells. Science *133*:196–197, 1961.
84. De Troyer A, Demanet JC: Correction of antidiuresis by demeclocycline. N. Engl. J. Med. *293*:915–918, 1975.
85. Frimpter GW, Timponelli AE, Eisenmenger WJ, et al.: Reversible Fanconi syndrome caused by degraded tetracycline. J.A.M.A. *184*:111–113, 1963.
86. Kalowski S, Nanra RS, Mathew TH, et al.: Deterioration in renal function in association with co-trimoxazole therapy. Lancet *1*:394–397, 1973.
87. Bailey RR, Little PJ: Deterioration in renal function in association with co-trimoxazole therapy. Med. J. Austr. *1*(Suppl.):914–916, 1976.
88. Lawson DH, Jick H: Adverse reactions to co-trimoxazole in hospitalized medical patients. Am. J. Med. Sci. *275*:53–57, 1978.
89. Hughes WT, Kuhn S, Chaudhary S, et al.: Successful chemoprophylaxis for *Pneumocystis carinii* pneumonitis. N. Engl. J. Med. *297*:1419–1426, 1977.
90. Western KA, Perera DR, Schultz MG: Pentamidine isethionate in the treatment of *Pneumocystis carinii* pneumonia. Ann. Intern. Med. *73*:695–702, 1970.
91. Walzer PD, Perl DP, Krogstad DJ, et al.: *Pneumocystis carinii* pneumonia in the United States. Ann. Intern. Med. *80*:83–93, 1974.
92. Burke BA, Good RA: *Pneumocystis carinii* infection. Medicine *52*:23–51, 1973.
93. Hughes WT, McNabb PC, Makres TD, et al.: Efficacy of trimethoprim and sulfamethoxazole in the prevention and treatment of *Pneumocystis carinii* pneumonitis. Antimicrob. Agents Chemother. *5*:289–293, 1974.
94. Lau WK, Young LS: Trimethoprim-sulfamethoxazole treatment of *Pneumocystis carinii* pneumonia in adults. N. Engl. J. Med. *295*:716–718, 1976.

Chapter 6

The Nephrotoxicity of Heavy Metals, Organic Solvents, Radiocontrast Agents, and Prostaglandin Inhibitors

by

William L. Henrich

In contrast to other chapters that focus on a single subject involving nephrotoxicity or hepatic toxicity, this chapter discusses the nephrotoxicity of several distinct and unrelated groups of therapeutic and diagnostic agents that have in common only their ability to reduce renal function. Heavy metals, organic solvents, radiocontrast agents, and prostaglandin inhibitors share few common features. For example, the agents included in this group of topics have been recognized as nephrotoxins for as long as centuries (in the case of mercury) or for only a short time (in the case of prostaglandin inhibitors). These agents also have clinical importance for such widely diverse purposes as diagnostic probes (e.g., radiocontrast agents) and as agents of attempted suicide (e.g., the poisons arsenic and ethylene glycol). The mechanisms of nephrotoxicity recognized as important for these agents also vary from direct tubular necrosis (heavy metals) to an alteration of kidney blood flow (prostaglandin inhibitors).

In view of these broad differences between these agents, each group will be considered individually. The clinical features and pathophysiology of each group of nephrotoxins will be discussed. The most clinically important agents have been selected from each group for detailed discussion.

DIRECT NEPHROTOXICITY OF HEAVY METALS

Heavy metal intoxication is generally regarded to produce a nephrotoxicity dominated by direct tubular damage. Clinically, this injury is manifest as acute renal failure, interstitial nephritis, and tubular dysfunction resulting in the Fanconi syndrome. The history of heavy metal damage to the kidneys spans several decades, reflecting the high frequency of heavy metal usage in industry, in the urban environment, and in medications.

PLATINUM

cis-Dichlorodiammineplatinum (*cis*-DDP) is a highly effective antitumor agent in humans, with greatest activity against testicular, ovarian, and bladder tumors, head and neck cancer, and malignant lymphoma. The atomic weight of platinum is 195; thus, it is quite close to mercury (201) in the periodic table. Platinum-containing agents have been recognized to possess potent antitumor properties for the last decade. The platinum compound with the greatest antitumor activity is *cis*-dichlorodiammineplatinum(II) [*cis*-DDP]. Interestingly, of the inorganic platinum compounds used clinically, only the *cis*-platinum complexes have nephrotoxic and antitumor potential.[1] The kidney is the major route of elimination for platinum and mercury and is a major site of concentration for these metals as well.[2] Nephrotoxicity will be produced by *cis*-DDP in approximately 30 per cent of patients treated with single courses of 2 mg/kg or 50 to 75 mg/m^2 body surface area. The toxicity of *cis*-DDP appears dose related. Greater decrements in renal function occur at higher doses. In general, the nephrotoxicity of *cis*-DDP is manifest as nonoliguric acute renal failure. Serum creatinine values peak at two to five times pretreatment levels. However, in many cases treated with higher dose *cis*-DDP, renal damage has been irreversible. Further, the cumulative dose of platinum is another determinant of nephrotoxicity.[3] Proximal tubular necrosis and interstitial fibrosis are the usual findings on light and electron microscopy in patients receiving *cis*-DDP courses.[4] Urinary cast formation, proteinuria, and a decrease in glomerular filtration rate may occur in the immediate post-treatment period and are often mild and reversible.[5] While the precise pathogenesis of *cis*-DDP nephrotoxicity is unknown, several maneuvers that increase solute excretion have been shown to reduce nephrotoxicity in animals and humans. Thus, saline loading,[5] mannitol-induced increases in solute excretion,[6] and furosemide[7] may all have salutory effects in obviating the toxicity of *cis*-DDP when given immediately prior to the *cis*-DDP injection. Conversely, the nephrotoxicity of this tubular toxin may be potentiated by the concomitant use of other recognized nephrotoxins, particularly the aminoglycoside antibiotics.[8] This is particularly relevant in view of the fact that immunosuppressed, hospitalized cancer patients often have serious infections with gram-negative organisms. Clearly, euvolemia is mandatory and an increase in solute excretion desirable if a maximum attempt to avoid nephrotoxicity from *cis*-DDP is to be undertaken.

One interesting and recently recognized consequence of *cis*-DDP therapy would appear to be hypomagnesemia secondary to a tubular defect in renal tubular magnesium reabsorption.[9, 10] The incidence of this occurrence was 52 per cent in one recent series.[9] Concomitant hypokalemia and secondary hypocalcemia may further complicate this event and correction of the serum magnesium has also resulted in correction of the hypocalcemia in at least one case.[10] In approximately half of patients who develop hypomagnesemia, the disturbance persists for several months, and in some cases, permanently.[9]

In summary, *cis*-DDP is an important antitumor agent that results in a demonstrable decline in glomerular filtration rate in approximately 30 per cent of patients receiving the agent. The drug is concentrated and excreted by the kidneys, and a dose-related nephrotoxicity is established for this agent. Nephrotoxicity is reduced by euvolemia and by measures that enhance solute excretion, and is potentiated by other nephrotoxins.

MERCURY

Mercurous chloride was used as a diuretic for centuries until it was replaced by the organomercurial mersalyl, which increased the range between the therapeutic and toxic dose.[11] The chief source of mercury at present is mercury sublimate, which is most commonly ingested accidently or in attempted suicide. Less than 0.1 gm of mercuric chloride by mouth may cause severe symptoms and 0.5 gm may prove fatal. Soluble mercury salts are quickly absorbed from the gastrointestinal tract or other mucous membranes. In patients receiving mercurial diuretics, the liver concentration of mercury may rise to 2600 μg per 100 ml and that of the kidneys to 27,500 μg per 100 ml.[12] Mercuric chloride concentrates in the distal portion of the proximal convoluted tubule and the loop of Henle and collecting tubules, but not in the glomeruli. Detectable amounts of mercury remain in the kidney for several months following intoxication.

Clinical features of acute intoxication include a bitter metallic taste, a sense of suffocation, abdominal pain, hypotension, and acute renal failure. Proteinuria, glycosuria, cellular casts, aminoaciduria, and oliguria are typical signs of acute mercury poisoning. Anuria is described frequently and may persist for 3 to 4 weeks in severe cases. Some evidence in experimental models of mercury-induced acute renal failure suggests that the hemodynamic changes (i.e., renal vasoconstriction) mediated by the renin-angiotensin system may be a cofactor in the genesis of acute renal failure in mercury intoxication.[13]

The pathology of the kidney is dominated by proximal tubular cell necrosis. Mercury combines with sulfhydryl groups of proteins in mitochondrial membranes and triggers the dissolution of the membrane and subsequent necrosis of the nuclei. The diagnosis of mercury intoxication is largely based on the clinical history. However, mercury may be detected in the urine, blood, and stool. A urinary excretion of 250 μg/L is evidence of excessive exposure, and clinical symptoms may appear with excretions of 300 to 500 μg/L. A blood concentration of inorganic mercury at 5 ppm has been associated with mild symptoms. With the alkyl mercury compounds 10 to 20 ppm appear to be safe. However, the likelihood of poisoning is quite high with concentrations above 65 ppm.

Treatment of acute ingestion includes immediate emesis followed by gastric lavage. Dimercaprol (BAL) should be administered to chelate mercuric ions. The dose of BAL is 2.5 to 3.0 mg/kg body weight every 4 hours up to six doses. Should anuria or oliguria ensue, BAL-mercury complexes are removable by hemodialysis.

LEAD

Chronic lead poisoning may be associated with renal dysfunction.[14–33] Childhood exposure usually occurs through oral ingestion (paint, soil, newsprint), while adult exposure occurs by inhalation (smelting and refining, casting of batteries, torch cutting and welding, and petroleum products) and by oral ingestion (moonshine liquor, improperly glazed pottery).[14-18] Acute lead intoxication is associated with proximal tubular dysfunction (bicarbonaturia, phosphaturia, renal glycosuria) with maintenance of glomerular filtration rate.[19] This syndrome appears to be responsive to chelation therapy. A number of reports have also suggested a form of chronic lead nephropathy in workers exposed to lead and in children and adults with excessive lead ingestion.[20-26] Several cases of chronic renal insufficiency occurring following long-term lead exposure have been reported. Small, granular contracted kidneys and marked hyperuricemia[27] are often present. In these cases, the history of chronic exposure, bone lead analysis, and basal and postchelation urinary lead excretion suggested the diagnosis of chronic lead nephropathy. However, the interstitial lesion of chronic lead nephropathy is nonspecific and increased renal tissue lead has not yet been documented. Moreover, a reproducible laboratory model of lead nephropathy remains to be established. Thus, although most observers feel that chronic lead exposure can induce a chronic nephropathy, the frequency, natural history, best means of diagnosis, and therapy remain open issues.[21-32]

The best means of diagnosing lead intoxication continues to be debated. Often, other clinical disorders (encephalopathy; neuropathy; colic; hypochromic, microcytic anemia with basophilic stippling) are present and are suggestive of the diagnosis. Serum lead levels greater than 80 μg/dl have been postulated to indicate definite toxicity.[21, 23, 26, 30, 33] However, the definition of normal values and difficulties in analysis of serum lead diminish the usefulness of this test. Moreover, the serum lead often demonstrates poor correlation with clinical illness and total body lead burden.

Since lead interferes with steps in the synthesis of heme, several hematologic parameters have been used to diagnose lead intoxication.[28, 30] Anemia occurs once serum lead levels exceed 100 μg/dl; thus, it is too insensitive to be diagnostically helpful. Basophilic stippling may be seen, but is nonspecific. Determination of aminolevulinic acid dehydratase (an enzyme inhibited by lead) provides "too sensitive" an assay, since inhibition occurs at lead levels of 15 μg/dl. Elevated urinary coproporphyrins are seen when lead levels exceed 35μg/dl. Similarly, elevated levels are seen in liver disease, alcoholism, and other disorders. Increased free erythrocytic protoporphyrins occur at lead levels of 25 to 50 μg/dl. The assay is technically difficult, and iron deficiency anemia also causes positive results.

Urinary lead levels are a practical and often utilized means to screen for lead intoxication.[26, 30] Urinary lead levels greater than 200 μg/L are suggestive of excess lead body burden. A 24-hour urinary lead level greater than 500 μg following three doses of EDTA (ethylenediaminetetraacetic acid) (25 mg/kg at 8-hour intervals) indicates excess total body lead burden.

Removal from further exposure is the first means of therapy. The major storage area of lead in the body is in bone. Chelating agents only slowly remove lead from bone.[31] Chelation therapy with EDTA (which may have some degree of nephrotoxicity) may be indicated (600 mg in 250 ml of 5 per cent dextrose in water over 1 hour). BAL therapy (2.5 to 3.0

mg/kg body weight) every 4 hours up to six doses may also be given. Oral penicillamine 1.0 to 1.5 gm/day can be utilized to chelate lead. Comparative studies on the efficacy:toxicity ratio of the various chelating drugs are not available.[25, 26, 33]

GOLD

Gold salts are valuable therapeutically in the treatment of rheumatoid arthritis. The form of gold in current widespread use is gold thiomalate, a compound in which gold makes up approximately 50 per cent of the total salt by weight. Gold agents are water soluble and are given by intramuscular injections only. A typical treatment plan would consist of 10 to 20 mg as a test dose for anaphylactic reactions, followed by 25 to 50 mg weekly until a total dose of 500 mg has been given. The dosage interval is then increased to 50 mg every 2 weeks and, finally, to 50 mg every 4 weeks, depending on the clinical response.

Gold has been implicated as a rare cause of acute tubular necrosis. However, the most commonly observed abnormality in renal function following gold therapy is proteinuria and the nephrotic syndrome.[34] This entity will be discussed in more detail in Chapter 7. The degree of proteinuria is not proportional to the gold blood or urine levels, the total dose administered, or the duration of treatment.[35] In one recent study, nephrotoxicity (defined as the onset of proteinuria) accounted for 19 per cent of the toxic reactions observed with gold therapy, and the mean duration of treatment to onset of proteinuria was 8 months.[36] However, patients who experienced a remission of arthritic symptoms with gold therapy and who had no adverse toxic reactions early in therapy were able to continue gold treatment for up to 3 years with an increasing margin of safety for renal toxicity.[36] The course of gold-induced proteinuria is generally regarded as benign, with a significant reduction in proteinuria occurring within 6 months following discontinuation of gold.[37]

The pathologic changes of gold nephropathy are those of membranous nephropathy.[38] Because of the poor correlation between total dose and degree of renal damage, and because of the varying temporal relationship between gold therapy and onset of proteinuria, the possibility that rheumatoid arthritis independently is associated with membranous nephropathy has been raised.[39] In many patients, however, the administration of gold results in proteinuria, although it is unknown whether or not this results from exacerbation of an underlying and unrecognized nephropathy that existed prior to therapy. The pathogenetic mechanism in gold-induced membranous nephropathy is unclear, but several theories exist. Gold particles are known to localize in the proximal tubular epithelial cells and interstitium.[40] Skrifvars has postulated that the damage to proximal tubular cells incites the formation of antitubular antibodies and, subsequently, immune complexes that ultimately localize in the glomerular basement membrane.[41] This hypothesis would explain the fact that membranous nephropathy is characterized by the existence of electron-dense particles (immune complexes) in the basement membrane, and immunofluorescence studies reveal prominent staining for anti-IgG and complement.[38, 40] Confirmation of this pathogenetic sequence is still lacking, however. Clearly, gold does not appear to be acting as a hapten in this process, given the absence of gold from the electron-dense deposits noted in glomeruli.

The treatment of acute gold toxicity is BAL 2.5 to 3.0 mg/kg. As noted previously, discontinuation of gold therapy is usually associated with resolution or a significant reduction of the proteinuria over a period of several months. No information on the ability of corticosteroids to alter the clinical course of gold nephrotoxicity is presently available.

OTHER HEAVY METALS

ARSENIC

Arsenic is a tasteless and odorless heavy metal which is a component of fertilizers, paint pigments, and some insect poisons. The fatal dose of arsenic is 100 to 200 mg, with as little as 20 mg occasionally being lethal. Arsenic is well absorbed orally and is concentrated in the kidneys. Symptoms of acute arsenic ingestion include profound hypotension, diarrhea, and vomiting. Tubular necrosis dominates the pathologic picture. BAL is a useful agent for chelating arsenic and preventing greater toxicity, but may be ineffectively excreted if oliguria or anuria has supervened. Hemodialysis is efficient in removing arsenic and arsenic-BAL complexes, accounting for a greater than 50 per cent reduction in serum arsenic levels in one dialysis of a poisoned patient.[42]

COPPER

Acute renal failure may also complicate copper ingestion. Gastrointestinal symptoms may follow ingestion of 500 mg of a copper salt. Hemolytic anemia is a key feature of intoxication, but tubular necrosis, particularly in the loop of Henle and distal convoluted tubules, is also observed. Usual sources of copper include corroded copper-containing hot water heaters or fungicide-contaminated seed grains. BAL constitutes the primary therapy.

BISMUTH

Bismuth was formerly an important cause of nephrotoxicity in patients treated for syphilis. Doses of 1.0 mg/kg of bismuth can produce proximal tubular necrosis and attendant acute renal failure. Yellow-colored inclusion bodies that have a refractile appearance are a characteristic finding of the nuclei of proximal convoluted tubules.

URANIUM

Soluble uranium compounds are also known to produce proximal tubular necrosis, and have been extensively utilized in experimental models of toxin-induced renal failure. The degree of functional impairment correlates best with alterations in renal hemodynamics induced by uranyl nitrate in experimental animals.[43]

ORGANIC SOLVENTS

Acute renal failure occurring as a consequence of organic solvent poisoning formerly occurred following heavy exposure to a number of industrial toxins. In recent years, however, organic solvent intoxication has been more frequently associated with both deliberate and inadvertent ingestion of organic compounds. For example, the utilization of many halogenated hydrocarbons (notably carbon tetrachloride) has been markedly restricted with increased recognition of toxicity. Conversely, the ingestion of glycols (particularly ethylene glycol) remains a common clinical circumstance, particularly in urban areas with large populations of alcoholics.

In this chapter, a tabulation of the organic solvents known to induce renal damage is provided in Table 6–1. Organic toxins of greater clinical importance will be discussed in greater detail.

TABLE 6–1. COMMON ORGANIC SOLVENTS CAUSING NEPHROTOXICITY

Glycols
Ethylene glycol
Diethylene glycol
Halogenated Hydrocarbons
Carbon tetrachloride
Trichloroethylene
Aromatic Hydrocarbons
Toluene
Aliphatic-aromatic Hydrocarbons
Gasoline and kerosene
Turpentine

Acute exposure to volatile solvents usually produces direct toxicity by inducing renal tubular cell necrosis.[44] This histologic damage is most often translated into a syndrome of acute renal failure characterized by anuria or oliguria. Recently, the possibility that organic solvent exposure may produce glomerular basement membrane damage with glomerulonephritis and proteinuria has been recognized.[45, 46] Finally, the possibility that chronic, lower-dose exposure to organic solvents results in chronic renal failure, of either interstitial or glomerular damage, is unresolved at present.

The route of entry of solvents may be by oral ingestion, inhalation, or absorption through the skin. Inhalation is a frequent route of access to the body, given the volatile characteristics of many of these compounds. Skin contact with a number of cleaning agents and industrial solvents usually results in only small amounts of absorption of the solvent.

Organic solvents are highly soluble in fat, and following absorption, significant quantities of the solvent are deposited unchanged in fat. A small percentage of the compound may be exhaled unaltered, while metabolites of these compounds begin to appear in the urine with time. Identification of the particular solvent may be made in the exhaled air during acute intoxication. Since most industrial solvents are provided as a mixture of several organic compounds, however, precise identification of a single agent is often impractical after industrial exposures. Thus, the medical history often is of the greatest diagnostic value in identifying the offending agent.

GLYCOLS

ETHYLENE GLYCOL

Ethylene glycol is a clear, odorless, and water-soluble liquid used as a substitute for glycerine in commercial products such as detergents, cosmetics, and paints. Primarily, ethylene glycol is utilized as a de-icer and as an antifreeze. This agent has a warm, sweet taste that may have enhanced its use as a suicide agent or as a substitute for alcohol.

The human minimum lethal dose for ethylene glycol is estimated at 100 ml.[47] The extreme toxicity of ethylene glycol makes prompt diagnosis and therapy imperative, and the delay in obtaining serum levels may compromise the clinical outcome. The diagnosis of ethylene glycol poisoning should be strongly suspected in the setting of anion gap metabolic acidosis when diabetic ketoacidosis has been excluded and (1) signs and symptoms of intoxication are present in the absence of alcohol odor, (2) coma is present, and (3) the urinalysis demonstrates calcium oxalate crystalluria.[48] However, many patients with ethylene glycol ingestion will not demonstrate calcium oxalate crystalluria.[47]

Several stages of clinical intoxication are recognized after ethylene glycol ingestion. Initially (first 12 hours), central nervous system manifestations, such as delerium, coma, convulsions, papilledema, and ophthalmoplegias, and metabolic acidosis dominate.[49] Cardiopulmonary failure with pulmonary edema then ensue 24 to 72 hours after ingestion. Renal failure is apparent approximately 48 hours following ingestion, and the clinical course is characterized by profuse crystalluria early (often with bilateral flank pain) that progresses to oliguric or anuric acute renal failure. Oliguria may occur as early as 12 hours after ingestion and last as long as 7 weeks.[50] Leukocytosis (10 to 40,000/mm^3), hypocalcemia (secondary to calcium chelation by oxalate), and metabolic acidosis (often with bicarbonate levels of 10 to 15 mEq/L) highlight the clinical picture. Microscopic sections of kidneys reveal dilated proximal tubules and degeneration of tubular epithelium as early as 72 hours after ingestion.[48] Intratubular calcium oxalate crystals may be prominent, although the exact role of these deposits in the pathogenesis of the renal failure is uncertain at present. Certainly, the cytotoxic effect of the ethylene glycol is of major importance in the development of the tubular damage.

The principal metabolic pathway of ethylene glycol is depicted in Figure 6–1, and is important in the understanding of appropriate therapy. The profound acidosis caused by ethylene glycol is due to its conversion to a series of toxic metabolites that may alter the redox potential of the cell as well as the primary production of lactic acid.[51, 52]

Therapy of ethylene glycol intoxication consists of several emergent steps: (1) the administration of a loading dose of I.V. ethanol (0.6 mg/kg as a 5 per cent solution) within 8 hours following ingestion to provide a substrate for alcohol dehydrogenase (Fig. 6–1), oral ethanol therapy may be substituted for I.V. therapy;[53] (2) if urine output is still present, promotion of an osmotic diuresis with mannitol or furosemide is beneficial in promoting ethylene glycol clearance and should be continued until crystalluria is reduced;[48] (3) immediate hemodialysis should be instituted for removal of ethylene glycol from the blood; and (4) vigorous treatment of metabolic acidosis (with bicarbonate and dialysis), hypocalcemia, and respiratory distress are necessary. In the majority of patients surviving the initial central nervous system toxicity who develop renal failure, recovery of renal function generally occurs.

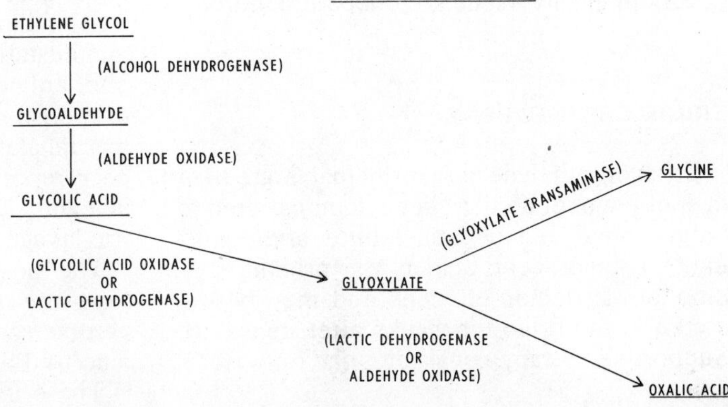

Figure 6–1. Metabolic pathway for ethylene glycol. Ethylene glycol and alcohol share a common degradative enzyme (alcohol dehydrogenase).

DIETHYLENE GLYCOL

Diethylene glycol is another water-soluble organic solvent used primarily as an antifreeze agent and as a solvent for dyes.[47] This agent has physical properties similar to ethylene glycol. Although the metabolic pathways of this agent are largely unknown, severe acidosis is not a predominant feature of intoxication. Diethylene glycol is a renal tubular toxin similar to ethylene glycol. Therapy is largely symptomatic and supportive following ingestion.

HALOGENATED HYDROCARBONS

CARBON TETRACHLORIDE

Carbon tetrachloride is a highly toxic solvent that is now used as an industrial solvent. It is no longer in widespread use as a household cleaning agent or in home fire extinguishers. Exposures most often occur via inhalation, although dermal and gastrointestinal absorption does occur.[54] A toxic dose is as little as 4 mg orally.[55] This agent is concentrated in body fat and is excreted via the lungs. When exhaled, carbon tetrachloride imparts a characteristic chemical odor to the breath. After ingestion, headache and intoxication symptoms are common and are followed by stupor and coma in severe cases. Nausea, vomiting, and emotional lability are usual. Acute intoxication with carbon tetrachloride leads to hepatic and renal tubular cell degeneration and necrosis. Although oliguria and anuria are the usual clinical occurrences, recovery of renal function is expected, provided overwhelming hepatic necrosis has not occurred. Therapy is largely supportive and includes the use of dialysis for renal failure. The mortality rate is approximately 30 per cent and occurs primarily because of hepatic failure.

TRICHLOROETHYLENE

Trichloroethylene is a principal ingredient in spot remover and has been demonstrated to induce renal and hepatic failure after sniffing.[56] Trichloracetic acid is the primary metabolite of trichloroethylene and may be excreted in the urine for weeks after ingestion. Supportive therapy constitutes the only treatment.

AROMATIC HYDROCARBONS

TOLUENE

Toluene is an organic solvent utilized in glue production and as a thinner for paints, lacquer, and adhesives. Ingestion may occur via dermal, gastrointestinal, and pulmonary pathways. Central nervous system (CNS) and renal tubular effects are the primary manifestations of toxicity resulting from excessive toluene inhalation. Usual symptoms of intoxication (which occur at concentrations of 600 to 800 ppm of air) are confusion, hallucinations, and vomiting. Hepatic and renal damage is less often reported than with other organic solvents. The recognition of distal renal tubular acidosis, hypokalemia, and systemic acidemia was reported in two patients sniffing toluene-containing glue.[57] In addition, a form of proximal renal tubular acidosis has also been recently observed following toluene sniffing.[58] When acute renal failure follows toluene inhalation or consumption, other factors, such as concomitant hepatic failure or myoglobinuria, may be present.[59] Thus, the ability of toluene alone to cause acute renal failure is limited.

ALIPHATIC-AROMATIC HYDROCARBONS

GASOLINE AND KEROSENE

Gasoline and kerosene are aliphatic-hydrocarbon mixtures that may be absorbed via the skin, lungs, or gastrointestinal tract. Acute intoxication produces gastric irritation if swallowed, followed by vomiting and gagging. CNS symptoms, such as drowsiness and stupor, then occur. Pulmonary damage with hemorrhage and hemoptysis is another frequent sign of acute ingestion. Although acute renal failure is not the predominant clinical manifestation of toxicity, it may occur even after only dermal exposure.[59] The acutely fatal oral dose of gasoline or kerosene is 20 to 30 ml; inhalation toxicity at 300 ppm has also been reported.[60] The treatment of acute gasoline and kerosene intoxication consists of gastric lavage followed by supportive care.

The possibility that chronic hydrocarbon exposure may lead to glomerulonephritis and chronic renal failure has been recently examined by Beirne et al. and other workers.[46, 61, 62] These investigators have found that excessive exposure to hydrocarbons is associated with anti-GBM antibody glomerulonephritis and idiopathic crescenteric glomerulonephritis in animal models and in human patients.[45,46,61,62] These results suggest that environmental exposure to hydrocarbons may be a predisposing factor in the development of glomerular diseases in some cases.

TURPENTINE

Turpentine is primarily used as a paint thinner and as a cleaning agent, and is usually absorbed through the skin. Symptoms of urethritis may accompany excretion of the agent. Turpentine produces renal tubular and hepatic necrosis when ingested in sufficient quantities (several ounces by mouth and 100 ppm in air). Therapy is similar to gasoline and kerosene intoxication.

RADIOCONTRAST-INDUCED ACUTE RENAL FAILURE

The fact that radiocontrast-induced acute renal failure is a significant cause of morbidity and mortality in hospitalized patients is verified by the proliferation of clinical reports regarding the incidence and characteristics of this problem. Despite the enhanced recognition of this form of acute renal failure, the incidence and pathogenesis remain unknown. Thus, a therapeutic plan aimed at prevention and treatment of the renal failure has not been forthcoming. This section focuses briefly on the pathophysiologic factors potentially responsible for acute renal failure from contrast agents, describes the clinical characteristics of the disease, and concludes with general guidelines for prevention as derived from the present literature.

CLINICAL CONSIDERATIONS

Radiocontrast-induced acute renal failure may occur after the parenteral or oral administration of radiocontrast material for any number of diagnostic procedures, including urography,[63] angiography,[64, 65] contrast-enhanced computerized tomography,[67] and, after repeated doses, cholecystography.[67] Some of the physical properties of several commonly used agents are listed in Table 6–2. Note that all of these agents are markedly hypertonic, which may play a pathophysiologic role in the induction of acute renal failure, particularly after intraarterial injections.

The incidence of radiocontrast-induced acute renal failure is difficult to ascertain, primarily because of differing diagnostic criteria and because most investigations have been performed retrospectively. A recent prospectively performed preliminary report on the spectrum of acute renal failure noted that contrast media accounted for 12 per cent of new cases of hospital-acquired acute renal failure.[68] The overall incidence of renal failure following administration of radiographic contrast material has ranged from 0 to 13 per cent[64, 69] and is heavily dependent on the characteristics of the patient population under study. For example, in a retrospective survey, Swartz et al. found a 12 per cent incidence of contrast agent–associated acute renal failure after angiography.[64] In contrast, no cases were

TABLE 6–2. CURRENTLY EMPLOYED CONTRAST AGENTS

Generic Name	Brand Name	Per Cent Iodine	Osmolality (mOsm/kg)
Sodium diatrizoate	Hypaque-NA	30%	1470
Meglumine diatrizoate	Renografin-M	28%	1400
	Hypaque Meglumine	28%	1350
Meglumine–sodium diatrizoate	Renografin-76	37%	1690
	Renografin-60	29%	1420
	Hypaque-M	37%	1780
Meglumine iothalamate	Conray-60	20%	1400

observed in a recent prospective study of 100 consecutive patients undergoing angiography.[70]

It is apparent from the pooled demographic descriptions of the clinical population that develops contrast-induced renal failure that several risk factors predispose to the illness. A partial list of these factors is provided in Table 6–3. Diabetes is clearly an important risk factor for the development of contrast-induced renal insufficiency. A number of studies have demonstrated a relatively high frequency of renal failure following use of contrast agents in patients with diabetes mellitus and underlying renal failure.[71-74] In addition, the dose of contrast media is also a risk factor in the diabetic. Perhaps the factor of greatest importance to the development of a decline in renal function after contrast exposure is preexisting renal disease.[64, 68, 71, 72] Of note is the fact that in the studies by Swartz et al.[65] and Byrd and Sherman,[69] the great majority of patients who developed contrast-induced renal failure had a combination of three or more risk factors noted in Table 6–3 at the time of study. The independent importance of hyperuricemia and proteinuria as clinical risk factors for this illness is probably minimal. Clearly, however, aging may adversely alter the response to hypertonic contrast agents via a loss of the kidneys to regulate vascular tone as precisely.

The clinical course of patients with contrast-induced renal failure is characterized by oliguria in approximately 70 per cent of cases,[63, 69] although a high urine output is not uncommon, occurring in 10 to 20 per cent of cases.[69] Oliguria most often begins within 48 hours of contrast administration, lasts for 2 to 3 days, and abates spontaneously. In the study by Byrd and Sherman[69] a mean increase of 3.4 mg/dl in the serum creatinine was observed with the onset of renal failure. The prognosis in this form of renal failure is generally good, with fully 70 to 90 per cent of patients recovering baseline renal function within 2 weeks.[50, 63, 64, 69, 71-75] Partial recovery to baseline serum creatinine values is reported to occur in 10 to 25 per cent of patients.[63] Although variable criteria are imposed for the indications for dialysis, a minority of patients with contrast-induced renal failure require dialysis during the course of their renal insufficiency (range: 9 per cent[71] to 46 per cent[65]). The overall death rate in most series of patients with contrast-induced renal failure is low,[65, 71] and higher death rates (8 per cent,[72] 11 per cent,[69] and 38 per cent[64]) may simply reflect the variable severity of underlying disease in the patients undergoing these procedures.

TABLE 6–3. CLINICAL RISK FACTORS IN THE DEVELOPMENT OF CONTRAST-INDUCED ACUTE RENAL FAILURE

Preexisting renal insufficiency
Greater than 60 years of age
Dehydration and extracellular fluid volume depletion
Diabetes mellitus
High dose of contrast and/or multiple contrast doses
Hypoalbuminemia
Proteinuria (>1 gm/24h)
Abnormal liver function
Multiple myeloma

PATHOPHYSIOLOGIC FACTORS IN CONTRAST-INDUCED ACUTE RENAL FAILURE

Table 6–4 lists several potential factors involved in the generation of contrast-induced acute renal failure. The intraarterial injection of the hypertonic contrast agents into the renal vasculature usually results in a decrease in renal blood flow. This acute effect of contrast agents would appear to be the result of the osmolality of the solutions utilized, since agents of lower osmolality decrease renal blood flow less.[76, 77] The importance of these high-osmolality solutions to provoke renal ischemia when they are injected into the venous circulation remains speculative at present, however.

The contribution of any microcirculatory alterations induced by these agents to impair renal perfusion is also unclarified. Alterations in red blood cell shape may promote sludging[78] and thereby worsen the decrease in renal function that occurs secondary to the effects of hyperosmolality to increase renal vascular resistance. The possibility that intratubular obstruction contributes to renal function deterioration after contrast agents seems small except in the presence of multiple myeloma. Diatrizoate and iothalamate are capable of precipitating Tamm-Horsfall mucoprotein *in vitro,*[79] although the importance of this observation in clinical terms is unknown. Several of the contrast agents are uricosuric (particularly

TABLE 6–4. POTENTIAL PATHOPHYSIOLOGIC FACTORS IN RADIOCONTRAST-INDUCED ACUTE RENAL FAILURE

Renal ischemia and microcirculation changes
Intratubular obstruction by protein, oxalate, or uric acid crystals
Immunologic reactions
Direct toxicity of the contrast agent

the cholecystographic agents Telepaque and Cholografin), thus providing another potential obstructive etiology in some patients. Similarly, the possibility that the increase in oxalate excretion seen in normal patients after diatrizoate injections could contribute to tubular obstruction awaits investigation.[80] However, it seems unlikely from most of the recent literature that acute urate or oxalate tubular obstruction is an independent pathogenetic factor of importance in the majority of cases.

Immunologic mechanisms may play a role in some cases of contrast-induced renal failure. Kleinknecht et al. noted circulating antibodies against contrast material in one patient developing renal failure after excretory urography.[81] A setting in which an immunologic mechanism may be of particular importance is in transplanted kidneys subjected to contrast agents. At least in some cases, the use of a contrast agent may have provoked transplant rejection, although the mechanism(s) responsible needs further clarification.[82] Thus, the role of immunologic mechanisms remains intriguing but unresolved at present.

Direct nephrotoxicity is at present believed to be the most important factor in contrast-induced toxicity. Contrast agents have been shown to cause glomerular and tubular proteinuria as well as tubular necrosis.[83] Diatrizoate and iothalamate have been further demonstrated to have the ability to alter tubular sodium transport.[84] Histologic studies by Lasser et al.[83] have incriminated the halogen portion of the contrast molecule as the important toxic factor. The contrast agents are excreted primarily via filtration without significant tubular reabsorption or secretion.[85] Tubular reabsorption of the organic iodide molecule probably does occur to a modest degree and other studies inferentially suggest that tubular damage may result from this reabsorption. The renal cortical accumulation and disappearance of iodide are currently unknown, however.

PROPHYLAXIS OF CONTRAST-INDUCED RENAL FAILURE

Based on the previously discussed risk factors and the potential pathogenetic mechanisms, several suggestions regarding the prevention of contrast-induced renal insufficiency are provided in Table 6–5. By avoiding volume depletion and dehydration (particularly in diabetic patients and others with markedly enhanced risk) a significant reduction in the incidence of this problem may be observed. Furthermore, careful monitoring of the amount of contrast administered and avoidance of serial repetitive studies should also be beneficial. Finally, as with all diagnostic procedures, the risk:benefit ratio for any of the routinely performed diagnostic contrast procedures must be meticulously assessed for each individual patient prior to study. Preliminary studies suggest that mannitol treatment (200 ml of 20 per cent solution) within 1 hour after radiocontrast media injection may decrease the occurrence of acute renal failure.

NEPHROTOXICITY OF PROSTAGLANDIN INHIBITORS

Prostaglandins are a group of ubiquitous substances that are formed from endogenous polyunsaturated fatty acids within virtually all cells in the body. These substances were originally discovered in seminal vesicle fluid over 40 years ago. Prostaglandins possess a heterogeneous spectrum of activity involving

TABLE 6–5. SUGGESTIONS FOR PREVENTION OF CONTRAST-INDUCED RENAL FAILURE

Use as low a dose of contrast agent as possible, and do not exceed recognized maximum doses (0.88 g iodine/kg or 65 ml/m^2).
Avoid dehydration and volume depletion, particularly with vigorous gastrointestinal preparations.
Avoid patients at the greatest risk for toxicity: preexisting renal insufficiency, >60 years of age, diabetes mellitus, and multiple myeloma.
Avoid serial contrast procedures if possible; if several procedures are required, they should be separated by the maximum amount of time allowable.
Avoid studies on patients with prior episodes of contrast-induced acute renal failure.
Infusion of 200 ml of 20 per cent mannitol within an hour after contrast exposure in high risk patients should be considered.

smooth muscle, the vasculature, renal function, uterine physiology, the gastrointestinal tract, myocardial performance, and blood platelets.

The kidneys are a major manufacturer of prostaglandins in response to a variety of stimuli. The prostaglandins are synthesized from arachidonic acid by a group of enzymes collectively called prostaglandin synthetase. A number of commonly used nonsteroidal anti-inflammatory agents (e.g., acetylsalicylic acid, indomethacin, ibuprofen) are capable of inhibiting prostaglandin synthesis. Prostaglandin synthesis occurs as a result of enhanced release of arachidonic acid from phospholipids following the activation of phospholipase. Corticosteroid drugs diminish prostaglandin formation through inhibition of phospholipase. Renal prostaglandin synthesis appears to be "compartmentalized." Thus, renal medullary interstitial cells and collecting duct epithelium are sites of prostaglandin biosynthesis. Prostaglandin E_2 (PGE_2) is the major renal prostaglandin found in this compartment. PGE_2 is a renal vasodilator and is antagonistic to the hydroosmotic effect of antidiuretic hormone. Prostaglandins are also synthesized in the walls of afferent arterioles and in the glomerulus. The main prostaglandin synthesized in renal arterioles is prostacyclin (or prostaglandin I_2, PGI_2), which is a potent renal vasodilator.[86] The kidneys also make small amounts of $PGF_2\alpha$, a substance that has little intrinsic renal activity, and thromboxane A_2, a potent vasoconstrictor.[86]

In focusing on the mechanisms of renal failure dysfunction induced by prostaglandin antagonists, this discussion will outline several aspects of the influence of prostaglandins on renal physiology. Next, several studies that bear directly on the importance of prostaglandins in experimental renal failure will be noted. Finally, the clinical experience with renal dysfunction following prostaglandin inhibition will be discussed.

BACKGROUND AND EXPERIMENTAL STUDIES ON PROSTAGLANDINS IN RENAL FAILURE

Renal prostaglandins, especially PGE_2 and PGI_2, are known to cause a prompt and dramatic increase in renal blood flow when infused intra-arterially. Moreover, renal vasoconstrictors, such as angiotensin II, norepinephrine, and renal nerve stimulation, are known to stimulate prostaglandin synthesis and release, an effect that opposes vasoconstriction. The physiologic importance of the relationship between vasoconstrictive stimuli and prostaglandins has been assessed in hypotensive hemorrhage studies demonstrating a marked enhancement of vasoconstriction induced by renal nerves and angiotensin II in the presence of prostaglandin inhibition.[87, 88] Thus, any increase in vasoconstrictive forces, such as may occur following hemorrhage, endotoxemia, anesthesia, extracellular volume depletion, and in high-renin conditions, would be expected to result in greater synthesis and release of prostaglandins as a modulating factor to counteract renal ischemia. Inhibition of prostaglandin synthesis in these conditions could potentially result in greater (unopposed) vasoconstriction and thereby lead to more profound renal ischemia.

Prostaglandin infusions generally result in a natriuresis in humans and in experimental animals. In many instances, the natriuresis associated with prostaglandin infusion is related to large increments in renal blood flow, although a direct effect of PGE_2 to inhibit sodium reabsorption across the collecting duct has been demonstrated.[89] Although controversy regarding the clinical importance of prostaglandins as natriuretic factors exists, it would appear that under conditions of decreased effective arterial volume, prostaglandins do play a natriuretic and hemodynamic role. For example, in 1978, Zia and colleagues documented a close correlation between plasma renin activity and 24-hour urinary PGE excretion; in this study, the highest PGE levels were noted in patients with cirrhosis and ascites.[90] Moreover, further studies in cirrhotic patients have shown that augmentation of PGE and sodium excretion occurs during the central volume expansion maneuver of water immersion to the neck.[91] These studies suggest that PGE is a determinant of renal function in patients with compromised effective arterial blood volumes. Similarly, the neck-immersion model has provided evidence that the natriuresis associated with central blood volume expansion in normal subjects is associated with a striking increase in renal PGE excretion that is attenuated by a prostaglandin inhibitor like indomethacin.[92] In these studies, the administration of indomethacin also blunted the natriuresis of neck immersion in sodium-depleted but not sodium-repleted subjects. Taken together, these studies suggest that PGE excretion is enhanced under conditions of effective volume depletion, sodium restriction, and other high-renin conditions, and that prostaglandin inhibition results in an antinatriuretic effect under these conditions. Prostaglandins also play a role in renal water excretion by exerting a negative feedback on the hydroosmotic effect of antidiuretic hormone. Thus, in the presence of prostaglandin inhibition, the water reabsorption stimulated by AVP has been demonstrated to be enhanced *in vivo*.[93] In summary, prostaglandin inhibition results in renal sodium and water retention, particularly in the setting of diminished effective circulating volume.

The interaction between renal prostaglandins and the renin-angiotensin-aldosterone system is highly complex. Prostaglandin infusions are known to stimulate renin release in humans and prostaglandin inhibition is associated with a lowering of basal plasma renin activity, possibly by interfering with the integrity of the renal baroreceptor.[94] As mentioned earlier, angiotensin II is a potent stimulus to prostaglandin synthesis, both directly and through vasoconstriction.

Several investigations into the possibility that prostaglandins moderate the development of experimental acute renal failure suggest that the hemodynamic effects of prostaglandins are of more than theoretical importance. Studies performed by Mauk and co-workers in 1977[95] demonstrated no protective effect of PGE administration to alter the renal failure induced by the nephrotoxin uranyl nitrate. In contrast, the administration of PGE prior to intra-arterial norepinephrine, was associated with a greater glomerular filtration rate following norepinephrine than kidneys not infused with PGE. Subsequent studies by Patak et al.[96] implicated the increase in osmolar excretion secondary to PGE_2 infusion as a mechanism of primary protective importance in this ischemic model of acute renal failure. PGE_2 infusions have also been shown to protect against the development of acute renal failure in other experimental models such as glycerol.[97] Conversely, *inhibition* of prostaglandin synthesis may enhance the incidence of and severity of glycerol-induced renal failure.[98]

Thus, the physiologic effects of prostaglandins to cause vasodilation and to induce a solute diuresis in the context of renal ischemia have been demonstrated to have a salutory effect on renal blood flow and glomerular filtration rate. Conversely, the inhibition of prostaglandin synthesis, particularly under the conditions of high-circulating renin and angiotensin, volume depletion, and sudden hypotensive stress will lead to enhanced vasoconstriction.

CLINICAL STUDIES OF NEPHROTOXICITY FOLLOWING PROSTAGLANDIN INHIBITION

The patient population at risk to develop renal insufficiency following prostaglandin inhibitors is incompletely defined, and the precise incidence of this occurrence is unknown. The spectrum of renal failure syndromes following prostaglandin inhibitors is currently evolving as enhanced recognition of the physiology of prostaglandins and wider use of the prostaglandin inhibitor agents increase. Several different types of renal dysfunction have been reported and are depicted in Table 6–6: (1) a hemodynamic deterioration in patients with enhanced PGE excretion who are dependent on prostaglandins for maintenance of renal function; (2) deterioration of renal function in patients with preexistent renal disease, particularly lupus; and (3) acute interstitial nephritis recognized primarily with nonsteroidal anti-inflammatory agents.

Acute renal failure due to enhanced renal vasoconstriction following prostaglandin inhibition has been reported in several disorders associated with low basal levels of renal blood flow, such as congestive cardiac failure, glomerulonephritis, and hepatic cirrhosis.[99-104] The clearest documentation of a patient with reduced effective blood volume dependent on

TABLE 6–6. POTENTIAL CLINICAL IMPLICATIONS OF PROSTAGLANDIN INHIBITION

Acute renal failure due to enhanced renal vasoconstriction in disorders with diminished basal levels of renal blood flow (hepatic cirrhosis, congestive heart failure, glomerulonephritis, shock states).
Direct nephrotoxicity with acute interstitial and glomerular inflammatory changes.
Suppression of the renin-angiotensin-aldosterone axis with resultant hyperkalemia.
Sodium and water retention; inhibition of action of diuretics with concomitant potential weight gain, hypertension, edema, and hyponatremia.

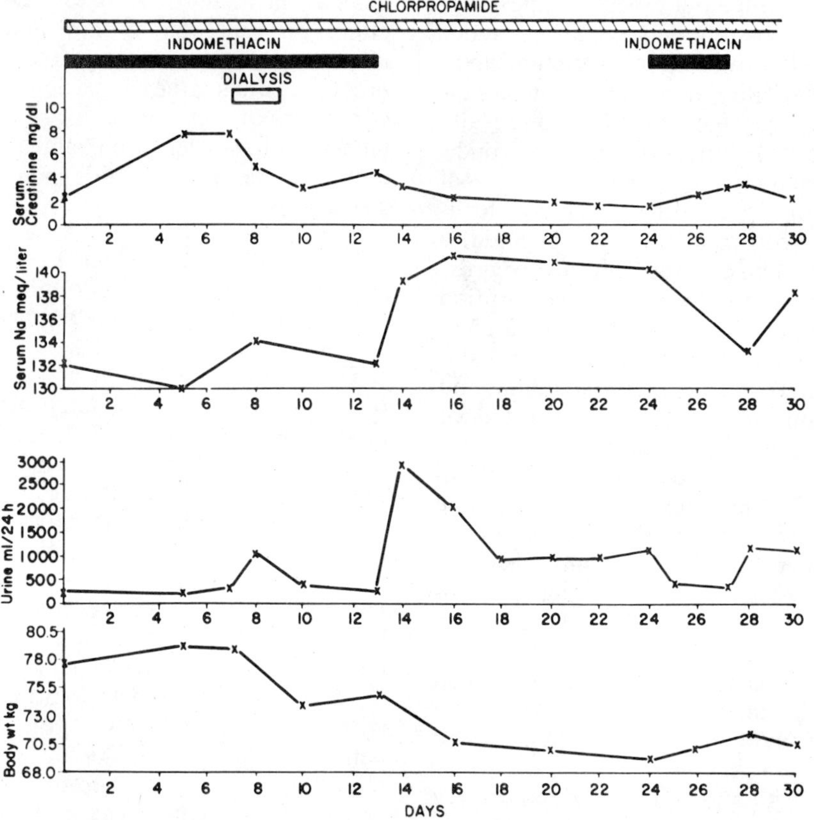

Figure 6–2. Clinical course in a patient with renal failure after indomethacin. Note the oliguria and rise in serum creatinine with indomethacin therapy. See text for details. (Reprinted from Walshe JJ, Venuto, RC: Acute oliguric renal failure induced by indomethacin; possible mechanism. Ann. Int. Med. 91:47–49, 1979, by permission.)

intact prostaglandin synthesis for maintenance of renal function was recently reported by Walshe and Venuto.[99] These authors described a patient with compensated congestive heart failure who received indomethacin and developed oliguric acute renal failure. Following discontinuation of the indomethacin and clinical recovery, the patient was rechallenged with indomethacin under supervised conditions (see Fig. 6–2). Urinary PGE excretion fell from 1058 mg/24h to 58 mg/24h as glomerular filtration and renal blood flow fell and the patient became oliguric. These authors also measured urinary PGE levels in five subsequent patients with congestive heart failure and noted a marked increase compared to normal (1534 ± 428 mg/24h vs. 377 ± 28 mg/24h, $p < 0.001$). Thus, patients with congestive heart failure, nephrotic syndrome, and volume depletion secondary to diuretics, gastrointestinal fluid loss, extensive burns, pancreatitis, and hemorrhage are particularly at risk for renal failure from prostaglandin inhibitors. Such an occurrence is compatible with the experimental studies described earlier in which prostaglandin inhibition greatly enhanced the vasoconstrictive forces already operant.[87, 88]

Another group of patients at risk for a decline in renal function from prostaglandin inhibitors are patients with preexistent renal disease, particularly those with lupus glomerulonephritis. Kimberly and Plotz reported on 13 lupus patients with active renal involvement who incurred decrements in renal function during treatment with aspirin.[100] This decrement in glomerular filtration rate was reversible on discontinuation of the drug. Subsequent studies in eight patients with lupus nephritis demonstrated elevated urinary PGE excretion in these patients that decreased when aspirin was administered. A concomitant decrease in glomerular filtration rate and renal blood flow and reversible elevation of the serum creatinine followed the reduction in urinary PGE excretion.[101] Other nonsteroidal anti-inflammatory agents that are propionic acid derivatives, such as ibuprofen, naproxen, and fenoprofen, have been implicated as causing similar effects to aspirin in patients with systemic lupus,[102] and even acute renal failure in one case.[103]

Another clinical setting often associated with increased urinary prostaglandin excretion and diminished basal levels of renal blood flow is advanced hepatic cirrhosis.[91] In this setting, removal of the vasodilating effect of prostaglandins with nonsteroidal antiinflammatory agents often precipitates acute renal failure.[104]

Two recent reports suggest that acute renal failure secondary to an acute interstitial nephritis may be induced by nonsteroidal anti-inflammatory agents. In the first report,[105] the patients suffered reversible acute renal failure and the nephrotic syndrome while ingesting either fenoprofen or naproxen. Renal biopsy revealed an intense interstitial inflammation similar to other allergic drug-induced interstitial processes. In the second report, a similar acute interstitial reaction with proteinuria and peripheral eosinophilia was reported in a patient taking fenoprofen.[106] In this case, treatment with corticosteroids resulted in resolution of the renal failure. Other similar cases of tubulointerstitial nephritis have also been documented recently.[107] In addition, indomethacin has been reported to be associated with induction of acute glomerulonephritis.[108]

Thus, in summary, the clinical manifestations of renal insufficiency secondary to prostaglandin inhibitors assume several distinct patterns. The deterioration of glomerular filtration rate and renal blood flow secondary to the loss of the compensatory vasodilatory activity of the prostaglandins constitutes a major risk in patients with reduced effective arterial blood volume (e.g., congestive heart failure, decompensated cirrhosis, or nephrotic syndrome). Secondly, some patients with preexistent renal disease, especially with systemic lupus, have elevated urinary excretion of PGE and appear to be at risk to develop a reversible decrease in renal function and even acute renal failure with prostaglandin inhibitors. The precise frequency of this occurrence and the relative risk of prostaglandin inhibitor–renal failure in patients with lupus nephritis is unknown. Finally, the newer nonsteroidal anti-inflammatory agents, particularly fenoprofen, appear capable of a third form of renal insult, an acute allergic type of interstitial nephritis characterized by a prompt decline in filtration and heavy proteinuria. This reaction may be independent of any effects on prostaglandin inhibition. Therefore, in order to avoid the deleterious effects of this group of agents, proper selection of patients to receive these agents and monitoring of renal function are required to avoid significant nephrotoxicity.

Additional fluid and electrolyte disturbances can be induced by prostaglandin inhibitors. Thus, the renin and aldosterone inhibition induced by indomethacin may result in hyperkalemia.[109] In 30 patients, a syndrome of hyporeninemic hypoaldosteronism with significant hyperkalemia was observed 1 week after starting indomethacin therapy. Hyperkalemia presented during therapy and was reversible when therapy was discontinued. Prostaglandin inhibition may also result in sodium and water retention with resultant weight gain, edema, and hypertension.[110] Finally, prostaglandin inhibition often antagonizes the natriuretic effect of several commonly used diuretic agents.[111] Taken together, it is obvious that prostaglandin inhibition can result in a number of disturbances of electrolyte metabolism. Patients with kidney and liver disease may be particularly susceptible to these adverse effects.

REFERENCES

1. Leonard BJ, Eccleston E, Jones D: Anti-leukemic and nephrotoxic properties of platinum compounds. Nature *234*:43–49, 1971.
2. Madias NE, Harrington JT: Platinum nephrotoxicity. Am. J. Med. *65*:307–314, 1978.
3. Maher JF: Toxic nephropathy. *In* The Kidney (BM Brenner and FC Rector, Jr, eds.). Philadelphia: W. B. Saunders Co., 1976, vol. 2, p. 1355.
4. Dentino M, Luft FC, Yum MN, Williams SD, Einhorn LH: Long term effect of cis-diamminedichloride platinum (CDDP) on renal function and structure in man. Cancer *41*:1274–1281, 1978.
5. Stark JJ, Howell SB: Nephrotoxicity of cis-platinum (II) dichlorodiammine. Clin. Pharmacol. Ther. *23*:461–466, 1978.
6. Rainer JM, Alberts DS: Safe, rapid administration schedule for cis-platinum-mannitol. Med. Pediatr. Oncol. *4*:371–375, 1978.
7. Ward JM, Grabin ME, Berlin E, et al.: Prevention of renal failure in rats receiving cis-diamminedichloroplatinum (II) by administration of furosemide. Can. Res. *37*:1238–1240, 1977.

8. Gonzales-Vitale J, Hayes DM, Cvitkovic E, et al.: Acute renal failure after cis-dichlorodiammine platinum (II) and gentamicin-cephalothin therapies. Can. Treat. Rep. *62*:693–698, 1978.
9. Schilsky RL, Anderson T: Hypomagnesemia and renal magnesium wasting in patients receiving cisplatin. Ann. Intern. Med. *90*:929–931, 1979.
10. Hill JB, Blachley JD, Trotter M: Hypomagnesemia, hypocalcemia, and hypokalemia with cis-platinum therapy. (Abstract.) Clin. Res. *26*:780A, 1978.
11. Kazantis G: Heavy metals and renal damage. Eur. J. Clin. Invest. *9*:3–4, 1979.
12. Thienes CH, Haley TJ: Kidney poisons. *In* Clinical Toxicology. Philadelphia, Lea and Febiger, 1972, p. 163.
13. DiBona GF, McDonald FD, Flamenbaum W, Dammin GJ, Oken DE: Maintenance of renal function in salt-loaded rats despite severe tubular necrosis induced by $HgCl_2$. Nephron *8*:205–220, 1971.
14. Browder A: The problem of lead poisoning. Medicine *52*:121, 1973.
15. Felton J: Heavy metal poisoning. Ann. Intern. Med. *76*:797, 1972.
16. Guinee V: Lead poisoning. Am. J. Med. *52*:283, 1972.
17. Haley T: Saturnism, pediatric and adult lead poisoning. Clin. Toxicol. *4*:11, 1971.
18. Hammond P: Exposure of humans to lead. Ann. Rev. Pharmacol. Toxicol. *17*:197, 1977.
19. Chisholm J: Aminoaciduria as a manifestation of lead intoxication. J. Pediatr. *60*:1, 1962.
20. Cramer K: Renal ultrastructure in lead toxicity. Br. J. Indus. Med. *31*:113, 1972.
21. Emerson B: Lead nephropathy. Kidney Int. *4*:1, 1973.
22. Goyar R: Lead and the kidney. Curr. Topics Pathol. *9*:147, 1971.
23. Lilis R: Nephropathy in chronic lead poisoning. Br. J. Indus. Med. *25*:196, 1968.
24. Morgan J: Nephropathy in lead poisoning. Arch. Intern. Med. *118*:17, 1966.
25. Morgan J: Chelation therapy in lead nephropathy. South. Med. J. *68*:1001, 1975.
26. Weeden R: Detection and treatment of occupational lead nephropathy. Arch. Intern. Med. *139*:53, 1979.
27. Ball G: Pathogenesis of hyperuricemia in saturine gout. N. Engl. J. Med. *280*:1199, 1969.
28. Chisholm J: Heme metabolites in relation to lead toxicity. Adv. Clin. Chem. *15*:225, 1978.
29. Delves H: Analytical techniques for blood lead measurements. J. Anal. Toxicol. *1*:261, 1977.
30. Morgan J: Comparative tests for the diagnosis of lead poisoning. Arch. Intern. Med. *130*:335, 1977.
31. Rabinowitz M: Kinetic analysis of lead metabolism in humans. J. Clin. Invest. *58*:260, 1976.
32. Vitab L: Blood lead — an inadequate measure of exposure. J. Occup. Med. *17*:155, 1975.
33. Hamman P: Effects of chelating agents in the tissue distribution of lead. Toxicol. Appl. Pharmacol. *18*:296, 1971.
34. Vaamonde CA, Hunt FR: The nephrotic syndrome as a complication of gold therapy. Arthritis Rheum. *13*:826–834, 1970.
35. Silverberg DS, Kidd EG, Shnitka TK: Gold neprhopathy: A clinical and pathological study. Arthritis Rheum. *13*:812–825, 1970.
36. Kean WF, Anastassiades TP: Long term chrysotherapy. Arthritis Rheum. *22*:495–501, 1979.
37. Husserl FE, Shuler SE: Gold nephropathy in juvenile rheumatoid arthritis. Am. J. Dis. Child. *133*:50–52, 1979.
38. Tornroth T, Skrifvars B: Gold nephropathy: Prototype of membranous glomerulonephritis. Am. J. Pathol. *75*:573–590, 1974.
39. Samuels B, Lee JC, Engleman EP, Hopper J, Jr: Membranous nephropathy in patients with rheumatoid arthritis: Relationship to gold therapy. Medicine *57*:319–327, 1977.
40. Katz A, Little AH: Gold nephropathy — an immunopathologic study. Arch. Pathol. *96*:133–136, 1973.
41. Skrifvars B: Hypothesis for the pathogenesis of sodium aurothiomalate (mycrosin) induced immune complex nephritis. Scand. J. Rheumatol. *8*:113–118, 1979.
42. Giberson A, Vaziri ND, Mirahamadi K, Rosen SM: Hemodialysis of acute arsenic intoxication with transient renal failure. Arch. Intern. Med. *136*:1303–1304, 1976.
43. Ryan R, McNeil JS, Flamenbaum W, Nagle R: Uranyl nitrate induced acute renal failure in the rat. Effect of varying doses and saline loading. Proc. Soc. Exp. Biol. Med. *143*:289–296, 1973.
44. Ehrenreich T: Renal disease from exposure to solvents. Ann. Clin. Lab. Sci. *7*:6–16, 1977.
45. Beirne GJ, Brennan JT: Glomerulonephritis associated with hydrocarbon solvents. Arch. Environ. Health *25*:365–371, 1972.
46. Kleinbrecht D, Morel-Maroger L, Callard P, et al.: Antiglomerular basement membrane nephritis after solvent exposure. Arch. Intern. Med. *140*:230–232, 1980.
47. Winek CL, Shingleton DP, and Shanov SP: Ethylene and diethylene glycol toxicity. Clin. Toxicol. *13*:297–324, 1978.
48. Parry MF, Wallach R: Ethylene glycol poisoning. Am. J. Med. *57*:143–150, 1974.
49. Ahmed MM: Ocular effects of antifreeze poisoning. Br. J. Ophthalmol. *55*:854–858, 1971.
50. Collins JM, Hennes DM, Holzgang CR, et al.: Recovery after prolonged oliguria due to ethylene glycol intoxication. Arch. Intern. Med. *125*:1059–1061, 1970.
51. Newman HW, Van Winkel W Jr, Kennedy NK, et al.: Comparative effects of propylene glycol, other glycols and alcohol on the liver directly. J. Pharmacol. Exp. Ther. *68*:194–199, 1970.
52. Bachmann E, Goldberg L: Reappraisal of the toxicology of ethylene glycol III. Mitochondrial effects. Food Cosmet. Toxicol. *9*:39–45, 1971.
53. Peterson CD, Collins AJ, Hines JM, et al.: Ethylene glycol poisoning. N. Engl. J. Med. *304*:21–23, 1981.
54. Maher JF: Toxic and irradiation nephropathies. *In* Strauss and Welt's Diseases of the Kidney (LE Earley and CM Gottschalk, eds.). Boston: Little, Brown and Co., 1979, pp. 1431–1472.
55. Thienes CH, Haley TJ: *Ibid.*, pp. 146–156.
56. Baerg RD, Kimberg DV: Centrilobular hepatic necrosis and acute renal failure in solvent sniffers. Ann. Intern. Med. *73*:713–715, 1970.
57. Taher SM, Anderson RJ, McCartney R, et al.: Renal tubular acidosis with toluene "sniffing." N. Engl. J. Med. *290*:765–768, 1974.
58. Moss AH, Gabow PA, Kaehny WD, et al.: Fanconi

syndrome and distal renal tubular acidosis after glue sniffing. Ann. Intern. Med. *92*:69–70, 1980.

59. Cohr KH, Stockholm J: Toluene. Scand. J. Work Environ. Health *5*:71–90, 1979.
60. Barrientos A, Ortuño MT, Morales JM, et al.: Acute renal failure after use of diesel fuel as shampoo. Arch. Intern. Med. *137*:1217, 1977.
61. Thienes CH, Haley TJ: *Ibid.*, p. 181, 1977.
62. Beirne GJ, Wagnild JP, Zimmerman SP, et al.: Idiopathic crescentic glomerulonephritis. Medicine *56*:349–380, 1977.
63. Alexander RD, Beckes SL, Abuelo JG: Contrast media-induced oliguric renal failure. Arch. Intern. Med. *138*:381–384, 1978.
64. Swartz RD, Rubin JE, Leeming BW, et al.: Renal failure following major angiography. Am. J. Med. *65*:31–37, 1978.
65. Weinrauch LA, Healey RW, Leland OS, Jr, et al.: Coronary angiography and acute renal failure in diabetic azotemic nephropathy. Ann. Intern. Med. *86*:56–59, 1977.
66. Henaway J, Black J: Renal failure following contrast injections for computerized tomography. J.A.M.A. *238*:2056, 1977.
67. Connales CO, Smith GH, Robinson JC, et al.: Acute renal failure after the administration of iopanoic acid as a cholecystographic agent. N. Engl. J. Med. *281*:89, 1969.
68. Bushinsky DA, Wish JB, Hou SH, et al.: Hospital acquired renal insufficiency (1978–1979).(Abstract.) Proc. Am. Soc. Nephrol. *12*:105A, 1979.
69. Byrd L, Sherman RL: Radiocontrast-induced acute renal failure. Medicine *58*:270–279, 1979.
70. Eisenberg RL, Bank WO, Hedgecock MW: Renal failure after major angiography. Amer. J. Med. *68*:43, 1980.
71. Kamdar A, Weidmann P, Makoff DL, et al.: Acute renal failure following intravenous use of radiographic contrast dyes in patients with diabetes mellitus. Diabetes *26*:643–649, 1977.
72. Ansari Z, Baldwin DS: Acute renal failure due to radiocontrast agents. Nephron *17*:28–40, 1976.
73. Van Zee BE, Hoy WE, Talley TE, Jaenike JR: Renal injury associated with intravenous pyelography in nondiabetic and diabetic patients. Ann. Intern. Med. *89*:51–54, 1978.
74. Harkoneon S, Kjellstrand CM: Exacerbation of diabetic renal failure following intravenous pyelography. Am. J. Med. *63*:939–942, 1977.
75. Anderson RJ, Linas SL, Berns AS, et al.: Nonoliguric renal failure: A prospective study. N. Engl. J. Med. *296*:1134–1138, 1977.
76. Russell SB, Sherwood T: Monomer/dimer contrast media in the renal circulation: experimental angiography. Br. J. Radiol. *47*:268–271, 1974.
77. Morris TW, Katzberg RW, Fisher HW: A comparison of the hemodynamic responses to metrizamide and meglumine/sodium diatrizoate in canine renal angiography. Invest. Radiol. *13*:74–79, 1978.
78. Schiantaielli P, Peroni F, Turone P, et al.: Effects of iodinated contrast media on erythrocytes. Invest. Radiol. *8*:199–204, 1973.
79. Berdon WE, Schwartz RH, Becker J, et al.: Tamm-Horsfall proteinuria: its relationship to prolonged nephrogram in infants and children with acute renal failure, following intravenous urography, and in adults with multiple myeloma. Radiology *92*:714–718, 1969.
80. Gelman ML, Rowe JW, Coggins CH, et al.: Effects of an angiographic contrast agent on renal function. Cardiovascular Med. *6*:313, 1979.
81. Kleinknecht D, Deloux J, Homberg JC: Acute renal failure after intravenous urography: detection of antibodies against contrast media. Clin. Nephrol. *2*:116–121, 1974.
82. Light JA, Perloff LJ, Etheredge EE, et al.: Adverse effects of meglumine diatrizoate on renal function in the early post-transplant period. Transplantation *20*:404–408, 1975.
83. Lasser EC, Lee SH, Fisher E, et al.: Some further pertinent considerations regarding the comparative toxicity of contrast materials for the dog kidney. Radiology *78*:240–243, 1962.
84. Ziegler TW, Ladens JH, Fanestil DD, et al.: Inhibition of active sodium transport by radiographic contrast media. Kidney Int. *7*:68–73, 1975.
85. Blaufox MD, Sanderson DR, Tauxe WN: Plasma diatrizoate I^{131} and glomerular filtration in the dog. Am. J. Physiol. *204*:536–542, 1963.
86. Dunn MJ, Hood VL: Prostaglandins and the kidney. Am. J. Physiol. *233*:169–184, 1977.
87. Vatner SF: Effects of hemorrhage on regional blood flow distribution in dogs and primates. J. Clin. Invest. *54*:225–235, 1974.
88. Henrich W, Anderson RJ, Berl T, et al.: Role of angiotensin II and prostaglandins in renal response to hypotensive hemorrhage. Am. J. Physiol. *235*:F46–51, 1978.
89. Stokes JB, Kokko JP: Inhibition of sodium transport by prostaglandin E_2 across the isolated, perfused rabbit collecting tubule. J. Clin. Invest. *59*:1099–1104, 1977.
90. Zia P, Zipser R, Speckart P, et al.: The measurement of urinary PGE in normal subjects and in high renin states. J. Lab. Clin. Med. *92*:415–422, 1978.
91. Epstein M, Lifschitz M, Preston S: Augmentation of renal PGE in decompensated cirrhosis. Implication for renal function. (Abstract.) Proc. Am. Soc. Nephrol. *12*:150A, 1979.
92. Epstein M, Lifschitz MD, Hoffman DS, et al.: Relationship between renal prostaglandin E and renal sodium handling during water immersion in normal man. Circ. Res. *45*:71–80, 1979.
93. Anderson RJ, Berl T, McDonald KM, et al.: Evidence for an *in vivo* antagonism between vasopressin and prostaglandin in the mammalian kidney. J. Clin. Invest. *56*:420–426, 1975.
94. Berl T, Henrich WL, Erickson AL, et al.: Prostaglandins in the beta adrenergic and baroreceptor-mediated secretion of renin. Am. J. Physiol. *236*:F472–477, 1979.
95. Mauk RH, Patak RW, Fadem SZ, et al.: Effect of prostaglandin E administration in a nephrotoxic vasoconstrictor model of acute renal failure. Kidney Int. *12*:122–130, 1977.
96. Patak RV, Fadem SZ, Lifschitz MD, et al.: Study of factors which modify the development of acute renal failure in the dog. Kidney Int. *15*:227–237, 1979.
97. Werb R, Clark WF, Lindsey RM, et al.: Protective effect of PGE in glycerol-induced acute renal failure. Clin. Sci. Mol. Med. *55*:505–507, 1978.
98. Torres VE, Strong CG, Romero JC, et al.: In-

domethacin enhancement of glycerol acute renal failure in rabbits. Kidney Int. *7*:170–178, 1975.

99. Walshe JJ, Venuto RC: Acute oliguric renal failure induced by indomethacin: possible mechanism. Ann. Intern. Med. *91*:47–49, 1979.
100. Kimberly RP, Poltz PH: Aspirin-induced depression of renal function. N. Engl. J. Med. *296*:418–424, 1977.
101. Kimberly RP, Gill JR, Bowden RE, et al.: Elevated urinary prostaglandins and the effects of aspirin on renal function in lupus erythematosus. Ann. Intern. Med. *89*:336–341, 1978.
102. Kimberly RP, Bowden RE, Keiser HR, et al.: Reduction of renal function by newer non-steroidal anti-inflammatory agents. Am. J. Med. *64*:804–807, 1978.
103. Kimberly RP, Sherman RL, Mouradian J, et al.: Apparent acute renal failure associated with therapeutic aspirin and ibuprofen administration. Arthritis Rheum. *22*:281–285, 1979.
104. Bayer TD, Zia P, Reynolds TB: Effect of indomethacin and prostaglandin A on renal function and plasma renin activity in alcoholic liver disease. Gastroenterology *77*:275, 1979.
105. Brezin JH, Katz SM, Schwartz AB, et al.: Reversible renal failure and nephrotic syndrome associated with nonsteroidal anti-inflammatory drugs. N. Engl. J. Med. *301*:1271–1273, 1979.
106. Curt GA, Kadany A, Whitley LG, et al.: Reversible rapidly progressive renal failure with nephrotic syndrome due to fenoprofen calcium. Ann. Intern. Med. *92*:72–73, 1980.
107. Wendland ML, Wagoner RD, Holley KE: Renal failure associated with fenoprofen. Mayo Clin. Proc. *55*:103–107, 1980.
108. Marsh FP, Almeyda JR, Levy IS: Nonthrombocytopenic purpura and acute glomerulonephritis after indomethacin therapy. Ann. Rheum. Dis. *30*:501, 1971.
109. Kutyrina IN, Androsova SO, Tareyara IE: Indomethacin induced hyporeninemic hypoaldosteronism. Lancet *1*:785, 1979.
110. Brater DC: Effect of indomethacin on salt and water homeostasis. Clin. Pharmacol. Ther. *25*:322, 1979.
111. Patak RV, Mookerjce BK, Bentzel CJ, et al.: Antagonism of the effect of furosemide by indomethacin in normal and hypertensive man. Prostaglandin *10*:649–659, 1975.

Chapter 7

Drug-Induced Immunologic-Renal Disease

by

David W. Knutson and Jack W. Coburn*

Many drugs cause renal damage through a direct toxic action. The administration of other drugs is associated with renal damage mediated by immunologic mechanisms. The first evidence for this was the finding that renal biopsies from certain cases of drug-associated renal disease showed histologic features similar to those in spontaneously occurring renal diseases that have a presumed immunologic pathogenesis. Thus, glomerulopathies with proteinuria and the nephrotic syndrome, interstitial nephritis, vasculitis, and acute glomerulonephritis each have been observed in association with drug therapy. It should be recognized that there is incomplete understanding of the pathogenesis of both drug-induced and spontaneously occurring immunologic-renal diseases. Nonetheless, the occurrence of these drug-induced lesions provides a unique opportunity for the study of immunologic-renal disease because the antigen or inciting agent, its dose and duration of exposure, as well as its physicochemical properties, are known and can be studied.

This chapter will briefly review general principles of diagnosis and treatment of drug-induced immunologic-renal injuries. Each major pattern or syndrome observed will then be reviewed. The best studied prototype drugs will be described in detail with a discussion of current concepts regarding the pathogenesis of the renal injury; information regarding less common and less well-studied associations will then be given.

*Dr. Knutson was supported by a Veterans Administration Research Associateship.

GENERAL PRINCIPLES OF DIAGNOSIS, PROGNOSIS, AND TREATMENT

The recognition and diagnosis of drug-induced immunologic-renal disease are dependent on the same clinical and laboratory parameters as is the case for spontaneous renal disease. Early and mild renal damage may have few clinical symptoms and signs; patients may note only nocturia due to the reversal of the diurnal pattern of urine excretion. Some patients may develop hypertension. Vasculitis is often accompanied by systemic symptoms due to involvement of other organs, and interstitial nephritis may be accompanied by an erythematous rash and peripheral eosinophilia. It is important to monitor patients at risk with periodic urinalyses and measurements of renal function, preferably levels of serum creatinine. Abnormalities should be further investigated with measurements of creatinine clearance and quantitative protein excretion. While certain drugs may cause tubular abnormalities, the measurement of urinary amino acids, glucose, phosphate, and uric acid is usually not helpful or necessary for the diagnosis of these immunologic renal disorders. The value of identifying eosinophils in the urine is discussed later under the section dealing with interstitial nephritis.

A knowledge of the temporal relationship between initial drug exposure and the onset of renal disease is important for the recognition of immunologic-renal disease in patients being treated with potentially injurious drugs. Vasculitis, acute glomerulonephritis, and interstitial nephritis usually appear after days to weeks of therapy; the nephrotic syndrome, however, tends to appear only after several months or even a year of treatment.

The specific therapies for different drug-associated renal disorders will be covered under the various sections. In many instances, the kidneys are capable of remarkable recovery when the offending drug is withdrawn. This may be true even when renal insufficiency is substantial, although some drugs have been associated with permanent renal damage and rare patients have even required dialysis. The latter observation underscores the importance of continued and careful monitoring of patients at risk.

In many clinical settings, a renal biopsy is not necessary to confirm the diagnosis. Thus, a patient with rheumatoid arthritis who develops mild to moderate proteinuria while receiving penicillamine or the patient who develops azotemia with skin rash and eosinophiluria while receiving methicillin are clinical examples in which the diagnosis does not require histologic confirmation. However, in complex situations or in patients with rapidly deteriorating renal function, a renal biopsy may disclose crescentic glomerulonephritis, which is not drug induced and which may suggest that the physician consider other treatment, such as plasmapheresis. In such cases, a renal biopsy may be helpful. When a renal biopsy is done, it is important that the biopsy be examined by appropriate immunofluorescence microscopy and, at times, electron microscopy in addition to standard light microscopy.

The risk of drug-associated immunologic-renal disease obviously varies from one drug to another. With many agents, these disorders are quite rare. The use of such drugs must include a consideration of potential benefit as well as the risk of this potential side effect. For some drugs, such as penicillamine and methicillin, the causal relationship between the drug and renal disease appears to be well established. Other associations may be based on only a limited number of case reports and there is the possibility that the development of renal disease in these patients was only fortuitous. Moreover, patients with drug-induced renal disease have frequently been exposed to multiple drugs, so it may be difficult to identify with certainty the drug responsible. In such cases, the most convincing evidence for the drug playing a pathogenic role is the recurrence of renal injury when patients receive an inadvertent repeated exposure to the drug in question. Finally, the list of drugs causing immunologic-renal disease is undoubtedly incomplete. Clinicians should be aware of this and be alert for renal disease that may result from drugs not discussed in this chapter.

DRUGS CAUSING PROTEINURIA AND THE NEPHROTIC SYNDROME

Numerous drugs can induce a clinical and pathologic syndrome that is nearly indistinguishable from early membranous nephropathy (Table 7–1). Heroin use may be associated with membranous nephropathy as well as other glomerular abnormalities and will be considered in a separate section.

MEMBRANOUS NEPHROPATHY

PENICILLAMINE AND GOLD

Penicillamine, a breakdown product of penicillin, is a chelating agent used in the treatment of cystinuria, Wilson's disease, heavy metal intoxication, and, more recently, rheumatoid arthritis.[1,2] Early reports had ascribed

TABLE 7–1. AGENTS ASSOCIATED WITH PROTEINURIA AND THE NEPHROTIC SYNDROME

Association strongly supported
Penicillamine
Gold
Mercury
Probable Association
Hydantoin anticonvulsants (trimethadione, paramethadione, and methylphenylethylhydantoin)
Captopril
Possible Association
Bismuth
Insect repellent
Meglumine diatrizoate
Perchlorate
Phenindione
Probenecid
Tolbutamide
Trichloroethylene

the nephrotic syndrome to the racemic form, DL-penicillamine;[3] however, it is clear from numerous other reports that D-penicillamine can cause the nephrotic syndrome.[4-7] Gold salts have long been used to treat rheumatoid arthritis[8] and more recently have been used to treat pemphigus.[9] Several different gold salts,[10] including sodium aurothiomalate,[11] aurothioglucose,[12] and aurothiosulfate,[12] have been associated with the nephrotic syndrome and/or membranous nephropathy.

Many of the cases of nephrotic syndrome associated with treatment with gold or penicillamine have developed in patients with rheumatoid arthritis, an immunologic disorder that might predispose to the renal lesion. However, several lines of evidence strongly suggest that these two drugs are directly responsible for renal disease: (1) The nephrotic syndrome is rare in patients with rheumatoid arthritis, but more common in those receiving these drugs.[13, 14] (2) Penicillamine treatment has been associated with nephrotic syndrome and membranous nephropathy in several nonimmunologic conditions, including Wilson's disease,[15, 16] lead poisoning,[17, 18] and cystinuria, although it may be less common in these disorders.[19] (3) Finally, penicillamine injected into monkeys[20] and rats[21] and gold salts injected into rats[22] have produced proteinuria and histologic features similar to those observed in afflicted human patients.

Incidence. With penicillamine treatment, the incidence of proteinuria varies from 7.4 per cent[23] to 20.0 per cent[24] in different series. The incidence of proteinuria and the nephrotic syndrome with gold therapy is clearly lower, but may have been underestimated by Hartfall et al.,[8] who found a 0.2 per cent incidence in a retrospective evaluation of patients with rheumatoid arthritis. The Research Subcommittee of the Empire Rheumatism Council places the incidence of nephrotic syndrome with gold therapy at 1 to 3 per cent,[13, 14] and proteinuria may be twice as common.

Clinical Features. The clinical picture is similar for both drugs. Significant proteinuria usually appears after several months of gold therapy, but it may appear as early as 6 weeks or as late as 1 year.[25, 26] For penicillamine, the highest incidence occurs at 4 to 12 months, but cases have been observed after as long as 3 years of therapy.[24] The glomerular injury probably antedates the appearance of proteinuria by weeks or even months, since the tubular maximum (Tm) for reabsorption of albumin is not reached until considerable amounts of protein leak through glomerular basement membrane. The urinalysis in patients with membranous nephropathy and proteinuria is usually devoid of significant cellular elements, although microscopic hematuria and occasional white cells may be seen.[23, 27]

The questions of whether or not relationships exist between the dosages of either penicillamine or gold and the development of proteinuria remain unanswered. Many patients with Wilson's disease have received penicillamine in doses as high as 2 gm/day for many years without developing proteinuria. Sternlieb[3] found no correlation between the quantity of proteinuria and the dosage of penicillamine in a large series of patients with rheumatoid arthritis and proteinuria. On the other hand, Day and Golding[24] found a correlation between the mean daily dosage and evidence of nephropathy, although one patient developed proteinuria with a mean dose of only 450 mg/day. It is possible that reducing the dose of penicillamine may control symptoms of rheumatoid arthritis and be associated with a lower incidence of proteinuria; however, a "safe" dose of penicillamine has not been established.

Gold is only slowly excreted, and the onset of proteinuria has been related to the total dose given. Transient, mild proteinuria has been described after initial injection of gold salts,[28] but membranous nephropathy with immunofluorescent deposits generally requires at least 6 weeks and usually longer to develop.[29, 30] Persistent proteinuria has been described after total injections of 235 to 3750 mg of gold salts.[12] Other patients have failed to develop nephropathy after doses as high as 6 gm. Such observations suggest that only certain patients are susceptible, but continued exposure may also be necessary before renal injury occurs. In patients who are susceptible, there may be a threshold mean daily dose of penicillamine or total dose of gold required to produce the renal lesion; however, it is likely that such a "threshold" dose is below the therapeutic amounts necessary to treat many of the diseases for which it is given.

Most authors view the full-blown nephrotic syndrome as an extension of asymptomatic proteinuria with greater quantities of urinary protein excreted; this leads to hypoalbuminemia, edema, and hyperlipidemia (hypercholesterolemia). Proteinuria associated with gold and penicillamine may be marked, with protein losses as high as 16 gm/day;[28] such cases have presumably resulted from late discovery and continued use of the offending drug after the onset of asymptomatic proteinuria. However, the nephrotic syndrome may occur rather quickly; we have observed the appearance of the nephrotic syndrome with protein excretion of 16 gm/day in a patient who had received penicillamine for 1 year; 6 weeks earlier the urinalysis had been negative. Because the condition is usually self-limiting and because the manifestations are easily monitored, the current policy of the Rheumatology Clinic at the UCLA Center for Health Sciences is to continue penicillamine at the lowest dose necessary to control symptoms of rheumatoid arthritis until proteinuria exceeds 1.5 to 2.0 gm/day. Others have continued to treat patients with low doses of penicillamine for up to 3 years after the appearance of mild proteinuria; the proteinuria persisted as long as the drug was given in the few reported cases. Generally, proteinuria of 0.5 gm/day or greater during gold therapy requires withdrawal of the drug, at least temporarily.

Proteinuria usually diminishes after penicillamine or gold is discontinued. On withdrawal of treatment with penicillamine, the nephrotic syndrome usually resolves and protein excretion falls below 3 gm/day by 3 to 6 months and below 1 gm/day after 12 months.[23] After the discontinuation of gold therapy, the resolution of proteinuria often follows a similar course, although it may persist beyond 1 year.[27] Remission of proteinuria after discontinuation of penicillamine can be followed by a recurrence of the nephrotic syndrome when the drug is reinstituted,[13] an observation providing further evidence of the cause-effect relationship for this drug. The occurrence of nephrotic syndrome during gold therapy usually precludes the further use of gold. Following lesser degrees of proteinuria, however, some rheumatologists would reinstitute gold therapy once the proteinuria has abated.

Renal excretory function is usually normal or near normal in most patients with mild to moderate proteinuria.[23, 28] Elevated levels of the serum creatinine and/or decreased creatinine clearances have been observed in patients with nephrotic syndrome associated with penicillamine[23] and gold.[27] However, the assessment of impaired renal function is difficult in the patient with hypoalbuminemia and hypovolemia. A reduction in circulating blood volume and consequent decrease in renal blood flow can reduce the glomerular filtration rate (GFR), and extreme hypoalbuminemia may lower the GFR to alarmingly low values. The GFR is usually restored to or near that of normal when either gold or penicillamine is discontinued and the nephrotic syndrome has resolved.[15, 27] Thus, gold and penicillamine do not ordinarily lead to permanent impairment of renal function. However, scarred glomeruli are sometimes seen with gold therapy, and a potential danger of permanent damage seems real for both drugs in spite of the absence of published reports.

Pathology. The histologic findings of renal biopsies have been remarkably similar in the nephropathies associated with gold and penicillamine, although certain minor differences between the two exist. Light microscopy usually reveals few abnormalities; slight swelling of epithelial cells and minimal thickening of the glomerular basement membrane have been described.[6, 20, 23] Focal mesangial proliferation has also been encountered.[23]

Histologic sections stained with silver methenamine or trichrome stains can show deposits that correlate with dense deposits seen with electron microscopy in the subepithelial spaces. These deposits are thought to represent antigen-antibody complexes. In idiopathic membranous nephropathy, "spikes" of glomerular basement membrane are often interposed between the deposits. Progression of the disease is accompanied by incorporation of the deposits into the basement membrane, which leads to thickening of the basement membrane and glomerular sclerosis. Such histologic features are less common in association with use of these two drugs, presumably because biopsies are obtained early in the disease. However, serial ultrastructural studies by Törnroth and Skrifvars have shown the development of spikes and subsequent incorporation of deposits into the glomerular basement membrane in gold nephropathy.[31]

The most characteristic changes in biopsies of drug-induced and idiopathic membranous nephropathy are seen with immunofluorescence microscopy. This technique uses fluorescein-coupled, specific antibodies to probe for the presence of immunoglobulins, components of complement, antigens, and other proteins in tissues. Granular deposits of IgG and the third component of complement (C_3) are usually seen in a monotonous pattern involving all the basement membranes of intact glomeruli, although early lesions may be focal. Occasionally, IgA and rarely IgM are present.[20] The microscopic lesions usually resolve after penicillamine is discontinued, but they may be detected in diminished quantities for up to a year.[25] Resumption of therapy may lead to prompt reintensification of the deposits.[20]

Gold-induced lesions may persist longer and require a year or more to resolve. Gold can be detected in the lysosomes of the proximal tubule with use of immunochemical or electron diffraction methods; there is slow loss of the gold from the proximal tubular cells when the therapy is discontinued.[34]

Pathogenesis. Overwhelming evidence supports the notion that idiopathic membranous nephropathy is caused by the deposition of antigen-antibody complexes in the subepithelial space of the glomerular basement membrane. The pathogenesis of the lesions is presumably similar for gold and penicillamine. The exact mechanisms of deposition are unclear and in dispute. The more classic concept is that soluble antigen-antibody complexes are formed in the circulation and filtered onto and into the glomerular basement membrane. It is also possible that antigen-antibody complexes can be formed *in situ*.[35] Certainly, the feasibility of the former mechanism has been established, and it probably accounts for most of *subendothelial* deposition of immune complexes in the glomeruli of patients with proliferative glomerulonephritis. However, the processes accounting for such deposition must be complicated, since patients with rheumatoid arthritis and certain malignancies often have circulating immune complexes in high levels but no renal damage. Presumably, differences in the physiochemical and immunologic properties of the immune complexes account for their propensity to localize in the glomeruli and cause injury. Variables that might affect the deposition of immune complexes include the availability of antigen in the circulation or within the glomerulus; the relative amounts of antigen and antibody; the physical properties of antigen and its immunologic valence, i.e., the number of antigenic determinants; and the class, affinity, and complement-fixing properties of the antibody.[36] It is also possible that drugs may cause a direct toxic damage of glomerular capillaries that renders these vessels more susceptible to the deposition of immune complexes. Finally, phagocytic cells, such as macrophages, epithelial cells, and possibly mesangial cells, are thought to remove and catabolize immune complexes deposited in the glomerulus. Failure of these mechanisms could contribute to the accumulation of pathogenic immune complexes in the glomerulus.

The exact relationship between the drug and the composition of immune deposits is not clear. The most straightforward theory is that the drug or one of its metabolites is the offending antigen. There is a conspicuous paucity of reports concerning the presence of antibodies to penicillamine or gold salts in afflicted patients.[37] On the other hand, the mere presence of circulating antibodies to these drugs would not prove that such antibodies contribute to the glomerular deposits. Attempts to demonstrate either gold or penicillamine within immune complexes in the glomeruli by immunofluorescence have so far been unsuccessful. This may be due to the "covering" of antigenic sites by endogenous antibodies.[38] Gold can be detected in proximal tubular cells but not in glomeruli by x-ray diffraction and histochemical techniques.[32-34,39] There are no reports of elution of drug-specific antibodies from the glomeruli of patients with nephropathy due to gold or penicillamine.

A second theory to explain drug-induced membranous nephropathy is that the offending drugs may damage proximal tubular cells and cause an abnormal release or altered composition of tubular antigens.[40] Antigen-antibody complexes then are formed and deposited in the glomeruli[10] in a manner analogous to Heymann nephritis in the rat.[41,42] Many of the drugs associated with nephrotic syndrome are known to be concentrated in the proximal tubules, and gold given in large doses to rats can cause acute tubular necrosis. However, antitubular cell antibodies have not been found in the sera of patients with drug-induced membranous nephropathy, and there is no direct evidence that immune deposits contain tubular antigens or antitubular antibodies.

The third theory is that complexes of immunoglobulins and anti-immunoglobulin antibodies form the major portion of immune deposits. McIntosh et al. have shown the presence of anti-immunoglobulin antibodies in the glomerular deposits of rabbits with experimental serum sickness induced with bovine serum albumin,[43] which supports the feasibility of such a mechanism. Antibodies to the Fc portion of IgG (rheumatoid factors) are frequently found in patients with rheumatoid arthritis, and normal subjects may have low titers of anti-IgG antibodies; thus, antibodies are present to contribute to the deposition of immune complexes. Moreover, treatment with gold was thought to induce rheumatoid factor in one patient with pemphigus vulgaris.[9] On the other hand, some authors have suggested that gold nephropathy may be more common in rheumatoid arthritis patients lacking anti-IgG antibodies, i.e., those who are "seronegative."[28, 29] In this theory, small amounts of drug-containing complexes might form a nidus that is crucial for the further disposition of anti-immunoglobulin antibody; when the drug is discontinued, the deposits might then resolve. Very small amounts of gold or penicillamine might be difficult to detect within the deposits. An attractive corollary of this hypothesis is that anti-idiotypic antibodies are responsible for the deposits. Much recent experimental work in immunology bears on the observation that antibodies to a given antigen themselves may elicit a second antibody response directed to the antigen-binding site of the first antibody. This second antibody, termed an anti-idiotypic antibody, can react with receptors on B lymphocytes and in this way may be immunoregulatory. Continued or recurrent exposure to the original antigen seems to be necessary for persistent production of both antibodies, but the antigen itself might not necessarily be contained in immune deposits. While this is an attractive theory, there is no direct evidence that anti-idiotypic antibodies or rheumatoid factor–type antibodies play an important role in either drug-induced or idiopathic membranous nephropathy.

In summary, there are several plausible theories concerning the deposition of immune complexes in the glomerular capillaries of drug-associated membranous nephropathy, but experimental evidence is incomplete for all of these. Kidney biopsies from patients with both gold-induced and penicillamine-induced nephrosis usually show immune deposits in the glomeruli. Occasionally, biopsies from patients with penicillamine-induced nephrotic syndrome have been negative by immunofluorescence; the mechanism of the nephrotic syndrome is unclear in such patients.

Penicillamine and gold may act on the immune system in other ways. Indeed, such effects may be the mechanism whereby their therapeutic benefit is derived. However, these other effects may also contribute to the development of nephrotic syndrome in an unknown manner. D-Penicillamine can suppress protein synthesis in certain viruses.[44] This seems to be a specific action, since L-penicillamine and other mercaptans do not have this effect. Penicillamine can impair the maturation of soluble collagen[45] and may thus affect the turnover of the glomerular basement membrane, a structure comprised largely of collagen. Penicillamine can also inhibit the mitogenic transformation of lymphocytes into blasts *in vitro*.[46]

Gold therapy can lead to a reduction of the titer of rheumatoid factor in patients with rheumatoid arthritis,[47, 48] and may also cause a decrease in the serum levels of certain immunoglobulins.[49, 50] Gold salts can also interfere with activation of complement by at least two mechanisms *in vitro*.[51] Other effects include inhibition of numerous cell-mediated immune responses to various mitogens and antigens,[51] impairment of phagocytosis by macrophages and polymorphonuclear leukocytes,[52, 53] and reduced migration of macrophages.[52]

OTHER DRUGS CAUSING PROTEINURIA AND THE NEPHROTIC SYNDROME

Mercury. Nephrotic syndrome has been associated with exposure to various mercury-containing compounds,[54] including mercurial diuretics[55-58] and skin creams containing ammoniated mercury[51] or amino mercuric chloride;[59, 60] moreover, mercuric chloride can induce immune deposits in the glomeruli of rats.[61-63] Most of the cases of the nephrotic syndrome were reported before the widespread availability of immunofluorescence techniques; however, membranous nephropathy with immune deposits has been demonstrated in isolated cases of nephrotic syndrome associated with mercurial diuretics[56] or amino mercuric chloride.[58] With this latter agent, a high incidence of nephrotic syndrome was found in black women in a nonmalarial region of Africa; this occurrence was traced to the use of skin lighteners containing amino mercuric chloride. In these cases, the glomeruli showed membranous nephropathy, and immunofluorescence was positive when performed. Careful reviews of reported cases of nephrotic syndrome in association with severe congestive heart failure disclosed that virtually all patients had received mercurial diuretics.[55, 64]

Hydantoin Anticonvulsants. Treatment with the hydantoin anticonvulsants, trimethadione,[65-68] paramethadione,[67, 69] and mesantoin,[70, 71] has been associated with proteinuria and nephrotic syndrome. The reported cases have usually occurred after the use of these drugs for a year or more. Light microscopy of the kidney has shown minimal glomerular changes, with some reports of mild thickening of the basement membrane. The few cases examined by immunofluorescence were negative by this technique. Many of the reported cases have occurred in children. Biopsies from children with the idiopathic nephrotic syndrome usually show minimal changes on light microscopy and immunofluorescence is often negative. Thus, it is possible that these cases represent the fortuitous occurrence of "lipoid nephrosis" during such therapy. However, there are other observations suggesting that the hydantoins are a real cause of the nephrotic syndrome. First, Heymann et al.[72] were able to induce marked proteinuria in some rats after treatment with trimethadione for more than 1 year. Second, reinstitution of therapy with trimethadione caused the nephrotic syndrome to reappear in two patients cited by Heymann; this happened twice in one case.[68] Finally, although immune deposits have not been documented, some cases had eosinophils infiltrating the glomeruli; this unusual histologic feature suggests a hypersensitivity reaction in the glomeruli that may be associated with these drugs.

Hydantoins can evoke other immunologic reactions, including exfoliative dermatitis, "allergic" mononucleosis, and lymphadenopathy that is associated with fever, rash, eosinophilia, and hepatosplenomegaly. The histology of the lymphadenopathy often cannot be distinguished from that of malignant lymphoma, and this has been termed "pseudolymphoma." Most of these cases have had a benign course, but whether hydantoins can cause a malignant lymphoma is unresolved.[73] It is of interest that nephrotic syndrome has occurred in association with spontaneous lymphomas; however, the renal histology in these cases usually shows the features of membranous nephropathy.[74]

Miscellaneous. Several other agents have been associated with nephrotic syndrome; these agents have been implicated in single-case reports, and the true association is not established. These agents include bismuth,[75] meglumine diatrizoate,[76] probenicid,[77-80] insect repellant,[81] perchlorate,[82] captopril,[83] methimazole,[84] and tolbutamide.[85]

HEROIN

Heroin addicts are thought to have an increased incidence of the nephrotic syndrome. The true incidence is difficult to assess because large numbers of addicts have not been carefully evaluated, and it is difficult to estimate the size of the population at risk. In an early study, Sapira[86] noted a 10 per cent incidence of glomerulonephritis in autopsies of addicts who died while institutionalized; however, details were not given in this report.[86] Thompson et al.[87] reported an 8.1 per cent incidence of proteinuria in 4164 addicts studied. On the other hand, Treser et al.[88] found no difference in the incidence of glomerular abnormalities in the kidneys of 45 addicts who died from overdose or trauma compared with age-matched controls. In a study by Arruda et al., the prevalence of proteinuria was also no different in 145 addicts compared with controls; however, three addicts did have proteinuria of greater than 0.4 gm/day and a renal biopsy of one of the three showed membranous nephropathy.[89] An incidence of nephrotic syndrome as high as 1 per cent could easily have been missed in these latter two reports. Heroin addiction may be associated with various infections, such as hepatitis, septicemia, endocarditis, malaria, and syphilis, which can themselves result in glomerulonephritis and/or the nephrotic syndrome. Therefore, one would expect an increased incidence of the nephrotic syndrome in heroin addicts *a priori*.

Numerous reports have described an increased incidence of glomerular focal and global sclerosis and hyalinosis ("focal sclerosis") in the renal biopsies from addicts with proteinuria[88, 90-97] compared with the incidence of this lesion in nonaddicts with the nephrotic syndrome. The incidence of focal sclerosis in addicts with the nephrotic syndrome is 28 to 100 per cent, whereas the incidence of focal sclerosis is about 12 per cent in adult nonaddicts with nephrotic syndrome.[74, 98] It has been suggested that heroin addiction may be associated with a specific nephropathy.[97] Others have questioned this because glomerular lesions other than focal sclerosis are seen in addicts who seem to be free of infections such as hepatitis and bacterial endocarditis.[94, 99, 100] However, the finding of a disproportionate incidence of focal sclerosis in addicts speaks strongly for either an unusual immunologic reaction in glomeruli to cause the nephrotic syndrome or a specific renal lesion in addicts superimposed on an increased incidence of nephrotic syndrome secondary to infections.

CLINICAL FEATURES

The clinical features of heroin-associated nephrotic syndrome have been remarkably similar in all reported series, regardless of the renal histology. Most patients tend to be in the third decade, and are male and black, observations that may reflect the population of addicts. Usually they have been addicted for 1 to 3 years, although occasionally patients have reported addiction for 15 to 25 years before developing the nephrotic syndrome.[88, 91, 101] Renal disease is usually discovered by routine urinalysis obtained when patients present to clinics for treatment of addiction or when painless edema or anasarca develops. Proteinuria frequently exceeds 10 gm/day. The urinalysis usually reveals many red blood cells with variable numbers of white cells and granular casts. Renal failure progresses rapidly; the majority of cases reach end-stage renal failure and require dialysis by 6 to 48 months after the diagnosis.[93, 96, 102] The combination of findings of hematuria and focal sclerosis in nonaddicted patients also may be associated with a poor prognosis.

It is uncertain whether or not discontinuing the use of heroin can affect the course of the renal disease. All the patients followed by Sreepada et al.[96] continued to use heroin; only two of 11 patients were found to have serum creatinine levels lower than 2 mg/dl during follow-up and one of these two patients was followed for only 2 months. Llach et al.[94] reported improved renal function and markedly lower protein excretion in four patients who claimed to have stopped using heroin.[94] Only one of these patients had focal sclerosis; the other three had focal proliferative glomerulonephritis or focal membranous glomerulonephritis. Nine addicts with focal sclerosis, who received renal transplants, discontinued the use of heroin and had no recurrence of proteinuria over 2 to 29 months of follow-up.[97] Six of these nine patients survived and had no rejection of their transplanted kidneys with serum creatinine levels ranging from 1.2 to 2.7 mg/dl. Two other addicts with functioning transplants continued to use heroin. One died of sepsis at 3 months; the other had proteinuria and renal failure at 20 months, and renal biopsy showed chronic rejection but no recurrence of focal sclerosis. In this regard, it should be noted that spontaneously occurring focal sclerosis often may recur in the transplanted kidneys of non-addicts.

PATHOLOGY

The histology in renal biopsies from heroin addicts has revealed a variety of glomerular abnormalities, including membranous nephropathy, focal glomerulonephritis, proliferative glomerulonephritis, focal sclerosis, and, in some cases, minimal abnormalities. The varied pathology encountered has been reviewed by Arruda and Kurtzman,[100] and has received emphasis in several series.[88, 90, 91, 94, 102] Renal histology in cases of focal sclerosis associated with heroin addiction has shown few distinguishing features from those of the focal sclerosis observed in nonaddicts. Segmental areas of the basement membrane become thickened and eventually sclerotic. There may be a slight increase in mesangial cellularity and in the amount of mesangial matrix. Deposits may be found in areas of segmental basement membrane thickening and, occasionally, in the mesangial matrix with electron microscopy; however, such deposits are usually scanty. Immunofluorescence microscopy usually reveals immunoglobulin and complement components that tend to localize in the areas of thickened basement membrane. IgM is most commonly present, although IgG and other immunoglobulin classes may be encountered. With advanced disease, glomeruli become totally sclerotic, the interstitium may contain mononuclear leukocytic infiltrates, and the renal tubules may atrophy or dilate.

PATHOGENESIS

As with membranous nephropathy, the primary pathogenic event in focal sclerosis associated with heroin abuse is thought to be the deposition of antigen-antibody complexes. The nature of the complexes is unknown. Some have postulated that contaminants in "street" heroin are the putative antigens.[88] However, the consistent tendency to develop focal sclerosis despite wide differences in both drug habits and in the composition of street heroin in different locales suggests that heroin itself is the common factor. Extracellular microparticles have been observed in the glomeruli of heroin users with nephrotic syndrome;[103] the pathogenic significance of these particles is unclear. Attempts to develop an animal model with morphine have resulted in tubular damage but no glomerular lesions.[104] The histologic features of focal sclerosis may represent an unusual immunologic response to a unique antigen or a unique response due to host factors in heroin addicts. There is no evidence available to support or disprove either explanation.

TREATMENT

Withdrawal of heroin has been practically impossible in most cases, as discussed in the previous section. No controlled trials of other therapy have been attempted. The few anecdotal cases treated with steroids alone or in combination with immunosuppressive drugs have not appeared to benefit.

OTHER RENAL DISEASES IN HEROIN ADDICTS

The renal consequences of narcotic abuse have been reviewed.[97, 100] Rhabdomyolysis with myoglobinuria and acute renal failure may occur in association with coma from drug overdoses. Rhabdomyolysis may occur as a consequence of muscle necrosis resulting from prolonged immobilization following heroin overdose or as a direct toxic effect of heroin on muscles. Rarely, tetanus may cause rhabdomyolosis in addicts. Infections such as hepatitis, endocarditis, and syphilis are common in addicts and may lead to glomerulonephritis or to interstitial nephritis when such infections are treated with certain antibiotics (see next section). Addicts may have necrotizing angiitis that has been attributed to intravenous amphetamines, and such vaculitis may affect the kidney (see section on vasculitis and glomerulonephritis).

ACUTE INTERSTITIAL NEPHRITIS

This disorder is a clinicopathologic entity characterized by an inflammatory process involving the interstitium of the kidneys with varying degrees of renal failure in patients exposed to one or more of a growing list of drugs (Table 7–2). The distinguishing features of acute interstitial nephritis include the clinical triad of fever, eosinophilia, and rash and the histologic finding of numerous eosinophils within the renal interstitium. Together, these features distinguish acute interstitial nephritis from acute pyelonephritis and from chronic interstitial disorders, such as analgesic nephropathy (see Chapter 8).

METHICILLIN

CLINICAL FEATURES

All age groups may develop acute interstitial nephritis with methicillin therapy. The incidence is unknown but may be more common in children, in whom a 13 per cent incidence of urinary abnormalities but little or no renal failure has been reported with methicillin therapy.[105] The clinical manifestations of 72 cases reported before 1977 were analyzed by Ditlove et al.:[106] A 3:1 predilection for males was noted. The likelihood of developing

TABLE 7-2. AGENTS ASSOCIATED WITH ACUTE INTERSTITIAL NEPHRITIS

Association Strongly Supported
Methicillin
Penicillin
Cephalothin
Ampicillin
Ibuprofen
Naproxen
Fenoprofen
Probable Association
Carbenicillin
Cephaloridine
Oxacillin
Sulfonamides
Phenindione
Rifampin
Thiazide diuretics
Furosemide
Association Poorly Supported
Tetracycline
Phenytoin

nephritis was not influenced by either the mean daily dose or the total dose of methicillin. The onset of the clinical syndrome usually appeared at 10 to 20 days of therapy, but was also observed after as few as 2 days to as long as 6 weeks. The most common findings were hematuria (97 per cent), which was often gross but sometimes only microscopic, proteinuria (93 per cent), sterile pyuria (92 per cent), fever (88 per cent), and eosinophilia (80 per cent). A transient rash, which was often generalized, morbilliform, and pruritic, was present in 20 per cent of cases. A fever of 39 to 40°C usually persisted until methicillin therapy was discontinued. Eosinophilia ranged from 7 to 66 per cent, and absolute counts ranged from 520 to 5500 eosinophils per cu mm. In a report from our institution, eosinophiluria was found in each of nine cases with urine examined by Wright's stain;[107] eosinophils accounted for a mean of 33 per cent of white cells in the urine, and the eosinophiluria tended to disappear as renal function improved in these patients. Eosinophiluria is unusual in other renal diseases;[109] it may occur during renal transplant rejection but usually does not exceed 5 per cent.[108] Wright's stain may fail to color the granules in eosinophils, possibly owing to the pH of urine; in such cases, eosinophils may be distinguished by their bilobed nuclei.[107] Renal scintiscans using gallium citrate were abnormal in each of three cases so studied by Linton and Lindsey.[110]

Renal function was highly variable in afflicted patients. Some patients, especially children,[105] had only abnormalities of the urinary sediment that cleared within days of stopping the methicillin. One mild case without renal insufficiency had renal tubular dysfunction manifested by salt wasting, hyperkalemia, and renal tubular acidosis.[111] Other patients had severe impairment of renal function and required dialysis. Over 90 per cent of afflicted patients were said to have recovered normal renal function. In our series, four to seven patients who did not receive prednisone treatment had persistent azotemia with serum creatinine levels remaining elevated at 2.0 to 3.7 mg/dl. Other rare cases with permanent renal impairment have been reported.[112] Six of our patients were treated with 60 mg of prednisone for an average duration of 9.6 days, and their course was compared with that of eight patients not given steroids. The treated patients attained a stable level of improved renal function more rapidly, and their ultimate serum creatinine levels were lower. They experienced no untoward side effects from the steroids. An example of the clinical course of such a patient is shown in Figure 7–1. Although our series was uncontrolled, prednisone was more often given to patients with more severe renal impairment. For these reasons, we advocate the use of steroids for a short period to treat patients with severe impairment in renal function. It should be noted that others have reported individual cases with no apparent benefit from steroid therapy.[106] An interesting syndrome has been described consisting of acute eosinophilic interstitial nephritis, granulomas of the marrow and lymph nodes, and anterior uveitis;[113] this condition might be confused with the drug-associated nephropathy.

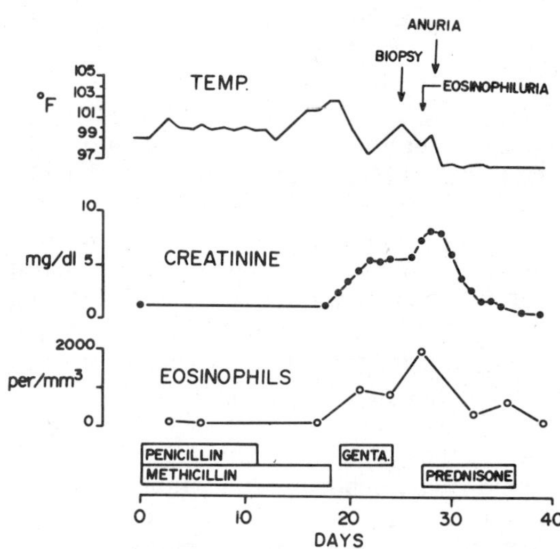

Figure 7–1. Clinical course of a patient who developed acute interstitial nephritis in association with therapy with methicillin (12 g/day) and penicillin (12 million units/day) therapy for pyoderma and cellulitis. The fever, azotemia and eosinophilia in the peripheral blood are typical of this syndrome; anuria is less commonly encountered. Numerous eosinophils were detected in the urine near the peak of the peripheral eosinophilia. A renal biopsy showed interstitial nephritis with a leukocytic infiltrate containing mononuclear cells and numerous eosinophils, findings which excluded gentamicin (GENTA) therapy as a cause of the renal damage. The clinical syndrome promptly remitted with a rapid diuresis concomitant with therapy with prednisone 60 mg/day for 7 days. (This case was included in the report by Galpin et al.[107])

PATHOLOGY

The interstitium of the kidney shows cellular infiltrates that may contain lymphocytes, macrophages, and, occasionally, polymorphonuclear granulocytes, but characteristically also includes varying numbers of eosinophils. Interstitial edema is also seen. Tubular cells may degenerate, desquamate, and occasionally form casts. Glomerular abnormalities are usually absent. Immunofluorescence microscopy may reveal linear deposition of IgG, C_3, and other immunoglobulins, but most cases are negative. Electron-dense deposits are usually not revealed by electron microscopy.

PATHOGENESIS

Several lines of evidence suggest that the interstitial nephritis developing in association with methicillin is mediated through an allergic-type immune reaction. The clinical triad of fever, rash, and eosinophilia and the interstitial infiltrates containing eosinophils and white cells support this view. The onset after 10 to 20 days of therapy is consistent with a primary immune response. The earlier onset or the rapid reappearance of interstitial nephritis, in some cases within hours of rechallenge with methicillin,[114] probably occurs on account of prior sensitization to methicillin or to a cross-reacting penicillin antigen (discussed later). Circulating IgE levels have been reported to be elevated in certain patients,[115] and antibodies to various penicillin antigens can be found in serum from other patients.[116, 117]

The results of renal biopsies utilizing immunofluorescence microscopy have been conflicting, with the majority of cases being negative by this technique. Isolated reports have described linear deposits of IgG and C_3 along the tubular basement membranes in the kidneys of patients with interstitial nephritis associated with methicillin therapy.[116, 117] In the one case studied by immunofluorescence, Baldwin et al.[116] demonstrated dimethoxyphenylpenicilloyl haptenic groups, the major antigen of methicillin, bound to the tubular basement membrane and also present in other sites in the kidneys.[116] Border et al.[117] also found methicillin antigen along the tubular basement membrane in a single case report. Antibodies to the tubular basement membrane but not to methicillin were found in this patient's serum. Antikidney antibodies were also found in the serum of other cases of interstitial nephritis associated with methicillin therapy.[118, 119] Delayed skin tests were positive with 0.1 M methicillin but negative with 0.1 M penicillin in two studies.[116, 117] It was posulated that either methicillin binds to the tubular basement membrane in certain patients and elicits an immune response or that the immune response is unique in susceptible patients, or that both may occur.[116, 117] The immune response might be mediated by antitubular basement membrane antibodies and/or by a cellular immune response to the methicillin bound in the kidneys, as shown by studies of experimental interstitial disease of the kidneys.[120, 122] The feasibility of such a mechanism was especially well demonstrated in an experimental model using fluorescein isothiocyanate as a hapten that can bind to structures in the kidneys.[122] Tamm-Horsfall protein has been detected in the interstitium in some cases,[123] and Hoyer has produced experimental interstitial nephritis in rats by immunization with Tamm-Horsfall protein.[124]

In spite of the positive findings on immunofluorescence cited previously, most cases of interstitial nephritis in association with methicillin therapy have been negative when studied by immunofluorescence. Moreover, linear immunofluorescence may be seen late but not early in the course of experimental interstitial nephritis in the rat. This observation suggests that IgG deposits on the tubular basement membrane may represent a secondary response and not the primary pathogenic mechanism. Thus, an immune reaction is almost certainly responsible for the interstitial nephritis, but it is not clear whether it is mediated through humoral or cellular mechanisms, either of which may involve eosinophils and/or lymphocytes.

Patients who develop acute interstitial nephritis while receiving treatment with methicillin often require further therapy with antibiotics. The question then arises whether or not another penicillin can be safely substituted. Cross sensitization between methicillin and other penicillins may occur with ampicillin,[114] cephalothin,[125, 126] and nafcillin[127] and cause a recurrence of acute interstitial nephritis. However, such cross sensitizations occur sporadically,[127, 129] and patients who develop interstitial nephritis with methicillin therapy may or may not incur a second episode of nephritis when another penicillin is substituted. The explanation for this observation may be that antibodies (or cellular immune responses) in different patients may be primarily directed at antigenic determinants that are *either* drug specific *or* shared among different penicillins. Drug-specific and cross-reacting antibodies for both penicillin G and cephalosporin are known to occur,[130] and the same kind of specificities have been inferred for methicillin.[116, 117] However, because cross sensitization is relatively uncommon and the resultant recurrence of interstitial nephritis is usually reversible, it may be justified to substitute another penicillin to treat certain patients who require further therapy with antibiotics.

Antigenically unrelated drugs, such as vancomycin,[106, 127] aminoglycosides,[118] and lincomycin,[127] can be substituted to treat persistent infections; however, the dosage of certain drugs may need adjustment because of the possibility of direct renal toxicity in patients whose interstitial nephritis may not have completely resolved.

OTHER PENICILLINS

Interstitial nephritis probably can occur with penicillin G and with other semisynthetic penicillins. Thus, the syndrome has been reported in association with treatment with carbenicillin,[131] cephalothin,[126, 132, 135] cephradine,[136] penicillin,[137, 139] ampicillin,[140, 143] and oxacillin.[144] In many of these reports, patients received other drugs that might explain the nephritis. We have encountered a single case of interstitial nephritis with the typical clinical features in a patient who received ampicillin and no other drug. One case associated with penicillin appeared after just 3 days of therapy; certain evidence suggests that complement had been activated by the alternative pathway in this patient.[145] The risk of interstitial nephritis is probably less with penicillin and ampicillin, which are used very commonly; yet, such cases are reported only rarely.[146] The relative risk with the less commonly used penicillins is difficult to estimate. The direct nephrotoxicity of cephaloridine and the possible synergistic toxicity of a combination of cephalothin and an aminoglycoside is well recognized,[132] as is discussed in Chapter 5.

SULFONAMIDES

Sulfonamide therapy has been associated with a variety of renal lesions, including tubular obstruction, acute tubular necrosis, interstitial nephritis, glomerular abnormalities, and vasculitis.[147, 148] A large number of reports appeared mainly in the 1940's,[146, 155] and it is difficult to abstract a clear notion of the immunopathology from the available data. Intrarenal obstruction was more common with earlier sulfonamide preparations that were less soluble in the tubular fluid. Some of the cases that were called interstitial nephritis were probably inflammatory reactions to necrotic tubules destroyed by obstruction due to the deposition of sulfa crystals. Renal histology in other cases revealed granulomatous lesions with mononuclear leukocytes, eosinophils, and polymorphonuclear granulocytes.[151, 154] More et al.[151] described eight such cases, five of which had similar granulomas in other organs, such as the liver and heart.[151] A review of autopsies at the Army Institute of Pathology described cases of interstitial nephritis and occasional glomerular lesions that were associated with sulfa drugs, but the details were not given.[147] The sheer number of cases reported lends support to the renal association between interstitial nephritis and sulfonamide use. The relative paucity of recent case reports is difficult to explain, but the reduced use of sulfonamides due to the advent of newer antibiotics is at least one factor.[156-160] Robison et al.[159] attributed one case of renal impairment to sulfa. Kalowski et al.[156] observed decreased renal function in 16 patients treated with sulfamethoxazole alone (two cases) or in combination with trimethoprim (14 cases). However, most of these patients had underlying renal disorders, so the pathogenic mechanism could not be explored. Two patients without previous renal disease showed acute tubular necrosis and interstitial inflammation. The onset of the clinical findings appeared at a mean of 10 days, and most patients recovered within 10 days of discontinuing the drug. However, permanent impairment of renal function was observed in three cases.

DIURETICS

There have been eight reported cases of interstitial nephritis attributed to thiazide and furosemide diuretics, both of which are sulfonurea derivatives.[161, 163] All but one of these cases[163] received at least one other drug that also has been associated with interstitial nephritis. However, the recurrence of the clinical syndrome on reinstitution of therapy with either thiazide or furosemide in two cases[162] and a second clinical episode with thiazide therapy in a patient who had initially developed acute interstitial nephritis with furosemide suggest that the association is real. However, it must be rare. It is of interest that in four of these cases the syndrome of interstitial nephritis developed in patients with preexisting nephrotic syndrome.[162] Because of possible increased susceptibility, the diagnosis of acute interstitial nephritis should be suspected when nephrotic patients who are being treated with these diuretics develop sudden worsening of renal function. All the reported cases recovered to their prior level of renal function on withdrawal of the diuretic; some patients were treated with steroids. Some of the clinical features were similar to those noted previously for acute interstitial nephritis associated with methicillin therapy; however, the disease appeared to be less acute in most cases, and renal insufficiency developed only over several months of treatment in some patients.

NONSTEROIDAL ANTI-INFLAMMATORY DRUGS

The development of the nephrotic syndrome and renal failure with histologic features of acute interstitial nephritis in the kidneys has been described in patients receiving ibuprofen, naproxen, or fenoprofen,[164-169] all of which have been recently introduced. The syndrome is distinct from the chronic interstitial nephritis that is observed in association with analgesics, such as aspirin and phenacetin (see Chap. 18), and also has features distinct from those of methicillin-associated interstitial nephritis. The renal failure has appeared acutely, but only after several months of treatment; some cases were oliguric and most required dialysis. The renal failure reversed within 2 to 7 weeks after discontinuation of the drug independent of whether or not steroids were used.[164, 168] Fever, rash, eosinophilia, eosinophiluria, and synovitis have been notably reported, but are usually absent. The risk of incurring this form of acute interstitial nephritis appears to be quite small.[165]

Renal biopsies have shown tubular necrosis and atrophy, disrupted tubular basement membranes, and inflammatory infiltrates of lymphocytes, plasma cells, and eosinophils in the interstitium with eosinophils present in moderate-to-large numbers. Immunofluorescence showed interstitial deposits of IgG and C_3 in one case, but was negative in two others. The glomeruli showed only minor abnormalities on light microscopy and fusion of foot processes on electron microscopy.

Most cases received other drugs that may be associated with renal abnormalities, including aspirin, thiazides, furosemide, or gold salts. However, the distinct clinicopathologic findings and the resolution of the renal failure on discontinuation of the drugs suggests a causal relationship in the few reported cases. The syndrome has only recently been described, and it is included because of the histologic similarities to methicillin-associated interstitial nephritis.

MISCELLANEOUS DRUGS ASSOCIATED WITH INTERSTITIAL NEPHRITIS

Therapy with allopurinol[170] and with a chemically related drug, azathioprine,[171] has been associated with interstitial nephritis in a few cases. Phenindione, an anticoagulant commonly used in Europe, has been implicated commonly.[172, 76] Phenytoin has also been associated with interstitial nephritis in two cases, both children.[177, 178] Hyman et al.[177] demonstrated the presence of phenytoin in the tubular basement membrane of cortical tubules, in the interstitium, and in the walls of small blood vessels.[177] Antibodies to tubular basement membranes were present in the serum, and IgG was demonstrated along the tubular basement membranes. Lymphocytes from two patients could be induced *in vitro* to undergo blast transformation with the addition of phenytoin, but not by other antigens;[177, 178] moreover, granulomas were observed in the renal interstitium. These observations are consistent with a cellular immune response being the pathogenic mechanism.

An interesting association of acute renal failure with *intermittent* rifampin therapy has been noted in several case reports.[179-185] An immune mechanism has been postulated because of the rapid appearance of fever, abdominal symptoms, and anuria that followed the ingestion of a single dose in some cases, and because symptoms have reappeared in sensitive patients who are reexposed to the drug. One case had eosinophilia in the peripheral blood; this case[180] and another[186] showed interstitial nephritis with eosinophils on renal biopsy. However, biopsies in other cases have shown acute tubular necrosis[185] or only sparse interstitial infiltrates of lymphocytes. Immunofluorescence has been negative when performed. Whether or not these cases represent acute tubular necrosis secondary to a systemic reaction to rifampicin or a specific immunologic renal lesion is unclear.

VASCULITIS AND GLOMERULONEPHRITIS

Treatment with certain drugs has been associated with a systemic vasculitis of the skin and other organs, such as the liver, heart, lungs, spleen, and kidneys (Table 7–3). When the kidneys are involved, there may be glomerular abnormalities accompanying vasculitis of the small- or medium-sized arterioles. In some cases, the renal manifestations may predominate. Whether drug-associated vasculitis ever occurs exclusively in the kidneys is unclear, but it certainly must be rare. Certain cases of microscopic polyarteritis in the kidneys may represent a hypersensitivity angiitis; no drugs have been identified as potential antigens, but hepatitis antigen has been suggested in some cases.[187]

Patients with a systemic vasculitis may have renal abnormalities that are *not* due to kidney involvement *per se*. Thus hemolysis can result in hemoglobinuria and lead to acute tubular necrosis in certain cases, and thrombocytopenia may cause bleeding into the urine from relatively minor abnormalities in the kidneys or urinary tract. Prerenal azotemia may occur from a variety of causes. In such cases, a renal biopsy might be helpful to discern the degree of kidney involvement. On the other hand, the findings of focal areas of vasculitis in the kidney of a patient with generalized vasculitis is neither surprising nor particularly helpful except in extreme cases. Moreover, a renal biopsy to document renal involvement is often not necessary before the clinician embarks on a course of therapy to treat the vasculitis in other involved organs.

TABLE 7–3. AGENTS ASSOCIATED WITH SYSTEMIC VASCULITIS THAT MAY INVOLVE THE KIDNEY

Penicillin
Methicillin
Allopurinol
Thiazides
Amphetamines
Hyperimmune antisera (e.g., antitetanus serum, antilymphocyte serum)
Toxoids
Hydrocarbons

PENICILLINS

Penicillin and methicillin have been associated with either acute glomerulonephritis or with diffuse vasculitis,[188-191] which was sometimes clinically similar to polyarteritis nodosa. However, most of these reports appeared before 1967, and there is a striking paucity of reports since the recognition of glomerulonephritis occurring in association with many bacterial and viral infections. Schrier et al. reported four cases and reviewed an additional 22 other cases in 1966.[188] Renal biopsies were not performed in all cases, and it is possible that some of the collected cases actually had interstitial nephritis, an entity that was not widely recognized at that time. A causal relationship between the penicillins and either glomerulonephritis or renal vasculitis, therefore, remains unproven.[193]

DRUGS CAUSING A LUPUS-LIKE SYNDROME

Therapy with numerous different drugs has been associated with a syndrome that resembles systemic lupus erythematosus (Table 7–4); several extensive reviews are available on this subject.[192-196] Renal involvement in drug-induced lupus with different drugs is uncommon to extremely rare. When the kidneys are involved, there may be proteinuria, cylindruria, microscopic hematuria, and/or azotemia. Such renal manifestations are generally mild and rapidly reversible when the offending drug is discontinued. Results from a few renal biopsies have been reported from such cases,[197-200] but only a few of these biopsies have shown histologic abnormalities that were typical for renal involvement with lupus erythematosus.

The majority of reported cases of drug-induced lupus have been attributed to three drugs; namely, hydralazine, procainamide, and isoniazid. Alarcon-Segovia incriminated these three drugs and certain anticonvulsants as drugs that induce a lupus-like syndrome as a consequence of sustained plasma levels,[193] i.e., as a function of dose and duration of therapy. It is of interest in this regard that these three drugs are all metabolized by the hepatic *N*-acetyltransferase system and that patients who are slow acetylators may be more prone to develop a lupus-like syndrome while ingesting these agents.

Other drugs that may induce a lupus-like

TABLE 7–4. AGENTS ASSOCIATED WITH A SYNDROME RESEMBLING SYSTEMIC LUPUS ERYTHEMATOSUS THAT MAY INVOLVE THE KIDNEY

Association Strongly Supported
Hydralazine
Procainamide
Isoniazid
Possible Association
D-Penicillamine
Hydantoin anticonvulsants
Ethosuximide
Thiouracils
Trimethadione
Doubtful Association
Reserpine
Quinidine

syndrome include *D*-penicillamine,[201] hydantoin anticonvulsants,[202, 203] ethosuximide,[204-206] thiouracils,[199, 207] and trimethadione.[197] The evidence implicating these drugs is less compelling than for hydralazine and procainamide. Therapy with most of these drugs is associated with an increased incidence of antinuclear antibodies. However, the risk of developing a full-blown lupus syndrome must be less for those latter drugs, as judged from the paucity of reported cases. Renal involvement has not been clearly documented for most, if not all, of these drugs; however, this may be owing to the small number of exposed patients, only a fraction of whom might be expected to develop renal involvement. Other drugs that had been reported to induce lupus were dismissed as potential causes in a critical review by Lee and Chase;[195] they are not discussed here, but are included in Table 7–4.

Whether these various drugs cause a specific syndrome or merely unmask lupus erythematosus in patients with a preexisting predisposition toward this disease is a question that may be unanswerable. However, several observations suggest that drug-induced lupus is a separate syndrome that may share certain pathogenic mechanisms with the naturally occurring disease. First, the age distribution of affected patients is different in drug-induced lupus. Second, the syndrome usually remits rapidly when the offending drug is withdrawn. Third, certain drugs, notably procainamide, can be associated with a high incidence of the syndrome when given in large doses for prolonged periods. Finally, experimental animals develop antinuclear antibodies in their serum when they are given these drugs.[197]

OTHER DRUGS AND TOXINS

Allopurinol and thiazides can be associated with the development of purpuric skin rashes and vasculitis elsewhere, including the blood vessels and glomeruli in the kidneys; however, only a few renal biopsies have been performed.[208-211] Citron et al.[212] reported 14 cases of necrotizing angiitis in drug abusers taking a variety of drugs, and usually more than one drug. Heroin and amphetamines or lysergic acid diethylamide (LSD) and amphetamines were the most common combinations of drugs taken; amphetamine was the only drug used by one patient. Five of these cases had evidence of renal involvement, with proteinuria, hematuria, azotemia, and/or renal failure. Renal histology showed arteritis in two of these patients.

Treatment with hyperimmune antisera can result in serum sickness. Examples include antitetanus antisera for the treatment of tetanus and the administration of antilymphocyte antisera to renal transplant recipients.[213] The systemic manifestations, such as fever, arthralgias, and skin rash, predominate. The glomerulonephritis that can occur is usually mild and self-limiting. Vaccination with toxoids can result in glomerular injury.[214, 215] In one extreme case, a nurse injected herself repeatedly with toxoids and developed glomerulonephritis that resolved after the injections were discontinued.[216]

Exposure to a variety of hydrocarbons has been linked with the occurrence of glomerulonephritis, especially glomerulonephritis due to antiglomerular basement membrane antibodies.[217-223] The data are difficult to interpret for several reasons: First, a wide variety of hydrocarbons have been included as possible etiologic agents, and no single compound or class of compounds has emerged as a potential toxin. Moreover, the types and duration of exposure have varied widely, and, in some cases, the exposure appears to have been quite remote from the development of glomerulonephritis. Second, nearly everyone living in a Western society encounters some environmental exposure to potentially toxic hydrocarbons, such as exhaust fumes and various solvents used as cleaning agents; despite this exposure, the development of glomerulonephritis is rare. Third, genetic factors probably play some role as evidenced by reports of exposure-related glomerulonephritis in twins[220] and in families.[219] Of interest, glomerulonephritis with antiglomerular basement membrane antibodies developed in one pair of identical twins within a few months of each other; both had encountered brief industrial exposure to different hydrocarbons. Finally, the same form of glomerulonephritis can occur in patients who have no clear history of exposure and no apparent genetic predisposition. Thus, multiple factors may play permissive or pathogenic roles. At present, the role of exposure to hydrocarbons is not clear.

REFERENCES

1. Sigler JW, Bluhm GB, Duncan H, et al.: Gold salts in the treatment of rheumatoid arthritis. Ann. Intern. Med. *80*:21–26, 1974.
2. Andrews FM, Golding DN, Freeman AM, et al.: Controlled trial of D-penicillamine in severe rheumatoid arthritis. Lancet *1*:275–280, 1973.
3. Sternlieb I: Penicillamine and the nephrotic syndrome. J.A.M.A. *198*:173–174, 1966.
4. Kean WF, Dwosh IL, Anastassiades TP, et al.: The toxicity pattern of D-penicillamine therapy. A guide to its use in rheumatoid arthritis. Arthritis Rheum. *23*:158–164, 1980.
5. Felts JH, Hing JS, Boyce WH: Nephrotic syndrome after treatment with D-penicillamine. Lancet *1*:53–54, 1968.
6. Jaffe IA, Treser, G, Suzuki Y, et al.: Nephropathy induced by D-penicillamine. Ann. Intern. Med. *69*:549–556, 1968.
7. Weiss AS, Markenson JA, Weiss MS, et al: Toxicity of D-penicillamine in rheumatoid arthritis. Am. J. Med. *64*:114–120, 1978.
8. Hartfall SJ, Garland HG, Goldie W: Gold treatment of arthritis, a review of 900 cases. Lancet *2*:828–842, 1937.
9. Penneys NS, Eaglestein WH, Frost P: Management of pemphigus with gold compounds. Arch. Dermatol. *112*:185–187, 1976.
10. Skrifvars B: Hypothesis for the pathogenesis of sodium aurothiomalate (Myocrisin) induced immune complex nephritis. Scand. J. Rheumatol. *8*(2):113–118, 1979.
11. Norton WL, Lewis DC, Eiff M: Electron dense deposits following injection of gold sodium thiomalate and thiomalic acid. Arthritis Rheum. *11*:436–443, 1968.
12. Silverberg DS, Kidd EG, Shnitka TK, et al.: Gold nephropathy: A clinical and pathologic study. Arthritis Rheum. *13*:812–825, 1970.
13. Empire Rheumatism Council, Research Subcommittee: Gold therapy in rheumatoid arthritis. Final report of multi-center controlled trial. Ann. Rheum. Dis. *20*:315–334, 1961.
14. Empire Rheumatism Council, Research Subcommittee: Gold therapy in rheumatoid arthritis. Report of a multi-center controlled trial. Ann. Rheum. Dis. *19*:95–119, 1960.
15. Adams DA, Goldman R, Maxwell MH, et al.: Nephrotic syndrome associated with penicillamine therapy of Wilson's disease. Am. J. Med. *36*:330–336, 1964.
16. Hirschman SZ, Isselbacher KJ: The nephrotic syndrome as a complication of penicillamine therapy for hepatolenticular degeneration (Wilson's disease). Ann. Intern. Med. *62*:1297–1300, 1965.
17. Goldberg A, Smith JA, Lockhead AC: Treatment of lead poisoning oral penicillamine. Br. Med. J. *1*:1270–1275, 1963.
18. Cramer K: D-Penicillamine and *N*-acetyl-D penicillamine in lead poisoning. Postgrad. Med. J. *50*:(Suppl. 2): 14–16, 1974.
19. Rosenberg LE, Hayslett JP: Nephrotoxic effects of penicillamine in cystinuria. J.A.M.A. *201*:128–129, 698–699, 1965.
20. Lange K: Nephropathy induced by D-penicillamine. Contrib. Nephrol. *10*:63–74, 1978.
21. Seelig HP, Seelig R, Fisher A, et al.: Glomerular immune-complex deposition in rats following oral application of D-penicillamine. Kidney Int. *11*:219, 1977.
22. Nagi AH, Alexander F, Barabas AZ: Gold nephropathy in rats: light and electron microscoic studies. Exp. Mol. Pathol. *15*:354–362, 1971.
23. Bacon PA, Tribe CR, Mackenzie JC, et al.: Penicillamine nephropathy in rheumatoid arthritis. Q. J. Med. *180*:661–684, 1976.
24. Day AT, Golding JR: Hazards of penicillamine therapy in the treatment of rheumatoid arthritis. Postgrad. Med. *50*:71–73, 1974.
25. Samuels B, Lee JC, Engleman EP, Hopper J, Jr.: Membranous nephropathy in patients with rheumatoid arthritis: Relationship to gold therapy. Medicine *57*:319–327, 1977.
26. Neild GH, Gärtner H-V, Bohle A: Penicillamine induced membranous glomerulonephritis. Scand. J. Rheumatol 28(Suppl.):79–90, 1979.
27. Vaamonde CA, Hunt FR: The nephrotic syndrome as a complication of gold therapy. Arthritis Rheum. *13*:826–834, 1970.
28. Skrifvars BV, Törnroth TS, Tallqvist GN: Gold induced immune complex nephritis in seronegative rheumatoid arthritis. Ann. Rheum. Dis. *36*:549–556, 1977.
29. Törnroth T, Skrifvars B: Gold nephropathy prototype of membranous glomerulonephritis. Am. J. Pathol. *75*:573–590, 1974.
30. Silverberg DS, Kidd EG, Shnitka TK, et al.: Gold nephropathy: A clinical and pathologic study. Arthritis Rheum. *13*:812–825, 1970.
31. Törnroth T, Skrifvars B: The development and resolution of glomerular basement membrane changes associated with subepithelial immune deposits. Am. J. Pathol. *79*:219–236, 1975.
32. Bran C, Olsen ST, Raaschon R, et al.: The localization of gold in the human kidney following chrysotherapy. Nephron *1*:265–276, 1964.
33. Watanabe I, Whittier FC, Moore J, et al.: Gold nephropathy. Ultrastructural, fluorescence and microanalytical studies of two patients. Arch. Path. Lab. Med. *100*:632–635, 1976.
34. Ganote CE, Beaver DL, Moses HL: Renal gold inclusions: A light and electron microscopic study. Arch. Pathol. *81*:429–438, 1966.
35. Couser WG, Steinmuller DR, Stilmant MM, et al.: Experimental glomerulonephritis in the isolated perfused rat kidney. J. Clin. Invest. *62*:1275–1287, 1978.
36. Barnett EV, Knutson DW, Chia D, et al.: The importance of circulating soluble immune complexes. Ann. Intern. Med. *91*:430–440, 1979.

37. Palosuo T, Provost TT, Milgram F: Gold nephropathy: Serologic data suggesting an immune complex disease. Clin. Exp. Immunol. *25*:311–318, 1976.
38. Wilson CB, Dixon FJ: Antigen quantitation in experimental immune complex glomerulonephritis. I. Acute serum sickness. J. Immunol. *105*:279–290, 1970.
39. Lee JC, Dushkin M, Eyring EJ, et al.: Renal lesions associated with gold therapy. Light and electron microscopic studies. Arthritis Rheum. *8*:1–13, 1965.
40. Stuve J, Galle P: Role of mitochondria in the handling of gold by the kidney. A study of electron microscopy and electron probe microanalysis. J. Cell Biol. *44*:667–676, 1970.
41. Edgington TS, Glassock RJ, Dixon RJ: Autologous immune complex nephritis induced with renal tubular antigen. J. Exp. Med. *127*:555–571, 1968.
42. Naruse T, Kitamura K, Miyakawa Y, et al.: Deposition of renal tubular epithelial antigen along the glomerular capillary walls of patients with membranous glomerulonephritis. J. Immunol. *110*:1163–1166, 1973.
43. McIntosh RM, Griswold WR, Chernack WB, et al.: Cryoglobulins III. Further studies on the nature, incidence, clinical diagnostic, prognostic and immunopathologic significance of cryoproteins in renal disease. Q. J. Med. *174*:285, 1975.
44. Jaffe IA, Merryman P, Hrenfeld EE: Further studies of the anti-viral effect of D-penicillamine. Postgrad. Med. *50*(Suppl. 2):50–55, 1974.
45. Francis MJO, Mowat AG: Effects of D-penicillamine on skin collagen in man. Postgrad. Med. *50*(Suppl. 2):30–33, 1974.
46. Roath S, Wills R: The effects of penicillamine on lymphocytes in culture. Postgrad. Med. J. *50*(Suppl. 2):56–57, 1974.
47. Gottlieb NL, Kiem IM, Penneys NS, et al.: The influence of crysotherapy on serum protein and immunoglobulin levels, rheumatoid factor, and antiepithelial antibody titers. J. Lab. Clin. Med. *86*:962–971, 1975.
48. Klinefelter HF, Achurra A: Effect of gold salts and antimalarials on the rheumatoid factor in rheumatoid arthritis. Scand. J. Rheumatol. *2*:177–182, 1973.
49. Bluestone R, Goldberg LS: Effect of D-penicillamine on serum immunoglobulins and rheumatoid factor. Ann. Rheum. Dis. *32*:50–52, 1973.
50. Stanworth DR, Hunneyball IM: Influence of D-penicillamine treatment on the humoral immune system. Scand. J. Rheumatol. *28*(S):37–46, 1979.
51. Harth M: Gold and modulations of the immune response. J. Rheumatol. *6*(S):7–11, 1979.
52. Vernon-Roberts B, Jessop JD, Doré J: Effects of gold salts and prednisolone on inflammatory cells. II. Suppression of inflammation and phagocytosis in the rat. Ann. Rheum. Dis. *32*:301–309, 1973.
53. Jessop JD, Vernon-Roberts B, Harris J: Effects of gold salts and prednisolone on inflammatory cells. I. Phagocytic activity of macrophages and polymorphs in inflammatory exudates studied by a "skin window" technique in rheumatoid and control patients. Ann. Rheum. Dis. *32*:294–300, 1973.
54. Kazantzis G, Schiller KFR, Asscher AW, et al.: Albuminuria and the nephrotic syndrome following exposure to mercury and its compounds. Q. J. Med. *31*:403–418, 1962.
55. Hilton PG, Jones NF, Tighe JR: Nephrotic syndrome with heart disease: A reappraisal. Br. Med. J. *3*:584–586, 1968.
56. Cameron JS, Trourre JR: Mebranous glomerulonephritis and the nephrotic syndrome appearing during mersalyl therapy. Guy's Hosp. Rep. *114*:101–107, 1965.
57. Becker CG, Becker EL, Maher JF, et al.: Nephrotic syndrome after contact with mercury: A report of five cases, three after use of ammoniated mercury ointment. Arch. Intern. Med. *110*:178–186, 1962.
58. Burston J, Darmady EM, Stranack F: Nephrosis due to mercurial diuretics. Br. Med. J. *1*:1277–1278, 1958.
59. Kibukamusoke JW, Davies DR, Hutt MSR: Membranous nephropathy due to skin lightening cream. Br. Med. J. *11*:646–647, 1974.
60. Barr RD, Rees PH, Cordy PE, et al.: Nephrotic syndrome in adult Africans in Nairobi. Br. Med. J. *1*:131–134, 1972.
61. Bariety J, Druet P: Glomerulonephritis with γ and β C-globulin deposits induced in rats by mercuric chloride. Am. J. Pathol. *65*:293–302, 1971.
62. Druet P, Druet E, Potdevin F, et al.: Immune type glomerulonephritis induced by $HgCl_2$ in the Brown Norway rat. Ann. Immunol. *120*:777–792, 1978.
63. Makker SP, Aikawa M: Mesangial glomerulonephropathy with deposition of IgG, IgM and C_3 induced by mercuric chloride: a new model. Lab. Invest. *41*(1):45–50, 1979.
64. Thayer JM, Glecker WJ, Holmes RO: The development of the nephrotic syndrome during the course of congestive heart failure: Case report and review of the literature. Ann. Intern. Med. *54*:1013–1025, 1961.
65. Bar-Khayim Y, Teplitz C, Garella S, et al.: Trimethadione (Tridione[R])-induced nephrotic syndrome. A report of a case with unique ultrastructural renal pathology. Am. J. Med. *54*:272, 1973.
66. Barnet HL, Simmons DJ, Wells RE, Jr.: Nephrotic syndrome occurring during Tridione therapy. Am. J. Med. *4*:760–764, 1948.
67. Heymann W: Nephrotic syndrome after use of trimethadione and paramethadione in petit mal. J.A.M.A. *202*:893–894, 1967.
68. Heymann W: Trimethadione (Tridione[R])-nephrosis. Pediatrics *22*:614–615, 1958.
69. Finkel FC, Israels S: Paradione nephrosis. Lancet *79*:243, 1959.
70. Von Hofle KH, Schoop W: Akutes nephrotisches syndrome bein mesantoin-behandlung. Dtsch. Med. Wochenschr. *84*:837, 1959.
71. Snead C, Siegel N, Hayslett J: Generalized lymphadenopathy and nephrotic syndrome as a manifestation of mephenytoin (mesantoin) toxicity. Pediatrics *57*:98–101, 1976.
72. Heymann W, Hackel DB, Hunter JLP: Trimethadion (Tridione[R]) nephrosis in rats. Pediatrics *25*:112–118, 1970.
73. Gams RA, Neal JA, Conrad FG: Hydantoin-induced pseudo-pseudolymphoma. Ann. Intern. Med. *69*:557–568, 1968.

74. Glassock RJ, Bennett CM: The Glomerulopathies. *In* The Kidney (BM Brenner and FC Rector, eds.). Philadelphia: W. B. Saunders Co., 1976.
75. Beattie JW: Nephrotic syndrome following sodium bismuth tartrate therapy in rheumatoid arthritis. Ann. Rheum. Dis. *12*:144–146, 1953.
76. Borra S, Hawkins D, Duquid W, et al.: Acute renal failure and nephrotic syndrome after angiocardiography with meglumine diatrizoate. N. Engl. J. Med. *284*:592–593, 1971.
77. Ferris TF, Morgan WS, Lenitin H: Nephrotic syndrome caused by probenecid. N. Engl. J. Med. *265*:381–382, 1961.
78. Sokal A, Brashner MH, Kun RO: Nephrotic syndrome caused by probenecid. J.A.M.A. *199*:101–102, 1967.
79. Hertz P, Yager H, Richardson JA: Probenecid-induced nephrotic syndrome. Arch. Pathol. *94*:241–243, 1972.
80. Scott JT, O'Brien PK: Probenecid, nephrotic syndrome and renal failure. Ann. Rheum. Dis. *27*:249–252, 1968.
81. Hoehn D: Nephrosis probably due to excessive use of "Sta-Way" insect repellent. J.A.M.A. *128*:513, 1945.
82. Lee RE, Ulstrom RA, Vernier RL: Nephrotic syndrome as a complication of perchlorate treatment of thyrotoxicosis. N. Engl. J. Med. *264*:1221, 1961.
83. Prins EJ, Hoorntje SJ, Weening JJ, et al.: Nephrotic syndrome in patient on captopril. Lancet *2*:306–307, 1979.
84. Reynolds LR, Bhthena D: Nephrotic syndrome associated with methimazole therapy. Arch. Intern. Med. *139*:236–237, 1979.
85. Schnall C, Winer, JS: Nephrosis during tolbutamide administration. J.A.M.A *167*:214–215, 1958.
86. Sapira JD: The narcotic addict as a medical patient. Am. J. Med. *45*:555–558, 1968.
87. Thompson AM, Antonouyeh T, Lin R, et al.: Focal membranoproliferative glomerulonephritis in heroin users. (Abstract.) Washington, D.C.: Am. Soc. Nephrol., 1973, p. 105.
88. Treser G, Cherubin C, Lonergan ET, et al.: Renal lesions in narcotic addicts. Am. J. Med. *57*:687–694, 1974.
89. Arruda JAL, Kurtzman NA, Veerasamy KG, et al.: Prevalence of renal disease in asymptomatic heroin addicts. Arch. Intern. Med. *135*:535–537, 1975.
90. Ekonyan G, Gyorkey, F, Dichoso C, et al.: Renal involvement in drug abuse. Arch. Intern. Med. *132*:801–806, 1973.
91. Salomon, MI, Pui Poon T, Goldblatt M, et al.: Renal lesions in heroin addicts. A study based on kidney biopsies. Nephron *9*:356–363, 1972.
92. Grishman E, Chung J: Focal glomerulosclerosis in nephrotic patients: An electron microscopy study. Kidney Int. *7*:111–112, 1975.
93. Kilcoyne MM, Daly JJ, Gocke DJ, et al.: Nephrotic syndrome in heroin addicts. Lancet *1*:17–20, 1972.
94. Llach F, Descoeudres C, Massry SG: Heroin associated nephropathy: clinical and histological studies in 19 patients. Clin. Nephrol. *11*:7–12, 1979.
95. McGinn JT, McGinn TG, Cherukin CE, et al.: Nephrotic syndrome in drug addicts. N.Y. State J. Med. *74*:92–95, 1974.
96. Sreepada TK, Nicastri AD, Friedman EA: Natural history of heroin associated nephropathy. N. Engl. J. Med. *290*:19–23, 1974.
97. Sreepada TK, Nicastri AD, Friedman EA: Renal consequences of narcotic abuse. Adv. Nephrol. *7*:261–290, 1970.
98. Earley LE, Forland M: Nephrotic syndrome. In Diseases of the Kidney (LE Early and CW Gottschalk, eds.) Boston: Little, Brown & Co., 1979, pp. 770.
99. Friedman, EA, Sreepada TK, Rao TK, et al.: Heroin associated nephropathy. Nephron *13*:421–426, 1974.
100. Arruda JAL, Kurtzman NA: Heroin addiction and renal disease. Contrib. Nephrology *7*:69–78, 1977.
101. Salomon MI, Pui Poon T, Goldblat M, et al.: Renal lesions in heroin addicts. A study based on kidney biopsies. Nephron *9*:356–363, 1972.
102. Matalon R, Katz L, Gallo G, et al.: Glomerular sclerosis in adults with nephrotic syndrome. Ann. Intern. Med. *80*:488–495, 1974.
103. Davis JS: Extracellular glomerular microparticles in nephrotic syndrome of heroin users. Arch. Pathol. *99*:278–282, 1975.
104. Marchand C, Catin M, Cote M: Evidence for the nephrotoxicity of morphine sulfate in rats. Can. J. Physiol. Pharmacol. *47*:649–655, 1969.
105. Sanjad SA, Haddad GG, Nassar VH: Nephropathy, an underestimated complication of methicillin therapy. J. Pediat. *84*:873–877, 1974.
106. Ditlove J, Weidmann P, Bernstein M, et al.: Methicillin nephritis. Medicine *56*:483–491, 1977.
107. Galpin JE, Shinaberger JH, Stanley TM, et al.: Acute interstitial nephritis due to methicillin. Am. J. Med. *65*:756–765, 1978.
108. Spencer ES, Posborg-Peterson V: The urinary sediment after renal transplantation. Acta Med. Scand. *182*:73–82, 1967.
109. Helgason S, Lindquist B: Eosinophiluria. Scand. J. Urol. Nephrol. *6*:257–259, 1972.
110. Linton AL, Lindsy RM: Antibiotic nephrotoxicity. Controver. Nephrol. *1*:549–559, 1979.
111. Cogan MC, Arieff AI: Sodium wasting, acidosis and hyperkalemia induced by methicillin interstitial nephritis. Am. J. Med. *64*:500–507, 1978.
112. Jensen HA, Halveg AB, Saunamaki KI: Permanent impairment of renal function after methicillin nephropathy. Br. Med. J. *4*:406, 1971.
113. Dobrin RS, Vernier RL, Fish AJ: Acute eosinophilic interstitial nephritis and renal failure with bone marrow-lymph node granulomas and anterior uveitis. Am. J. Med. *59*:325–333, 1975.
114. Gilbert DN, Gourley B, d'Agastino A, et al.: Interstitial nephritis due to methicillin, penicillin and ampicillin. Ann. Allergy *28*:378–385, 1970.
115. Ooi BS, Pesce AS, First MR, et al.: IgE levels in interstitial nephritis. Lancet *1*:1254–1256, 1974.
116. Baldwin DS, Levine BB, McCluskey RT, et al.: Renal failure and interstitial nephritis due to penicillin and methicillin. N. Engl. J. Med. *279*:1245–1252, 1968.
117. Border WA, Lehman DH, Eagan JD, et al.: Antitubular basement membrane antibodies in methicillin-associated interstitial nephritis. N. Engl. J. Med. *291*:381–384, 1974.
118. Mayaud C, Kanfer A, Kourlfisky O, et al.: Interstitial nephritis after methicillin. N. Engl. J. Med. *292*:1132–1133, 1975.

119. Olsen S, Asklund M: Interstitial nephritis with acute renal failure following cardiac surgery and treatment with methicillin. Acta Med. Scand. *199*:305–310, 1973.
120. Steblay RW, Rudofsky U: Renal tubular disease and autoantibodies against tubular basement membrane induced in Guinea pigs. J. Immunol. *107*:589–594, 1971.
121. Baldamus CA, Kachel G, Knoch C, et al.: Cellular immune mechanisms in experimental tubulo-interstitial nephritis. Contrib. Nephrol. *16*:141–146, 1978.
122. Domoto DT, Askenase PW, Kashgariara M: Tubulo-interstitial nephritis (TIN) due to fluorescein isothiocynate (FITC). A possible hapten-immunologially mediated reaction. Kidney Int. *12*:512, 1977.
123. Cotran RS, Galvanek E: Immunopathology of human tubulo-interstitial diseases: Localization of immunoglobulins complement and Tamm-Horsfall protein. Contrib. Nephrol. *16*:126–131, 1979.
124. Hoyer JR: Auto-immune tubulo-interstitial nephritis induced in rats by immunization with Tamm-Horsfall glycoprotein. Kidney Int. *10*:554(A), 1976.
125. Alexander MR, Ensey R: Methicillin nephritis. Drug Intell. Clin. Pharmacol. *8*:115, 1974.
126. Engle JE, Drago J, Carlin B, et al.: Reversible acute renal failure after cephalothin. Ann. Intern. Med. *83*:232–233, 1975.
127. Parry MF, Ball WD, Conte JE, et al.: Nafcillin nephritis. J.A.M.A. *225*:2178, 1973.
128. Doyle WF, Davey FR, Chojnacki RE: Interstitial nephritis associated with methicillin therapy: Case report. Milit. Med. *139*:384–387, 1974.
129. London RD: Hematuria associated with methicillin therapy. J. Pediatr. *70*:285–286, 1967.
130. Petz LD: Immunologic cross-reactivity between penicillins and cephalosporins: A review. J. Infect. Dis. *137*(Suppl.):S74–S79, 1978.
131. Appel GB, Woda BA, Neu HC, et al.: Acute interstitial nephritis associated with carbenicillin therapy. Arch. Intern. Med. *138*:1265–1267, 1978.
132. Barza M: The nephrotoxicity of cephalosporins: An overview. J. Infect. Dis. *137*:S60–S73, 1978.
133. Carling PC, Idelson BA, Casano AA, et al.: Nephrotoxicity associated with cephalothin administration. Arch. Intern. Med. *135*:797–801, 1975.
134. Burton JR, Lichenstein NS, Calvin RB, et al.: Acute renal failure during cephalothin therapy. J.A.M.A. *229*:679–682, 1974.
135. Barrientos A, Bellow I, Gutierrez-Millet V, et al.: Renal failure and cephalothin. Ann. Intern. Med. *84*:612, 1979.
136. Wiles CM, Assem ESK, Cohen SL, et al.: Cephradine-induced interstitial nephritis. Clin. Exp. Immunol. *36*:342–346, 1979.
137. Calvin RB, Burton JR, Hyslop HE, Jr, et al.: Penicillin-associated interstitial nephritis. Ann. Intern. Med. *81*:404–405, 1974.
138. Orchard RT, Rooker G: Penicillin-hypersensitivity nephritis. Lancet *1*:689, 1974.
139. Geller M, Kriz RJ, Zimmerman SW, et al.: Penicillin-associated pulmonary hypersensitivity reaction and interstitial nephritis. Ann. Allergy *37*:183–190, 1976.
140. Woodroffe AJ, Weldon M, Meadows R, et al.: Acute interstitial nephritis following ampicillin hypersensitivity. Med. J. Aust. *1*:65–68, 1975.
141. Ruley ES, Lisi L: Interstitial nephritis and renal failure due to ampicillin. J. Pediatr. *84*:878–881, 1974.
142. Lee HA, Hill CF: The use of ampicillin in renal disease. Brit. J. Clin. Pract. *22*:354–357, 1968.
143. Maxwell D, Szwed JJ, Wahle W, et al.: Ampicillin nephrotoxicity. J.A.M.A. 230:586–587, 1974.
144. Burton, JR, Lichtenstein NS, Colvin RB, et al.: Acute interstitial nephritis of oxacillin. Johns Hopkins Med. J. *134*:58–61, 1974.
145. Walter L, Rosen S, Schur PH: Allergic interstitial nephritis: Report of a case with activation of complement by the alternate pathway. Clin. Nephrol. *3*:153–159, 1975.
146. Kancin, LM, Tuazon CU, Cardella TA, et al.: Comparison of methicillin and nafcillin in the treatment of staphylococcal endocarditis. Clin. Res. *24*:24A, 1976.
147. French AJ: Hypersensitivity in the histopathological changes associated with sulfonamide chemotherapy. Am. J. Pathol. *22*:679–701, 1946.
148. Minetti L, Barbiano-de'Belgioloso G, Busnach G: Immunohistological diagnosis of drug-induced hypersensitivity nephritis. Nephron *11*:526–533, 1975.
149. Murphy FD, Wood WD: Acute nephritis and the effects of sulfonamide on the kidney. Ann. Intern. Med. *18*:999–1005, 1943.
150. Bakken K: The allergic reaction of the kidney to sulfonamide medication. J. Pathol. Bacteriol. *59*:501–504, 1947.
151. More RH, McMillan GC, Lyman-Duff G: The pathology of sulfonamide allergy in man. Am. J. Pathol. *22*:703–725, 1946.
152. Simon MA: Pathologic lesions following the administration of sulfonamide drugs. Am. J. Med. Sci. *205*:439–454, 1943.
153. Prien EL: The mechanism of renal complication in sulfonamide therapy. N. Engl. J. Med. *232*:63–71, 1945.
154. Merkel WC, Crawford RC: Pathologic lesions produced by sulfathiozole: A report of four fatal cases. J.A.M.A. *119*:770–776, 1942.
155. Black-Schaffer B: Pathology of anaphylaxis due to sulfonamide drugs. Arch. Pathol. *39*:301–314, 1945.
156. Kalowski S, Nara RS, Mathew TH, et al.: Deterioration in renal function in association with co-trimoxazole therapy. Lancet *1*:394–397, 1973.
157. Dry J, Leynadier F, Herman D, et al.: Complication immunoallergique de l'association sulfaméthoxazole-triméthoprime: thrombopénie, néphropathie interstitielle aigué, anomalie électrophorétique. Therapie *30*:705–712, 1975.
158. Fialk MA, Romankieioicz J, Pemone F: Allergic interstitial nephritis with diuretics. Ann. Intern. Med. *81*:403–404, 1974.
159. Robson M, Levi J, Dolberg L, et al.: Acute tubulo-interstitial nephritis following sulfadiazine therapy. Isr. J. Med. Sci. *6*:561–566, 1970.
160. Saltissi D, Pusey CD, Rainford DJ: Recurrent acute renal failure due to antibiotic-induced interstitial nephritis. Br. Med. J. *1*:1182–1183, 1979.
161. McMenamin RA, Davies LM, Craswell PW: Drug

induced interstitial nephritis, hepatitis and exfoliative dermatitis. Aust. NZ J. Med. *6*:583–587, 1976.
162. Lyons H, Puin VW, Cortell S, et al.: Allergic interstitial nephritis causing reversible renal failure in four patients with idiopathic nephrotic syndrome. N. Engl. J. Med. *288*:124–128, 1973.
163. Fuller TJ, Barcenas CG, White MG: Diuretic induced interstitial nephritis. J.A.M.A., *235*:1998–1999, 1976.
164. Brezin JH, Katz SM, Schwartz AB, et al.: Reversible renal failure and nephrotic syndrome associated with non-steroidal anti-inflammatory drugs. N. Engl. J. Med. *301*:1271–1273, 1979.
165. Emmerson JL, Gibson WR, Pierce EC, et al.: Preclinical toxicology of fenoprofen. Toxicol. Appl. Pharmacol. *25*:444, 1973.
166. Cartwright KC, Trotter TL, Cohen ML: Naproxen nephrotoxicity. Ariz. Med. *36*:124–126, 1979.
167. Kimberly RP, Bowden RE, Keiser HR, et al.: Reduction of renal function by newer non-steroidal anti-inflammatory drugs. Am. J. Med. *64*:804–807, 1978.
168. Wendland ML, Wagoner RD, Holley KE: Renal failure associated with fenoprofen. Mayo Clin. Proc. *55*:103–107, 1980.
169. Johnson WJ: Nephrotoxicity of non-steroidal anti-inflammatory drugs. Mayo Clin. Proc. *55*:120, 1980.
170. Gelbart DR, Weinstein, AB, Fajardo LF: Allopurinol-induced interstitial nephritis. Ann. Intern. Med. *86*:196–208, 1977.
171. Sloth K, Thomsen AC: Acute renal insufficiency during treatment with azathioprine. Acta Med. Scand. *189*:145–148, 1971.
172. Srear JD, Beaufits P, Maroger LM, et al.: Néphrite interstitielle chronique due á la phenylindanedione faisant siute á une insuffisance rénate aigue. Nouv. Presse Med. *1*:193–196, 1972.
173. Wright JS: Phenindione sensitivity with leukemoid reaction and hepatorenal damage. Postgrad. Med. *46*:452–455, 1970.
174. Baker SB de C, Williams RT: Acute interstitial nephritis due to drug sensitivity. Br. Med. J. *1*:1655–1658, 1963.
175. Heptinstall RH: Interstitial nephritis. Am. J. Pathol. *83*:214–236, 1976.
176. Nicholls MG, Heale WF: Phenindione sensitivity and acute renal failure. Aust. N. Z. J. Med. *71*:214–216, 1970.
177. Hyman LR, Ballow M, Knieser MR: Diphenylhydantoin interstitial nephritis. Roles of cellular and humoral immunologic injury. J. Pediatr. *92*:915–920, 1978.
178. Sheth KJ, Caspen JT, Good TA: Interstitial nephritis due to phenytoin hypersensitivity. J. Pediatr. *91*:438–441, 1977.
179. Poole G, Stadling P, Worlledge S: Potentially serious side effects of high-dose, twice weekly rifampicin. Br. Med. J. *3*:343–347, 1971.
180. Ramgopal V, Leonard G, Bhathena D: Acute renal failure associated with rifampicin. Lancet *1*:1195–1196, 1973.
181. Seufert CD: Acute renal failure after rifampicin therapy. Scand. J. Respir. Dis. *84*(Suppl.):174–179, 1973.
182. Minetti L, de Belgioioso GB, Civati C, et al.: Drug induced hypersensitivity nephritis. Proc. Eur. Dial. Transplant Assoc. *11*:526–533, 1975.
183. Flynn CT, Rainford DJ, Hope E: Acute renal failure and rifampicin: Danger of unsuspected intermittent dosage. Br. Med. J. *2*:482, 1974.
184. Rothwell DL, Richmond DE: Hepatorenal failure with self-initiated intermittent rifampicin therapy. Br. Med. J. *2*:481–482, 1974.
185. Campese VM, Marzullo F, Schena FP, et al.: Acute renal failure during rifampicin therapy. Nephron *10*:256–261, 1973.
186. Kleinknecht D, Homberg JC, Decroix G: Acute renal failure after rifampicin. Lancet *1*:1238–1239, 1972.
187. Grocke DJ, Hsu K, Morgan C, et al.: Vasculitis in asociation with Australia antigen. J. Exp. Med. *134*:330S–336S, 1971.
188. Schrier RW, Bulger RJ, Van Ardsel PP: Nephropathy associated with penicillin and homologues. Ann. Intern. Med. *64*:116–127, 1966.
189. Peters GA, Moskowitz RW, Prickman LE, et al.: Fatal necrotizing angiitis associated with hypersensitivity to penicillin O and iodides: Report of a case. J. Allergy *31*455–467, 1960.
190. Kiellbo H, Stakeberg H, Mellgren J: Possibly thiazide-induced renal necrotising vasculitis. Lancet *1*:1034–1035, 1965.
191. Kovnat P, Labovitz E, Levison S: Antibiotics and the kidney. Med. Clin. North Am. *57*:1045–1063, 1973.
192. Lee SL, Rivero I, Siegel M: Activation of SLE by drugs. Arch. Intern. Med. *117*:620–626, 1966.
193. Alarcon-Segovia D: Drug-induced lupus syndromes. Mayo Clin. Proc. *44*:664–681, 1969.
194. Dorfmann H, Kahn MD, deSeze S: Les lupus iatrogenes: etat actuel de la question. Nouv. Presse Med. I. *1*:2907–2912, II. 2967–2970, 1972.
195. Lee SL, Chase PH: Drug-induced systemic lupus erythematosus: A critical review. Semin. Arthritis Rheum. *5*:83–103, 1975.
196. Holley HL: Drug therapy and the etiology of SLE. Ann. Intern. Med. *55*:1036–1039, 1961.
197. Rallison MJ, Carlisle JW, Lee RE, Jr, et al.: Lupus erythematosus and the Stevens-Johnson syndrome. Am. J. Dis. Child. *101*:725–738, 1961.
198. Thoenes W, Thoenes G, Ansorge R: Drogeninduzierte lupus-nephritis. Lichtelektronen-und immunofluorescenzmikroskopische utersuchungen. Verh. Dtsch. Ges. Pathol. *6*:346–352, 1972.
199. Amrhein JA, Kenny RM, Ross D: Granulocytopenia, lupus-like syndrome and other complications of propylthiouracil therapy. J. Pediatr. *76*:54–63, 1970.
200. Whittingham, S, Mackay IR: Systemic lupus erythematosus induced by procainamide. Australas. Ann. Med. *19*:358–361, 1970.
201. Harpey JP, Caille B, Moulias R, et al.: Lupus-like syndrome induced by D-penicillamine in Wilson's disease. Lancet *1*:292, 1971.
202. Benton JW, Tynes B, Register HB, Jr, et al.: Systemic lupus erythematosus occurring during anticonvulsive drug therapy. J.A.M.A. *180*: 115–118, 1962.
203. Dano P: Connective tissue disease following antiepileptic therapy. Epilepsia *10*:481–486, 1969.
204. Livingston S, Rodriguez H, Greene CA, et al.: Systemic lupus erythematosus. Occurrence in association with ethosuximide therapy. J.A.M.A. *204*:731–732, 1968.
205. Alter BP: Systemic lupus erythematosus and ethosuccinimide. J. Pediatr. *77*:1093–1094, 1972.

206. Dabbours IA, Idriss HM: Occurrence of systemic lupus erythematosus in association with ethosuccimide therapy: Case report. J. Pediatr. *76*:617–620, 1970.
207. Best MM, Duncan CH: A lupus-like syndrome following propylthiouracil administration. J. Ky. Med. Assoc. *62*:47–49, 1964.
208. Young JL, Jr, Boswell RB, Nies NS: Severe allopurinol hypersensitivity. Association with thiazides and prior renal compromise. Arch. Intern. Med. *134*:533–558, 1974.
209. Jarzobski J, Femy J, et al.: Vasculitis with allopurinol therapy. Am. Heart J. *79*:116–121, 1970.
210. Mills RM, Jr.: Severe hypersensitivity reactions associated with allopurinol. J.A.M.A. *216*:799–802, 1971.
211. Kantor GL: Toxic epidermal necrolysis, azotemia and death after allopurinol therapy. J.A.M.A. *212*:478–479, 1970.
212. Citron BP, Halpern M, McCarron M, et al.: Necrotizing angiitis associatied with drug abuse. N. Engl. J. Med. *283*:1003–1011, 1970.
213. Monaco AP, Wood ML, Russell PS: Some effects of purified heterologous antihuman lymphocyte serum in man. Transplantation *5*:1106–1114, 1967.
214. Peeler RN, Kadull PJ, Cluff LE: Intensive immunization of man: evaluation of possible adverse consequences. Ann. Intern. Med. *63*:44–57, 1965.
215. Joekes AM, Gabriel JRT, Goggin MJ: Renal disease following prophylactic inoculation. Nephron *9*:162–170, 1973.
216. Boulton-Jones JM, Sissons JGP, Naish PF, et al.: Self-induced glomerulonephritis. Br. Med. J. *3*:387–390, 1974.
217. Beirne GJ, Brennan JT: Glomerulonephritis associated with hydrocarbon solvents mediated by antiglomerular basement membrane antibody. Arch. Environ. Health *25*:365–369, 1972.
218. D'Apice AJF, Kincaid-Smith P, Becker GJ, et al: Goodpasture's syndrome in identical twins. Ann. Intern. Med. *88*:62–72, 1978.
219. Ehrenreich T, Yunis SL, Chung J: Membranous nephropathy following exposure to volatile hydrocarbons. Environ. Res. *14*:35–45, 1977.
220. LaGrue G: Hydrocarbon exposure and chronic glomerulonephritis. Lancet *1*:1191, 1976.
221. Ravnskov U, Forsberg B, Skerfuing S: Glomerulonephritis and exposure to organic solvents. Acta Med. Scand. *205*:575–579, 1979.
222. Ravnskov U: Acute glomerulonephritis and exposure to organic solvents in father and daughter. Acta Med. Scand. *205*:581–582, 1979.
223. Zimmerman SW, Groehler K, Beirne GJ: Hydrocarbon exposure and chronic glomerulonephritis. Lancet *2*:199–201, 1975.

Chapter 8

Drug-Induced Chronic Renal Failure

by

Antoine de Torrenté and Robert J. Anderson

Exposure to a number of pharmacologic agents can induce severe chronic renal insufficiency. The best example is analgesic abuse nephropathy. In some countries, including the United States, chronic nephropathy due to analgesic abuse affects a substantial number of individuals and is thus a major public health problem. Additional drugs that may induce a chronic nephropathy include CCNU/BCNU (1-[2-chloroethyl]-3-[4-methyl cyclohexyl]-1-nitrosourea/1,3-bis(2-chloroethyl)-1-nitrosourea), lithium, and amphotericin B. Rarely, permanent renal insufficiency results from *cis*-platinum and other heavy metals, aminoglycoside antimicrobial agents, radiographic contrast material, and drugs that injure the kidneys through immunologic mechanisms. This chapter will discuss drug-induced chronic renal failure with emphasis on analgesic abuse nephropathy and the controversy regarding chronic nephropathy associated with lithium.

ANALGESIC NEPHROPATHY

An association between chronic renal failure and heavy consumption of analgesic drugs was suspected in 1950 and confirmed by 1953 by Spühler and Zollinger.[1] These pathologists noticed the heavy consumption of phenacetin-containing drugs in a series of autopsy patients who died of renal failure. After a lag period of some years, an increasing number of publications began to appear, mainly from Scandinavian countries, confirming the association between analgesic consumption and renal damage.[2] Later, workers from other countries, including Australia, Great Britain, Canada, and subsequently the United States, began to recognize the disease.[3-11] Today, although the nature of the chemical substance causing damage is debated, the reality of the disease is accepted by almost everybody. The thousands of cases described, the characteristic clinical syndrome, the typical anatomic lesions, and the frequent improvement in renal function on cessation of analgesic use constitute strong evidence for such an entity.

Analgesic nephropathy is not only a disease of the kidneys, it is also an example of a self-induced disease that could be checked by appropriate legislation. Legislative action aimed at removal of phenacetin and its derivatives from over-the-counter sale has been taken in some countries, such as Sweden, Canada, and Great Britain, with some success.[12] However, Kincaid-Smith feels that restriction of phenacetin availability has not reduced the frequency of analgesic abuse nephropathy in Australia.[13] In Switzerland, where 20 per cent of all patients in dialysis or transplant programs suffer from analgesic abuse nephropathy,[14-16] phenacetin and acetaminophen are still components of dozens of analgesic preparations sold over-the-counter. This disease could indeed be classified as well under social as under medical problems. The similarities between analgesic addiction and alcoholism are striking.

Analgesic nephropathy is an especially important entity for the practicing physician to recognize, since the downhill course of a good proportion of patients can be stabilized or even reversed if the intake of the offending drug is discontinued.[8, 13, 17, 18] For example, in one study of 52 patients followed for several years after stopping analgesics, 50 per cent improved, 35 per cent remained stable, and 15 per cent deteriorated with regard to renal function.[13]

DEFINITION AND BREADTH OF THE PROBLEM

The definition of what constitutes analgesic abuse is difficult. There is still doubt about the offending agent(s) and the duration of exposure required to produce the renal lesion. Almost all patients with definite renal lesions have consumed more than 1 kg of phenacetin (up to 50 kg). In a series of 31 patients studied by Mihatsch et al., the mean duration of abuse was 22 years ± 11.5 (SD).[14, 15] A good working definition is the one adopted internationally of 1 gm of phenacetin per day for more than 3 years, or 1 kg of phenacetin as the total dose consumed.[19]

The work of Spühler and Zollinger was only an indication that a causal link between analgesic abuse and renal failure might exist. Almost a decade elapsed between the original work and an excellent epidemiologic study.[2] In this study, two small Swedish towns, about 300 km apart, were examined. The populations were similar, with most inhabitants employed in industrial work. The main difference between the two towns was the amount of phenacetin consumed per capita, per year, i.e., 54 gm in Huskvarna and 5.3 gm in Fagersta. The habit of analgesic consumption in Huskvarna started in 1918, during the influenza pandemic, when a respected physician prescribed a powder of his composition to relieve severe myalgias caused by the disease. The "Hjorton Powder" contained 150 mg caffeine, 500 mg of phenazone, and 500 mg of phenacetin. The remarkable effects of this powder on the well-being and mood of those who took it led to a staggering increase in its consumption, especially among factory workers. The consumption of analgesic drugs remained at an acceptable level in Fagersta. Comparing the deaths from renal failure in the two towns, Grimlund found 6.5 per cent in Huskvarna as compared to 2 per cent in Fagersta.[2] Thirty per cent of the male factory workers in Huskvarna taking the powder had a severe renal concentrating defect and 34 per cent had a serum creatinine level above 1.5 mg/100 ml. Only 2.4 per cent of the workers denying the use of the powder had a concentrating defect or an abnormal serum creatinine.

Another major epidemiologic study was conducted in Switzerland by Dubach et al.,[20] who followed longitudinally more than 1200 female factory workers. The intake of phenacetin or aspirin was checked by the chemical determination of acetaminophen (the major metabolite of phenacetin) or salicylate in the urine. A study (abusers) and a control group (nonabusers) were defined, matched for age, parity, and social conditions, and followed with urinalysis and serum creatinine concentrations for four years. A concentrating defect appeared in 3.8 per cent of abusers and in 0.8 per cent of the control group. The incidence of raised serum creatinine was also significantly higher in the study group (2.9 vs. 0.4 per cent). If the study group was divided into high and low intake groups, the differences became even more pronounced. These epidemiologic studies, combined with more than 4000 described cases since the original work, demonstrate clearly the link between heavy analgesic consumption and renal damage.

In the United States, however, there has always been an atmosphere of prudent skepticism. Goldberg has to be credited for popularizing the disease in the United States. He and Bluemle first demonstrated that acetaminophen is concentrated at the papillary tip, affording some explanation for the association of analgesic nephropathy with papillary necrosis.[21] He then published with Murray[9] a report of a series of 101 patients suffering from chronic interstitial nephritis, in which they were able to demonstrate that analgesic abuse was the primary cause in 20 per cent of these patients, drawing the attention of the general internist to the disease (Table 8–1). More recently, these authors have emphasized that analgesic abuse neophropathy is recognized throughout the United States.[22]

In some countries, the impact of analgesic nephropathy on public health is enormous. In Australia and Switzerland about 20 per cent of the patients entering a dialysis-transplant program do so because of analgesic nephropathy.[16] The estimated number of phenacetin abusers currently living in Switzerland (6 million population) is 20,000 to 40,000.[12] As a whole, in Europe, 3 per cent of all dialysis and transplant patients are analgesic abusers. In Canada, an incidence of 50 cases per million population has been projected.[11] In England

TABLE 8–1. ETIOLOGIC FACTORS IN 101 CASES OF CHRONIC INTERSTITIAL NEPHRITIS*

Factor	Primary Causes† (No.)	Secondary Factor‡ (No.)
Anatomic abnormalities	31	0
Analgesic abuse	20	0
Hyperuricemia	11	0
Nephrosclerosis	10	7
Stones	9	3
Sickle cell disease (SS)	1	1
Renal tuberculosis	1	0
Bacterial urinary tract infection	0	27
Multiple	7	
Idiopathic or indeterminate	11	

*Reproduced with permission from Murray T, Goldberg M: Chronic interstitial nephritis: etiologic factors. Ann. Intern. Med. *82*:453–459, 1975.

†Only or initial etiologic factor present in indicated number of patients.

‡Occurred subsequent to primary cause (see text).

and Wales, as many as 450 new cases per year may appear.[23]

PATHOLOGY

Over the years, a clear picture of the anatomic lesions in analgesic nephropathy has appeared. The gross lesion is decreased kidney size with scarring of the surface. The cut section shows whole segments of shrunken cortex with necrosis of the underlying papilla. The cortex is pale and sometimes of tough texture. The papilla may be pale in cases of early necrosis or frankly dark brown in more advanced cases. Some calcification may be present. Sometimes, the papillae lie freely in the calyces or they may be missing altogether. If no infection is complicating the picture, the calyces and pelvis are usually normal. The Bertin columns may be hypertrophied.

Microscopically, there is an interstitial fibrosis and a peculiar necrobiosis or sclerosis of the vasa recta described as "analgesic microangiopathy."[24-26] The papilla shows coagulation necrosis with little cellular infiltration. The time course of the papillary necrosis (acute vs. chronic) changes the histologic picture with regard to degree and extent of cellular infiltration. A brownish lipofuscin-like pigment is deposited in the tubular cell cytoplasm. The cortical tubules show atrophy if they drain into a necrotic papilla. The glomeruli may be normal or totally hyalinized. Papillary necrosis is distinctly unique in its frequency among analgesic abusers, with a frequency varying from 6 to 94 per cent. Figure 8–1 illustrates the gross appearance of papillary necrosis. Figure 8–2 shows the peculiar capillary vascular lesions of analgesic abuse.

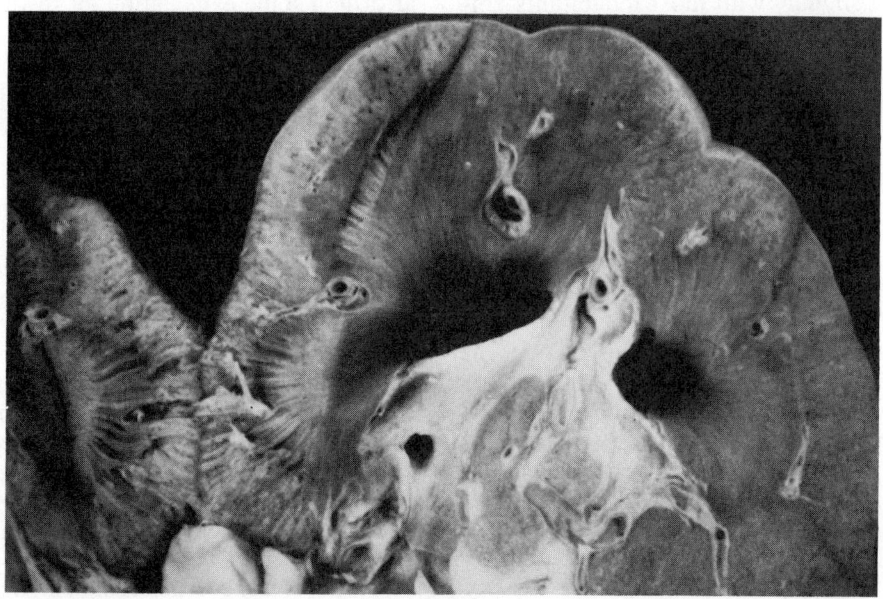

Figure 8–1. Kidney of 48-year-old woman with long-term phenacetin abuse. The figure shows two *in situ* necrotic papillae with a characteristic brown-black discoloration. (Courtesy of Professor F. Chatelanat. Institut de Pathologie, Université de Geneve, Switzerland.)

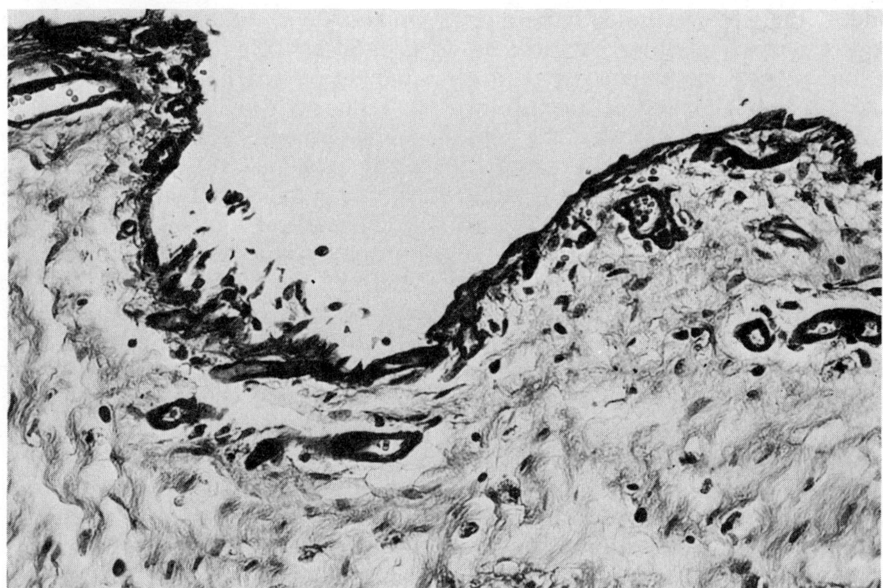

Figure 8–2. Calyceal wall with well-demonstrated submucosal capillary sclerosis in 32-year-old woman. PAS × 220. (Courtesy of Professor F. Chatelanat. Institut de Pathologie, Université de Geneve, Switzerland.)

CLINICAL ASPECTS OF ANALGESIC NEPHROPATHY

Analgesic nephropathy is not an easy diagnosis to establish. Similarly to alcoholics, patients who abuse analgesics greatly minimize their intake. Often, they hide tablets or powders in different locations. Direct questioning is usually met with anxiety, vigorous denial, or simply failure to return for the next appointment. A gentle, sometimes very indirect approach is preferable. Faced with compatible clinical and radiologic findings, but with a negative history, measurement of salicylate or acetaminophen in two or three urine specimens is needed. A quick "screen" can be obtained for urinary salicylates by use of the ferric chloride impregnated urinalysis "dipstick." The urine specimens should be voided at the physician's office because if the patients are asked to bring in their urine, they may refrain from their habit that day with consequently negative results. Some of these patients also develop low-level sulfhemoglobinemia or methemoglobinemia.

The motivations for taking analgesic drugs are numerous, but headaches are often cited as a main reason. Other people complain of various musculoskeletal pains. Some need the analgesic for its mild stimulating and depression-relieving properties: "I cannot start the day without two pills" or "I need a pick-me-up in the middle of the morning" are frequently heard reasons. Just simple imitation of a fellow worker who seems so much better after a "pill-break" is also very frequent. The intake of analgesics has been on a steady rise in almost all countries, as has been the intake of alcohol and other psychoactive drugs.

Analgesic nephropathy is mainly a disease of middle-aged females (Table 8–2). Only two series show a male predominance — the one

TABLE 8–2. CLINICAL FEATURES IN PATIENTS WITH ANALGESIC NEPHROPATHY*

FEATURE	
Age	29–72 yr.
Females	50–85%
Headache	35–100%
Anemia	60–90%
Gastrointestinal symptoms	40–60%
Hypertension	15–70%
Urinary tract infection	30–60%
Abnormal urogram	85–95%
Papillary necrosis	25–85%
Pyuria	50–100%

*Reproduced with permission from Murray T, Goldberg M: Analgesic abuse and renal disease. Ann. Rev. Med. *26*:537, 1975.

by Grimlund in 1963,[2] who studied only male factory workers, and the other by Nordenfelt,[27] who studied the same patient population as Grimlund after the removal of phenacetin from the "Hjorton Powder." In all other published material, the female-to-male ratio is usually 3:1 to 2:1. The peak age incidence is between 40 and 60 years of age, and the disease is distinctly rare before age 30.

General medical problems are encountered with high frequency in patients with analgesic abuse, the most common of which is anemia. Linton observed that 60 per cent of his cases had a hemoglobin level below 11 gm/dl.[8] The anemia is usually normochromic and normocytic, but can also be hypochromic and microcytic. At least three different factors may play a role in the genesis of the anemia of analgesic abuse: (1) Renal failure, if severe enough, can contribute to hyporegenerative anemia. (2) Chronic ingestion of analgesics containing aspirin may induce gastrointestinal bleeding and lead to iron deficiency. Moreover, peptic ulcer disease is common in analgesic nephropathy and frank gastrointestinal hemorrhage occurs. (3) As many as 17 per cent of one series of patients abusing analgesics had a hemolytic anemia, probably induced by phenacetin or related metabolites.[8] The presence of methemoglobinemia or sulfhemoglobinemia is characteristic and is probably caused by phenetidine (a phenacetin metabolite) or acetic-4-chloranilid, a manufacturing contaminant.

As noted, gastrointestinal complaints are frequent. Frank duodenal or gastric ulcers have been observed in more than 20 per cent of the patients and up to 50 per cent in Wilson's series had x-ray proven ulcer disease.[11] The chronic digestive complaints might even be one of the alleged reasons why people take the analgesic.

Some investigators, notably Kincaid-Smith, have suggested that severe accelerated atherosclerotic disease may complicate the course of analgesic abuse. Thus, myocardial infarction is a common cause of death,[13] and atheromatous plaques in the renal arteries may be encountered with high frequency.[13]

Premature aging can also be a striking feature in some patients who abuse analgesics. Thus, excessive wrinkling, loss of elasticity, and thinning of the skin, as well as early graying of the hair are commonly noted.[13]

A number of authors have described psychiatric or psychologic problems in patients abusing analgesic drugs. Murray suggested that organic dementia could be induced by analgesic abuse.[28] He showed the histopathologic changes of Alzheimer's disease in 6 of 7 patients with analgesic abuse and electroencephalographic changes. Moreover, as already explained, the alleged reason for analgesic use in many patients is headache.

The earliest clinical sign of analgesic nephropathy is a decrease in the concentrating ability of the kidney.[2] This results in polyuria and nocturia and may be explained by the early lesions in the vasa recta, which are required for maintenance of high corticopapillary interstitial solute gradient. An extremely common laboratory finding is sterile pyuria present in 50 per cent of patients. In many centers, analgesic nephropathy has replaced tuberculosis as the most frequent cause of sterile pyuria. The incidence of associated bacteriuria varies widely from 15 to 65 per cent.[4, 8]

There has been much debate as to the responsibility of urinary tract infection in the decline of renal function of analgesic abusers. It is possible that the damage induced by the analgesic abuse predisposes the kidney to infection, especially in patients obstructed by debris of shed papillae. Nevertheless, it seems clear that bacterial infection is not required for deterioration in renal function in this disorder.[29] However, urinary tract infection or frank pyelonephritis frequently complicates this disorder and can accentuate the degree of renal failure.[30]

The fall in the glomerular filtration rate in many patients occurs late in the disease. The incidence of some diminution of renal function at the time of diagnosis varies from 75 to 90 per cent of patients, and over 25 per cent may have severe renal insufficiency with serum creatinine above 3 mg/dl at presentation. Hematuria occurs in 30 to 40 per cent of cases and can be related either to the sloughing of renal papillae, to urinary tract infection, or to the development of cancer of the urinary tract, which is another potential complication of chronic analgesic abuse.[31] These uroepithelial tumors occur much more frequently in analgesic abusers than in the normal population. The prognosis is poor and metastases to the bones, liver, and lungs occur.[31, 32]

Proteinuria is often present in association with analgesic nephropathy. However, the magnitude of the proteinuria is usually less than 2 gm/24 hours. In some patients, high-grade ($>$ 4 gm/day) proteinuria may be observed. When kidneys exhibiting high-grade proteinuria are examined histologically, focal glomerulosclerosis will be observed.[13] Hypertension may be present in up to 70 per cent of patients and may contribute to deterioration in renal function. As with other renal diseases affecting the renal medulla and interstitium, some patients suffer from distal renal tubular acidosis and nephrogenic diabetes insipidus. The renal tubular acidosis may contribute to the medullary calcification, which is sometimes seen in analgesic nephropathy. Episodes of renal colic, obstruction, and infection may supervene during the course of the disease, thereby accelerating the downhill course.

Analgesic nephropathy is often accompanied by a distinctive radiologic picture, i.e., papillary or medullary necrosis. An excretory urogram is abnormal in more than 90 per cent of patients who demonstrate either a diminished concentrating ability or an elevated serum creatinine.[8] Thus, this exmaination is necessary in assessment of the disease. In the early stages, the kidneys may be of normal shape and contour with swollen papillae. This may correspond to necrosis *in situ*. Later, the calyceal margin becomes irregular, the papilla demarcates itself, becomes loose in the calyx (the so-called "ring-sign"), and can even be found in the pelvis or ureter. The calyx then becomes clubbed, and usually a cortical depression forms containing the nephrons that previously drained into that papilla. The medullary necrosis starts with small foci in the medulla, which then becomes confluent. The focus of medullary necrosis finally communicates with the calyx, but the papilla is retained. Medullary calcifications are common. These different forms of papillary and medullary necrosis are schematized in Figure 8–3. Once papillary necrosis supervenes, there is usually a reduction in kidney size with irregular cortical outlines. However, cortical scarring is sometimes less frequent in analgesic nephropathy than in chronic pyelonephritis owing to anatomical defects of the urinary tract. The pelvis, ureter, and bladder must be carefully examined so as not to miss a uroepithelial tumor.

ETIOLOGY/PATHOPHYSIOLOGY

An enormous amount of effort has been devoted to elucidate the etiology of analgesic nephropathy. To find "the cause" would obviously facilitate the removal of the toxic substance from analgesic drugs and potentially eradicate the disease. Unfortunately, much disagreement exists as to the primary cause of this process. Historically, phenacetin was first thought to be responsible. Subsequent epidemiologic data buttress the concept that phenacetin is the main toxic substance. After the early work of Grimlund and others, phenacetin was removed from over-the-counter drugs in Sweden and the Scandinavian countries in 1961. At the same factory in Huskvarna where workers formerly abused a mixture of phenacetin, phenazone, and caffeine, the number of deaths from renal failure

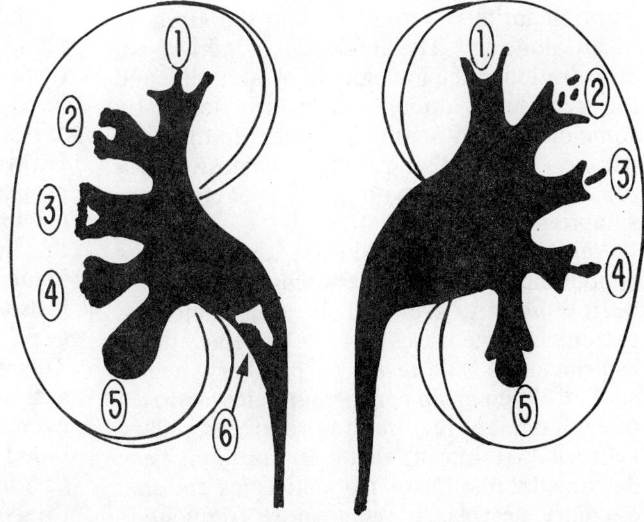

Figure 8–3. Schematic representation of radiographic manifestations of papillary necrosis following analgesic abuse.

has diminished sharply since 1967.[27] In Sweden, Bengtsson noted a steady fall in the percentage of cases of analgesic nephropathy from 58 per cent of all pyelonephritides in 1961 to 25 per cent in 1965.[31] The number of cases of papillary necrosis coming to autopsy in Denmark dropped by 50 per cent from 1959 to 1967. The same trend was published by Murray in 1971 in western Scotland.[28]

Aspirin is usually a component of analgesic mixtures, especially in Australia and North America. It was, therefore, natural that it was considered a possible cause of analgesic nephropathy. Indeed, in animal studies, aspirin may be more toxic than phenacetin.[13] Kincaid-Smith claimed no decline in the number of patients with papillary necrosis in Australia after the removal of phenacetin from the National Service Listing.[7, 13] However, acetaminophen (which is the main metabolite of phenacetin) has been substituted for phenacetin in Australia, and this may explain the failure to detect less papillary necrosis. In 10 cases, papillary necrosis was apparently induced by aspirin consumption alone.[13] There is no doubt that aspirin may be toxic to the kidneys if taken in gram quantities per day. It provokes enzymuria and sometimes hematuria and excretion of renal tubular cells. It clearly diminishes the creatinine clearance in some patients already suffering from renal diseases.[33, 34] When administered in therapeutic doses to healthy volunteers, a 5 to 10 per cent decrease in endogenous creatinine clearance and inulin clearance can be observed.[35] However, there are studies pointing toward the relative innocuousness of aspirin, even if taken for a long period of time, and in kilogram quantities, provided that the drug is taken alone.[36-39] The influence of periods of dehydration in the hot climate of Australia and the very large amounts of aspirin taken by some of Kincaid-Smith's patients (up to 30 gm per day) may explain cases of analgesic nephropathy occurring without phenacetin consumption.[13]

Animal experimentation has also been disappointing, and a consistent animal model has been difficult to establish. In animal models, extremely large doses of either phenacetin or aspirin alone will result in papillary necrosis.[40, 41] When given concurrently, lower doses of each one are required to produce papillary necrosis.[40] It appears that dehydration is very detrimental to animals fed analgesics and that papillary necrosis is much more frequent in rats allowed to become dehydrated while receiving phenacetin and other analgesic compounds.[40, 41]

There is no doubt that in Europe phenacetin is felt to be a major and important offending drug in analgesic abuse nephropathy. It is entirely possible that combining phenacetin and phenazone with aspirin constitutes a more detrimental combination than each drug taken separately. As Koutsaimanis and de Wardener have emphasized,[23] "the hypothesis that phenacetin can destroy [the papilla] only in the presence of some other substance has to explain why such different substances as caffein, phenazone, aspirin, aminopyrine and codeine all appear to be effective. These doubts should not obscure the overriding fact that it is the presence of phenacetin with which the destruction of the renal papilla in man is associated."

Careful histologic examination of the kidneys of analgesic abusers suggests the presence of a slow ischemic process responsible for the papillary necrosis. A specific histopathologic change of capillary sclerosis is demonstrable in the lower urinary tract as well as in the vasa recta of the renal medulla[26] (see Fig. 8–2). The papilla is exceedingly sensitive to ischemic processes, being already underperfused in normal conditions. Additional episodes of dehydration with diminution of the renal blood flow may further curtail papillary perfusion and may explain some acute episodes of papillary necrosis.[38] How and why phenacetin or mixtures of analgesics containing phenacetin provoke this peculiar vascular necrosis is unknown. Phenacetin is a strong oxidant and is concentrated along the papilla of the dog's kidney. The maximal value of phenacetin at the papillary tip exceeds by tenfold the renal cortical concentration.[21] Such a differential tissue concentration mechanism does not exist for the salicylate ion. However, salicylate could enhance the toxic properties of phenacetin by inhibition of hexose monophosphate shunt activity, a pathway that normally protects renal tissue from oxidants.[21] The role of the local inhibition of prostaglandin synthesis in the lesions of analgesic nephropathy has not yet been clarified. This inhibition, induced by many nonsteroidal anti-inflammatory drugs, could result in an even further curtailment of renal papillary blood flow. Indeed, preliminary reports suggest that agents that inhibit prostaglandin synthesis may also result in papillary necrosis.[41]

A more detailed review of the renal effects of prostaglandin inhibition is presented in Chapter 6.

THERAPY

The diagnosis of analgesic nephropathy is extremely important to establish. A substantial proportion of patients will stabilize or improve kidney function with cessation of analgesic abuse[8, 28, 43, 44] (Fig. 8–4). This goal is most achievable in patients who are not yet at the end stage of their disease. Conversely, if the abuse continues unabated in a patient with diagnosed analgesic nephropathy, the result will be end-stage failure in most cases. This is illustrated in Figure 8–4. The single most important step in the treatment of analgesic abuse is to have the patient understand the link between the constant intake of analgesic compounds and the renal disease. The number of patients who, if properly educated and motivated by their physician, can stop their ingestion is quite high. Reassurance and psychologic support are essential and a punitive attitude is not warranted. Sometimes, a mild tranquilizer will help the patient through the period of detoxification. Regular checks of acetaminophen and salicylate in the urine are sometimes needed to ensure that the patient has stopped the abuse. Unfortunately, not every patient will respond with an increase in renal function to discontinuation of their habit.[13] In approximately 20 to 30 per cent of patients, scarring and shrinkage of the renal mass will continue, with loss of the renal function.

Between 15 and 70 per cent of patients have high blood pressure. Appropriate treatment of this condition will certainly help slow down the decrease in renal function. A stepwise treatment with diuretics and antihypertensive agents is indicated. Brisk diuresis induced by potent loop diuretics, however, should be avoided, since these patients have a low tolerance for rapid extracellular fluid volume depletion owing to renal sodium wasting. Gentle blood pressure reduction is vastly preferable to drastic measures. The patient should be checked regularly for urinary tract infection and treated with adequate antimicrobial therapy according to the sensitivity of the organism and to renal function.

An acute deterioration in renal function complicating the course of analgesic nephropathy should always raise suspicion of intravascular volume depletion due to renal salt wasting or acute obstructive uropathy (ureteral obstruction due to a sloughed papilla or uroepithelial tumor). Every effort should be made to diagnose these conditions. Volume depletion is rapidly remedied and surgical intervention is mandatory if obstructive uropathy does not clear in 3 to 5 days or if acute infection intervenes. Slower obstruction of the urinary tract can also result from uroepithelial tumors, which are especially frequent among analgesic abusers.

OTHER AGENTS

LITHIUM

Lithium salts are widely prescribed for the treatment of manic-depressive psychosis. Recently, a number of reports have appeared

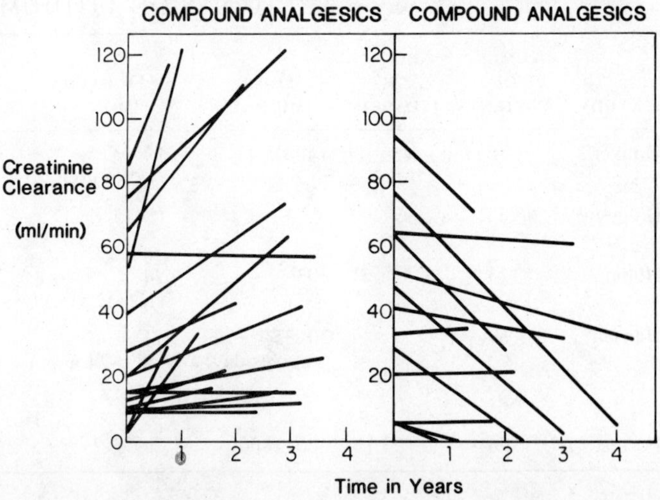

Figure 8–4. Sequential changes in renal function in patients who stopped (left) or continued (right) analgesics (Reproduced with permission from Linton AL: Renal disease due to analgesics. I. Recognition of the problem. Canad. Med. Assoc. J. *107*:749, 1972.)

suggesting that chronic lithium therapy can be associated with significant renal disease. The renal disorders felt to be induced by lithium include acute renal failure,[45-49] nephrogenic diabetes insipidus,[50-57] renal tubular dysfunction with hypocalciuria and impaired renal acidification,[58] and chronic renal insufficiency.[59-69] Considering the large numbers of patients at risk for development of lithium nephropathy, a review of the subject is appropriate.

Two clinical studies have suggested that chronic lithium therapy may lead to a chronic interstitial nephropathy.[59, 60] In 1977, Hestbeck and colleagues described 14 patients with chronic nephropathy felt to be due to lithium.[59] All patients had either marked polyuria or acute, severe lithium intoxication. Mild to moderate diminution in glomerular filtration rate and impaired maximal renal concentration were usually present. Thirteen of these 14 patients had renal histopathologic abnormalities consisting of chronic focal tubular atrophy, interstitial fibrosis, and sclerotic glomeruli. Since this study was heavily weighted toward patients with lithium overdose, a subsequent study was performed on outpatients taking lithium for at least 2 years.[59] In these patients, mildly elevated serum creatinine values were observed in eight of 69 patients.[60] No cause other than lithium could be found to explain the decreased renal function. Fifteen of these 69 patients, including the eight with elevated serum creatinine, also had daily urine volumes of more than 3 L/day. Renal biopsy specimens obtained on 14 of these 15 patients again demonstrated sclerotic glomeruli, increased interstitial fibrous tissue, and atrophic tubules. In addition, six of 14 biopsy specimens contained cysts lined with cuboidal epithelium. Similar histologic changes following chronic lithium therapy have been observed in other patients and in lithium-treated rats.[63-66] Other renal pathologic studies have also observed striking distal tubular cells ballooning with vacuolation of the cytoplasm in five patients treated with lithium for 4 months to 9 years.[67, 68] Taken together, these histopathologic and clinical observations suggest a role for lithium to induce a chronic nephropathy. However, appropriate control populations have not been reported in these studies.

Three additional studies have addressed the issue of lithium nephropathy[52, 61, 62] (see Table 8–3). In these studies, glomerular filtration rate and urinary excretion of beta$_2$ microglobulin were studied in 219 patients treated chronically with lithium. Five per cent of patients were felt to have lithium-induced diminution in glomerular filtration rate. The decreased glomerular filtration rate resulted in a slight (10 to 20 per cent) increase in serum creatinine. Although these studies suggest a small but significant potential for lithium to induce a chronic nephropathy, no age, sex, and psychotropic-medication matched control data were presented.

A number of isolated case reports of lithium-associated acute renal failure have appeared.[45-49] In all of these cases, several factors known to reduce renal function were present. However, series of patients with acute, severe lithium intoxication demonstrate a 25 to 30 per cent frequency of associated acute renal failure.[67] Thus, acute lithium intoxication appears to be frequently associated

TABLE 8–3. STUDIES ON LITHIUM NEPHROPATHY

Study	Number of Patients	Mean Age (Years)	Dose (mg/day)	Duration (months)	Polyuria	Decreased GFR	Other
Donker[52]	30	45	1400	39 (1/2–6 yrs)	8/30	0/30	Normal urinary beta$_2$ microglobulin
Hällgren[61]	66	49	?	(1–15 yrs.)	?	4/66 (mild)	2/66 increased urinary beta$_2$ microglobulin
Hullin[62]	123	55	803	74 (1/2–12 yrs.)	6/106	6/106	Normal urinary beta$_2$ microglobulin
Hansen[60]	69	?	30–35 (mmoles/day)	71 (all >24 mos.)	15/69	8/69	18/69 with diminished maximum Uosm; 14/14 with interstitial nephritis on biopsy
Forrest[50]	96	?	900–1800	?	11/96	?	?

with acute renal failure. Lithium is eliminated from the body predominantly by renal excretion. Any decrease in renal function, in the face of continued lithium intake, will, therefore, result in raised increments in plasma lithium leading to potential neurotoxicity.

The most common renal effect of lithium is polyuria (see Table 8–3). Approximately 10 to 20 per cent of patients on chronic lithium therapy produce more than 3 L of urine per day.[50-57] This polyuria is due to a vasopressin-resistant nephrogenic diabetes insipidus. The mechanism of this defect has been studied by several investigators. Antidiuretic hormone increases water permeability in the distal tubule and collecting duct by activating adenylate cyclase and cyclic AMP production. Lithium interferes with the action of activated adenylate cyclase to increase cyclic-AMP formation.[69] In some cases, a primary increase in thirst secondary to the psychiatric disorder may induce polyuria during lithium treatment.[70] Usually, the polyuria is reversible on discontinuation of lithium therapy. However, several cases of persistent nephrogenic diabetes insipidus following long-term lithium therapy have been reported.[50-54] Pathologic examination of kidneys from these patients demonstrates interstitial fibrosis.[59, 60] The polyuria rarely exceeds 4 L/day and usually does not require therapy.

Recently, it has been suggested that the mechanism of lithium-induced polyuria involves prostaglandins. Prostaglandins have been demonstrated to antagonize the hydroosmotic effect of antidiuretic hormone. In the rat and in humans, lithium therapy increases urinary prostaglandin excretion.[71, 72] Moreover, prostaglandin inhibition with indomethacin can lower urinary volume and increase urine osmolality in patients with lithium-induced polyuria.[72] This increased urinary concentrating ability following indomethacin occurs despite constancy of glomerular filtration rate and solute excretion. These provocative preliminary communications, if confirmed, suggest an important pathogenic mechanism of prostaglandins underlying lithium-induced polyuria.

There is solid evidence that lithium induces substantial changes in other aspects of renal tubular function as well. Thus, lithium-induced renal tubular acidosis,[58] hypocalciuria,[58] and hypercalcemia[73] have been well documented (see Chap. 9). Recently, two reports have suggested that lithium may induce minimal-change nephrotic syndrome.[74, 75] In one of these cases, nephrotic syndrome disappeared after withdrawal of the drug and reappeared after reinstitution of lithium.[64]

The following conclusions regarding lithium and the kidney seem appropriate:

1. Mild to moderate polyuria due to nephrogenic diabetes insipidus is the most common renal lesion observed during chronic lithium treatment. This lesion usually requires no therapy and is generally reversible after discontinuation of lithium. However, reports of lithium-induced permanent nephrogenic diabetes insipidus are appearing with increasing frequency.

2. No prospective, controlled series are available to address the issue of lithium-induced chronic tubulointerstitial nephropathy. At present, the risk of significant tubulointerstitial nephritis appears to be low. However, patients with lithium overdose may be at high risk for this lesion. Also, the presence of persistent nephrogenic diabetes insipidus identifies lithium-treated patients with a high likelihood of renal interstitial lesion. Although only mild renal failure has been reported, long-term follow-up studies on patients with this lesion are not available.

3. There appears to be a high incidence of acute renal failure that complicates the course of acute lithium intoxication.

4. Lithium may occasionally be associated with mild distal renal tubular acidosis, hypocalciuria, and hypercalcemia.

Taken together, these observations suggest that periodic (6- to 12-month intervals) determinations of both urine volume and renal function should be obtained in patients on chronic lithium therapy.

NITROSOUREAS

Recently, three reports have appeared suggesting that some nitrosourea compounds may induce chronic renal insufficiency. In monkeys receiving CCNU (1-[2-chloroethyl]-3-[4-methyl cyclohexyl]-1-nitrosourea) at doses larger than 120 mg/sq m, acute interstitial nephritis occurred as a dose-limiting toxic effect.[76] In a recent 3- to 6-year follow-up of 17 children treated with CCNU, all six children treated with more than 1500 mg of CCNU per sq m body surface area had severe chronic renal failure.[77] In some patients receiving smaller doses of CCNU, a progressive diminution in renal size occurred, but early death prevented long-term follow-up. The renal failure following CCNU usually did not become apparent until 1 to 2 years following drug administration. Renal tissue examination revealed glomerular sclerosis, interstitial fibrosis, and focal tubular atrophy. These results are in agreement with a preliminary communication of Schacht and Baldwin.[78] These workers observed chronic nephropathy in 14 of 106 patients treated with either CCNU or BCNU (1,3-bis(2-chloroethyl)-1-nitrosourea). Chronic renal failure developed in 14 of 17 patients who received more than 1200 mg/sq m and in all nine who received more than 1800 mg total dose. Signs and symptoms of renal insufficiency appeared only after cessation of therapy. Interstitial fibrosis and glomerular sclerosis were present on biopsy in five cases. Taken together, these observations[76-79] suggest that exposure to more than 1200 to 1500 of CCNU or BCNU per sq m body surface area leads to a high incidence of chronic renal failure. Until this nephrotoxicity has been better clarified, cumulative doses of CCNU and BCNU should not exceed 1500 mg/sq m.

AMPHOTERICIN B

A variety of nephrotoxic reactions to amphotericin B have been reported.[80-88] In both humans and the dog, amphotericin B decreases renal blood flow.[84] A variety of histologic abnormalities associated with amphotericin B have been described, including nonspecific glomerular abnormalities and calcification in the proximal and distal convoluted tubules and the ascending limb of Henle.[85, 86] Impaired renal function with resultant increases in serum creatinine and decreases in creatinine clearance occurs in most patients receiving the drug.[80, 82, 87] This impaired renal function usually returns to pretreatment levels. However, failure to return to basal levels with resultant chronic renal failure has been observed in elderly patients and patients receiving total doses of more than 4 gm. Distal renal tubular acidosis also frequently follows amphotericin B therapy.[87-90] This renal tubular defect can be associated with significant potassium wasting and nephrocalcinosis. The defect is usually mild, associated with only mild systemic acidosis, and clears within 6 months after cessation of therapy. Urinary concentration defects and renal sodium, potassium, and magnesium wasting have also been observed following amphotericin B therapy. Although these renal tubular defects are usually transient, permanent defects have been observed.

A prospective clinical study reported in 1976 has provided a current overview of amphotericin nephrotoxicity.[89] In this study, 11 patients received 1 mg/kg amphotericin B on alternate days until 2 gm were administered. Half of the patients served as controls while the other half were given 1 gm/kg of isotonic mannitol concomitant with the amphotericin. Mannitol was utilized because this agent appeared to exert a protective effect on renal function when amphotericin was given to dogs[91] and humans.[92] This latter study[92] was neither prospective nor contained control patients. In the most recent study,[89] all patients' inulin clearance declined from 2 to 80 per cent of basal levels. Mean decrement in inulin clearance was 30 per cent and was not affected by mannitol therapy. Abnormal renal concentrating ability was observed in five of 11 patients, while diminished urinary acidification was noted in three of 11. In 10 patients undergoing renal biopsy, a peculiar vacuolation of arteriolar walls was noted in all cases. Extensive, diffuse renal tubular calcification was observed in nine of 10 patients. No light or immunofluorescent microscopic abnormalities were observed in the glomeruli. Mannitol therapy did not affect either renal histology or renal function.

At present, careful monitoring of renal function and plasma electrolytes is indicated in all patients receiving amphotericin B. Alternate-day dosage and diminution in either dosage or frequency of administration once serum creatinine increases to greater than 2.5 mg/dl are widely thought to minimize nephrotoxicity. Avoidance of renal hypoperfusion and concomitant administration of other potential nephrotoxins (radiographic contrast agents, aminoglycosides and other antimicrobials) should be undertaken when amphotericin B is administered.

MISCELLANEOUS AGENTS

Rarely, lack of recovery from acute renal failure complicating aminoglycoside antimicrobial agents, *cis*-platinum, and radiographic contrast agents (see Chaps. 6 and 7) is noted. This appears to be an unusual occurrence. About 1 per cent of all patients maintained on chronic hemodialysis in Utah and Colorado have had an episode of drug-induced acute renal failure with lack of recovery. In general, lack of recovery occurs when large doses of the nephrotoxin have been administered and when therapy is continued despite development of severe renal failure. Several heavy metals have been utilized as therapeutic agents and may induce a chronic nephropathy as discussed in Chapters 6 and 7. Lead nephropathy is the prototype in this group. Chronic nephropathy associated with parenteral drug abuse (heroin) occurs and is detailed in Chapter 7. Chronic renal failure due to retroperitoneal fibrosis with obstructive uropathy occasionally complicates the course of methysergide therapy and possibly alphamethyldopa.[93, 94]

CONCLUSION

The potential public health implications of drug-induced chronic, end-stage renal disease are best emphasized by analysis of the European dialysis and transplantation experience.[95] In 1977, 9.5 per cent of all new European end-stage renal disease patients suffered from some form of drug-induced chronic nephropathy. This represents a threefold increase in prevalence of drug-induced nephropathy since 1970.[94] Chronic abuse of analgesic drugs is by far the most common form of drug-related chronic renal disease. A high index of suspicion of this disorder is necessary, since renal function may improve with cessation of analgesic ingestion. Some patients on long-term lithium therapy may develop a chronic nephropathy. Periodic assessment of renal function should be undertaken in this population until this clinical entity is better defined. Large-dose nitrosourea therapy also appears to predispose to chronic renal failure. Thus, doses greater than 1200 to 1500 mg/sq m should be avoided.

REFERENCES

1. Spühler O, Zollinger HU: Die chronische interstitielle nephritis. Z. Klin. Med. *151*:1–50, 1953.
2. Grimlund K: Phenacetin and renal damage at a Swedish factory. Acta Med. Scand. *174*(S):405, 1963.
3. Abel JA: Analgesic nephropathy. A review of the literature 1967–1970. Clin. Pharm: Ther. *12*:583–598, 1971.
4. Fellner SK, Tuttle EP: The clinical syndrome of analgesic abuse. Arch. Intern. Med. *124*:379–382, 1969.
5. Gault MH, Rudwal TC, Engles WD, Dossetor JB: Syndrome associated with the abuse of analgesics. Ann. Intern. Med. *68*:906–924, 1968.
6. Kennedy A: Analgesic nephropathy. J. Clin. Pathol. *28*(S) 9:14–23, 1975.
7. Kincaid-Smith P: Analgesic nephropathy. A common form of renal disease in Australia. Aust. N.Z. J. Med. *6*:498–508, 1976.
8. Linton AL: Renal disease due to analgesics. I. Recognition of the problem of analgesic nephropathy. Can. Med. Assoc. J. *107*:749–751, 1972.
9. Murray T, Goldberg M: Chronic interstitial nephritis: etiologic factors. Ann. Intern. Med. *82*:453–459, 1975.
10. Stewart JH, Gallery EDM: Analgesic abuse and kidney disease. Aust. N.Z. J. Med. *6*:498–508, 1976.
11. Wilson DR: Analgesic nephropathy in Canada. Can. Med. Assoc. J. *107*:752–755, 1972.
12. Gault MH, Wilson DR: Analgesic nephropathy in Canada: Clinical syndrome, management and outcome. Kidney Int. *13*:58–63, 1978.
13. Kincaid-Smith P: Analgesic abuse and the kidney. Kidney Int. *17*:250–260, 1980.
14. Mihatsch MJ, Hofer HO, Gutzwiler F, Brunner FP, Zollinger HU: Phenacetinabusus I. Häufigkeit, Pro-Kopf-Verbrauch und Folgkosten. Schweiz. Med. Wochenschr. *110*:108–115, 1980.
15. Mihatsch MJ, Schmidlin P, Brunner FP, Hofer HO, Six P, Zollinger HU: Phenacetinabusus II. Die chronische renale insuffizienz im basler autopsiegut. Schweiz. Med. Wochenschr. *110*:116–124, 1980.
16. Societe Suisse De Nephrologie: Analgesiques et atteinte renal. Bull. Médecins Suisses *60*:2555–2556, 1979.
17. Burry AF, Axelsen RA, Trolov P: Analgesic nephropathy: Its present contribution to the renal mortality and morbidity profile. Med. J. Austral. *1*:31–36, 1974.
18. Murray RM: Analgesic nephropathy: Removal of phenacetin from proprietary analgesics. Br. Med. J. *4*:131–132, 1972.
19. Nanra RS, Stuart-Taylor J, McLeon AH, White KH: Analgesic nephropathy: Etiology, clinical syndrome and clinicopathologic correlations in Australia. Kidney Int. 13:79–84, 1978.
20. Dubach UC, Levy PS, Rosner B, Baumeler HR, Müller A, Peier A, Ehrensperger T: Relation between regular intake of phenacetin-containing analgesics and laboratory evidence for uro-renal disorders in a working female population of Switzerland. Lancet *1*:539–543, 1975.
21. Bluemle LW, Goldberg M: Renal accumulation of salicylate and phenacetin: Possible mechanisms in the nephropathy of analgesic abuse. J. Clin. Invest. *47*:2507–2514, 1968.
22. Murray TG, Goldberg M: Analgesic-associated nephropathy in the USA: Epidemiologic, clinical and pathogenetic features. Kidney Int. *13*:64–71, 1978.
23. Koutsaimanis KG, de Wardener HE: Phenacetin nephropathy, with particular reference to the effect of surgery. Br. Med. J. *4*:131–134, 1970.
24. Abrahams C: Cause of analgesic-induced renal papillary necrosis. Lancet *2*:346–347, 1976.
25. Abrahams C, Furman KI, Salant D: Analgesic abuse and microvascular changes. Am. Heart J. *95*: 268–269, 1978.
26. Mihatsch MJ, Torhorst J, Steinmann E, Zollinger HU: The morphologic diagnosis of analgesic

(phenacetin) abuse. Pathol. Res. Pract. *164*:68–79, 1979.
27. Nordenfelt O: Deaths from renal failure in abusers of phenacetin-containing drugs. Acta Med. Scand. *191*:11–16, 1972.
28. Murray RM, Lawson DH, Linton AL: Analgesic nephropathy: Clinical syndrome and prognosis. Br. Med. J. *1*:479–482, 1971.
29. Gault MH, Blennerhassett J, Muehrcke RC: Analgesic nephropathy. A clinicopathological study using electromicroscopy. Am. J. Med. *51*:740–756, 1971.
30. Barker LR, Cattell WR, Fry IK, Mallinson WJ: Acute renal failure due to bacterial pyelonephritis. Q. J. Med. *68*:603, 1979.
31. Bengtsson U: Phenacetin and renal pelvic carcinoma. Clin. Nephrol. *2*:123–126, 1974.
32. Hultengren N, Lagergren C, Ljungquist A: Carcinoma of the renal pelvis in renal papillary necrosis. Acta Chir. Scand. *130*:314–320, 1968.
33. Kimberly RP, Poltz PH: Aspirin-induced depression of renal function. N. Engl. J. Med. *296*:418–424, 1977.
34. Kimberly RP, Plotz PH: Aspirin-induced depression of renal function. N. Engl. J. Med. *296*:418–424, 1975.
35. Muther RS, Bennett WM: Effects of aspirin on glomerular filtration rate in normal humans. Ann. Int. Med. *92*:386–387, 1980.
36. Kimberly RP: Renal prostaglandins in ischemic lupus erythematosus. Lancet *2*:553–555, 1978.
37. Macklon AF, Craft AW, Thompson M, Kerr DNS: Aspirin and analgesic nephropathy. Br. Med. J. *1*:597–600, 1974.
38. Nanra RS, Hicks JD, McNamara JH, Lie JT, Leslie DW, Jackson B, Kincaid-Smith P: Seasonal variation in the post-mortem incidence of renal papillary necrosis. Med. J. Austral. *1*:293–296, 1970.
39. New Zealand Rheumatism Association Study: Aspirin and the kidney. Br. Med. J. *1*:593–596, 1974.
40. Molland EA: Experimental renal papillary necrosis. Kidney Int. *13*:5–14, 1978.
41. Nanra RS, Chirawong P, Kincaid-Smith P: Renal papillary necrosis in rats produced by aspirin, A.P.C. and other analgesics. *In* Renal Infection and Renal Scarring (P Kincaid-Smith and KF Fairley, eds.) Melbourne: Mercedes Publishing Service, 1971, pp. 347–358.
42. Nanra RS, Kincaid-Smith P: Experimental renal papillary necrosis (RPN) with non-steroid anti-inflammatory analgesics. *In* Problems on Phenacetin Abuse (H Haschek, ed.). Vienna: Facta Publications, 1973, p. 67.
43. Gault MH: The clinical course of patients with analgesic nephropathy. Can. Med. Assoc. J. *113*:204–207, 1975.
44. Haschek H, Schmidt W: Nierenschaden durch phenacetinabusus. Med. Klin. *70*:313–321, 1975.
45. Lavender S, Brown JN, Burrell WT: Acute renal failure and lithium intoxication. Postgrad. Med. J. *49*:277–279, 1973.
46. Amdisin A, Skaldborg H: Hemodialysis for lithium poisoning. Lancet *2*:213, 1969.
47. Hawkins JB, Darkin PR: Lithium. Lancet *1*:839, 1969.
48. Deas N, Hacken AG: Oligiuric acute renal failure complicating lithium carbonate therapy. Nephron *10*:246–249, 1972.
49. Schau M, Amdisin A, Trap-Jensen J: Lithium poisoning. Am. J. Psychiatry *125*:520, 1963.
50. Forrest JN, Cohen AD, Torretti J, Himmelhock JM, Epstein FH: On the mechanisms of lithium-induced diabetes insipidus in man and the rat. J. Clin. Invest. *53*:1115–1123, 1974.
51. Robin EZ, Garston RG, Weir RV, Posen GA: Persistent nephrogenic diabetes insipidus association with long-term lithium carbonate treatment. Can. Med. Assoc. J. *121*:194–198, 1979.
52. Donker AJ, Prins E, Meyer S, Sluiter WJ, Van Berkestyn JW, Dols LC: A renal function study in 30 patients on long-term lithium therapy. Clin. Nephrol. *12*:254–262, 1979.
53. Price TR, Beisswenger PJ: Lithium and diabetes insipidus. Ann. Intern. Med. *88*:576–577, 1978.
54. Lee RV, Jampol LM, Brown WV: Nephrogenic diabetes insipidus and lithium intoxication — complications of lithium carbonate therapy. N. Engl. J. Med. *284*:93–94, 1971.
55. Ramsey TA, Mendels J, Stokes JW, Fitzgerald RG: Lithium carbonate and kidney function. J.A.M.A. *219*:1446–1449, 1972.
56. Cattell WR, Coppen A, Bailey J, Rama Roa VA: Impairment of renal concentrating capacity by lithium. Lancet *2*:44–45, 1978.
57. Bucht G, Wahlin A: Impairment of renal concentrating capacity by lithium. Lancet *1*:778–779, 1978.
58. Miller PD, Dubovsky SL, McDonald KM, Katz FH, Robertson GL, Schrier RW: Hypocalciuric effect of lithium in man. Mineral Eelectrolyte Metab. *1*:3, 1978.
59. Hestbeck J, Hansen HE, Amdisin A, Olsen S: Chronic renal lesions following long-term treatment with lithium. Kidney Int. *12*:204–213, 1977.
60. Hansen HE, Hestbeck J, Sorensen JL, Norgaard K, Heilskov J, Amdisin A: Chronic interstitial nephropathy in patients on long-term lithium therapy. Q. J. Med. *48*:577–591, 1979.
61. Hällgren R, Alm PO, Hellseny K: Renal function in patients on lithium treatment. Br. J. Psychiatry *135*:22–27, 1979.
62. Hullin RP, Caley VD, Birch NJ, Thomas TH, Morgan DB: Renal function after long-term treatment with lithium. Br. Med. J. *1*:1457–1459, 1979.
63. Lindop GBM, Padfield PL: The renal pathology in a case of lithium-induced diabetes insipidus. J. Clin. Pathol. *28*:472–475, 1975.
64. Thomsen K: Toxic effects of lithium on the kidney. *In* Lithium: Controversies and Unresolved Issues (TB Cooper, S Gershon, N Kline, et al., eds.). Amsterdam: Excerpta Medica, 1979, p. 619.
65. Schou M: Lithium studies. 1. Toxicity. Acta Pharmacol. Toxicol. *15*:70–84, 1958.
66. Evan AP, Ollerich DA: The effect of lithium carbonate on the structure of the rat kidney. Am. J. Anat. *134*:97–106, 1972.
67. Hansen HE: Lithium intoxication. Report of 23 cases and review of the literature. Q. J. Med. *47*:123–144, 1972.
68. Burrows GD, Davies B, Kincaid-Smith P: Unique tubular lesion after lithium. Lancet *1*:1310, 1978.
69. Martinez-Maldonado M, Stavroulaki-Tsapara A, Tsaparas N, Suki WN, Eknoyan G: Renal effects of lithium administration in rats: alterations in water and electrolyte metabolism and the response to vasopressin and cyclic-adenosine monophosphate during prolonged administration. J. Lab. Clin. Med. *86*:445–461, 1975.
70. Miller PD, Dubovsky SL, McDonald KM, Katz FH, Robertson GL, Schrier RW: Central, renal and

adrenal effects of lithium in man. Am. J. Med. *66*:797–803, 1979.

71. Nally JV, Rutecki GW, Ferris TF: The acute effect of lithium on renal renin and prostaglandin E synthesis in the dog. Circ. Res. *46*:737–744, 1980.
72. Walker RM, Stoff JS, Brown JS, Epstein FH: The relation of renal prostaglandins to urinary dilution in lithium induced nephrogenic diabetes insipidus and normal subjects. Clin. Res. *28*:463A, 1980.
73. Christenson TA: Lithium, hypercalcemia and hyperparathyroidism. Lancet *2*:413, 1976.
74. Duflot JP, Dore C, Fellion G: L'utilisation du carbonate de lithium dans une institution psychiatrique. Ann. Med. Psychol. (Paris) *131*:311–321, 1973.
75. Richman AV, Masco HL, Rifkin SI, Acharya MK: Minimal-change disease and the nephrotic syndrome associated with lithium therapy. Ann. Int. Med. *92*:70–72, 1980.
76. Schaeppi U, Fleischman RW, Phelan RS: CCNU (NSC-79037): preclinical toxicologic evaluation of a single intravenous infusion in dogs and monkeys. Cancer Chemother. Rep. Part 3 5:53–64, 1974.
77. Harmon WE, Cohen JH, Scheeberger EE, Grupe WE: Chronic renal failure in children treated with methyl CCNU. N. Engl. J. Med. *300*:1200–1203, 1979.
78. Schacht RG, Baldwin DS: Chronic interstitial nephritis and renal failure due to nitrosourea (NU) therapy. Kidney Int. *14*:661, 1978.
79. Morton DL: CCNU nephrotoxicity following sustained remission in oat cell carcinoma. Cancer Treat. Rep. *63*:226–227, 1979.
80. Miller RP, Bates JH: Amphotericin B toxicity. Ann. Intern. Med. *71*:1090–1095, 1969.
81. Bell NH, Andriole VT, Sabesin SM: On the nephrotoxicity of amphotericin B in man. Am. J. Med. *33*:64–69, 1962.
82. Burgess JL, Birchall R: Nephrotoxicity of amphotericin B, with emphasis on tubular function. Am. J. Med. *53*:77–84, 1972.
83. Butler WT, Hill GJ, Swzed CF, Knight V: Amphotericin B renal toxicity in the dog. J. Pharmacol. Exp. Ther. *143*:47–56, 1964.
84. Wertlake PT, Butler WT, Hill GJ, Utz JP: Nephrotoxic tubular damage and calcium deposition following amphotericin B therapy. Am. J. Pathol. *43*:449–458, 1963.
85. Hill GJ: Amphotericin B toxicity: Changes in renal morphology. Ann. Intern. Med. *61*:349–354, 1964.
86. Butler WT, Bennett JE, Alling DW, Wertlake PT, Utz JP, Hill GJ: Nephrotoxicity of amphotericin B. Ann. Intern. Med. *61*:174–187, 1964.
87. McCurdy DK, Frederic M, Elkington JR: Renal tubular acidosis due to amphotericin B. N. Engl. J. Med. *278*:124–131, 1968.
88. Patterson RM, Ackerman GL: Renal tubular acidosis due to amphotericin B nephrotoxicity. Arch. Intern. Med. *127*:241–244, 1971.
89. Bullock WE, Luke RG, Nuttall CE, Bhathena D: Can mannitol reduce amphotericin B toxicity? Antimicrob. Agents Chemother. *10*:555–563, 1976.
90. Bhathena DB, Bullock WE, Nuttall CE, Luke RG: The effects of amphotericin B therapy on the intrarenal vasculature and renal tubules in man. A study of renal biopsies by light, electron and immunofluorescence microscopy. Clin. Nephrol. *9*:103–110, 1978.
91. Hellebusch AA, Salana F, Eodie E: The use of mannitol to reduce the nephrotoxicity of amphotericin B. Surg. Gynecol. Obstet. *134*:241, 1972.
92. Olivero JJ, Logans-Mendez J, Ghafary EM, Ebnoyan G, Suki WN: Mitigation of amphotericin B nephrotoxicity by mannitol. Br. Med. J. *1*:550–551, 1975.
93. Koep L, Zuidema GD: The clinical significance of retroperitoneal fibrosis. Surgery *81*:250, 1977.
94. Lepor H, Walsh PC: Idiopathic retroperitoneal fibrosis. J. Urol. *122*:1, 1979.
95. Wing AJ, Brunner FP, Brynger H, et al.: Combined report on regular dialysis and transplantation in Europe, VIII, 1977. Proc. Eur. Dial. Transplant Assoc. *15*:3–76, 1978.

Chapter 9

Drug-Induced Fluid and Electrolyte Disorders

by

Pravit Cadnapaphornchai and Saadi Taher

Life-threatening fluid, electrolyte, and acid-base disturbances can be induced by numerous drugs. Awareness of these side effects and the clinical circumstances in which they occur is essential for prevention and proper management. Moreover, patients with kidney and liver disease may be especially prone to develop drug-induced fluid, electrolyte, and acid-base disturbances. This chapter will, therefore, provide a comprehensive review of drug-induced disturbances of fluid, electrolyte, and acid-base metabolism.

DRUG-INDUCED DISORDERS OF SERUM SODIUM

HYPONATREMIA (Table 9–1)

Hyponatremia, defined by a serum sodium level of less than 135 mEq/L, is the result of increased water intake at a time when there is a concomitant impairment in renal water excretion. The impairment of the renal water excretion can be due to intrarenal factors such as a decreased delivery of glomerular filtrate to the ascending limb of Henle's loop (where solute-free water is generated), or to a decrease in sodium chloride reabsorption in the same nephron segment. The major factor involved in impaired renal water excretion is the persistent presence of antidiuretic hormone (ADH — arginine vasopressin in humans), with resultant increased water-permeability of the collecting duct. Drugs that cause hyponatremia must, therefore, interfere with one or all of these mechanisms. The antihistamines, anticholinergics, antipsychotics, and tricyclic antidepressants can cause dry mouth and may, therefore, stimulate drinking. In addition, the anticholinergic effect of these drugs may cause urinary retention, particularly in the elderly male. These drugs, however, do not cause hyponatremia unless there is a concomitant impairment in renal water excretion. The use of these drugs in patients with decompensated psychosis may be associated with hyponatremia, since decompensated psychosis is often associated with increased ADH secretion.[1-3]

Mannitol and glycerol are osmotic agents sometimes utilized to diminish cell swelling and to induce a diuresis.[5] Since these substances do not freely cross cell membranes, their presence in large quantities in the plasma and interstitium osmotically moves water from the intracellular into the extracellular space and thereby lowers the serum sodium concentration.[5] In this setting, the decrease in serum sodium concentration is not accompanied by a concomitant decrease in plasma osmolality.

The use of diuretics is commonly associated with hyponatremia, hypokalemia, and metabolic alkalosis.[4] Several factors that may be responsible for the diuretic-induced hyponatremia are (1) decreased delivery of the glomerular filtrate to the diluting segment resulting from hypovolemia, (2) interference with

TABLE 9–1. DRUGS THAT MAY INDUCE HYPONATREMIA

Drugs that Stimulate Thirst
Antihistamines, anticholinergics, phenothiazines, butyrophenones, thioxanthene derivatives, tricyclic antidepressants

Drugs that Interfere with Renal Tubular Sodium Reabsorption
Thiazides, chlorthalidone, furosemide, ethacrynic acid, mercurials, mannitol, glucose, glycerol, urea

Drugs that Stimulate Antidiuretic Hormone Release
Acetylcholine, barbiturates, carbamazepine, clofibrate, isoproterenol, morphine, nicotine, vincristine

Drugs that Enhance Antidiuretic Hormone–Like Actions
Chlorpropamide, tolbutamide, phenformin, oxytocin, nonsteroidal anti-inflammatory agents, acetaminophen

Drugs Impairing Renal Dilution—Acting by Unknown Mechanisms
Cyclophosphamide, amitriptyline, thiothixene, fluphenazine, monamine oxidase inhibitors, ACTH

sodium chloride reabsorption in the distal diluting segments, (3) increased ADH release resulting from hypovolemia, and (4) shift of sodium from the extracellular compartment into the potassium-depleted cells. The thiazides, chlorthalidone, and the loop diuretics (furosemide and ethacrynic acid) are some of the more commonly used diuretics associated with hyponatremia.

Drugs that increase ADH activity may do so by stimulating ADH release or enhancing the hydroosmotic action of ADH at the level of the renal tubule.[6] Drugs that have been shown to increase endogenous ADH release and may be associated with hyponatremia include morphine, carbamazepine,[7, 8] and vincristine.[9] Other drugs that stimulate ADH release but have not been reported to be associated with clinical hyponatremia are acetylcholine, barbiturates, clofibrate, nicotine, and isoproterenol. Chlorpropamide and tolbutamide enhance the action of ADH, and clinical hyponatremia has been reported to be associated with the use of these agents.[10] Other drugs, such as acetaminophen, indomethacin, and phenformin, also potentiate the hydroosmotic effect of ADH. However, clinical hyponatremia has not yet been reported with these drugs. The mechanism for cyclophosphamide-induced hyponatremia[15] is still not well defined. Both enhanced release and end-organ enhancement of the hydroosmotic effect of ADH have been postulated.

A number of other drugs, including amitriptyline,[12] thiothixene, monamine oxidase inhibitors,[13] and fluphenazine,[14] have been associated with hyponatremia. It has been suggested that these drugs increase ADH release. However, interpretation of these data[12, 13, 14] is difficult, since many of the patients studied were psychotic and some were undergoing electroconvulsive therapy, factors that may have been responsible for ADH release. Further study of these drugs is needed. Infusion of adrenocorticotropic hormone (ACTH) has been associated with severe hyponatremia.[11] Although the mechanism of ACTH-induced hyponatremia is not clear, it has been suggested that the ACTH used may have been contaminated with vasopressin.

The physician must be aware of hyponatremic complications when using the abovementioned drugs. The diagnosis and treatment of clinical hyponatremia have been reviewed recently.[16] Since patients with renal, hepatic, and cardiac disease often have impaired renal water excretion, they may be especially prone to develop drug-induced hyponatremia. The symptoms and signs of hyponatremia include confusion, lethargy, weakness, and seizures. Diagnosis is established by measurement of serum electrolytes and exclusion of other causes of hyponatremia.[16] Treatment consists of withholding the offending agent and water restriction. In life-threatening cases of hyponatremia, administration of hypertonic saline and furosemide may be indicated. In patients with diuretic-induced hyponatremia, reexpansion of volume with sodium chloride and administration of potassium, if hypokalemia is present, will usually return plasma sodium to normal after cessation of the diuretic.

HYPERNATREMIA (Table 9–2)

Hypernatremia may result from inadequate water intake, excessive water loss, or an abrupt hypertonic salt load. By far, the most common cause of hypernatremia appears to be inadequate water intake in older patients residing in care homes or in patients with cerebrovascular accidents. Drugs that increase water loss may do so through the gastrointestinal (GI) tract, skin, and kidneys or into the peritoneal cavity. An agent that enhances GI water loss is lactulose, which is used for the treatment of hepatic encephalopathy. Since lactulose is poorly absorbed from the gut, it acts as an osmotic cathartic, and in the absence of adequate water intake hypernatremia may result.[17] Cholestyramine, a basic anionic

TABLE 9–2. DRUGS THAT MAY INDUCE HYPERNATREMIA

Drugs that Induce Water Loss
- Gastrointestinal tract loss (lactulose, high-solute infant formulas, tube feedings)
- Skin loss (povidone-iodine [Betadine])
- Peritoneal loss (hypertonic dialysate)
- Kidney loss (osmotic diuresis [high protein tube feeding, cholestyramine, mannitol, glucose, urea], suppression of antidiuretic hormone release [alcohol, phenytoin], suppression of antidiuretic hormone action on renal tubules [lithium, demeclochlortetracycline, methoxyflurane, isophosphamide, glyburide, propoxyphene])

Drugs Causing Rapid Sodium Gain
- Hypertonic NaCl, $NaHCO_3$, Na_2SO_4, salt tablets, massive doses of sodium penicillin G

exchange resin, has been used in intractable diarrhea secondary to cholestatic liver disease and for therapy in hypercholesterolemic states. Each gram of cholestyramine adds 5 mOsm of solute load for renal excretion, and this osmotic diuresis increases renal water losses. Inadequate water intake in such cases can result in hypernatremia.[18, 19] The topical use of large quantities of providone-iodine in burned patients may cause hypernatremia. Since this preparation has an osmolality greater than 1000 mOsm/kg water, excessive loss of water through the skin occurs in patients who have no eschar.[20] The use of hypertonic peritoneal dialysate (7 per cent glucose) has been reported to cause hypernatremia owing to water loss into the peritoneal cavity and addition of hypertonic saline into the patient's vascular compartment.

Increased loss of water through the kidneys can be due either to an osmotic diuresis or to lack of vasopressin action. In the absence of adequate water intake, the use of mannitol and hypertonic glucose may cause hypernatremia by greater renal loss of water than sodium. However, these two substances may also shift fluid from the cells into the extracellular space and result in hyponatremia rather than hypernatremia. Thus, the level of water intake, renal water losses, and intracellular water shifts into the extracellular fluid (ECF) compartment combine to determine whether or not low, normal, or high serum sodium concentration occurs. High protein tube feeding may result in urea diuresis and hypernatremia.[21]

Drugs that suppress ADH release or antagonize its renal tubular action may cause water loss and polyuria.[22] Inadequate replacement of water during the administration of these drugs can result in hypernatremia. Owing to an intact thirst mechanism and ready access to water, clinical hypernatremia, however, is rarely associated with such agents. To date, hypernatremia has not been observed with agents that suppress pituitary release of ADH, such as alcohol and phenytoin. Drugs that antagonize the renal hydroosmotic effect of ADH appear to interfere with ADH–cyclic AMP system interaction. Such agents include lithium and demeclochlortetracycline; these drugs are capable of producing large urinary losses of hypotonic fluid. Either lack of fluid intake or replacement of urinary losses by more hypertonic solutions could result in hypernatremia. Indeed, hypernatremia has been reported in patients receiving lithium therapy with concomitant sodium chloride infusion.[23]

Probably the most common cause of medication-related hypernatremia is rapid administration of high concentrations of sodium salts. Thus, hypernatremia has been observed following hypertonic sodium chloride for abortion,[24] in patients receiving hypertonic sodium bicarbonate during cardiac resuscitation,[25] and in patients receiving sodium sulfate for treatment of hypercalcemia. The use of massive doses of penicillin G sodium in patients with impaired renal function may also result in severe hypernatremia.

The diagnosis of drug-induced hypernatremia depends on the awareness of this potential adverse effect. Signs and symptoms of hypernatremia involve evidence of central nervous system dysfunction. Demonstration of high serum sodium and/or hyperosmolality rapidly confirm the diagnosis. The treatment of hypernatremia must be aimed at the cause. Removal of the offending agent in the initial step and replacement of water is usually needed. In cases of hypernatremia resulting from rapid salt loads, the use of diuretics and administration of water is appropriate.

DRUG-INDUCED DISORDERS OF SERUM POTASSIUM

HYPOKALEMIA (Table 9–3)

Hypokalemia is frequently drug related. Several mechanisms are involved in drug-induced hypokalemia. The low serum potassium may be due to redistribution of potassium; a shift of potassium to the intracellular space occurs in metabolic or respiratory alkalosis in

TABLE 9-3. MECHANISMS INVOLVED IN DRUG-INDUCED HYPOKALEMIA

Intracellular Shift of Potassium
- Drug-induced alkalosis (see Table 9–7)
- Glucose and insulin
- Soluble barium salts

Increased Urinary Losses of Potassium
- Diuretics
- Mineralocorticoid preparations (ACTH, fludrocortisone, 9α-fluoroprednisolone nasal spray, licorice, tobacco)
- Drug-induced renal tubular acidosis (see Table 9–6)
- Poorly reabsorbed anions (carbenicillin disodium, sodium penicillin, nafcillin, sodium sulfate)
- Drug-induced hypomagnesemia (gentamicin, *cis*-platinum)
- L-Dopa

exchange for H^+. Drugs that induce alkalosis will be discussed later. The administration of glucose and insulin will cause the entry of potassium into cells and may cause significant hypokalemia, especially if the patient is potassium deficient. The ingestion of soluble barium has been reported to cause hypokalemia, flaccid paralysis, respiratory failure, hypertension, and cardiac arrhythmias.[26] The hypokalemia in this setting also appears to be secondary to the intracellular shift of potassium.[26]

Increased urinary potassium excretion (urine potassium greater than 20 mEq/L in the face of hypokalemia) is a major cause of hypokalemia. The most frequent cause of excessive urinary losses is diuretic administration. All diuretics that act proximal to the distal nephron site of potassium secretion will increase the secretion and thus excretion of potassium. This effect to enhance potassium secretion is mediated by increasing the tubular fluid flow and sodium delivery to the distal nephron. Secondary hyperaldosteronism caused by diuretic-induced volume depletion may also play a role in increasing renal potassium excretion following diuretic usage. Diuretics that cause hypokalemia include agents that act in the proximal tubule (aminophylline, carbonic anhydrase inhibitors, and osmotic agents), the medullary portion of Henle's limb (furosemide, ethacrynic acid, mercurials), and the cortical portion of Henle's limb (thiazides, chlorthalidone, and ticrynafen).

In one report, less than 5 per cent of nonedematous patients receiving chronic oral diuretics developed hypokalemia.[27] In none of these patients was the hypokalemia of serious clinical consequence. The routine administration of potassium supplements was, therefore, not recommended in the nonedematous patient receiving diuretics, e.g., hypertensive patients. However, potassium supplementation should be considered when the abovementioned potassium-losing diuretics are administered to edematous patients who generally have secondary aldosteronism. In addition, when diuretics are administered acutely in large doses (e.g., in the treatment of hypercalcemia with furosemide and normal saline), to patients receiving digoxin or to patients with liver disease who are prone to hepatic coma, potassium supplementation should be considered.

Recently, in Italy, hypokalemia, metabolic alkalosis, and hypertension were observed to result from the use of 9α-fluoroprednisolone nasal spray.[28] Enough of this steroid with mineralocorticoid properties was absorbed to cause sodium retention, hypertension, and marked renal potassium wasting. Both hypertension and the metabolic problems were reversed on cessation of use of the nasal spray.

Drugs causing proximal and distal renal tubular acidosis (RTA) are also associated with renal potassium wasting (Table 9–6). Severe hypokalemia (serum potassium, <1.1 mEq/L) and both proximal and distal renal tubular acidosis have been reported following toluene (e.g., glue or paint) sniffing. In proximal RTA, the administration of sodium bicarbonate usually worsens the renal potassium losses by increasing the delivery of bicarbonate sodium and tubular flow to the distal potassium secretory sites. Thus, potassium bicarbonate replacement is more appropriate than sodium bicarbonate in such patients. Treatment of distal RTA with bicarbonate can reduce the renal potassium wasting, although some may still be present after correction of the metabolic acidosis.

The ingestion of large amounts of black licorice may induce severe life-threatening hypokalemia. The potassium wasting is mediated by the mineralocorticoid activity of glycyrrhizic acid contained in some forms of black licorice.[29] Carbenoxolene, a drug used to treat gastric ulcer, also has mineralocorticoid activity and thus may produce hypokalemia.[30] Recently, swallowing large amounts of chewing tobacco has been shown to produce renal potassium wasting, also through a mineralocorticoid-like mechanism.[31]

Carbenicillin and other poorly absorbable anions increase urinary potassium excretion by increasing distal tubular lumen negativity and/or flow rate, thus enhancing the movement of potassium from the renal tubule cells into the lumen.[32] Carbenicillin-induced renal potassium wasting is rapidly reversible on cessation of drug administration.

Magnesium depletion also may cause renal potassium wasting and hypokalemia. In this setting, the mechanism of the renal potassium wasting is not known.[33] *Cis*-platinum and aminoglycoside antimicrobials can result in renal potassium and magnesium wasting. This tubular defect is reversible with magnesium repletion.[34, 35]

Hypokalemia has been observed in 10 per cent of Parkinsonian patients treated with L-dopa.[36] The drug increased the urinary excretion of potassium, an effect blocked by the administration of the peripheral inhibitor dopa decarboxylase. The mechanism of this renal potassium wasting remains to be elucidated.

Gastrointestinal losses of potassium may follow the excessive use of enemas or laxative abuse. In addition to the loss of 50 to 60 mEq of potassium per liter in the stools, secondary hyperaldosteronism may have a role in the hypokalemia by increasing urinary potassium wasting. It is now recognized that many patients will not admit to laxative abuse and thus may present with idiopathic hypokalemia. These patients may mimic patients with Bartter's syndrome with volume depletion, hypokalemia, hyperaldosteronism, juxtaglomerular cell hyperplasia, and resistance to the pressor effect of exogenous angiotensin II. The accompanying acid-base disturbance is, however, metabolic acidosis rather than metabolic alkalosis, because of stool bicarbonate losses.

Hypokalemia may be manifested clinically as paresthesias, muscle cramps, proximal muscle weakness, and even paralysis. These symptoms are usually seen when serum potassium is less than 2.5 mEq/L. Respiratory failure secondary to intercostal muscle paralysis, urinary retention, and ileus are occasionally seen in severely hypokalemic patients. Polyuria, secondary to both nephrogenic diabetes insipidus and increased thirst, is another major symptom of hypokalemia. ECG changes include depressed ST segment, flat or inverted T waves, U waves, prolonged QT interval, and atrial and ventricular arrhythmias. For modest hypokalemia, the oral administration of potassium chloride, 40 to 60 mEq/day, may be sufficient; however, in some instances, amounts of 300 to 400 mEq/day may be needed. Intravenous potassium therapy may be indicated with severe hypokalemia, especially if there are serious cardiac or neuromuscular manifestations.

HYPERKALEMIA

The drugs that may be associated with hyperkalemia are listed in Table 9–4. Drugs may induce hyperkalemia through a shift of potassium from the intracellular to the extracellular compartment. Thus, serum potassium increases during both respiratory and metabolic acidosis induced by drugs. The increase in hydrogen ion in extracellular fluid is thought to lead to the entry of hydrogen ion into the cells to be buffered in exchange for potassium. There is some recent evidence that the decrease in bicarbonate level *per se* in metabolic acidosis may also mediate this increase in serum potassium.[37] In certain types of metabolic acidosis (lactic acidosis), hyperkalemia may be absent despite severe acidosis.[38] This may be because the movement of hydrogen ion into the intracellular compartment is accompanied by an anion, thus not obligating the exit of a potassium ion to maintain electrical neutrality. The causes of drug-induced acidosis are listed in Tables 9–5 and 9–6.

Massive digoxin overdosage has been asso-

TABLE 9–4. MECHANISMS INVOLVED IN DRUG-INDUCED HYPERKALEMIA

Extracellular Shift
- Respiratory and metabolic acidosis (see Tables 9–6 and 9–7)
- Release of cellular potassium (succinylcholine, digitalis overdosage, hyperglycemia)
- Arginine infusion
- Beta-adrenergic inhibitors, aldosterone deficiency, insulin deficiency

High Intake
- Salt substitutes
- Intravenous potassium (potassium penicillin, transfusion of old stored blood)

Infusion of Hypertonic Solutions
- Mannitol, hypertonic glucose in diabetics

Decreased Urinary Excretion of Potassium
- Drug-induced acute and chronic renal failure
- Hypoaldosteronism (indomethacin, heparin)
- Potassium-sparing diuretics (spironolactone, triamterene, amiloride)

ciated with severe hyperkalemia and death. This is probably related to the inhibition of the Na-K ATPase pump interfering with the uptake of potassium into cells.[39] Another drug that causes a slight increase in serum potassium is the depolarizing muscle relaxant succinylcholine.[40] This increase is due to release of potassium from the muscle during cellular depolarization. Patients with trauma, neuromuscular disease, paraplegia, tetanus, or renal failure may have an exaggerated hyperkalemic response to succinylcholine with resultant dangerous hyperkalemia.[40] Marked fatal hyperkalemia has been reported during the infusion of arginine monohydrochloride.[41] The hyperkalemia is the result of displacement by the amino acid of potassium in the intracellular compartment. The potassium that moves into the extracellular compartment is promptly excreted by the kidney, unless renal impairment is present. Infusion of 30 to 60 gm of arginine monohydrochloride into human subjects during 30 minutes will only increase serum potassium by 1 mEq/L. Since the degree of hyperkalemia is directly related to plasma arginine levels, patients with liver disease may be more susceptible to hyperkalemia owing to their inability to metabolize arginine.[41]

Patients with impaired renal function may develop dangerous hyperkalemia if their potassium intake is high. Drugs inducing hyperkalemia due to increased potassium loads include salt "substitutes" (733 mg potassium/½ tsp of salt),[42] potassium penicillin (1.6 mEq/million units), and old, stored blood.[43]

The intravenous injection of hypertonic glucose to insulin-dependent diabetics may induce dangerous hyperkalemia.[44] The glucose-induced rise in plasma osmolality enhances osmotic water movement accompanied by the shift of potassium from the intra- to extracellular compartment.

Drug-induced acute or chronic renal failure is usually associated with hyperkalemia only when urine output is less than 500 ml/day. The drug-induced causes of renal failure are discussed in Chapters 5, 6, 7, and 8.

Some patients, mostly with diabetes mellitus, may have only mild renal impairment and good urine flow, yet demonstrate hyperkalemia and impaired urinary potassium excretion. The majority of these patients exhibit the syndrome of hyporeninemic hypoaldosteronism. Rare cases of selective hypoaldosteronism and hyperkalemia have been described after prolonged heparin therapy.[45] This effect is probably mediated through the reduction of aldosterone secretion.[46] More recently, the prostaglandin synthetase inhibitor indomethacin has been reported to cause hyperkalemia by inducing a state of hyporeninemic hypoaldosteronism.[47] In 30 patients, the syndrome was observed 1 week after starting indomethacin, persisted during treatment, and was reversible on discontinuing the treatment.

Treatment with potassium-sparing diuretics, e.g., spironolactone, triamterene, or amiloride, does not usually induce hyperkalemia unless renal insufficiency is present or potassium supplements are ingested. Diabetic patients are highly susceptible to hyperkalemia with usage of potassium-sparing diuretics, even in the absence of renal impairment.[48, 49]

In addition to muscle weakness, hyperkalemia is associated with electrocardiographic abnormalities and cardiac arrhythmias. The ECG changes do not always correlate with the serum potassium level. The need for treatment of hyperkalemia depends both on the level of hyperkalemia and on ECG changes. If there is prolongation of QRS complexes, heart block, or ventricular arrhythmias, the IV administration of calcium gluconate followed by IV glucose and insulin or sodium bicarbonate should be administered. These procedures antagonize the neuromuscular effects of hyperkalemia and move potassium into cells, respectively. In addition, removal of potassium should be instituted by the administration of exchange resins (sodium polystyrene sulfonate [Kayexalate]) or the use of dialysis, depending on the clinical situation.

DRUG-INDUCED ACID-BASE DISORDERS

ANION GAP METABOLIC ACIDOSIS (Table 9–5)

Metabolic acidosis can result either from the loss of base from the body or from the gain of acid. For the ease of clinical approach, metabolic acidosis, therefore, can be classified into high anion gap (acid gain) or normal anion gap (base loss) acidosis. The anion gap (AG) is calculated from the equation $AG = Na - (Cl + HCO_3)$. The normal gap is 8 to 12 mEq/L. Except for renal failure, in which the acidosis is due to the failure of the excretion of normally produced organic acids, the high anion gap metabolic acidosis is due either to the exogenous ingestion or the endogenous production of acids. Tetracyclines, because of

TABLE 9–5. DRUGS ASSOCIATED WITH HIGH ANION GAP METABOLIC ACIDOSIS

Drugs Increasing Uremic Acidosis
Tetracycline

Drugs Increasing Ketoacidosis
Salbutamol, alcohol, diazoxide

Drugs Increasing Lactic Acid Formation
Phenformin, metformin, alcohol, streptozotocin, isoniazid, sodium nitroprusside, povidone-iodine ointment, fructose, xylitol, sorbitol

Drugs Increasing Other Organic Acids
Salicylate, methanol, ethylene glycol, paraldehyde, toluene, nalidixic acid, high doses of carbenicillin, methenamine mandelate or hippuric acid salts

their antianabolic effect, may increase BUN and worsen the metabolic acidosis in patients with renal failure.[50] The severity of the acidosis depends on the dosage, the duration of treatment, and the level of the underlying renal function. Symptoms usually develop after a few days of therapy. Cases of tetracycline-induced metabolic acidosis have also been reported in patients who have impairment of liver function.[51]

Salbutamol, a selective $beta_2$-adrenergic agonist, is used in the treatment of premature labor and asthma. When given intravenously to normal individuals, there is a rapid rise in free-fatty acids, ketones, insulin, glucose, and lactate. Diabetics who lack endogenous insulin may be especially prone to salbutamol ketoacidosis.[52] Diabetic ketoacidosis has also been reported in patients receiving intravenous diazoxide for hypertension, because of the drug's hyperglycemic effect.[53]

The homeostasis of lactate has recently been reviewed.[54] Lactic acidosis represents the imbalance between lactate production and metabolism or excretion by the liver and the kidneys.[54] It is, therefore, not uncommon to see lactic acidosis in patients with renal or hepatic failure. Drugs that increase lactic acid formation result in clinically significant lactic acidosis, predominantly in patients with kidney and liver disease. Phenformin, a biguanide, is one of the most common causes of lactic acidosis.[55] The drug depletes glycogen stores and increases lactate production. Its use in diabetes mellitus has resulted in severe lactic acidosis and, at times, death. The reported incidence of lactic acidosis ranges from 1.5 to 77 per cent.[55] Most of the cases reported are associated with renal failure and liver impairment. Phenformin is no longer commercially available in the United States. In contrast to phenformin, metformin, another biguanide, has rarely been reported to cause lactic acidosis.[56, 57] Ethanol-induced lactic acidosis was first noted by Himwich et al.[58] Subsequent studies suggested that hyperlactemia is common after alcohol ingestion.[59] The acidosis is usually mild, although severe lactic acidosis has been reported. The increase in blood lactate after alcohol ingestion is due to a decreased hepatic uptake rather than increased production. It is more likely to occur in the diabetic patient and it occasionally is associated with ketoacidosis. A case of lactic acidosis associated with the use of streptozotocin in a patient with an oat cell carcinoma of the lung has been reported.[60] The acidosis developed within 24 hours after the administration of the drug. It was suggested that the drug may have interfered with the metabolism of lactate. It should, however, be pointed out that the patient also had renal failure and hepatic impairment. The occurrence of metabolic acidosis associated with isoniazid (INH) overdose has been reported.[61] The acidosis was thought to be due to the inhibition by INH of the conversion of lactate to pyruvate. In both cases, serum glutamic-oxaloacetic transaminase (SGOT) and lactic dehydrogenase (LDH) were elevated. Metabolic acidosis can develop in patients receiving sodium nitroprusside for control of hypertension.[62-64] The acidosis is associated with infusion of large doses for a long period of time. The mechanism is not clear but may be related to the accumulation of cyanide that inhibits mitochondrial–cytochrome oxidase. Discontinuation of the drug is associated with the correction of the acidosis.

Povidone-iodine ointment is used for topical therapy of burns. The ointment contains 1 per cent available iodine in a water-soluble base containing 10 per cent povidone-iodine with a pH of 2.43 and an osmolality of 1000 mOsm/L. As already discussed, its use has been associated with hypernatremia through the excessive loss of water through the skin.[20] In addition, high anion gap metabolic acidosis has been reported[55]; the mechanism for the acidosis is not clear. In one case, serum lactate was elevated. A case of lactic acidosis also was reported in a woman after the ingestion of an unknown quantity of Lugol's solution, which consists of 5 per cent iodine and 10 per cent potassium iodine solution.[66] In addition to lactic acidosis, mild renal failure and impaired renal acidification were also present. Fructose has been used as an intravenous nutrient in patients with diabetic ketoacidosis and hepatic failure. The association between fructose infusion and lactic acidosis has recently been reviewed by Cohen and Woods.[67] Similar findings have been reported with xylitol administration. Sorbitol, which is converted to fructose, may also be associated with lactic acidosis. The diagnosis of lactic acidosis is not difficult once the physician is alerted to the potential of drug-induced lactic acidosis and the finding of a high anion gap metabolic acid.

The treatment of lactic acidosis consists of removing the offending agents and, if necessary, administration of $NaHCO_3$ to correct the severe acidosis. Dialysis using bicarbonate or acetate bath may be helpful.

In a study done in 1978, aspirin intoxication was associated with simple respiratory alkalosis in 22 per cent and a mixed respiratory alkalosis and metabolic acidosis in 56 per cent of the patients.[68] The acidosis is unlikely to be due to salicylic acid alone. Ketoacidosis, lactic acidosis, and perhaps other organic acids may also be responsible. Ingestion of methanol and ethylene glycol is associated with severe "anion gap" metabolic acidosis. The responsible acids are formic acid and glycolic acid in methanol and ethylene glycol intoxications, respectively. A high index of suspicion of methanol and ethylene glycol is needed when a markedly increased anion gap metabolic acidosis is associated with a high osmolar gap (difference between the calculated and the measured plasma osmolality), blurred vision and retinitis (methanol), and the presence of hippuric and oxalate crystals in the urine (ethylene glycol). Direct drug assays confirm the diagnosis. Treatment consists of administration of ethanol, which is selectively metabolized, preventing formation of the toxic metabolites of methanol and ethylene glycol. In addition, correction of acidosis with bicarbonate and removal of the toxin with dialysis is necessary.[69]

The metabolic acidosis due to administration of paraldehyde is related to the presence of various organic acids. The diagnosis, again, can be made from the history of ingestion and the presence of a typical pungent smell in the patient's breath. Because of its low pH, high doses of carbenicillin have been associated with increased anion gap metabolic acidosis.

NONANION GAP METABOLIC ACIDOSIS

Normal anion gap metabolic acidosis (Table 9–6) may result from intestinal loss or renal loss of bicarbonate, decreased renal hydrogen ion secretion, or administration of agents containing hydrochloric acid. Intestinal fluid contains large quantities of HCO_3. For example, the bicarbonate content of bile (45 mEq/L), pancreatic juice (92 mEq/L), ileal fluid (29 mEq/L), and cecal fluid (22 mEq/L) is substantial. Excessive loss of these fluids, therefore, may result in hyperchloremic acidosis. Chronic abuse of laxatives is one of the most common causes. Laxatives increase intestinal fluid secretion with resulting diarrhea. Drugs that damage absorbing mucosa may also lead to diarrhea with loss of bicarbonate. These drugs include alcohol, colchicine, neomycin, antimetabolites, and certain antibiotics, such as clindamycin and ampicillin. Cholestyramine is an anion exchange resin. It is nonreabsorbable and exchanges its chloride for endogenous HCO_3. The resultant fall in bicarbonate then results in hyperchloremic acidosis.[70]

Impaired urinary acidification may be induced by several drugs (Table 9–6). In addition to nonanion gap metabolic acidosis, other aspects of the clinical and biochemical presentation depend on the type of acidosis. In the proximal (type II) renal tubular acidosis (RTA), renal bicarbonate wasting (>20 per cent of filtered HCO_3 load), often with other tubular dysfunction (aminoaciduria, glycosuria, hyperuricosuria and phosphaturia), is

TABLE 9–6. DRUGS ASSOCIATED WITH NORMAL ANION GAP METABOLIC ACIDOSIS

Drugs Inducing Intestinal HCO_3^- Loss
- Laxatives (bisacodyl, cascara, dioctyl sodium sulfosuccinate, oxyphenisatin, phenolphthalein, castor oil)
- Alcohol, colchicine, antimetabolites, antibiotics
- Cholestyramine chloride

Drugs Inducing Impaired Urinary Acidification
- Proximal RTA (outdated tetracyclines, carbonic anhydrase inhibitors, some sulfonamides, 6-mercaptopurine, toluene)
- Distal RTA (amphotericin B, toluene, lithium)
- Spironolactone, heparin

Drugs Increasing HCl Acid
- NH_4Cl, $CaCl_2$
- Cationic amino acids (arginine, lysine, histidine)

Miscellaneous
- Flower of sulfur

seen. The urine pH is inappropriately high (>5.3) unless the systemic acidosis is severe (serum bicarbonate <12 mEq/L), at which time urine pH becomes appropriately low. Outdated tetracyclines have been reported to cause proximal RTA and Fanconi's syndrome. These patients developed hyperphosphaturia, hypercalciuria, hyperuricosuria, glycosuria, and aminoaciduria. In addition to hyperchloremic acidosis, these patients were hypokalemic, hypouricemic, and hypophosphatemic. The acidosis may last several months before complete recovery. This syndrome is not currently seen because citric acid, which causes tetracycline degradation resulting in nephrotoxic products,[71] is no longer used as a tetracycline preservative.

Drugs that inhibit the enzyme carbonic anhydrase, e.g., acetazolamide, induce a prompt increase in the urinary excretion of bicarbonate. Acetazolamide administration is associated with a mild degree of hyperchloremic acidosis and hypokalemia (serum bicarbonate approximately 21 mEq/L). Sulfamylon (mefenide hydrochloride or acetate), when used topically in burns, may cause a similar problem owing to its absorption from damaged skin and conversion to *p*-carboxybenzine, which is a potent carbonic anhydrase inhibitor.[72] The acidosis is mild or absent because the drug stimulates the respiratory center, thus producing respiratory alkalosis that counteracts the hyperchloremic acidosis.[72]

Amphotericin B induces a dose-related nephrotoxicity. Over 80 per cent of patients receiving a total dose of more than 4 gm develop a decrease in glomerular filtration rate with microscopic hematuria, pyuria, and cylindruria. Mild distal RTA with renal potassium wasting may be seen at a much lower total dose.[73] This defect appears to be due to the passive diffusion of secreted hydrogen ion from the lumen back into the distal tubular cells.[74] The defect is transient and recovery occurs within three months. When this tubular defect is encountered, the dose of amphotericin need not be reduced. The decision whether or not to continue amphotericin depends on the severity of infection and the degree of decrease in glomerular filtration rate.

Inhalation of toluene, which may be done by deliberately sniffing glue or paint to achieve a "high," may produce severe, transient RTA and severe hypokalemia.[75, 76] The mechanism of this acidification defect is not yet clear, although a similar tubular defect as produced by amphotericin B has been suggested. A recent report indicates that toluene may cause proximal as well as distal tubular dysfunction.[75, 76] Lithium carbonate at normal therapeutic levels has been reported to induce incomplete distal renal tubular acidosis (impaired urinary acidification without overt clinical acidosis).[77, 78] The mechanism of the defect has not been defined.

Spironolactone, an aldosterone antagonist, impairs renal potassium secretion and acidification. In 1979, Gabow et al.[79] reported reversible hyperchloremic acidosis in cirrhotic patients treated with spironolactone. NH_4Cl has been used in diet pills and as a urinary acidifying agent for detection of a renal acidification defect. Since NH_4Cl is converted to NH_3 and HCl, excessive use may lead to acidosis.[70-81] To avoid ammonia intoxication with NH_4Cl, oral $CaCl_2$ has been used for detection of renal acidification defect in patients with cirrhosis. In the gut, however, $CaCl_2$ reacts with $NaHCO_3$ to form HCl; therefore, metabolic acidosis may result. Hyperchloremic acidosis also has been observed in patients receiving total parenteral nutrition (containing mixtures of synthetic L-amino acids, particularly the cationic amino acids arginine, lysine, and histidine),[80] and after oral ingestion of ammonium chloride.[81] The acidosis is not due to infusion of preformed H^+, but is due to the metabolism of cationic amino acids into excessive H^+ ions. A case of hyperchloremic acidosis associated with sulfur ingestion has been reported by Blum and Coe.[82] In this setting, sulfur is oxidized to sulfide and then sulfate.

METABOLIC ALKALOSIS (Table 9–7)

The generation and maintenance of metabolic alkalosis have been previously reviewed.[83] Metabolic alkalosis can result from a gain of alkali or a loss of acid from the extracellular fluid. Administration of bicarbonate or its precursors is the most common cause of alkali excess. Precursors of bicarbonate include lactate, citrate, and acetate, all of which are converted to bicarbonate. However, this rarely produces significant alkalosis unless there is impairment of kidney function. For example, the administration of massive amounts of commercially available human plasma proteins (containing 42 and 40 mM/L of acetate in Protenate and Plasmatein, respectively)[84] or massive blood transfusions

TABLE 9-7. MECHANISMS INVOLVED IN DRUG-INDUCED METABOLIC ALKALOSIS

Gain of Exogenous Base – Drugs Causing Excessive Load of Bicarbonate or Its Precursors
Sodium bicarbonate, citrate, lactate, acetate, human plasma protein with high acetate content, massive blood transfusions

Loss of Hydrogen Ion
Drugs causing gastric loss of acid (magnesium oxide, combined Kayexalate and magnesium hydroxide)
Drugs causing renal loss of acid (hormones with mineralocorticoid activity – aldosterone; large doses of hydrocortisone, DOCA, diuretics, carbenoxolone, licorice, tobacco, carbenicillin, ticarcillin, massive doses of sodium penicillin)

(containing 17 mEq of citrate per unit of whole blood) to patients with renal failure has resulted in severe metabolic alkalosis.

Loss of acid from extracellular fluid can be due either to gastric loss or to renal loss. In the kidney, for each milliequivalent of acid excreted, 1 mEq of bicarbonate is added to the blood. The increase in renal H^+ secretion can be due to two mechanisms: (1) an increase in sodium and fluid delivery to the distal tubule with simultaneous increase in the stimulus for distal Na-H exchange, and (2) an increase in the delivery of a nonreabsorbable anion to the distal tubule.

Drugs inducing gastric loss of acid through vomiting are rare, since the drugs are usually promptly discontinued. A case of metabolic alkalosis was reported in a patient receiving massive doses of magnesium oxide.[85] It was suggested that MgO was converted to $MgCl_2$, which was converted to magnesium carbonate or bicarbonate, thereby causing metabolic alkalosis. This speculation remains to be confirmed. A similar case of alkalosis developed in a patient receiving sodium polystyrene sulfonate (Kayexalate) and magnesium hydroxide.[86, 87] In this case, the magnesium chloride produced from the interaction of magnesium hydroxide with hydrochloric acid was removed by the resin, and the free bicarbonate was reabsorbed, producing metabolic alkalosis.

Chronic administration of aldosterone results in very little change in the serum bicarbonate level when dietary intake is normal.[88] However, when serum potassium decreases, metabolic alkalosis develops until the serum potassium is replenished again. The alkalosis produced by the administration of hydrocortisone and desoxycorticosterone acetate (DOCA) are also related to the degree of hypokalemia. The alkalosis-producing effect of hydrocortisone is believed to reflect the mineralocorticoid property of the hormone. The administration of diuretics may also be associated with hypokalemia and metabolic alkalosis. The alkalosis is the result of increased sodium delivery to the distal tubule in the face of high levels of aldosterone. There is an increase in the Na-H exchange that results in the loss of acid and, therefore, metabolic alkalosis. Similarly, the mineralocorticoid-like activity of carbenoxolone may produce hypokalemic metabolic alkalosis in 10 per cent of cases.[30] In addition, carbenoxolone produces sodium retention and may result in edema, hypertension, and congestive heart failure. As already discussed, abuse of licorice can produce a syndrome similar to mineralocorticoid excess, since the licorice contains glycyrrhizic acid, which has mineralocorticoid activity.[29] Carbenicillin and massive doses of penicillin have been shown to produce severe hypokalemic metabolic alkalosis.[89, 90] Both carbenicillin and penicillin behave as poorly reabsorbable anions.[32, 90] In order to preserve electroneutrality, hydrogen and potassium ions move down the electrochemical gradient from the blood to renal tubular lumen, resulting in an increased urinary excretion of acid and potassium, and, consequently, metabolic alkalosis and hypokalemia.

The diagnosis of drug-induced metabolic alkalosis is confirmed by the presence of high plasma pH and bicarbonate or total CO_2 content. The urine Cl concentration can be helpful in differentiating between metabolic alkalosis produced by gastric loss or renal loss of acids. In metabolic alkalosis produced by gastric losses, the urine Cl is less than 10 mEq/L (sodium chloride responsive), whereas in alkalosis produced by renal loss, the urine Cl is greater than 20 mEq/L (sodium chloride resistant). The urine chloride is not helpful in patients with renal failure, since they may not be able to maximally conserve Cl. The treatment of metabolic alkalosis depends on the cause. Removal of the offending agents and sodium chloride and potassium supplementation are sufficient in those cases with gastric acid loss, whereas with excess mineralocorticoid-like activity and renal acid loss, removal of the drug is the primary treatment in these sodium chloride–resistant cases.

DRUG-INDUCED DISORDERS OF CALCIUM, PHOSPHORUS, AND MAGNESIUM

HYPERCALCEMIA (Table 9–8)

Vitamin D–induced hypercalcemia is due to both increased bone resorption and increased intestinal absorption of calcium.[91] It occurs in patients receiving vitamin D or one of its metabolites. Individuals vary in the dose of vitamin D and duration required for the production of hypercalcemia. Factors accounting for this variability include body fat content, hepatic metabolism, and protein binding of the vitamin D. Recovery from the hypercalcemia usually takes 2 to 3 months after cessation of the drug, but may take as long as 22 months. For the metabolites, the half-time for reversal of hypercalcemia and hypercalciuria is much shorter:

1,25 $(OH)_2$ cholecalciferol: 1.5 ± 0.2 days
1,α(OH) cholecalciferol: 3.4 ± 0.4 days
Califerol: 25.5 ± 9.1 days
Dihydroxytachysterol: 44 days

The half-time is independent of the dose given and duration of therapy. It is apparent that the rapidly reversible hypercalcemia makes 1,25$(OH)_2$ vitamin D preferable to the other agents in patients who develop hypercalcemia.

Ingestion of large doses of vitamin A may cause hypercalcemia, skeletal pains, bone resorption, and periosteal calcification.[93] The minimum daily requirement of vitamin A is 3000 IU for children and 5000 IU for adults. Patients may, however, ingest large amounts of the vitamin, 50,000 to 200,000 IU daily, as a nutritional supplement, to improve night vision, or to treat acne vulgaris. It is these doses that may be associated with hypercalcemia. Recovery from the hypercalcemia usually takes 2 to 4 weeks. The exact mechanism of the hypercalcemia is unclear, but probably involves increased bone reabsorption.

TABLE 9–8. DRUGS THAT MAY INDUCE HYPERCALCEMIA

Vitamin D and Metabolites 1,25 $(OH)_2$ cholecalciferol, 1 (OH) cholecalciferol, dihydroxytachysterol
Vitamin A
Lithium Carbonate
Thiazide Diuretics
Chlorthalidone
Calcium salts
Tamoxifen

The ingestion of large quantities of milk and soluble alkali (sodium bicarbonate) over several years may cause hypercalcemia without hypercalciuria or hypophosphatemia. The original six patients described by Burnett[94] had peptic ulcer and had taken large amounts of milk and absorbable alkali over a period of 3 to 30 years. They were markedly azotemic with mild alkalosis and tissue calcinosis, especially in the cornea. The serum phosphate, alkaline phosphatase, and urine calcium levels were normal. Three of these patients died of renal failure. Upon the reduction of excessive milk and alkali intake, the serum calcium returned to normal in one patient, fell to hypocalcemic levels in association with further decrease in renal function in two patients, and improved but still remained at hypercalcemic levels in the other three patients. Subsequently, a similar syndrome was described within one week after starting therapy for peptic ulcer disease with calcium carbonate, milk, and cream.[95] Serum calcium concentrations as high as 18 mg/dl were noted. The hypercalcemia, azotemia, and alkalosis were reversible when the antacid, milk, and cream were discontinued. The presenting clinical symptoms are largely related to the hypercalcemia, i.e., nausea, vomiting, anorexia, weakness, headache, mental confusion, ataxia, and stupor.

The exact mechanism of hypercalcemia in the milk alkali syndrome is not established. It has been suggested that continued calcium intake, milk with associated vitamin D intake, impaired renal function and thus excretion of calcium, and vomiting-induced extracellular fluid volume contraction all contribute to the hypercalcemia.

Thiazide diuretics may cause hypercalcemia in normal subjects, in patients with high bone turnover rates, such as primary hyperparathyroidism, and in vitamin D–treated patients with hypoparathyroidism and juvenile osteoporosis. In normal subjects, the hypercalcemia is mild (usually less than 11 mg/dl) and transient. Thus, normal homeostatic mechanisms with feedback suppression of parathyroid hormone secretion prevent severe hypercalcemia. Sustained hypercalcemia, however, is seen in patients with persistently high levels of parathyroid hormone or in patients with increased bone resorption with or without high circulating parathyroid hormone. The incidence of hypercalcemia in 1034 hypertensive patients receiving thiazides was 1.9 per cent (20 patients). Of these 20 patients, 15 (75 per cent) had parathyroid adenomas when explored surgically.[96]

The mechanism of the thiazide-induced hypercalcemia may involve several factors, including (1) decreased urinary excretion of calcium secondary to extracellular fluid volume contraction with enhanced proximal reabsorption of calcium, (2) potentiation of the effects of parathyroid hormone on bone and renal tubules, and (3) a possible direct effect on the renal tubule. Evidence for potentiation of the action of parathyroid hormone on bone is suggested by the hypercalcemia produced in hemodialyzed patients treated with thiazides; this observation, however, has not been confirmed. Chlorthalidone has a nephron site of action similar to the thiazide diuretics. Of 39 patients receiving the drug, six (15 per cent) developed hypercalcemia. The hypercalcemia was completely reversible on cessation of the drug.[97]

Long-term lithium carbonate therapy for manic-depressive psychosis is occasionally associated with hypercalcemia, even with a normal therapeutic range of serum lithium concentration. In these patients, the serum parathyroid level may be inappropriately high for the degree of hypercalcemia. Christianson reported 14 of 96 patients treated with lithium had high parathyroid hormone (PTH) levels and hypercalcemia.[98] When the parathyroid glands were explored, an adenoma was found in every patient. Thus, it appears that lithium may unmask primary hyperparathyroidism, perhaps secondary to the hypocalciuric effect of lithium.[78]

Tamoxifen, an antiestrogenic drug, has been associated with hypercalcemia in about 1 per cent of patients with advanced metastatic breast cancer. The hypercalcemia occurs shortly after initiation of therapy and is usually mild and transient; however, two cases of severe hypercalcemia (17 to 21 mg/dl) have been reported.[99] In both, the hypercalcemia resolved with cessation of tamoxifen, hydration, and administration of steroids and mithramycin. Readministration of tamoxifen with steroids at a later date did not cause hypercalcemia, thus raising a question about the drug's role in causing the hypercalcemia.

HYPOCALCEMIA (Table 9–9)

Drug-induced hypocalcemia may present as paresthesias, tetany, and Jacksonian or grand mal seizures. Nonspecific neuropsychiatric systems, such as irritability, emotional instability, and hallucinations, may occur. These symptoms are especially pronounced with acute, severe hypocalcemia. Deep tendon reflexes are diminished or absent.

Drug-induced hypomagnesemia secondary to gentamicin or *cis*-platinum administration may be associated with severe symptomatic hypocalcemia.[34, 35] The mechanisms include skeletal resistance to PTH, decreased release of PTH, and increased movement of calcium from the extracellular compartment into the bone. The hypocalcemia is resistant to calcium administration unless the hypomagnesemia is corrected.

Hypocalcemia and osteomalacia have been documented following the prolonged administration of phenytoin and phenobarbital. These drugs may induce hepatic microsomal P-450 enzyme activity, which then is responsible for the hydroxylation of vitamin D in an abnormal fashion whereby biologically inactive steroids are produced. A 1977 study[100] reported normal levels of 1,25 $(OH)_2$ vitamin D_3, suggesting that the anticonvulsants may also interfere with the action of the active form of the hormone on the bone or intestine.

In the treatment of hypercalcemia or hypophosphatemia, the rapid infusion of potassium or sodium phosphate (> 50 mM — 1550 mg — in < 3 hours) has been reported to cause severe hypocalcemia.[101] This response is especially pronounced in patients with renal im-

TABLE 9–9. MECHANISMS INVOLVED IN DRUG-INDUCED HYPOCALCEMIA

Reduced Action of PTH
- Drug-induced hypomagnesemia (see Table 9–11)
  - *Cis*-platinum
  - Gentamicin
- Cimetidine
- Propranolol

Reduced Action of Vitamin D
- Drug-induced malabsorption (cholestyramine)
- Anticonvulsants (phenytoin, barbiturates)

Miscellaneous
- Rapid phosphate infusion
- EDTA infusion
- Citrate infusion

pairment. A similar effect has been reported following phosphate enemas.[102]

The infusion of ethylenediaminetetraacetic acid (EDTA) complexes calcium and causes a transient hypocalcemia. A similar response is seen following transfusion of a large number of units of citrated blood. Mithramycin, commonly used to treat cancer-related hypercalcemia, lowers serum calcium within hours, occasionally to hypocalcemic levels. The effect is probably due to inhibition of bone resorption.[103]

HYPOPHOSPHATEMIA (Table 9–10)

Selective hypophosphatemia due to decreased intake of phosphate is extremely rare, since phosphate is ubiquitous in most foods.[104] The chronic ingestion of aluminum or magnesium hydroxide and aluminum carbonate antacids may lead to severe hypophosphatemia, especially in malnourished alcoholics or dialyzed subjects. These antacids bind phosphates in the gut, thus leading to selective malabsorption of phosphate.[105]

Parenteral or enteral hyperalimentation, when used without phosphate supplements, may cause severe hypophosphatemia. This is due to the shift of phosphate from the extracellular to the intracellular space during the anabolic process that occurs in the absence of adequate phosphate intake.

Drug-induced alkalosis, especially respiratory alkalosis (as with salicylate intoxication), may cause profound hypophosphatemia.[104]

TABLE 9–10. MECHANISMS INVOLVED IN DRUG-INDUCED HYPOPHOSPHATEMIA

Decreased Absorption
Antacids
Transcellular Shifts
Respiratory alkalosis
Androgens
Catecholamines
Glucagon and fructose administration
Lactate administration
Hyperalimentation
Increased Urinary Loss
Diuretics
Glucagon
Osmotic diuresis
Multiple Mechanisms
Chronic alcohol intake

This effect relates to increased glycolysis due to increased intracellular pH and activity of phosphofructokinase that cause a shift of phosphate into the cells. For the same degree of extracellular alkalosis, the intracellular pH is higher in respiratory than metabolic alkalosis owing to the rapid equilibration of CO_2 across cell membranes compared to the slow equilibration of bicarbonate. Mild transient hypophosphatemia is occasionally seen in catabolic patients receiving androgens and following epinephrine administration. In both circumstances, the mechanism is thought to be secondary to an intracellular shift of phosphate.

The administration of glucose, by stimulating insulin release, will enhance the entry of both phosphates and glucose into the muscle and hepatic cells. The resulting hypophosphatemia is mild, except in the starved or cirrhotic patient in whom severe hypophosphatemia may occur. The intravenous administration of fructose may also induce hypophosphatemia, which may be more marked than that associated with glucose administration because of the unregulated uptake of fructose by the liver.

The acute administration of acetazolamide, thiazides, and large doses of furosemide increase the urinary excretion of phosphate.[104] This phosphaturic effect is probably mediated through the carbonic anhydrase–inhibiting action of these diuretics. Osmotic diuretics also will increase the urinary excretion of phosphate. The hypophosphatemia is transient if the urinary losses of sodium and water are not replaced, since ECF volume contraction occurs and leads to increased reabsorption of phosphate, sodium, and water in the proximal tubule.

Moderate hypophosphatemia due to increased urinary excretion of phosphate may follow glucagon administration, perhaps secondary both to renal losses and to an intracellular shift of phosphate.[104]

Chronic alcoholism is associated with hypophosphatemia in at least 50 per cent of hospitalized alcoholic patients.[106] It is usually seen approximately 24 to 48 hours after admission and coincides with the administration of glucose, respiratory alkalosis, hypomagnesemia, and, occasionally, sepsis. The evidence that alcohol *per se* increases urinary phosphate loss is not convincing.

Severe hypophosphatemia (serum phosphate less than 1 mg/dl) can result in major clinical problems. Proximal myopathy, rhabdomyolysis, bone pain, and joint stiffness are well documented. The rhabdomyolysis may lead to myoglobinuria-induced acute renal failure. In addition, decreased red blood cell oxygen release due to decreased 2,3-diphosphoglycerate (2,3-DPG) and decreased white blood cell and platelet functions are frequently observed.[104] Encephalopathy, cardiomyopathy, hemolytic anemia, respiratory paralysis, and worsening liver function have also been described.

Most hypophosphatemic patients respond well to skim milk, 1 to 2 q/day. High caloric intake should be avoided, since enhanced phosphorylation of glucose may worsen hypophosphatemia. Severe hypophosphatemia with muscle paralysis or seizures requires intravenous phosphate therapy (potassium phosphate, 40 mEq three times a day).

HYPOMAGNESEMIA (Table 9–11)

Hypomagnesemia may result from either gastrointestinal or renal losses of magnesium. Drugs that increase gastrointestinal magnesium loss are those associated with diarrhea or malabsorption. It has been suggested that drugs causing steatorrhea may lead to magnesium depletion by the formation of magnesium soaps. Neomycin depresses fat absorption by binding and precipitating the fatty acids important in the formation of micelles. In addition, neomycin has a toxic effect on the mucosa of the small intestine. High doses of colchicine may be associated with steatorrhea and vitamin B_{12} malabsorption. Cholestyramine increases fat excretion in normal persons; the steatorrhea is considerably worse when cholestyramine is given to patients with ileal resection. Para-aminosalicylic acid can also cause steatorrhea, but the mechanism is unknown. Chronic abuse of laxatives containing phenolphthalein, bisacodyl, cascara, and oxyphenisatin may lead to steatorrhea. Hypokalemia and metabolic acidosis are also frequently observed in patients with cathartic abuse.

TABLE 9–11. DRUGS THAT MAY INDUCE HYPOMAGNESEMIA

Drugs Increasing Gastrointestinal Loss
Neomycin, kanamycin, para-aminosalicylic acid, colchicine, cholestyramine, colestipol, laxatives

Drugs Increasing Renal Loss
Ethanol
Diuretics (mannitol, benzothiadiazine diuretics, furosemide, ethacrynic acid, mercurial diuretics)
Aminoglycosides (viomycin, capreomycin, gentamicin, tobramycin, amikacin, sisomicin)
Hormones (aldosterone, DOCA, fludrocortisone)
Antineoplastic agents (*cis*-platinum)
Antifungal agents (amphotericin B)
Acidifying agents (NH_4Cl)

Hypomagnesemia was observed in 25 per cent of patients requiring admission for alcoholism.[106] Many factors may be responsible, including poor intake, vomiting, and diarrhea. In addition, ingestion of alcohol causes a profound increase in urinary magnesium loss.[107] The mechanism whereby alcohol inhibits tubular reabsorption of magnesium is unclear. Although acetazolamide inhibits solute reabsorption in the proximal tubule, it has minimal effect on renal magnesium excretion. Administration of loop diuretics and mannitol increases magnesium as well as sodium and calcium excretion, probably by inhibition of tubular water absorption in the ascending limb of the loop of Henle.[108] Chronic administration of benzothiadiazine diuretics also results in magnesium depletion.[109,110] Spironolactone does not cause an increase in renal magnesium excretion. On the contrary, a decrease in magnesium excretion is observed in primary hyperaldosteronism. Early reports indicated that capreomycin and viomycin caused hypomagnesemia.[111,112] More recently, other aminoglycosides have been incriminated.[113] Bar et al. reported two cases of hypomagnesemia associated with massive doses of gentamicin.[34] In addition to the hypomagnesemia, hypocalcemia, hypokalemia, and metabolic alkalosis also developed with gentamicin use. Drug-induced increases in magnesium and potassium excretion are probably responsible for the hypomagnesemia. The hypocalcemia probably results from a state of functional hypoparathyroidism and end organ unresponsiveness to PTH in response to the magnesium depletion.[114-116] *Cis*-platinum, an anticancer agent active against solid tumors, has been reported to be associated with hypomagnesemia in 23 of 44 patients receiving a mean dose of 467 mg.[35] Renal magnesium wasting was documented in four patients. Other agents that may cause hypomagnesemia include mineralocorticoid hormones, NH_4Cl, and amphotericin B.

The diagnosis of drug-induced hypomagnesemia can be suspected by the associated symptoms and signs. These include muscle

TABLE 9-12. SODIUM AND MAGNESIUM CONTENT OF VARIOUS DRUGS

Drug	Sodium	Magnesium
Antimicrobials		
Ampicillin	3.1 mEq/gm	
Carbenicillin	4.7 mEq/gm	
Cephalothin	2.4 mEq/gm	
Chloramphenicol	2.3 mEq/gm	
Cloxacillin	2.3 mEq/gm	
Dicloxacillin	2.1 mEq/gm	
Erythromycin	12.0 mEq/gm	
Methicillin	2.4 mEq/gm	
Nafcillin	3.2 mEq/gm	
Oxacillin	2.6 mEq/gm	
Penicillin G potassium	0.3 mEq/gm	
Penicillin G sodium	1.7 mEq/gm	
Antacids		
Alka-Seltzer	23.0 mEq/tab	0
Aludrox	0.2 mEq/5 ml	3.5 mEq/5 ml
Amphagel	0.3 mEq/5 ml	0
Basaljel	0.4 mEq/5 ml	0
Di-Gel	0.2 mEq/5 ml	10.0 mEq/5 ml
Eno-Salts	32.0 mEq/tsp.	0
Gelusil	0.3 mEq/5 ml	5.7 mEq/5 ml
Maalox	0.3 mEq/5 ml	7.0 mEq/5 ml
Milk of magnesia	0	10.0 mEq/5 ml
Mylanta	7.0 mEq/tab	6.9 mEq/5 ml
Antacids (Continued)		
Phosphajel	0.6 mEq/5 ml	0
Riopan	0.3 mEq/5 ml	6.5 mEq/5 ml
Robalate	0.4 mEq/5 ml	0
Rolaids	2.0 mEq/tab	0
Titralac	0.5 mEq/5 ml	0
Miscellaneous		
Amigen 5%	35.0 mEq/L	
Aminosol 5%	10.0 mEq/L	
Dilantin sodium	3.8 mEq/gm	
Fleets phosphosoda	24.0 mEq/5 ml	
Fleet enema	47.0 mEq/oz	
Fizrin	29.0 mEq/pack	
Heparin	1.5 mEq/10 ml	
Hypaque M 75%	8.7 mEq/20 ml	
Hypaque M 90%	9.6 mEq/20 ml	
Kayexalate	4.4 mEq/gm	
Mucomyst	12.0 mEq/10 ml	
Oragrafin	0.8 mEq/cap	
Phenergan exp.	2.5 mEq/5 ml	
Probanthine w/ Dartal	5.0 mEq/tab	
Sodium salicylate	2.1 mEq/gm	
Skiodan 40%	16.0 mEq/10 ml	
Vivonex HN	33.5 mEq/L	

weakness, tremor, athetoid movements, fasciculation, tetany, irritability, psychosis, mental depression, and positive Chvostek and Trousseau's signs. More recently, dysphagia and nystagmus have also been reported with hypomagnesemia. Magnesium supplementation, along with discontinuation of the causative drug, is usually adequate to treat these manifestations of hypomagnesemia.

MISCELLANEOUS

Drug-induced hypermagnesemia is uncommon when renal function is normal. However, when renal function is impaired, administration of magnesium-containing substances may be hazardous and lead to severe hypermagnesemia.[35, 117] The symptoms of hypermagnesemia are hypotension, central nervous system depression, hyporeflexia, suppression of respiration, coma, and even cardiac arrest. Drugs containing high magnesium content are listed in Table 9–12. Table 9–12 also lists the sodium content of various drugs.

Lastly, drugs that induce sodium and water retention are listed in Table 9–13. These drugs induce positive sodium balance and can thereby elevate blood pressure and induce edema. These drugs act to induce sodium retention by several mechanisms: (1) aldosterone-related enhanced renal tubular sodium reabsorption, (2) inhibition of the effect of renal prostaglandins, and (3) lowering of renal perfusion pressure (Table 9–13). Drugs that induce either release of ADH or renal response to ADH (see Table 9–1) impair renal water excretion and thereby lead to weight gain. Patients with kidney and liver disease may be especially susceptible to the sodium and water retention properties of these agents. Drugs that may increase blood urea nitrogen (BUN) and/or serum creatinine are listed in Table 9–14.

TABLE 9–13. DRUGS INDUCING SODIUM AND WATER RETENTION

Hormones
Estrogen, progesterone, aldosterone, glucocorticoids, DOCA, fluohydrocortisone, licorice, carbenoxolone, tobacco

Nonsteroidal Anti-Inflammatory Agents
Indomethacin, phenylbutazone, oxyphenbutazone, ibuprofen, fenoprofen, naproxen, tolemetin sodium

Antihypertensive Agents

Drugs Stimulating Vasopressin Release or Enhancing Vasopressin Action
See Table 9–1

TABLE 9-14. DRUGS INCREASING BUN AND/OR CREATININE

Increased Catabolism or Decreased Anabolism
Tetracycline
Glucocorticoids
Drugs That Interfere with Creatinine Secretion
Cimetidine
Trimethoprim

SUMMARY

Patients with renal and hepatic disease are often uniquely susceptible to drug-induced fluid, electrolyte, and acid-base disorders. An awareness of potential drug-induced metabolic abnormalities combined with careful clinical and laboratory monitoring can prevent these complications.

REFERENCES

1. Hobson JA, English JT: Self-induced water intoxication. Case study of a chronically schizophrenic patient with physiological evidence of water retention due to inappropriate release of antidiuretic hormone. Ann. Intern. Med. *58*:324–332, 1963.
2. Dubovsky SL, Grabon S, Berl T, et al.: Syndrome of inappropriate secretion of antidiuretic hormone with exacerbated psychosis. Ann. Intern. Med. *79*:551–554, 1973.
3. Cadnapaphornchai P, Taher S, McDonald FD: Syndrome of inappropriate secretion in chronic schizophrenia. (Abstract.) Kidney Int. *14*:647A, 1978.
4. Fichman MP, Vorherr H, Kleeman CR, et al.: Diuretic-induced hyponatremia. Ann. Intern. Med. *75*:853–863, 1971.
5. Sears ES: Non-ketotic hyperosmolar hyperglycemia during glycerol therapy for cerebral edema. Neurology *26*:89–94, 1976.
6. Moses AN, Miller M: Drug-induced dilutional hyponatremia. N. Engl. J. Med. *291*:1234–1239, 1974.
7. Henry DA, Lawson DH, Reavey P, et al.: Hyponatremia during carbamazepine treatment. Br. Med. J. *1*:83–84, 1977.
8. Rado JP: Water intoxication during carbamazepine treatment. Br. Med. J. *3*:479, 1973.
9. Rosenthal S, Kaufman S: Vincristine neurotoxicity. Ann. Intern. Med. *80*:733–737, 1974.
10. Piters K: Chlorpropamide-induced hyponatremia. J. Clin. Endocrinol. Metab. *43*:1085–1087, 1976.
11. Sheeler LR, Schumacher OP: Hyponatremia during ACTH infusions. Ann. Intern. Med. *19*:798–799, 1979.
12. Luzecky MH, Burman KD, Schultz ER: The syndrome of inappropriate secretion of antidiuretic hormone associated with amitriptyline administration. South. Med. J. *67*:495–497, 1974.
13. Peterson JC, Plack RW, Mahoney JJ, et al.: Inappropriate antidiuretic hormone. Secondary to a monoamine oxidase inhibitor. J.A.M.A. *239*:1422–1423, 1978.
14. DeRivera JLG: Inappropriate secretion of antidiuretic hormone from fluphenazine therapy. Ann. Intern. Med. *82*:811–812, 1975.
15. DeFronzo RA, Braine H, Colvin M, et al.: Water intoxication in man after cyclophosphamide therapy: Time course in relation to drug activation. Ann. Intern. Med. *78*:861–869, 1973.
16. Berl T, Anderson RJ, McDonald KM, et al.: Clinical disorders of water metabolism. Kidney Int. *10*:117–132, 1976.
17. Kaupke C, Sprague T, Gitnick GL: Hypernatremia after the administration of lactulose. Ann. Intern. Med. *86*:745–746, 1977.
18. Primack WA, Gartner LM, McGurk HE, et al.: Hypernatremia associated with cholestyramine therapy. Pediatrics *90*:1024–1025, 1977.
19. Runeberg L, Miettinen TA, Mikkila EA: Effect of cholestyramine on mineral excretion in man. Acta Med. Scand. *192*:71–76, 1972.
20. Scoggin C, McClellan JR, Gary JM: Hypernatremia and acidosis in association with topical treatment of burns. Lancet *1*:959, 1977.
21. Gault MH, Dixon ME, Dayle M, et al.: Hypernatremia, azotemia and dehydration due to high protein tube feeding. Ann. Intern. Med. *68*:778–791, 1968.
22. Singer I, Forrest JV: Drug induced states of nephrogenic diabetes insipidus. Kidney Int. *109*:82–95, 1976.
23. Mann J, Branton LJ, Larkins LG: Hyperosmolality complicating recovery from lithium toxicity. Br. Med. J. *2*:1522–1523, 1978.
24. DeVillota ED, Cavanilles JM, Stein L, et al.: Hyperosmolality crisis following infusion of hypertonic sodium chloride for purposes of therapeutic abortion. Am. J. Med. *55*:116–122, 1973.
25. Mattar JA, Weil MH, Shubin H, et al.: Cardiac arrest in the critically ill. II. Hyperosmolar states following cardiac arrest. Am. J. Med. *56*:162–168, 1974.
26. Diengott D, Rozsa O, Levy N, et al.: Hypokalemia in barium poisoning. Lancet *2*:343–344, 1964.
27. Lawson DH, Boddy K, Gray JMB, et al.: Potassium supplements in patients receiving long-term diuretics for oedema. Q. J. Med. *45*:469–478, 1976.
28. Ghione S, Glerico A, Fommei E, et al.: Hypertension and hypokalaemia caused by 9 alpha-fluoroprednisolone in a nasal spray [letter]. Lancet *1*:1301, 1979.
29. Conn JW, Rovner DR, Cohen EL: Licorice-induced pseudoaldosteronism. J.A.M.A. *205*:492, 1968.
30. Davies GJ, Rhodes J, Calcraft BJ: Complication of carbenoxolone therapy. Br. Med. J. *3*:400–402, 1974.
31. Blachley JD, Knochel JP: Tobacco chewers hypokalemia: licorice revisited. N. Engl. J. Med. *302*:784, 1980.
32. Lipner HI, Ruzany F, Dasgupta M, et al.: The behavior of carbenicillin as nonreabsorbable anion. J. Lab. Clin. Med. *86*:183–194, 1975.
33. Shils ME: Experimental human magnesium depletion. Medicine (Baltimore) *48*:61–85, 1969.
34. Bar RS, Wilson HE, Massaferri EL: Hypomagnesemic hypocalcemia, secondary to renal magnesemia wasting: A possible consequence of high-

dose gentamicin therapy. Ann. Intern. Med. *82*:646–649, 1975.
35. Schilsky RL, Anderson T: Hypomagnesemia and renal magnesium wasting in patients receiving cisplatin. Ann. Intern. Med. *90*:929–931, 1979.
36. Granerus AK, Jagenburg R, Savanborg A: Kaliuretic effect of L-dopa treatment in Parkinsonian patients. Acta Med. Scand. *201*:291–297, 1977.
37. Fraley DS, Adler S: Isohydric regulation of the plasma potassium by bicarbonate in the rat. Kidney Int. *9*:333–343, 1976.
38. Orringer CE, Eustace JC, Wunsch CD, et al.: Natural history of lactic acidosis after grand mal seizure. N. Engl. J. Med. *297*:796–799, 1977.
39. Smith TW, Willerson JT: Suicidal and accidental digoxin ingestion. Circulation *44*:29, 1971.
40. Cooperman LH: Succinylcholine-induced hyperkalemia in neuromuscular disease. J.A.M.A. *213*:1867–1871, 1970.
41. Bushinsky DA, Gennari J: Life-threatening hyperkalemia induced by arginine. Ann. Intern. Med. *89*:632–634, 1978.
42. Snyder EL, Dixon T, Bresnitz E: Abuse of salt "substitute." N. Engl. J. Med. *292*:320, 1975.
43. Simon GE, Bov JR: The potassium load from blood transfusion. Postgrad. Med. *49*:61–64, 1971.
44. Vibarti GC: Glucose-induced hyperkalemia: a hazard for diabetics? Lancet *1*:690–691, 1978.
45. Wilson D, Goetz FC: Selective hypoaldosteronism after prolonged heparin administration. Am. J. Med. *36*:535–539, 1964.
46. Schlatmann RJ, Jansen AP, Prenen H, et al.: The natriuretic and aldosterone-suppressive action of heparin and some related polysulfated polysaccharides. J. Clin. Endocrinol. Metab. *24*:35–47, 1964.
47. Kutyrina IN, Androsova SO, Tareyera IE: Indomethacin-induced hyporeninemic hypoaldosteronism. Lancet *1*:785, 1979.
48. McDonald CJ: Use of computer to detect and respond to clinical events: its effect on clinician behavior. Ann. Intern. Med. *84*:162–167, 1976.
49. Walker BR, Capuzzi DM, Alexander F: Hyperkalemia after triamterene in diabetic patients. Clin. Pharmacol. Ther. *13*:643–651, 1972.
50. Shils ME: Renal disease and the metabolic effects of tetracycline. Ann. Intern. Med. *58*:389–408, 1963.
51. Kunelis CT, Peters J, Edmondson HA: Fatty liver of pregnancy and its relationship to tetracycline. Am. J. Med. *38*:359–377, 1965.
52. Thomas DJB, Gill B, Brown T, Stubbs WA: Salbutamol-induced diabetic ketoacidosis. Br. Med. J. *3*:438, 1977.
53. Updike SJ, Harrington AR: Acute diabetic ketoacidosis. A complication of intravenous diazoxide treatment of refractory hypertension. N. Engl. J. Med. *280*:768, 1969.
54. Relman AS: Lactic Acidosis, Acid-base and Potassium Homeostasis. New York: Churchill Livingstone, 1978, pp. 65–100.
55. Misbin RI: Phenformin-associated lactic acidosis: pathogenesis and treatment. Ann. Intern. Med. *87*:591–595, 1977.
56. Lebacq EG, Terzmalis A: Metformin and lactic acidosis. Lancet *1*:314–315, 1972.
57. Hayat JC: The treatment of lactic acidosis in the diabetic patient by peritoneal dialysis using sodium acetate. A report of two cases. Diabetologia *10*:485–487, 1974.
58. Himwich HE, Nahum LH, Rakieten N, et al.: The metabolism of alcohol. J.A.M.A. *100*:651, 1933.
59. Kreisberg RA, Owen WC, Siegal AN: Alcohol-induced hyperlactic acidemia, inhibition of lactate utilization. J. Clin. Invest. *50*:166–174, 1971.
60. Narins RG, Blumenthal SA, Fraser BW, et al.: Streptozotocin-induced lactic acidosis. Am. J. Med. Sci. *265*:455–461, 1973.
61. Bear ES, Hoffman PF, Siegel SR, et al.: Suicidal ingestion of isoniazid: an uncommon cause of metabolic acidosis and seizures. South. Med. J. *69*:31–32, 1976.
62. Greiss L, Trembay NAG, Davies DW: The toxicity of sodium nitroprusside. Can. Anesth. Soc. J. *23*:480–485, 1976.
63. McDowall DE, Keaney NP, Turner JN, et al.: The toxicity of sodium nitroprusside. Br. J. Anesth. *46*:327–332, 1974.
64. Humphrey SH, Nash DA, Jr.: Lactic acidosis complicating sodium nitroprusside therapy. Ann. Intern. Med. *88*:58–59, 1978.
65. Pietsch J, Meakins JL: Complications of povidone-iodine absorption in topically treated burn patients. Lancet *1*:280–282, 1976.
66. Dyck RF, Bear RA, Goldstein NB, et al.: Iodine-iodide toxic reaction: Case report with emphasis on the nature of the metabolic acidosis. Can. Med. Assoc. *120*:704–706, 1979.
67. Cohen RD, Woods HF: Clinical and Biochemical Aspects of Lactic Acidosis. Oxford: Blackwell Scientific Publications, 1976.
68. Gabow PA, Anderson RJ, Potts DE, et al.: Acid-base disturbances in the salicylate-intoxicated adult. Arch. Intern. Med. *138*:1481–1484, 1978.
69. Parry MF, Wallach R: Ethylene glycol poisoning. Am. J. Med. *57*:143–150, 1974.
70. Kleinman PK: Cholestyramine and metabolic acidosis. N. Engl. J. Med. *290*:861, 1974.
71. Fulop M, Draphin A: Potassium depletion syndrome secondary to nephropathy apparently caused by "outdated tetracycline." N. Engl. J. Med. *272*:986–989, 1965.
72. Asch MJ, White MG, Pruitt BA, Jr.: Acid-base changes associated with topical sulfamylon therapy. Ann. Surg. *172*:946–950, 1970.
73. Butler WT, Bennett JE, Alling DW, et al.: Nephrotoxicity of amphotericin B. Early and late effects in 81 patients. Ann. Intern. Med. *61*:175–187, 1964.
74. Steinmetz PR, Alawqati Q, Lawton WJ: Renal tubular acidosis. Am. J. Med. Sci. *271*:41–54, 1976.
75. Taher S, Anderson RJ, McCartney R, et al.: Renal tubular acidosis associated with toluene sniffing. N. Engl. J. Med. *290*:765–768, 1974.
76. Moss AH, Gabow PA, Kaehny WD, et al.: Fanconi's syndrome and distal renal tubular acidosis after glue sniffing. Ann. Intern. Med. *92*:69–70, 1980.
77. Perez GO, Oster JR, Vaamonde CA: Incomplete syndrome of renal tubular acidosis induced by lithium carbonate. J. Lab. Clin. Med. *86*:386–394, 1975.
78. Miller PD, Dubovsky SI, McDonald KM, et al.: Central, renal and adrenal effects of lithium in man. Am. J. Med. *66*:787–803, 1979.
79. Gabow PA, Moore S, Schrier RW: Spironolactone-

induced hyperchloremic acidosis in cirrhosis. Ann. Intern. Med. *90*:338–340, 1979.

80. Heird WC, Dell RB, Driscoll JN, Jr., et al.: Metabolic acidosis resulting from an intravenous alimentation mixture containing synthetic amino acids. N. Engl. J. Med. *287*:943–948, 1972.
81. Relman AS, Shelburn PF, Talman A: Profound acidosis resulting from excessive ammonium chloride in previously healthy subjects. N. Engl. J. Med. *264*:848–852, 1961.
82. Blum JE, Coe FL: Metabolic acidosis after sulfur ingestion. N. Engl. J. Med. *297*:869–870, 1977.
83. Seldin DW, Rector FC, Jr.: The generation and maintenance of metabolic alkalosis. Kidney Int. *1*:306–321, 1972.
84. Rahilly GT, Berl T: Severe metabolic alkalosis caused by administration of plasma protein fraction in end-stage renal failure. N. Engl. J. Med. *301*:824–826, 1979.
85. Urakabe S. Nakata K, Ando A, et al.: Hypokalemia and metabolic alkalosis resulting from overuse of magnesium oxide. Jpn. Circ. J. *39*:1136–1137, 1975.
86. Ziessman HA: Alkalosis and seizure due to a cation exchange and magnesium hydroxide. South. Med. J. *69*:497–499, 1976.
87. Schroeder ET: Alkalosis resulting from combined administration of a "non-systemic" antacid and a cation-exchange resin. Gastroenterology *56*:868–874, 1968.
88. Kassirer JP, London AM, Goldman M, et al.: On the pathogenesis of metabolic alkalosis in hyperaldosteronism. Am. J. Med. *49*:306–315, 1970.
89. Klastersky J, Vanderkelen B, Daneau D, et al.: Carbenicillin and hypokalemia. Ann. Intern. Med. *78*:774–775, 1973.
90. Brunner FP, Frick PG: Hypokalemia, metabolic alkalosis, and hypernatremia due to "massive" sodium penicillin therapy. Br. Med. J. *4*:550–552, 1968.
91. Lee DB, Zawada ET, Kleeman CR: The pathophysiology and clinical aspects of hypercalcemic disorders. West. J. Med. *129*:278–320, 1978.
92. Karris JA, Russell RGG: Rate of reversal of hypercalcemia and hypercalciuria induced by vitamin D and its 1-α-hydroxylated derivatives. Br. Med. J. *1*:78–81, 1977.
93. Frame B, Jackson CE, Raynols WA, et al.: Hypercalcemia and skeletal effects in chronic hyper vitaminosis A. Ann. Intern. Med. *80*:44–48, 1974.
94. Burnett CH, Commons RR, Albright F, et al.: Hypercalcemia without hypercalciuria or hypophosphatemia. Calcinosis and renal insufficiency: a syndrome following prolonged ingestion of milk and alkali. N. Engl. J. Med. *240*:787–794, 1949.
95. Wenger J, Kirsner JB, Palmer WL: The milk alkali syndrome: hypercalcemia, alkalosis and azotemia following calcium carbonate and milk therapy for peptic ulcer. Gastroenterology *33*:745–769, 1957.
96. Christensson T, Helstrom K, Wengel B: Hypercalcemia and primary hyperparathyroidism prevalence in patients receiving thiazides as detected in health screen. Arch. Intern. Med. *137*:1138–1142, 1977.
97. Leemnuis MP, van Damme KJ, Struyvenberg A: Effects of chlorthalidone on serum and total body potassium in hypertensive patients. Acta Med. Scand. *200*:37–45, 1976.
98. Christianson TAT: Lithium, hypercalcemia and hyperparathyroidism. Lancet *2*:144, 1976.
99. Spooner D, Evans BD: Tamoxifen and life-threatening hypercalcemia. Lancet *2*:413, 1979.
100. Jubiz W, Haussler MR, MCCain TA, et al.: Plasma 1,25-dihydroxy vitamin D levels in patients receiving anti-convulsant drugs. J. Clin. Endocrinol. Metab. *44*:617–621, 1977.
101. Shackney S, Hasson J: Precipitous fall in serum calcium, hypotension and acute renal failure after intravenous phosphate therapy of hypercalcemia. Ann. Intern. Med. *66*:906–916, 1967.
102. Davis RF, Eichner JM, Bleyer WA, et al.: Hypocalcemia, hyperphosphatemia and dehydration following a single hypertonic phosphate enema. J. Pediatr. *90*:484–485, 1977.
103. Kiarp DT, Lokan MK, Kennedy BJ: Mechanism of the hypocalcemia effect of mithramycin. J. Clin. Endocrinol. Metab. *48*:341–344, 1979.
104. Knochel JP: The pathophysiology and clinical characteristics of severe hypophosphatemia. Arch. Intern. Med. *137*:203–220, 1977.
105. Lotz M, Zisman E, Barter FC: Evidence for a phosphorus depletion syndrome in man. N. Engl. J. Med. *278*:409–415, 1968.
106. Heaton FW, Pyrah LN, Beresford CC, et al.: Hypomagnesemia in chronic alcoholism. Lancet *2*:802–805, 1962.
107. Kalbfleisch JM, Lindeman RD, Ginn HE, et al.: Effects of ethanol administration on urinary excretion of magnesium and other electrolytes in alcoholics and normal subjects. J. Clin. Invest. *42*:1471–1475, 1963.
108. Duarte CG: Effects of ethacrynic acid and furosemide on urinary calcium, phosphate and magnesium. Metabolism *17*:867–876, 1968.
109. Smith WO, Kyriakopoulos AA, Hammersten JF: Magnesium depletion induced by various diuretics. J. Okla. State Med. Assoc. *55*:248–250, 1962.
110. Wacker WEC: Effect of hydrochlorothiazide on magnesium excretion. J. Clin. Invest. *40*:1086, 1961.
111. Holmes AM, Hesling CM, Wilson TM: Drug-induced secondary aldosteronism in patients with pulmonary tuberculosis. Q. J. Med. *39*:299–315, 1970.
112. Holmes AM, Hesling CM, Wilson TM: Capreomycin-induced serum electrolyte abnormalities. Thorax *25*:608–611, 1970.
113. Keating MJ, Sethi MR, Body GP, et al.: Hypocalcemia with hypoparathyroidism and renal tubular dysfunction associated with aminoglycoside therapy. Cancer *39*:1410–1414, 1977.
114. Anast CS, Winnacker JL, Forte LR, et al.: Impaired release of parathyroid hormone in magnesium deficiency. J. Clin. Endocrinol. Metab. *42*:707–717, 1976.
115. Reddy CR, Coburn JW, Hartenbower DC, et al.: Studies on mechanism of hypocalcemia of magnesium depletion. J. Clin. Invest. *52*:3000–3010, 1973.
116. Chase LR, Slatopolsky E: Secretion and metabolic efficacy of parathyroid hormone in patients with severe hypomagnesemia. J. Clin. Endocrinol. Metab. *38*:363–371, 1974.
117. Randall RE Jr, Cohen MD, Spray CC, Jr., et al.: Hypermagnesemia and renal failure. Etiology and toxic manifestations. Ann. Intern. Med. *61*:73–88, 1964.

Chapter 10

Drug-Induced Hepatitis

by

Lawrence E. Feinberg

Drug-induced liver injury has emerged as one of the important causes of acute and chronic liver disease among adults. The physician must be alert to this problem because unrecognized drug-induced hepatitis can be particularly severe and can progress to hepatic failure and death. In recent years, one out of four cases of fulminant hepatic failure in the United States has been caused by therapeutic drugs. The large number of therapeutic agents introduced during the past 25 years has led to successive waves of drug-induced hepatic injury. Between 1950 and 1960, the focus was on jaundice induced by androgens and phenothiazines. Then halothane-induced hepatitis and liver disease induced by tetracycline and erythromycin prompted many reports. During the 1970's, hepatic injury caused by isoniazid and acetaminophen attracted attention. Most recently, the entity of drug-induced chronic liver disease has been increasingly recognized.

The problem of serious drug-induced liver disease continues. In May of 1979, American physicians began to prescribe the apparently safe diuretic, ticrynafen (Selacryn), but by March of 1980, 363 reported cases of liver damage, including 24 fatal cases, had been associated with its use. This experience demonstrates once again that a drug can be released for general use before the first hepatotoxic reactions are seen. This is because the incidence of hepatotoxic reactions to drugs is very low; many drugs cause liver disease in less than one in a thousand persons exposed. Yet the incidence and severity of hepatotoxic reactions can be minimized by the thoughtful use of drugs and by an informed clinical approach to patients with possible drug-induced liver disease.

PATHOGENESIS[1-4]

REASONS FOR LIVER SUSCEPTIBILITY TO TOXIC INJURY

The liver contains a system of drug-metabolizing enzymes that biotransform drugs generally to metabolites with reduced pharmacologic effects when compared to the parent drug. The initial phase of drug metabolism (phase I) is carried out by a system of microsomal enzymes referred to as mixed function oxidases. The terminal oxidase of this system, cytochrome P-450, binds drug, oxygen, electrons, and cofactors, such as nicotinamide adenosine dehydrogenase (NADH), and transforms the parent drug into a generally more polar compound. These compounds may undergo a second phase of synthetic reactions that conjugate the altered drug with glucuronides, sulfates, and amino acids to further enhance water solubility (Fig. 10–1). These hepatic enzymatic reactions are dependent on access to various cofactors, an important example of which is glutathione. These cofactors may actually serve as tissue protective molecules because of their ability to bind to reactive and potentially toxic drug metabolites (Fig. 10–2).

Many factors underlie the liver's susceptibility to injury by drugs. The central role of the liver in converting lipid-soluble drugs to water-soluble products in order to facilitate drug excretion results in high drug concentra-

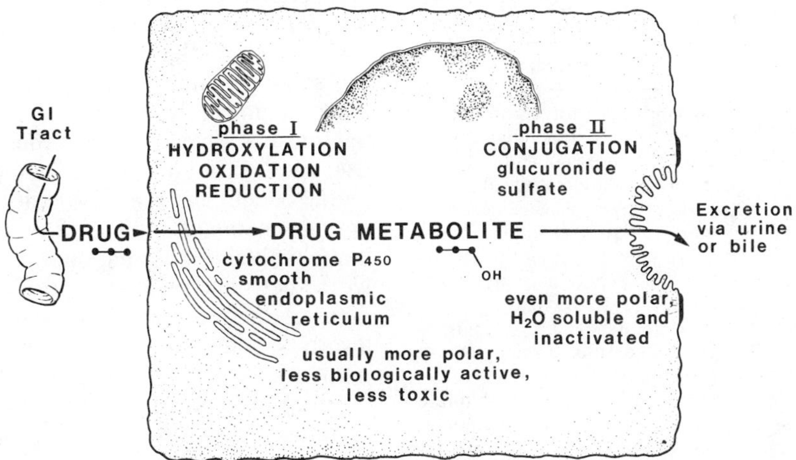

Figure 10–1. Overview of hepatic drug metabolism. Most drugs are converted by hepatic enzymes to inactivated and increasingly water soluble metabolites.

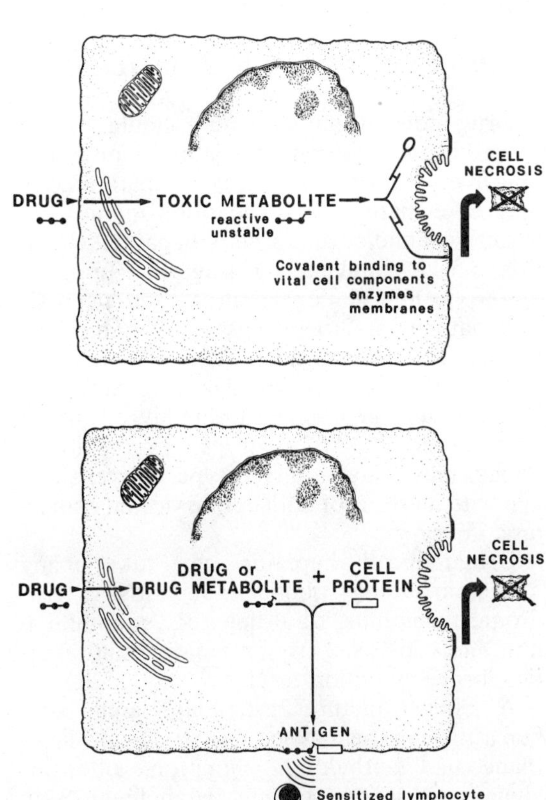

Figure 10–2. Models of drug hepatotoxicity. Reactive metabolites are formed in amounts which exceed the detoxifying capacity of the liver → toxic metabolites bind to tissue macromolecules → membrane damage and cell necrosis (above). In some cases, a drug binds to cell proteins to form an immunogenic complex → host immunological response results in lymphocyte or immune complex-mediated injury to hepatocyte (below).

tions in the liver. Moreover, the liver is exposed to high levels of orally ingested compounds because of portal vein delivery from the gut. Finally, the liver's conversion of drugs to reactive metabolites and the excretion of these agents in the bile further contributes to drug exposure and to chemical injury. However, liver injury caused by therapeutic agents is generally dose-independent, unpredictable, and often related to variations in the way individual patients metabolize drugs or dispose of their active metabolites. For example, genetically determined differences in the rate of formation of drug metabolites may be an important factor in determining susceptibility to isoniazid-induced hepatitis (Table 10–1). Thus, many cases of drug-induced liver disease depend on an unusual susceptibility or idiosyncrasy of the host rather than on the intrinsic toxicity of the agent.

Since liver damage caused by therapeutic agents may be severe, it is important to recognize multiple additional factors that increase the likelihood and severity of hepatic drug reactions (Table 10–1). Continued drug use after development of hepatitis, advanced age, and female sex may all increase susceptibility to drug-induced hepatitis. Poor nutrition may contribute to drug toxicity by diminishing the hepatocyte store of "protective substances" such as glutathione. Moreover, the chronic ingestion of ethanol and barbiturates often results in induction of hepatic microsomal enzymes important in drug metabolism. The resultant increased capacity to metabolize

TABLE 10–1. FACTORS AFFECTING THE INCIDENCE AND SEVERITY OF HEPATIC DRUG REACTIONS

Factor	Comment
Dose	Threshold dose for certain drugs exists (e.g., tetracycline > 1.5 gm/day, intravenously).
Duration of use	Continuation after onset of symptomatic liver disease leads to more severe liver injury.
Age	Persons over age 40 are most susceptible; hepatotoxic drug reactions are rare in children.
Sex	Increased incidence of idiosyncratic hepatotoxic reactions has been reported in women.
Other drugs	Chronic ethanol and barbiturate ingestion leads to induction of microsomal enzymes; this induction could potentially result in increased production of "toxic metabolites" (isoniazid, acetaminophen).
Nutrition	Poor nutrition and alcoholism may deplete hepatocyte-protective molecules, such as glutathione, thereby increasing susceptibility to drug injury (acetaminophen).
Genetic make-up	Undefined, genetically determined differences in drug metabolism may increase individual suscepibility to drug toxicity.
Preexisting liver disease	There is minimal evidence to suggest that susceptibility to hepatotoxicity is enhanced by underlying liver disease.

drugs in this setting can lead to high concentrations of toxic metabolites. Such a mechanism has been proposed to enhance hepatotoxicity following the use of acetaminophen and isoniazid. Thus, a number of clinically recognizable factors may predispose to drug-induced hepatitis.

Other agents may cause hepatic injury by interfering with vital metabolic processes of the hepatocyte, leading to fatty infiltration and cell necrosis. Fatty infiltration caused by methotrexate or high-dose parenteral tetracycline is presumed to occur because of the drugs' interference with assembly of the lipoprotein complex required for transport of lipid from the liver.

The means of exposure to potential hepatotoxic drugs deserves comment. The list of therapeutic agents that have potential to induce hepatic injury continues to grow (Table 10–2). Many of the agents included in this list are among the most common drugs currently prescribed in the United States. Fortunately, the frequency of hepatotoxic reactions to most of these agents is quite low and has been estimated to be less than one in 1000. However, some agents, such as methotrexate and L-asparaginase, have known significant potential for hepatotoxicity. With these agents, drug use involves a clinical decision regarding potential benefit and risk of toxicity. Exposure to potent chemical toxins often occurs in the home (solvents), recreational (mushrooms), or work (petrochemicals) environment. Unfortunately, the individual exposed is often unaware of potential hepatotoxicity. Finally, hepatotoxicity may be encountered in the setting of drug overdose, as with acetaminophen. Taken together, the potential for exposure to hepatotoxic compounds covers a large segment of our population.

DRUG-INDUCED ACUTE HEPATITIS

CLINICAL AND BIOCHEMICAL FEATURES

Drug-induced hepatic injury should be suspected in every patient with jaundice or abnormal liver function tests. Drug hepatotoxicity may take many forms and often mimics obstructive jaundice and/or viral hepatitis. Hepatitis can be simulated by drugs that promote cytotoxic injury, degeneration, and necrosis of hepatocytes. Other drugs, such as chlorpromazine, cause impairment of bile flow (cholestasis), with little if any damage to hepatocytes. These latter agents are thoroughly discussed in Chapter 11. Many drugs, e.g., sulfonamides, may cause a mixed type of liver damage with features of both cytotoxic and cholestatic injury.

Drug-induced hepatitis can take many forms, including fulminant hepatitis, a syndrome resembling viral hepatitis, granulomatous hepatitis, and asymptomatic abnormalities in liver function tests.

A clinical picture resembling acute viral hepatitis can be caused by isoniazid, halothane, and methyldopa. Symptoms often include malaise and fatigue. High fever, skin rash, and eosinophilia occur in a minority of cases, but are characteristic features of hepatitis caused by other agents such as allopurinol, sulfonamides, and phenytoin.[6] Other extrahepatic manifestations encountered with these latter drugs may include peripheral blood cytopenias, "atypical" lymphocytosis, lymph-

TABLE 10–2. CAUSES OF DRUG-INDUCED HEPATITIS*

Category of Drug	
Anesthetics	Halothane (H)
	Methoxyflurane (H)
Anticonvulsants	Carbamazepine (C)
	Phenytoin (HC)[g]
	Trimethadione (H)
	Valproic acid (H)
Antihypertensive Agents, Diuretics	Chlorthalidone (C)
	Methyldopa (HC)
	Metolazone (H)[g]
	Thiazides (C)
Antimicrobial Agents	Amoxicillin (H)
	Ampicillin (H)
	Carbenicillin (H)
	Cephalexin (H)[g]
	Chloramphenicol (HC)
	Clindamycin (H)
	Erythromycins (C)
	5-Fluorocytosine (H)
	Griseofulvin (HC)
	Isoniazid (H)
	Nitrofurantoin (HC)
	Oxacillin (H)[g]
	Para-aminosalicylate (HC)
	Penicillin (HC)[g]
	Piperazines (C)
	Quinacrine (H)
	Rifampin (H)
	Sulfonamides (HC)[g]
	Tetracyclines (H)[f]
	Thiobendazole (C)
Antirheumatic Drugs, Analgesics, Muscle Relaxants	Acetaminophen (H)
	Allopurinol(H)
	Carisoprodol (H)
	D-Penicillamine (C)
	Dantrolene (H)
	Diazepam (C)
	Gold (C)
	Ibuprofen (H)
	Indomethacin (H)
	Naproxen (C)
	Oxyphenbutazone (H)[g]
	Phenylbutazone (H)[g]
	Probenecid (H)
	Propoxyphene (C)
	Salicylates (H)
	Sulindac (C)
Cardiovascular	Aprindine (H)
	Papaverine (HC)
	Procainamide (HC)[g]
	Quinidine (HC)[g]
	Warfarin (C)
Chemotherapeutic Immunosuppressive Agents[14]	Azathioprine (HC)
	Busulfan (C)
	Corticosteroids[f]
	Cytosine arabinoside (H)
	L-Asparaginase (H)[f]
	6-Mercaptopurine (HC)
	Methotrexate (H)
	Mithramycin (H)
	Mitomycin (H)[f]
	Nitrosoureas (H)
	Procarbazine (HC)[g]
Hormonal Agents Drugs Used in Metabolic Disorders	Anabolic steroids (C) (C-17 alkylated)
	Bromocriptine (H)[15]
	Chlorpropamide (C)
	Clofibrate (HC)[g]
	Contraceptives, oral (C)
	Estrogens (C)
	Methimazole (C)
	Nicotinic acid (C)
	Propylthiouracil (HC)
	Tolazamide (C)
	Tolbutamide (C)
Psychotropic Drugs	Chlordiazepoxide (C)
	Diazepam (C)
	Flurazepam (C)
	Haloperidol (C)
	MAO-inhibitors (H)
	Phenothiazines (C)
	Tricyclic antidepressants (HC)
Miscellaneous	Cimetidine (HC)[16]
	Disulfiram (H)
	Danthron (H)
	Methoxsalen (H)
	Phenazopyridine (H)

H = Hepatocellular necrosis; C = Cholestasis; HC = Necrosis and/or cholestasis; g = Granulomas reported in some cases; f = Fatty change

*Table lists currently available therapeutic drugs that have been reported to cause hepatic injury; the predominant type of injury is shown in parentheses. The reader is urged to examine the original reports of these drug reactions; most are cited in references 2, 13, and 20.

adenopathy, and renal disease. Liver function abnormalities observed in drug-induced acute hepatitis include increased serum aminotransferase levels. Aspartate aminotransferase (AST) is the new internationally standardized term for glutamic oxalacetic transaminase; alanine aminotransferase (ALT) is the new term for glutamic pyruvic transaminase. With acute drug-induced hepatitis these enzymes may be 10 to 100 times that of the upper limit of normal with usually just modest increases in serum alkaline phosphatase. The degree of hyperbilirubinemia is variable, but deep jaundice (> 25 mg/dl) and prolonged prothrombin time indicate extensive hepatic necrosis.

More extensive drug-induced liver diseases result in submassive (bridging) necrosis of the liver.[7] The clinical and biochemical picture suggests severe hepatitis. The biopsy feature of bridging necrosis describes zones of confluent liver cell necrosis that bridge adjacent portal triads and central veins (Fig. 10–3*A*). Submassive or massive hepatic necrosis can result in fulminant hepatic failure, usually within 3 to 30 days after the onset of a typical hepatitis prodrome. Signs of hepatic failure include encephalopathy (lethargy → unresponsive coma), asterixis, fetor hepaticus, coagulopathy, acid-base imbalance, cerebral edema, and progressive renal failure. The mortality rate associated with massive hepatic necrosis exceeds 50 per cent. This lesion is pictured in Figure 10–3*B*.

In contrast to these severe, life-threatening forms of hepatitis, certain drugs tend to promote milder hepatic injury accompanied by an inflammatory response that contains granulomas.[8] These are rounded formations of lymphocytes surrounding a core of epithelioid cells (Fig. 10–3*C*). The drugs most frequently associated with granulomatous hepatitis include quinidine, phenylbutazone, allopurinol, sulfonamides, and sulfonylurea hypoglycemic

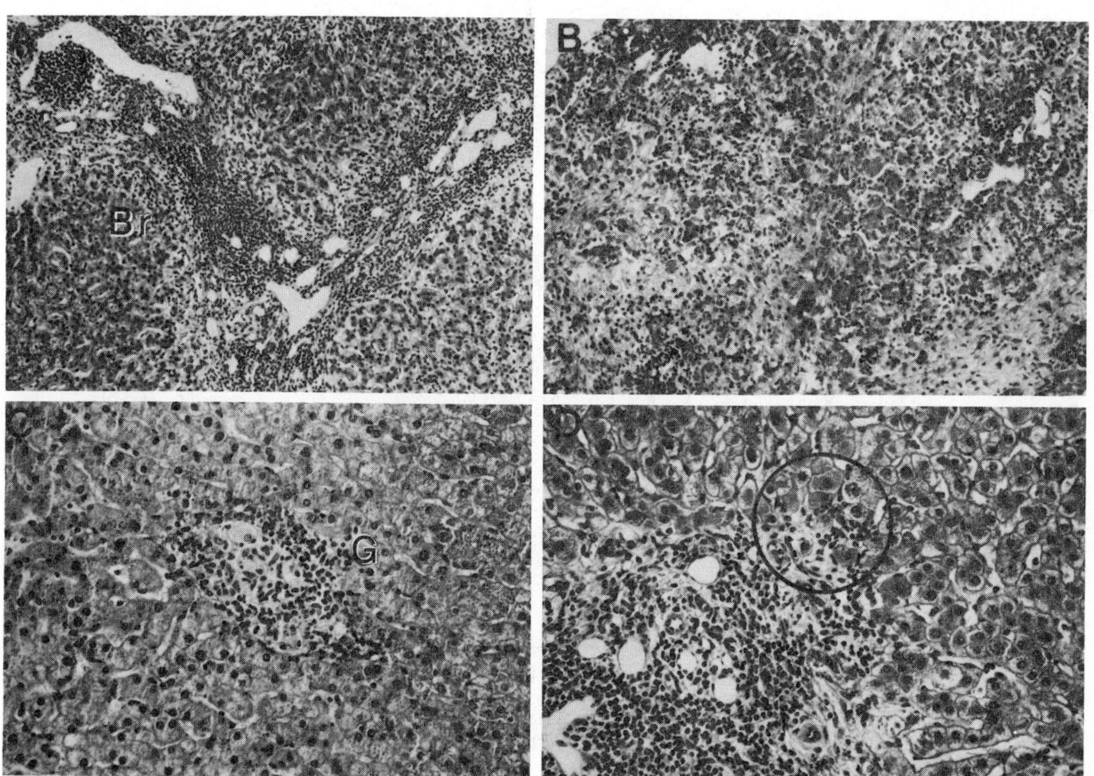

Figure 10–3. Examples of drug-induced hepatic injury. *A,* Bridging necrosis. Intense mononuclear cell inflammation associated with confluent liver cell necrosis that bridges (Br) adjacent portal tracts and central vein → lobular collapse. Methyldopa (× 95). *B,* Massive hepatic necrosis. Cell degeneration, necrosis, and drop-out with diffuse inflammatory infiltrate. Halothane (× 95). *C,* Granuloma. Lymphocytes surround a focus of transformed macrophages (epithelioid cells). Phenytoin (× 240). *D,* Chronic active hepatitis. Inflamed portal tract with mononuclear cells extending outward into the parenchyma, promoting hepatocyte degeneration and piecemeal necrosis. Methyldopa (× 240).

agents. There are isolated case reports of granulomatous hepatitis associated with phenytoin, oxacillin, procainamide, and other drugs. Penicillin and hydralazine have caused granulomas within the liver, but these have not been accompanied by other signs of liver disease. The clinical picture of granulomatous hepatitis is typically that of a relatively mild drug-induced hepatitis with accompanying skin rash, eosinophilia, lymphadenopathy, and other systemic manifestations. Biochemical tests often reveal comparable elevations of AST and alkaline phosphatase, indicative of a mixed injury. Occasionally, hepatic granulomas are associated with a predominantly cholestatic injury (high alkaline phosphatase, minimal elevations in AST, and no parenchymal necrosis on biopsy).

Focal hepatitis is another mild form of drug-induced hepatic injury. The underlying focal disease is mirrored by AST elevations up to four to five times that of normal among drug recipients who remain asymptomatic and well. Isoniazid, the best studied example, promotes AST elevations greater than two times that of normal in 10 to 20 per cent of patients taking this medication.[9, 10] These abnormalities reflect subclinical hepatic injury that most often completely resolves or improves despite continuation of the drug. There is no indication that these patients develop serious and irreversible liver disease while remaining asymptomatic.[11] However, progression to a more diffuse and overt hepatitis can occur and is heralded by prodromal symptoms.

Proper diagnosis of subclinical or overt drug-induced hepatitis starts with the basic consideration that a drug taken by the patient can cause the observed liver damage. A sophisticated knowledge of drug-induced liver disease is not necessary; what is necessary is the nearly reflex inquiry by the physician: "Could a drug be causing or aggravating this patient's condition?" If the clinician is uncertain about a particular drug's record of hepatotoxicity, a summary of such drug reactions can be consulted (Table 10–2 and references 2, 12, and 13). If drug-induced hepatitis remains a possibility, the suspected drug(s) should be withdrawn. In so doing the clinician will have instituted the most definitive therapy available for drug-induced liver disease.

Acute drug-induced hepatitis almost always occurs within the first year and typically within the initial 3 to 6 months of continuous drug use. For example, more than 80 per cent of cases of acute hepatitis attributed to methyldopa occur by the eighth week of therapy[17, 18]; more than 90 per cent of icteric cases of isoniazid-induced hepatitis will occur within nine months.[9, 10, 19] Acute hepatitis accompanied by skin rash, high fever, eosinophilia, and other systemic features usually occurs between 1 and 5 weeks after the drug has been started. Earlier onset of hepatic injury is rare but may reflect past exposure and sensitization. Rarely, drug-induced hepatitis will not appear until 7 to 10 days after the responsible drug treatment has been completed.[20]

DIAGNOSTIC LIMITATIONS

There are few procedures that can definitively confirm drug-induced hepatitis. Thus, the diagnosis usually depends on circumstantial evidence. Although signs of hepatitis might appear while a drug is being taken and disappear after the drug is withdrawn, the diagnosis of an adverse drug reaction often remains insecure. This is because patients have coexisting, complex, and changing medical problems, multiple drug regimens, and a susceptibility to coincidental viral hepatitis. Tests that we might expect to be definitive, such as liver biopsy and drug rechallenge, turn out to have major limitations.

Liver biopsy is rarely conclusive in establishing that the drug in question is responsible for the patient's liver disease. Upon examination of drug-induced cases, the pathologist observes hepatocyte degeneration and necrosis along with infiltration of the hepatic lobule and portal tracts by inflammatory cells. The range of severity extends from mild, patchy hepatitis to submassive necrosis with bridging and lobular collapse. These histologic changes are totally nonspecific and must be interpreted in light of the patient's history, clinical features, and biochemical changes. Liver biopsy is more often performed to assess the extent of liver damage rather than to incriminate a drug as a possible cause of the damage. There are, however, several histologic features that should arouse suspicion of drug toxicity in patients manifesting an acute hepatitis picture. These signals for the clinician and pathologist are listed in Table 10–3.[21] Liver biopsy is advocated for patients with severe hepatitis with features suggesting bridging necrosis ($\uparrow$ prothrombin time, deep jaundice, protracted course, age > 40), particularly if the suspected drug is con-

TABLE 10–3. SUGGESTIVE HISTOLOGIC FEATURES OF DRUG-INDUCED ACUTE HEPATITIS

Severe degree of necrosis out of proportion to patient's clinical condition and biochemical changes
Fatty change in the fully developed stage of hepatitis
Granuloma formation
Infiltration by many eosinophils
Periportal cholestasis early in the course of illness
Bile duct damage

sidered uniquely important to the patient's welfare. If, however, the hepatic injury is of mild to moderate severity and the offending drug treatment can be readily replaced, then a biopsy is not routinely indicated. In these latter cases, specific diagnostic yield is low and the procedure's therapeutic and prognostic implications are usually negligible. The modest risk of percutaneous liver biopsy is not acceptable in this setting. Of course, many patients, particularly those with multiple possible causes of hepatitis, will require an individualized approach.

Drug rechallenge is the most definitive way of confirming a drug-induced hepatitis, as the recurrence of hepatic dysfunction after a test dose offers specific support for this diagnosis. Although rechallenge is generally safe, a single test dose of a drug known to cause cytotoxic injury may cause serious and fatal hepatitis. Such testing is, therefore, rarely warranted and employed only with indispensable drugs that the patient should, if at all possible, receive again.

If drug rechallenge is to be undertaken, the patient should be hospitalized. Baseline observations, informed consent, and monitoring studies should be obtained according to the protocol of the National Institutes of Health.[22] Failure to develop AST abnormalities after planned or inadvertent rechallenge does not preclude the diagnosis of drug-induced hepatitis, since only about 50 per cent of patients with otherwise typical drug-induced jaundice will demonstrate signs of hepatic dysfunction after a test dose. A drug such as isoniazid, which appears to damage the liver via a toxic metabolite, may reproduce hepatic injury only after weeks of repeat administration.

Considering the limitations of drug rechallenge and liver histology, it is disappointing to note that there is currently no reliable and readily available *in vitro* test or serum assay that can definitively confirm a suspected hepatic drug reaction. *In vitro* testing for drug-dependent lymphocyte transformation has been most widely utilized for this purpose,[23] but these and other studies must still be considered investigational procedures.

DIFFERENTIAL DIAGNOSIS (Table 10–4)

If a patient exposed to a drug develops acute hepatitis and the drug is known to cause liver disease, then the diagnosis of drug-induced hepatitis must be considered. This is a sensible approach because the diagnostic choices often narrow down to drug-induced and viral hepatitis. Since specific therapy is lacking for viral disease, the added emphasis on recognizing a drug etiology is appropriate.

Both drug-induced and viral hepatitis can present with similar clinical and biochemical features. A viral etiology may be suggested by epidemiologic factors and confirmed by serologic tests. Recent blood transfusion, parenteral drug abuse, male homosexual activity, or membership in a family cluster or wider outbreak of acute hepatitis all suggest viral disease rather than hepatitis caused by drugs. Initial testing that reveals an acute phase antibody to the hepatitis A virus, anti-HAV (IgM), or a positive hepatitis B surface antigen (HB_sAg) would obviously support a diagnosis of acute viral hepatitis. The physician must be aware that detection of HB_sAg does not confirm unequivocally that hepatitis B infection is responsible for the patient's acute liver disease. Patients at high risk for hepatitis B exposure, such as hemodialysis and transplant patients, male homosexuals, and natives of Asia and Africa (12 per cent of current Indo-Chinese refugees are HB_sAg–positive) may have been unrecognized symptomless HB_sAg carriers prior to the current episode of acute (and possibly drug-induced) hepatitis.

TABLE 10–4. DIFFERENTIAL DIAGNOSIS OF ACUTE HEPATITIS

Drug-induced
Toxic
Viral
Anoxic liver injury (shock, hepatic congestion)
Acute biliary tract disease
Exacerbation of chronic liver disease
Miscellaneous (toxemia and fatty liver of pregnancy, parenteral nutrition, and bacterial sepsis)

Another cause of acute hepatitis is toxic liver injury caused by compounds other than therapeutic drugs. The term is also applied to liver damage caused by therapeutic drugs when taken as a massive overdose. Halogenated hydrocarbons, toxic mushrooms, and acetaminophen overdosage appear to cause most isolated cases of toxic hepatitis. Hepatotoxic chemicals exclusively used by industry or research laboratories are not addressed here and the reader should consult Zimmerman's work[2] (pp. 277–345). Chlorobenzene and related chemicals present in insecticides, mothballs, and other household products may be responsible for inadvertent toxic liver injury.[2, 24] Serious hepatic damage may also follow ingestion of *Amanita* mushroom species. These instances of wild mushroom poisoning occur in the summer and autumn.[25] Ingestion of massive doses of acetaminophen usually reflects a suicide attempt. Inhalation of volatile chemicals in poorly ventilated rooms or glue sniffing (trichloroethylene and toluene) by euphoria seekers can also result in hepatic injury. After a brief latent period, these toxins characteristically promote severe gastrointestinal disturbances, including nausea, vomiting, abdominal pain, and diarrhea. Neurologic signs of lethargy, confusion, convulsions, and coma may follow. Early evidence of renal failure should also suggest a toxic injury (Table 10–5).

Acute hepatitis may be simulated by circulatory failure.[26] Patients who experience shock, particularly if accompanied by hypoxemia and passive congestion of the liver, may develop anoxic liver damage and manifest extremely high AST values and mild jaundice. Patients with isolated left ventricular failure have also been reported to manifest this hepatitis-like picture.[27] During such a confusing episode of jaundice or a rise in AST, careful scrutiny would be directed at any potentially hepatotoxic drugs taken by the patient.

TABLE 10–5. FEATURES SUGGESTIVE OF TOXIC HEPATITIS

Abrupt violent GI disturbances
Early cerebral dysfunction
Obvious toxin exposure at home or work place
Ongoing depression, suicidal intent
Associated renal failure early in the course of liver disease
Zonal necrosis and fatty infiltration on liver biopsy

Jaundice and transiently high AST levels may be early signs of acute biliary tract disease, particularly choledocholithiasis. Any form of cholangitis can promote discrete AST elevations that peak above 1000 IU/ml, but the rapid decline of AST and the presence of abdominal pain, rigors, high fever, or leukocytosis should point to biliary tract disease.

The presentation of a previously occult chronic liver disease may correspond by chance to the institution of a new drug and falsely lead the clinician to diagnose an adverse drug reaction. The misleading chronic disease is most often alcoholic hepatitis. Marked hepatic enlargement and spider angiomata are expected when alcoholic liver disease is severe enough to mimic drug-induced hepatitis. The relatively low AST and ALT levels (90 per cent < 300 IU) and the consistently higher elevation of AST compared to ALT are also of assistance in diagnosing alcoholic liver disease.[28] An exacerbation of chronic active hepatitis must also be considered in the differential diagnosis of an acute hepatitis picture.

Fatty liver and toxemia must be considered in pregnant women with acute liver disease. Severe bacterial sepsis and parenteral nutrition are other factors that can promote a mixed liver injury among hospitalized patients.

Hepatic injury caused by drugs will promptly resolve after the offending agent is stopped. Most patients will be free of symptoms within two to three weeks and will clear jaundice and AST abnormalities within two months. Persistence of active liver disease beyond this time should suggest another diagnosis.

SELECTED DRUGS THAT MAY CAUSE ACUTE HEPATITIS

Five hepatotoxic agents (isoniazid, methyldopa, halothane, aspirin, phenytoin) are emphasized in this section. Acetaminophen hepatotoxicity is discussed in the following section. The use of the first three agents has been modified because of the threat of liver disease. Fatal liver disease occurs with all these agents except aspirin. Aspirin is included because its hepatotoxicity in therapeutic dosage is a relatively new discovery. Since phenytoin often plays an absolutely essential role in seizure management, its pattern of hepatic injury should be familiar so that unrelated liver disease will not inadvertently be attributed to the drug.

ISONIAZID

Isoniazid[9, 10, 19, 24] causes elevations of serum AST above twice that of normal in 10 to 20 per cent of persons taking the drug. These abnormalities are usually transient and represent a mild focal hepatitis. The incidence of overt hepatitis is approximately 1 per cent and 20 per cent of these individuals will die of hepatitis. The majority of affected persons have been over the age of 50. Alcoholism and preexisting liver disease are probably risk factors. The average duration of isoniazid treatment prior to the onset of jaundice is three months, and almost all clinical hepatitis occurs within six months. Virtually all patients experience prodromal symptoms. The longer isoniazid is continued after the onset of symptoms, the more severe the liver damage. The histopathologic lesions are indistinguishable from the picture of acute viral hepatitis and may include bridging and multilobular necrosis.

The hepatic injury is mediated by a reactive acetylated metabolite of isoniazid, acetylhydrazine. Recent clinical studies do not confirm a higher prevalence of liver injury among rapid acetylators, and the current view of isoniazid metabolism suggests that the toxic metabolite, monoacetylhydrazine, is also eliminated more rapidly in these individuals via conversion to diacetylhydrazine, a nontoxic product.[30] There is also little evidence that rifampin significantly alters isoniazid metabolism or that the isoniazid plus rifampin regimen is substantially more hepatotoxic than isoniazid alone.

The preventive benefit of isoniazid must outweigh the risk of hepatitis.[31] Individuals who clearly merit isoniazid preventive treatment are close contacts of diagnosed cases of active tuberculosis, positive skin test reactors with chest x-ray evidence of quiescent tuberculosis (typically upper lung zone fibronodular disease; not granulomas alone) and patients with present or past reactivity to PPD (purified protein derivative of tuberculin) who are now immunocompromised owing to renal failure or neoplasia and must receive immunosuppressive therapy.

Patients taking isoniazid must be taught to immediately report symptoms compatible with an adverse reaction. Fatigue, weakness, nausea, vomiting, or unexplained fever of three or more days duration must prompt investigation. Further aspects of patient surveillance are detailed on pages 150 and 151.

METHYLDOPA

Methyldopa[11, 17, 18] remains the twelfth most commonly prescribed drug in the United States. Its use will be maintained by the proven survival benefit associated with treating even mildly hypertensive persons. Methyldopa causes mild to moderate elevations of AST in 3 to 6 per cent of patients taking the drug. These abnormalities usually disappear despite continued drug administration. Symptomatic hepatitis is uncommon and it promptly resolves after drug withdrawal. However, severe, even fatal, liver disease may result when the drug is continued despite symptoms. Prodromal symptoms, such as fatigue, anorexia, and nausea, occur in all patients with severe liver disease and usually begin three to four weeks prior to the onset of jaundice. Almost all reported cases of acute methyldopa-induced hepatitis occur within three months after starting the drug and most between one and six weeks. The corresponding liver pathology spans the same range between patchy hepatitis and submassive necrosis that is observed with isoniazid.

Considering the added risk of liver disease for older women and the availability of other sympatholytic agents, methyldopa is not a favored drug for hypertensive women over age 50. Patients with active liver disease should also not receive this agent. Methyldopa-induced hepatitis is not more likely to occur in this setting, but its role in promoting liver damage could be more readily overlooked. Routine monitoring of liver function tests is rarely warranted. The patient's well-being should be closely monitored as outlined on pages 150 and 151.

HALOTHANE

Halothane[2, 32] anesthesia rarely causes overt hepatic damage. Overall, approximately 7 per 10,000 persons who have two or more exposures to halothane will experience clinical hepatitis. Obese women are particularly susceptible. Additional cases have been reported among hospital personnel after repeated sniffing of halothane to produce a drug "high." The delay between exposure and the onset of fever is between 7 and 21 days after a first exposure. Jaundice usually appears 2 to 3 days later. If jaundice develops, the mortality is high, 10 to 50 per cent. Mild anicteric liver injury may be more common than previously thought. Prevention of potentially dangerous halothane exposure is the clinician's aim. Patients who have experienced unexplained fever, jaundice, or high AST levels after previous halothane anesthesia should not receive this agent again.

ASPIRIN

Aspirin causes hepatic injury in rabbits and behaves as a dose-dependent hepatotoxin in man.[33, 34] This applies to choline and sodium salicylate as well as to acetylsalicylic acid. The prevalence of acetylsalicylic acid–induced liver injury can be as high as 50 per cent among patients taking high dosage (3 to 5 gm/day) with corresponding high blood salicylate levels (> 25 mg/dl). Hepatotoxicity may be manifest as early as five days after the start of treatment. Symptoms of anorexia, nausea, and abdominal distress are accompanied by a 10- to 40-fold increase in AST with normal or minimally increased alkaline phosphatase. Hyperbilirubinemia is uncommon, and no overt jaundice has been reported. Almost all reported cases have involved patients with systemic lupus erythematosus, juvenile and classic rheumatoid arthritis, acute rheumatic fever, or other connective tissue disorders. This problem has, however, occurred among individuals taking high doses of acetylsalicylic acid for other reasons. Symptoms and AST elevation rapidly subside after withdrawal of acetylsalicylic acid; the drug can be instituted at lower dosage without causing illness or elevated aminotransferase levels.

PHENYTOIN

The incidence of hepatic injury caused by phenytoin[2, 6, 35] is fortunately very low, but the mortality associated with phenytoin-induced jaundice is approximately 50 per cent. Eighty per cent of cases are seen in adults. The hepatic injury is invariably part of a systemic hypersensitivity-type reaction that consistently occurs after one to five weeks of taking the drug. Fever, skin rash, lymphadenopathy, elevated white blood cell count with lymphocytosis (60 per cent), and eosinophilia (20 per cent) accompany signs of acute hepatitis. Aminotransferase values reach five to 20 times normal with variable levels of jaundice, and occasionally, high alkaline phosphatase levels. This increased alkaline phosphatase may be of hepatic origin if associated with elevated levels of gamma-glutamyl transpeptidase (GGT). However, an isolated increase in alkaline phosphatase should not prompt drug discontinuation. Rather, investigation of possible phenytoin-induced osteomalacia should be undertaken.[36]

TOXIC DRUG OVERDOSAGE DUE TO ACETAMINOPHEN

Suicidal or accidental ingestion of drug overdoses may cause acute hepatic injury. Ferrous salts, aspirin, and phenylbutazone have caused severe liver damage when ingested in this way, typically by unsupervised children. Acetaminophen hepatotoxicity deserves special emphasis because this readily available agent can be lethal, yet aggressive treatment can virtually eliminate the occurrence of fatal liver damage.

Acetaminophen-induced hepatic necrosis[37] has become a major cause of acute hepatic failure in Great Britain and appears to be an increasingly common mode of attempted suicide in the United States. Most severe cases of liver damage involve ingestion of more than 15 gm, although single doses of 8 to 12 gm have also proved harmful. Lower doses of acetaminophen taken over a longer time span, such as 8 gm/day for 4 days and 5 to 6 gm/day for 3 weeks have been reported to cause hepatic injury. A toxic overdose of 10 to 15 gm involves ingestion of as little as 30 to 45 regular tablets or 20 to 30 extra strength acetaminophen tablets.

Symptoms of nausea and vomiting have a gradual onset within the first 12 to 24 hours after an overdose. These symptoms then disappear within another 24 hours and the patient may feel well. After 48 to 96 hours, biochemical evidence of liver injury may be seen (AST over 1000 U). Overt liver disease becomes evident about 4 to 6 days after acetaminophen ingestion. Mild to moderate jaundice may be accompanied by metabolic acidosis, hypo-

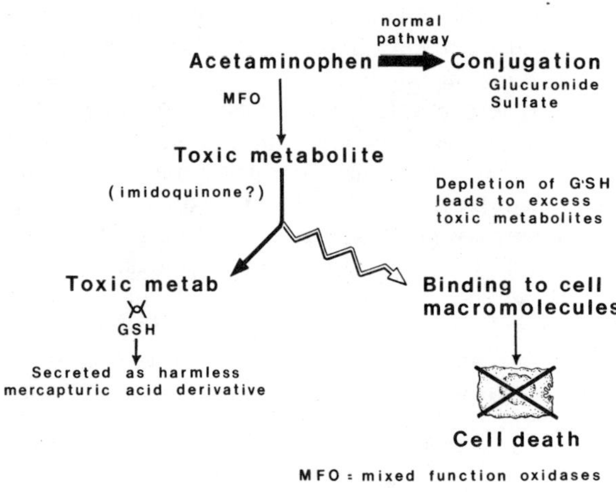

Figure 10–4. Proposed mechanism of acetaminophen hepatotoxicity. Excessive amounts of toxic metabolite overwhelm protective stores of intracellular glutathione → cell necrosis.

prothrombinemia, and acute tubular necrosis. The hepatic necrosis is most marked at the central zones of the hepatic lobule with minimal inflammation and no fatty change. Persons who do not receive aggressive treatment within 24 hours and later develop signs of hepatic failure evidence a mortality rate of 5 to 20 per cent.

Massive acetaminophen ingestion saturates the normal conjugation processes of acetaminophen metabolism and leads to excessive levels of toxic oxidation products (Fig. 10–4). These toxic metabolites bind covalently with proteins in the cytosol and endoplasmic reticulum, thereby contributing to hepatic necrosis. Patients with poor nutrition and those who regularly take microsomal enzyme-inducing drugs, such as barbiturates or ethanol, appear to be more susceptible to acetaminophen-induced liver injury.[38]

Prompt recognition and treatment of acetaminophen intoxication can be life-saving. Gastric lavage, activated charcoal, and other supportive measures should be undertaken. A plasma acetaminophen level should be obtained promptly. If a major overdose is suspected, *N*-acetylcysteine (Mucomyst) should be administered. A simple semilogarithmic plot of plasma acetaminophen level versus time after ingestion is constructed to guide therapy (Fig. 10–5). If this nomogram predicts possible liver damage, *N*-acetylcys-

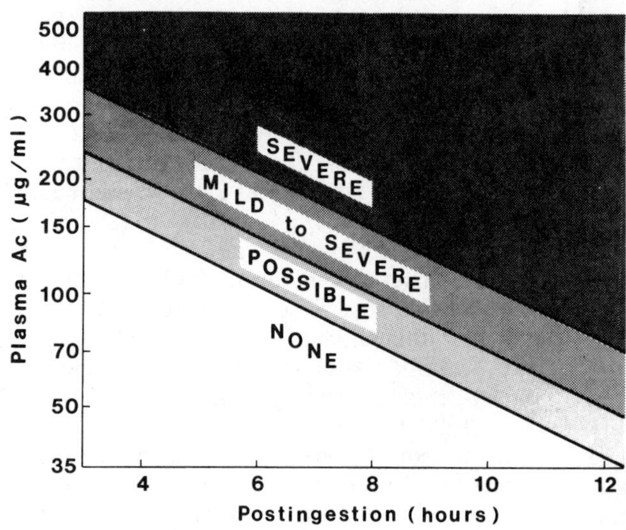

Figure 10–5. Nomogram for treatment of acetaminophen (Ac) overdosage. If the plot of plasma level versus time after ingestion predicts mild or severe liver damage, *N*-acetylcysteine therapy is indicated. Therapy is also suggested for patients whose plasma acetaminophen level predicts "possible" liver damage.

teine should be continued. Use of this agent within 24 hours after ingestion has reduced the fatality rate to zero. The treatment regimen consists of *N*-acetylcysteine, 20 per cent solution, diluted 1:3 in fruit juice, 140 mg/kg body weight, given orally or via nasogastric tube. This solution can be given intravenously, but this is rarely necessary. Acetylcysteine should be administered as 70 mg/kg p.o. q4h for a total of 72 hours, unless the initial blood level plot indicates negligible risk for liver damage. In that event, treatment can be discontinued. The rationale for the use of acetylcysteine in management of acetaminophen intoxication is based on the observations that a metabolite of acetaminophen is the hepatotoxin.[1] This metabolite is usually bound to glutathione and rendered nontoxic. With massive acetaminophen overdose, depletion of hepatic glutathione occurs. In this circumstance, acetylcysteine serves as a "surrogate glutathione" and supplies sulfhydryl groups that bind the toxic metabolite.

DRUG-INDUCED CHRONIC HEPATITIS

CLINICAL ASPECTS

Prolonged exposure to certain therapeutic agents can result in subtle, continuous injury to the liver.[7, 39] This type of ongoing hepatic necrosis can lead to a clinical and pathologic picture of chronic active hepatitis (CAH). Drug-induced CAH, such as that caused by methyldopa or nitrofurantoin, may be indistinguishable from other etiologies of CAH (Table 10–6) can can manifest the same evolution to postnecrotic cirrhosis. Cirrhosis can also evolve after drug-induced submassive (bridging) hepatic necrosis.

CAH most commonly presents with progressive fatigability and anorexia. Abdominal discomfort, nausea, vomiting, and arthralgias are less consistent presenting features. Hepatomegaly is the most reliable physical finding; scleral icterus and splenomegaly may be evident. Physical signs of advanced liver disease, such as ascites, are rarely observed in these cases. Aminotransferase levels are elevated, usually five to 15 times that of normal. Prothrombin time is normal, but serum albumin may be depressed. Hypergammaglobulinemia is noted in 50 per cent of cases and the gamma globulin fraction may exceed 3.0 gm/dl.

TABLE 10–6. DIFFERENTIAL DIAGNOSIS OF CHRONIC ACTIVE HEPATITIS

Viral (B, non-A, non-B)
Idiopathic – "Autoimmune"
Drug-induced
Wilson's disease
Alpha-1-antitrypsin deficiency
Chronic cholangiolitic hepatitis (primary biliary cirrhosis, early stages)

Histologic examination of the liver shows chronic inflammatory cells infiltrating the portal tracts, extending outward into the parenchyma from the limiting plate, and participating in piecemeal necrosis of hepatocytes (Fig. 10–3*D*). This biopsy evidence of drug-induced chronic hepatitis has generally been obtained from patients who have been ill for less than three months. This relatively brief time span does not conform to the clinician's definition of CAH; namely, symptomatic or biochemical signs of hepatitis of at least four to six months duration.[40] Most reported cases of drug-induced CAH have, therefore, been pathologic diagnoses, yet the relevant points for the clinician remain the same: (1) Patients regularly taking a drug for months or years may experience the insidious onset of symptomatic liver disease caused by the drug. (2) A liver biopsy showing portal inflammation and piecemeal necrosis may prompt the pathologic diagnosis of chronic active ("aggressive") hepatitis, even though the patient has only been clinically ill for weeks. (3) Drug-induced CAH is usually clinically, biochemically, and histologically indistinguishable from CAH of other etiologies. (4) The longer the drug is continued after the onset of symptoms, the more severe will be the liver damage. (5) Virtually all patients will show resolution of all signs of active liver disease after the inciting drug is withdrawn; some patients may be left with an inactive cirrhosis.

These aspects of drug-induced chronic hepatitis were exemplified by the experience with the laxative, oxyphenisatin. Reynolds' 1971 report of seven patients with apparent "autoimmune" CAH who achieved remission after withdrawal of oxyphenisatin[41] was the first convincing documentation of drug-induced CAH. Subsequent reports from Denmark and Australia[41a, 41b] suggested that this drug-induced variety of CAH was common and that oxyphenisatin might have played a role in up to one third of their collected patients with CAH. How had the drug's harmful role been overlooked for so many years? Presumably, this oversight reflected the rare idiosyncratic occurrence of these cases, but, in retrospect, it also reflected an inadequate approach to patients with obscure liver disease. Did the clinician ask: "Could a drug be causing or aggravating this patient's condition?" At least 10 therapeutic agents have since been implicated in the causation of liver disease fitting the CAH-cirrhosis spectrum. These include methyldopa, nitrofurantoin, isoniazid, halothane, acetaminophen, aspirin, phenylbutazone, propylthiouracil, sulfonamides, and dantrolene.

SELECTED DRUGS THAT MAY CAUSE CAH

METHYLDOPA

Methyldopa can present with insidious progression of anorexia, malaise, and jaundice associated with biopsy evidence of CAH[11, 39]; symptoms are usually seen within two to six months of starting the drug. Patients become clinically well after discontinuation of the drug, but residual postnecrotic cirrhosis has been reported.

NITROFURANTOIN

Almost 30 case reports of nitrofurantoin-associated CAH, including two fatal cases, have been reported.[42, 43] Patients, exclusively women thus far, have regularly or intermittently used this drug for six or more months before the onset of fatigue, anorexia, and, often, jaundice. Aminotransferase levels are typically over 400 and low albumin and hypergammaglobulinemia are usually present. Typical CAH is observed on liver biopsy. Clinical and biochemical improvement occurs within 12 weeks after drug withdrawal. At least five cases of residual inactive cirrhosis have been documented.

ACETAMINOPHEN

Two patients, ages 53 and 59, ingesting 2.9 to 3.9 gm/day of acetaminophen for 1 year, have been reported to develop CAH.[44, 45] In these cases, anorexia, fatigue, and/or tender hepatomegaly were the initial symptoms. Aminotransferase levels were in the 200 to 600 range. Liver biopsies showed portal inflammation with mononuclear cells, piecemeal and bridging necrosis, and fibrosis throughout hepatic lobules. An etiologic role for acetaminophen was confirmed by rechallenge. After withdrawal of acetaminophen, one patient became asymptomatic with a normal AST level. The other patient showed a normal AST level but continued CAH by histologic examination, subsequently improved in association with prednisone-azathioprine therapy. The popularity of acetaminophen combined with its hepatotoxic potential suggest that this form of drug-induced chronic hepatitis will be increasingly recognized.

METHOTREXATE

Methotrexate-induced hepatotoxicity is observed most often during long-term treatment of severe psoriasis.[46, 47] Up to 10 to 20 per cent of such patients may be affected. Larger doses of methotrexate at weekly intervals are less likely to cause liver disease than smaller daily doses. Liver damage following methotrexate correlates with the total duration of therapy. Alcoholism probably predisposes to methotrexate-induced hepatic injury. The hepatic lesion can progress through stages of fatty liver and fibrosis to micronodular cirrhosis. Methotrexate-associated cirrhosis can evolve without any deviation in standard "liver function tests." Therefore, screening for liver damage at present requires liver biopsy. A pretreatment liver biopsy is mandatory for regular ethanol users and for patients with other indications of liver disease. In other patients, liver biopsy should be considered 12 to 24 months after therapy. If liver histology remains normal after two years, a formal program of regular, but less frequent tissue sampling can be followed thereafter. If liver histology demonstrates mild hepatic changes consistent with methotrexate toxicity, serious consideration must be given to withdrawing methotrexate and employing alternate therapy. Within recent years, photochemotherapy with psoralens and ultraviolet light has become an alternative to methotrexate treatment of severe psoriasis. Although occasional elevations of serum AST have been reported with psoralens and ultraviolet therapy, there is no firm evidence of histologic liver damage caused by this regimen.

ETHANOL

A detailed discussion of alcohol-induced clinical liver disease is beyond the scope of this chapter. However, this toxic liver disease must be considered a diagnostic possibility in virtually all adults with acute and chronic liver disease. The three main forms of liver disease in the alcoholic patient include fatty liver, alcoholic hepatitis, and cirrhosis. Fatty liver is found in 70 to 100 per cent of patients ingesting excessive amounts of alcohol. Hepatomegaly is often the only abnormal physical finding. Mild hyperbilirubinemia (usually below 2.5 mg/dl) is noted in about 20 per cent of patients. AST values are normal or minimally raised, while serum alkaline phosphatase is usually increased. More severe hyperbilirubinemia or signs of hepatic failure and portal hypertension suggest the presence of alcoholic hepatitis and possible cirrhosis. The laboratory picture associated with alcoholic hepatitis often includes anemia and leukocytosis. AST levels rarely exceed 300 IU (normal <25 to 40). Unlike most cases of acute and chronic hepatitis caused by therapeutic drugs, the AST level is higher than the ALT in 90 to 95 per cent of patients with alcoholic hepatitis. Hypoalbuminemia is common and hypergammaglobulinemia may be seen in 50 per cent of cases. The characteristic histologic picture involves fatty infiltration, accumulation of hyalin, and focal hepatocellular necrosis with aggregates of neutrophils. A diffuse centrilobular fibrosis and micronodular cirrhosis are seen in many patients. These "distinctive" pathologic changes have also been observed following prolonged use of perhexilene (an antianginal drug available in Europe) and have been recently described in patients who are typically middle-aged, obese, diabetic, and hypertriglyceridemic (and presumably not hidden abusers of ethanol).[47a, 47b] The key aspects of alcoholic liver disease relevant to differential diagnosis include:

1. Ethanol use has been long-standing and excessive.
2. Hepatomegaly, often massive, is a consistent finding.
3. Spider angiomata and palmar erythema are observed in most patients.
4. ALT and AST levels are not markedly elevated; AST is usually increased more than ALT.
5. Fatty liver change is regularly observed in the liver biopsy of actively drinking patients with alcoholic liver disease.

TREATMENT AND PREVENTION

TREATMENT

Simple guidelines exist for the treatment of drug-induced acute and chronic hepatitis. The physician should be alert to this problem, stop the responsible agent, and provide supportive care. The more promptly the problem is recognized and the drug is withdrawn, the less severe is the resultant hepatic injury. This trend was clearly evident among the initial cases of hepatitis caused by isoniazid and methyldopa. Patients with submassive necrosis had taken these drugs for about twice as long after the onset of prodromal symptoms (4 weeks vs. 2 weeks) as had patients who displayed mild hepatitis. Most reported cases of fatal hepatic necrosis have occurred among patients who were ill for weeks before seeing a physician and who, unfortunately, were continued on the responsible agent.

Drug-induced hepatic injury should be suspected in every patient with jaundice, in every patient with an illness consistent with early hepatitis, and in every patient with abnormal "liver function tests." Persons with overt jaundice should discontinue the use of potentially hepatotoxic drugs, at least until an alternate diagnosis is confirmed. If vital drugs are continued in this setting, an adjustment in dosage may be necessary.

Patients who experience symptoms consistent with the prodromal phase of hepatitis require an individualized approach. Symptoms of nausea, vomiting, loss of appetite, malaise, abdominal distress, or fever that persist beyond 3 to 5 days, particularly if noted during the initial months of drug therapy, demand that the physician make efforts to exclude drug-induced liver disease. At the minimum, this would require checking a serum AST level. Accompanying skin rash, tender hepatomegaly, or an office urine test positive for bilirubin should prompt immediate withdrawal of the drug. A newly elevated AST level should prompt the same action.

After the offending drug is stopped, most patients with mild to moderate degrees of hepatitis demonstrate prompt improvement. The patient's well-being improves while fever and skin rash, if present, subside within 5 to 10 days. Liver function tests normalize over a longer period, typically 3 to 6 weeks. Antiemetics and antihistamines can be safely used to minimize vomiting and pruritus, respectively. Corticosteroid therapy is inappropriate because most patients will improve spontaneously after withdrawal of the offending drug.

Unfortunately, once jaundice develops, there is a significant incidence of progressive liver failure and death despite withdrawal of the inciting agent. These seriously ill patients require hospitalization and intensive care. Since effective artificial liver support systems are not yet available, general supportive measures are most important. An aggressive approach to management includes provision of adequate calories, correction of any blood pH and electrolyte abnormalities, antacid prophylaxis against stress gastritis, administration of lactulose or neomycin, and vigorous treatment of infection. These and other aspects of managing patients with fulminant hepatic failure are detailed elsewhere.[48]

Corticosteroids are often employed in the treatment of severe fulminant drug-induced hepatitis. This practice has no proven value. Steroid therapy could potentially be detrimental. In this regard, in severe viral hepatitis, corticosteroid therapy is associated with impaired survival.[49] Nevertheless, at least two respected clinicians experienced in dealing with severe drug-induced hepatitis advocate empiric high-dose corticosteroid therapy, particularly for patients with encephalopathy, deep jaundice, or prothrombin time prolonged more than 6 seconds.[2, 20] Overall, corticosteroid therapy is rarely indicated and is only considered for patients with signs of hepatic failure or for patients with severe hepatitis who show continuing deterioration 1 to 2 weeks after the responsible drug has been discontinued. Patients with hepatitis and signs of a severe systemic hypersensitivity reaction are also candidates for corticosteroid therapy. Methylprednisolone 10 to 20 mg every 6 hours represents one steroid regimen to be employed in these rare situations.

Treatment of chronic active hepatitis caused by therapeutic drugs is straightforward. Withdrawal of the responsible agent is usually sufficient. If a patient with drug-induced CAH is unimproved or has progressive illness after 10 to 14 days off the harmful drug, then short-term corticosteroid therapy should be considered.

PREVENTION

Preventive efforts to reduce incidence and severity of hepatotoxic drug reactions include thoughtful drug prescribing, careful surveillance of high-risk patients, and prompt reporting of unusual reactions. Many cases of drug-induced hepatitis occur so rarely (from 1 in 500 to 1 in 10,000 or more exposures) that current protocols of drug testing may not detect this potential problem. For example, despite an excellent safety record in clinical trials, ticrynafen was associated with liver damage in 1 per 1000 recipients during its eight months on the American market.

Since new advances in drug therapy will continue to involve some risk of liver damage, the physician should be particularly selective in the use of new drugs. An established drug with comparable efficacy, cost, and convenience, but with an excellent long-term safety record, is always the preferred agent. Even more preferred is patient care that is well accomplished without the use of medication. In some circumstances, management that includes careful observation, reassurance, education, and change in life style, diet, or psychological support may be successful and eliminate the risk of drug reactions altogether. Once again, the recent ticrynafen experience is illustrative. Most persons who received this drug, and presumably several who died as a result, were treated to prevent or correct asymptomatic hyperuricemia associated with diuretic therapy. Unfortunately, this indication was considered to be inappropriate even prior to recognition of the drug's hepatotoxicity.[50]

Once drug therapy is begun, special attention should be given to patients who receive newly marketed drugs or drugs that are known to cause serious liver disease. A baseline AST should be obtained, but symptoms, not serum enzymes, should be the focus of patient education and surveillance during the initial months of treatment. In high-risk situations, such as isoniazid therapy in the elderly, there is no substitute for routine assessment of the patient's clinical status. This is accomplished via brief office visits, telephone calls, or pharmacy visits to refill drug supplies that have been purposely limited. Routine monitoring of aminotransferase levels is not advocated, with the exception of women over age 40 who are started on isoniazid or methyldopa. Monthly AST determinations for the initial four months represent an added precautionary measure for these high-risk individuals. If routine monitoring or incidental tests detect an abnormal AST level, the patient's well-being should be reassessed. If a decline in energy or appetite is elicited, the drug should be discontinued. If the patient is truly well, the drug can be continued despite AST values up to five times normal. Higher AST levels among asymptomatic patients should prompt drug withdrawal, but an individualized approach is necessary for drugs, such as isoniazid, for which few alternatives exist.

Another way to prevent hepatic drug reactions involves reporting to the manufacturer or to the U.S. Food and Drug Administration of any possible cases of drug-induced liver damage. Active case reporting of ticrynafen-associated liver disease was given credit for the prompt recognition of this problem and the likely avoidance of further morbidity and mortality. All physicians are urged to follow this example of reporting unusual or unprecedented cases of drug-induced hepatitis. This recommendation obviously applies to old drugs as well as new ones and to the reporting of all types of adverse drug reactions, not just examples of hepatic injury.

REFERENCES

1. Mitchell JR, Jollow DJ: Metabolic activation of drugs to toxic substances. Gastroenterology *68*:392–410, 1975.
2. Zimmerman HJ: Hepatotoxicity — The Adverse Effects of Drugs and Other Chemicals on the Liver. 1st ed. New York: Appleton-Century Crofts, 1978.
3. Black M: Hepatotoxicity: pathogenesis and therapeutic intervention. Clin. Gastroenterol. *8*:89–104, 1979.
4. Sherlock S: Hepatic reactions to drugs. Gut *20*:634–648, 1979.
5. Mihas AA, Goldenberg DJ, Slaughter RL: Sulfasalazine toxic reactions: hepatitis, fever and skin rash with hypocomplementemia and immune complexes. J.A.M.A. *239*:2590–2591, 1978.
6. Hurada F: Phenytoin hypersensitivity. Neurology *29*:1480–1485, 1979.
7. Spitz RD, Keren DF, Boitnott JK, et al.: Bridging hepatic necrosis: etiology and prognosis. Am. J. Dig. Dis. *23*:1076–1078, 1978.
8. Ishak KG, Kirschner JP, Dhar JK: Granulomas and cholestatic hepatocellular injury associated with phenylbutazone. Report of two cases. Am. J. Dig. Dis. *22*:611–617, 1977. (Complete bibliography.)
9. Mitchell JR, Zimmerman HJ, Ishak KG, et al.: Isoniazid liver injury: clinical spectrum, pathology and probable pathogenesis. Ann. Intern. Med. *84*:181–192, 1976.
10. Byrd RB, Horn BR, Solomon DA, et al.: Toxic effects of isoniazid in tuberculosis chemoprophylaxis. J.A.M.A. *241*:1239–1241, 1979.
11. Maddrey WC, Boitnott JK: Drug-induced chronic liver disease. Gastroenterology *72*:1348–1353, 1977.
12. Klatskin G: Drug-Induced Hepatic Injury. *In* The Liver and Its Diseases (F Schaffner, S Sherlock and CM Leevy, eds.) New York: Intercontinental Medical Book Corp., 1974, pp. 163–178.
13. Ludwig J: Drug effects on the liver: a tabular compilation of drugs and drug-related hepatic diseases. Dig. Dis. Sci. *24*:785–796, 1979.
14. Menard DB, Gisselbrecht C, Marty M, et al.: Antineoplastic agents and the liver. Gastroenterology *78*:142–164, 1980.
15. Teychenne PF, Jones EA, Ishak KG, et al.: Hepatocellular injury with distinctive mitochondrial changes induced by lergotrile mesylate: a dopaminergic ergot derivative. Gastroenterology *76*:575–583, 1979.
16. Villeneuve JP, Warner HA: Cimetidine hepatitis. Gastroenterology *77*:143–144, 1979.
17. Maddrey WC, Boitnott JK: Severe hepatitis from methyldopa. Gastroenterology *78*:351–360, 1975.
18. Rodman JS, Deutsch DJ, Gutman SI: Methyldopa hepatitis. A report of six cases and review of the literature. Am. J. Med. *60*:941–948, 1976.
19. Black M, Mitchell JR, Zimmerman HJ, et al.: Isoniazid-associated hepatitis in 114 patients. Gastroenterology *69*:289–302, 1975.
20. Klatskin G: Toxic and drug-induced hepatitis. *In* Diseases of the Liver (L Schiff, ed.). Philadelphia: J. B. Lippincott, 1975, pp. 604–710.
21. Scheuer PJ, Bianchi L, et al.: Guidelines for diagnosis of therapeutic drug-induced liver injury in liver biopsies. Lancet 1:854–857, 1974.
22. Davidson CS, Leevy CM, Chamberlayne EC: Guidelines for Detection of Hepatotoxicity due to Drugs and Chemicals. U.S. Department of Health, Education, and Welfare. National Institutes of Health Publication 79–313.
23. Warrington RJ, Tse KS, Gorski BA, et al.: Evaluation of isoniazid-associated hepatitis by immunological tests. Clin. Exp. Immunol. *32*:97–104, 1978.
24. Arena JM: Poisoning. Chemistry-Symptoms-Treatment. 2nd ed. Springfield, Ill.: Charles C Thomas, 1974.
25. Becker CE, Tong TG, Boerner U, et al.: Diagnosis and treatment of amanita phalloides-type mushroom poisoning. West. J. Med. *125*:100–109, 1976.
26. Novel O, Henrion J, Bernuau J, et al.: Fulminant hepatic failure due to transient circulatory failure in patients with chronic heart disease. Dig. Dis. Sci. *25*:49–52, 1980.
27. Cohen JA, Kaplan MM: Left-sided heart failure presenting as hepatitis. Gastroenterology *74*:583–587, 1978.
28. Cohen JA, Kaplan MM: The SGOT/SGPT ratio — an indicator of alcoholic liver disease. Dig. Dis. Sci. *24*:835–838, 1979.
29. Kopanoff DE, Snider DE, Caras GJ: Isoniazid-related hepatitis: A U.S. Public Health Service cooperative surveillance study. Am. Rev. Resp. Dis. *117*:*991*–1001, 1978.
30. Weber WW, Hein DW: Clinical pharmacokinetics of isoniazid. Clinical Pharmacokinetics *4*:401–422, 1979.
31. Comstock GW, Edwards PQ: The competing risks of tuberculosis and hepatitis for adult tuberculin reactors. Am. Rev. Resp. Dis. *111*:573–577, 1975.
32. Moult P, Sherlock S: Halothane-related hepatitis. Q. J. Med. *44*:99–114, 1975.
33. Wolfe JD, Metzger AL, Goldstein RC: Aspirin hepatitis. Ann. Intern. Med. *80*:74–76, 1974.

34. Seaman WE, Plotz PH: Effect of aspirin on liver tests in patients with RA or SLE and in normal volunteers. Arthritis Rheum. *19*:155–160, 1976.
35. Parker WA, Shearer CA: Phenytoin hepatotoxicity: a case report and review. Neurology *29*:175–178, 1979.
36. Hahn TJ: Bone complications of anticonvulsants. Drugs *12*:201–211, 1976.
37. Black M: Acetaminophen hepatotoxicity. Gastroenterology *78*:382–392, 1980.
38. Licht H, Seeff LB, Zimmerman HJ: Apparent potentiation of acetaminophen hepatotoxicity by alcohol. Ann. Intern. Med. *92*:511, 1980.
39. Zimmerman HJ: Drug-induced chronic hepatic disease. Med. Clin. North Am. *63*:567–582, 1979.
40. Boyer JL: Chronic hepatitis — a perspective on classification and determinants of prognosis. Gastroenterology *70*:1161–1171, 1976.
41. Reynolds TB, Peters RL, Yamada S: Chronic active and lupoid hepatitis caused by a laxative, oxyphenisatin. N. Engl. J. Med. *285*:813–820, 1971.
41a. Goldstein GB, Lam KC, Mistilis SP: Drug-induced active chronic hepatitis. Am. J. Dig. Dis. *18*:177–184, 1973.
41b. Dietrichson O: Chronic active hepatitis. Aetiological considerations based on clinical and serologic studies. Scand. J. Gastroenterol. *10*:617–624, 1975.
42. Black M, Rabin L, Schatz N: Nitrofurantoin-induced chronic active hepatitis. Ann. Intern. Med. *92*:62–64, 1980.
43. Sharp JR, Ishak KG, Zimmerman HJ: Chronic active hepatitis and severe hepatic necrosis associated with nitrofurantoin. Ann. Intern. Med. *92*:14–19, 1980.
44. Johnson GK, Tolman KG: Chronic liver disease and acetaminophen. Ann. Intern. Med. *87*:302–304, 1977.
45. Bonkowsky HL, Mudge GH, McMurtry RJ: Chronic hepatic inflammation and fibrosis due to low doses of paracetamol. Lancet *1*:1016–1018, 1978.
46. Podurgiel BG, McGill DB, Ludwig J, et al.: Liver injury associated with methotrexate therapy for psoriasis. Mayo Clinic Proc. *48*:787–792, 1973.
47. Nyfors A: Liver biopsies from psoriatics related to methotrexate therapy. Acta Pathol. Microbiol. Scand. Sect. A, *85*:511–518, 1977.
47a. Ludwig J, Viggiano TR, McGill DB, et al.: Nonalcoholic steatohepatitis. Mayo Clin. Proc. *55*:434–438, 1980.
47b. Adler M, Schaffner F: Fatty liver hepatitis and cirrhosis in obese patients. Am. J. Med. *67*:811–816, 1979.
48. Auslander MO, Gitnick G: Vigorous medical management of acute fulminant hepatitis. Arch. Intern. Med. *137*:599–601, 1977.
49. European Association for the Study of the Liver: Randomized trial of steroid therapy in acute liver failure. Gut *20*:620–623, 1979.
50. Kosman ME: Evaluation of a new uricosuric diuretic — ticrynafen. J.A.M.A. *242*:2876–2878, 1979.

Chapter 11

Drug-Induced Cholestasis

by

Joel S. Levine

A generally accepted definition of cholestasis is an arrest in the liver's flow of bile.[1] For the clinician faced with a jaundiced patient, the most important consideration is whether the jaundice is due to anatomic obstruction of the extrahepatic biliary tree or to hepatic disease impairing the flow of bile (intrahepatic cholestasis). The answer to this question will determine whether a therapeutic laparotomy is undertaken. Such a laparotomy relieves obstruction of the extrahepatic biliary tree but may be detrimental in patients with intrahepatic cholestasis.

Drugs can cause a spectrum of hepatotoxic injuries that lead patients to consult their physician because of jaundice. Since the pathogenesis, differential diagnosis, and consequences of drug-induced hepatocellular necrosis are different than those of drug-induced cholestasis, it is appropriate that these major subgroupings be discussed separately (see Chap. 10). It is important to note, however, that a mixed necrosis-cholestasis biochemical profile is often found in many drug-induced hepatotoxic reactions. This chapter will provide an approach for evaluating jaundiced patients who have been exposed to pharmaceutic agents and focus on drug-induced cholestasis.

PATHOGENESIS

Since it was initially appreciated that drugs could induce cholestasis, investigators have attempted to understand the mechanisms of the impaired bile secretion. Initially, work centered on clinical observations that sporadic, drug-induced cholestasis commonly had a short latent period and presented with fever and eosinophilia. To many workers, this suggested that an immune reaction to a drug-hapten immunogen (hypersensitivity) was the direct cause of the liver damage.[2] This hypothesis, however, did not explain the identical cholestatic lesions that occur in the absence of clinical findings of hypersensitivity. In the past decade, the ability to isolate and purify hepatocyte membranes has allowed an examination of the direct effects of therapeutic agents on bile secretion. Extensive studies are available on two prototypic drugs, chlorpromazine and estrogens (C-17 alkylated hormones), that often are incriminated in drug-induced cholestatic reactions.

CHLORPROMAZINE

Chlorpromazine (CPZ) is the prototype of drugs that have been thought to induce cholestasis by an immunologic mechanism. Less than 1 per cent of those taking CPZ develop jaundice. In 90 per cent of patients taking CPZ who develop jaundice, onset of jaundice is within five weeks of starting the drug. Fever and eosinophilia are common (50 to 70 per cent), and a chronic syndrome resembling primary biliary cirrhosis has been reported.[3] Although these observations are compatible with a hypersensitivity reaction, recent *in vitro* observations suggest a direct hepatotoxic effect of either CPZ or its metabolites. Although the mechanism of CPZ-induced cholestasis has not been definitely determined, CPZ is an amphilic cationic detergent that can be incorporated into the lipid bilayer of cell membranes. After exposure to microsomal enzymes, CPZ also forms free radicals within hepatocytes. In recent studies, these CPZ free radicals have been shown to markedly inhibit Na^+K^+–ATPase in isolated hepatocyte membranes[5] and to polymerize actin that is present in the hepatocyte microfilament cytoskeleton.[6] Both effects have been associated with decreased bile flow.

A possible reason for the infrequency of clinical cholestasis complicating CPZ use is the intrinsic protective mechanism of the hepatocyte. For example, oxygenation of the free radical of CPZ, with formation of stable CPZ-sulfoxide, may protect from CPZ-induced membrane injury. In addition, conjugation of CPZ radicals with intracellular sources of glutathione may also protect against CPZ-induced damage (Fig. 11–1). Thus, individual *idiosyncrasy* in drug metabolism may be an important variable that explains the sporadic nature of CPZ-induced cholestasis. In the light of these findings, the relative importance of *hypersensitivity* in causing CPZ-induced jaundice must be reexamined. It is possible, however, that the CPZ free radicals change canalicular membrane structure so that it becomes antigenic and thus initiates a *secondary* immunologic reaction.

C-17 ALKYLATED HORMONES

In contrast to CPZ (and essentially all other drugs that cause cholestasis), hormone-associated cholestasis is rarely, if ever, associated with clinical signs of hypersensitivity. However, clinical jaundice is still sporadic, and the latent period is usually less than three months. There is evidence that some of these steroidal hormones cause a predictable and reversible reduction in the formation of bile.

The characteristic structural prerequisite for hormones to cause hepatic dysfunction is the presence of an alkyl group at the C-17 position.[8] This applies for both estrogenic (e.g., ethinyl estradiol, mestranol) and androgenic (e.g., oxymetholone, methyltestosterone) sex steroids. The hepatotoxic effects of the C-17 alkylated steroids are present whether the drug is administered orally or parenterally. Studies of estrogen in humans and rats are consistent with a dose-dependent, diffuse effect on surface hepatocyte and bile canalicular membranes (Fig. 11–1). In addition to reducing basal bile flow and membrane Na^+K^+–ATPase, estrogens decrease the maximum capacity of hepatocytes to excrete Bromsulfophthalein, bilirubin, and bile acids. These transport abnormalities appear to be related primarily to a decrease in membrane fluidity rather than to any change in active transport.[7]

With direct hepatotoxicity demonstrable, what explains the rarity of liver disease in the large number of women taking oral contraceptives? It appears that the majority of individuals who become jaundiced while using oral contraceptives have a preexisting abnormality in biliary excretory capacity.[9] Normally, the liver has a large excretory reserve, and serum bilirubin levels do not rise until excretory capacity has been reduced below 10 per cent

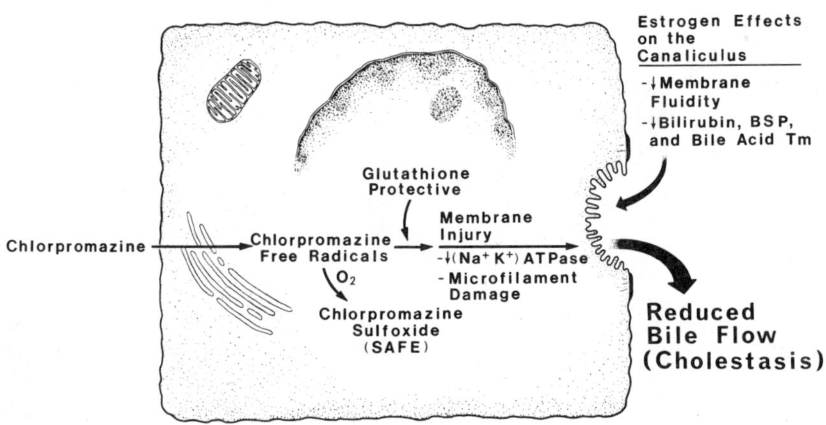

Figure 11–1. Schematic representation of possible mechanisms leading to cholestasis after the administration of chlorpromazine and estrogen. (After Samuels and Carey,[5] Elias and Boyer,[6] and Simon.[7])

of normal. Thus, only in the setting of reduced bile excretion will jaundice appear after oral contraceptive use. Consistent with this hypothesis is the fact that about 50 per cent of individuals who develop jaundice while using oral contraceptives have had intrahepatic cholestasis of pregnancy.[10] Patients with intrahepatic cholestasis of pregnancy often have pruritus during the second half of pregnancy. In some cases, jaundice and cholestatic liver function abnormalities are also present. Pruritus and liver function abnormalities disappear after parturition. Although considered an inherited disorder, the pathogenesis of intrahepatic cholestasis of pregnancy is unknown.

CLINICAL PRESENTATION

GENERAL FEATURES

On the basis of their differing clinical presentations and pathogenesis, drug-induced cholestasis has been separated into two groups, termed hepatocanalicular ("sensitivity") and canalicular ("steroid")[11] (Table 11–1). This division documents the spectrum of disease observed. In practical terms, it must be emphasized that *all* reported cases of drug-induced cholestasis have the hepatocanalicular "type," except for those associated with the 17-alkylated androgens and contraceptive steroids, which are the only known drug causes of canalicular jaundice. The hepatocanalicular reactions are commonly associated with symptoms and signs of "hypersensitivity," which may provide the only evidence suggesting that the jaundice is drug induced. The most important feature suggesting drug-induced disease is short duration of pharmaceutical exposure prior to onset of cholestasis. If the exposure has been for longer than three months, drug-induced jaundice is rare. Other signs of hypersensitivity, such as fever, rash, and eosinophilia, are seen in approximately 50 per cent of cases and are important if present. Abdominal pain, pruritus, and anorexia are common features in cholestasis of any etiology, and are thus frequently seen in drug-induced disease. There is no evidence that underlying structural liver disease predisposes to drug-induced liver toxicity.

TABLE 11–1. TYPES OF DRUG-INDUCED CHOLESTASIS*

FINDINGS	HEPATOCANALICULAR ("SENSITIVITY")	CANALICULAR ("STEROID")
Clinical		
Onset	5 weeks of ℞	Early or late
Anorexia, abdominal pain, fever	40–80%	No
Pruritus	50%	≅ 100%
Hepatic failure	No	No
Biochemical†		
Eosinophilia	40–70%	No
AST/ALT	< 8×↑	< 3×↑
Alk Phos	> 3×↑	Nl to 3×↑
Liver Biopsy	Cholestasis, portal inflammation, mild necrosis	Cholestasis
Complications		
Mortality	<<< 1%	Negligible
"Primary" biliary cirrhosis	Rare	No
Adenoma/hepatocarcinoma	No	Yes (rare)
Examples	Chlorpromazine (essentially *all* sporadic cases of drug cholestasis)	C-17 alkylated anabolic and contraceptive steroids

*Modified with permission from Zimmerman HJ: Hepatoxicity—Adverse Effects of Drugs and Other Chemicals on the Liver. 1st ed. New York: Appleton-Century-Crofts, 1978, p. 66.

†AST = Aspartate aminotransferase (SGOT); ALT = Alanine aminotransferase (SGPT); Alk Phos = Alkaline Phosphatase

BIOCHEMICAL FEATURES

The diagnosis of cholestasis is usually made by finding an alkaline phosphatase level increased three times above normal in a patient with direct hyperbilirubinemia. An hepatic rather than an osseous source of the elevated alkaline phosphatase level can be confirmed by finding increases in other liver enzymes, such as 5′-nucleotidase or gamma-glutamyl transpeptidase (GGT). Also, fractionation of alkaline phosphatase into its isoenzymes can determine the source of increased alkaline phosphatase. Since the GGT can be easily measured on multichannel autoanalyzers, it is commonly present on biochemical screens offered by clinical pathology laboratories. Unfortunately, this enzyme can be elevated by a number of environmental and pharmaceutical agents that increase liver microsomal enzyme function, such as alcohol, phenytoin, and phenobarbital.[13, 14] This may limit its usefulness as a reliable sign of cholestasis in individual cases. Canalicular lesions (17-alkylated sex hormones) often have minimal elevations of alkaline phosphatase despite bilirubin levels greater than 5 mg/dl.

The use of more sensitive methods for evaluating hepatic excretory function, such as Bromsulfophthalein (BSP) excretion or serum bile salts should be restricted to special clinical circumstances. For practical purposes, these tests are always abnormal in the icteric patient and rarely add new diagnostic information. An exception is the rare Dubin-Johnson syndrome in which the alkaline phosphatase, BSP, and serum bile salts are normal in the presence of direct hyperbilirubinemia. Determination of the serum bile salt level may be helpful to document cholestasis in the nonicteric, pruritic patient taking oral contraceptives with a normal or only slightly increased alkaline phosphatase level.

The further direction of diagnostic evaluation depends on whether cholestasis with hepatocellular necrosis or pure cholestasis is the cause of the jaundice. This differential can usually be based on the results of initial liver function tests.[12] In general, cholestasis with hepatocellular necrosis is associated with increases in aspartate aminotransferase (AST) and alanine aminotransferase (ALT) levels of two to four times normal. All causes of jaundice due to severe hepatocellular necrosis are associated with AST and ALT levels more than eight times normal. Thus, in drug-induced jaundice, AST and ALT levels above eight times normal indicate short-term (hepatic failure) and long-term (chronic active hepatitis) risks that are not seen with pure cholestasis or cholestasis with minimal to mild hepatocellular necrosis.

LIVER BIOPSY FINDINGS

Once a cholestatic biochemical profile has been found in the appropriate clinical setting of drug-induced cholestasis, an attempt to obtain a definitive diagnosis by performing a liver biopsy may be considered. In general, liver biopsy should be considered if (1) extrahepatic biliary obstruction has been made less likely by a normal ultrasound or computed tomographic (CT) scan; (2) cholestasis has persisted after stopping the drug or the medication cannot be stopped; and (3) cholestasis has not been previously reported to occur with the medication under question. The clinician obtaining a liver biopsy should understand that although the histologic appearance may strongly suggest that drug therapy is responsible for a lesion, it rarely, if ever, provides conclusive evidence.[15]

The overall risks of liver biopsy are low (1/600 bleeding, 1/6000 death). However, in the patient with cholestasis, there is often concern that puncturing a dilated ductal system could induce bile peritonitis. This concern is diminished by Morris and co-workers,[16] who reported that only one case of bile peritonitis requiring operation occurred in a series of 127 liver biopsies in patients with proven extrahepatic obstruction. The cost of the biopsy procedure, if the patient is hospitalized, can be substantial ($499–$700).[17]

The most common drug-induced lesion in icteric patients is cholestasis (defined as bile pigment in tissue sections) with cellular inflammation and necrosis. Chlorpromazine produces such a lesion. Initially, the histologic picture is dominated by centrilobular cholestasis (Fig. 11–2A) and expansion of portal tracts by mononuclear cell infiltration. This infiltrate ultimately disappears, even in patients running a more chronic course. In time, necrosis and swelling ("ballooning degeneration") (Fig. 11–2*B*) of hepatocytes is seen in the areas of cholestasis. If jaundice persists for three to four weeks, the cholestasis will become partly periportal in location and accompanied by substantial liver cell swelling.[15] Portal triad or sinusoidal eosinophilia is helpful in the diagno-

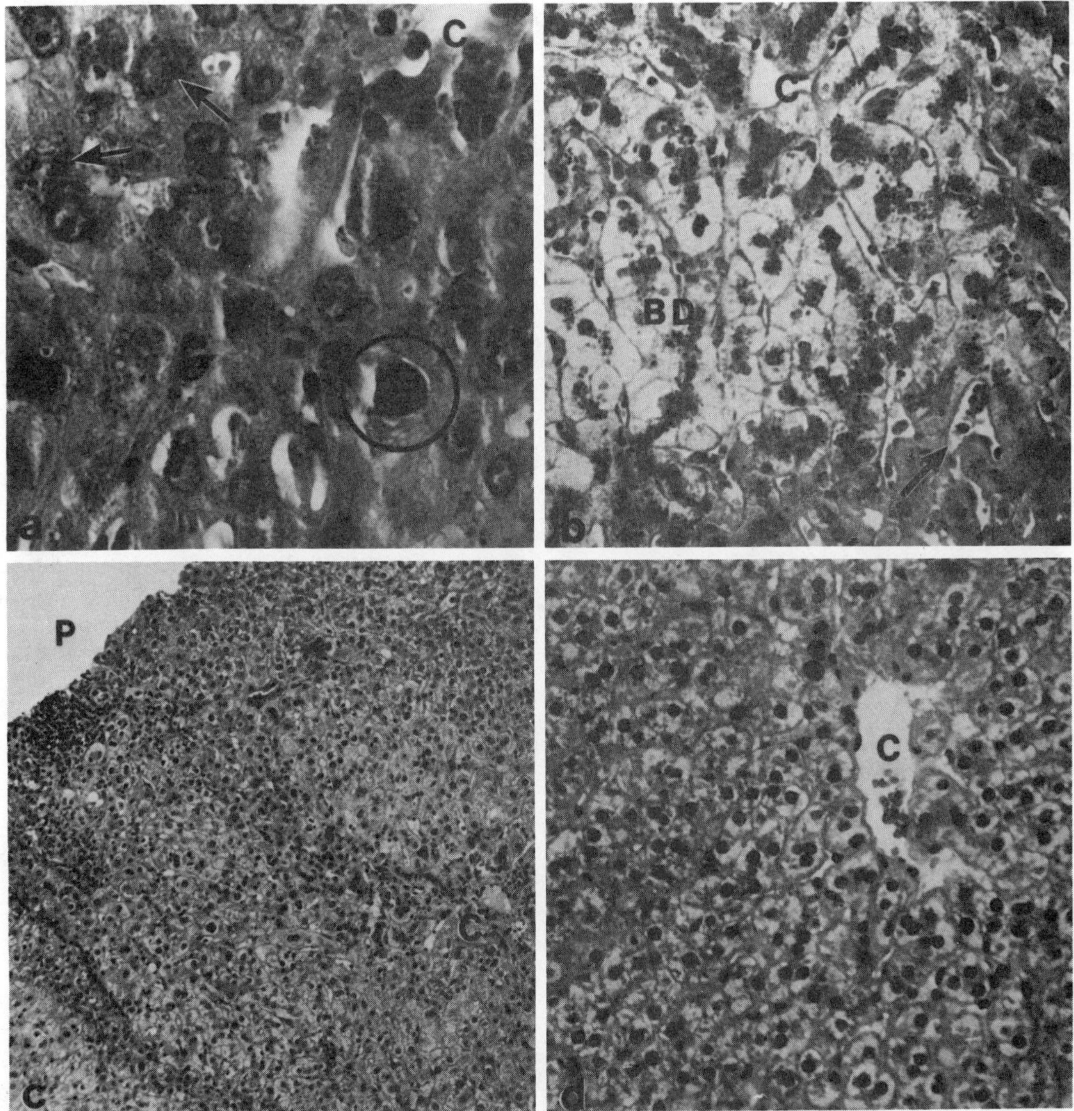

Figure 11–2. Liver biopsies from patients with drug-induced *(a,b,d)* and obstructive (*c*) cholestasis. *a*, Chlorpromazine jaundice × 1 week showing essentially normal hepatic parenchyma in centrizonal area with bile plug (circled) and bile pigment within hepatocytes (arrows), × 420. *b*, Chlorpromazine jaundice × 4 weeks with ballooning degeneration (BD) and sinusoidal dilatation (arrow), × 260. *c*, Extrahepatic obstruction showing centrizonal cholestasis identical to *a*, but also neutrophilic inflammation in portal area (P) and within bile ducts, × 100. *d*, Contraceptive jaundice × 1 week showing very mild cholestasis and normal parenchyma, × 260. All hematoxylin and eosin. C = central vein.

sis. Unfortunately, the infiltration is patchy, often absent, and is, occasionally, seen in viral hepatitis and extrahepatic obstruction. Bile-duct proliferation, scattered neutrophils near bile ducts, portal tract edema, and bile infarcts favor extrahepatic obstruction as the cause of cholestasis (Fig. 11–2*C*).[18]

Pure cholestasis (Fig. 11–2*D*) is characterized by centrilobular cholestasis without inflammatory cell infiltration or significant hepatocyte necrosis. The icteric patient with elevated alkaline phosphatase who is taking anabolic or contraceptive steroids will typically have this morphological picture.

A number of patients with drug toxicity and a cholestatic biochemical profile have been found to have granulomas (see Chap. 10), with and without cholestasis or necrosis, which disappear after drug withdrawal. The distribution or appearance of the granulomas does not allow separation from other causes of granulomatous hepatitis.

There is strong circumstantial evidence that the long-term use of contraceptive[19] and anabolic steroids[20] may lead to development of hepatic adenomas or hepatocellular carcinoma. Relative risk has not been assessed, but most believe the relationship to be real. In general, the adenomas are asymptomatic unless they bleed and cause hemoperitoneum. Industrial exposure to vinyl chloride[21] and medical exposure to Thorotrast[22] have been associated with the remote development of hepatic angiosarcomas.

PROGNOSIS AND THERAPY

The only apparent adverse sequelae of acute drug-induced cholestasis are the consequences of invasive diagnostic tests (percutaneous cholangiogram) or inadvertent laparotomy. Indeed, there are well-documented instances in which cholestasis abated during continued drug use, suggesting that the liver can compensate for the injury in some patients. Rarely (perhaps a total of 35 cases), drug-induced cholestasis has become chronic and has led to a syndrome resembling primary biliary cirrhosis.

Therapy, other than discontinuation of the implicated drug, is rarely necessary. However, in cases of protracted jaundice with severe pruritus, therapeutic intervention may be appropriate. Pruritus may be alleviated by giving a bile salt–binding agent, such as cholestyramine, orally. Since the taste of this agent frequently limits patient compliance, using one 4-gm packet prior to breakfast only (when the majority of the bile salt pool is in the gallbladder after the overnight fast) may suffice. Phenobarbital has been reported to reduce jaundice and pruritus,[23] but the dosage employed (120 to 250 mg/day) usually induces excessive sedation.

DRUGS THAT CAUSE CHOLESTASIS (Table 11–2)

Individual drugs or groups of drugs that have been commonly reported to induce cholestasis will be briefly reviewed. For more extensive reviews of individual drugs as well as a listing of drugs that can induce cholestasis, the reader is referred to Table 11–2 and other sources.[11, 24–26]

PHENOTHIAZINES

In selected populations, phenothiazines can be a common cause of jaundice. For example, phenothiazines account for 15 to 20 per cent of jaundice encountered in geriatric and psychiatric hospitals. The overall incidence of phenothiazine jaundice appears to be less than 1 per cent. Chlorpromazine (CPZ) has been most closely studied,[3] but most phenothiazine derivatives can produce cholestatic jaundice.

Ninety per cent of those who ultimately become jaundiced taking CPZ have a latent period after starting the drug of less than five weeks. Fever (70 per cent), pruritus (60 per cent), anorexia (50 per cent), and mild abdominal pain (50 per cent) are seen commonly, but 20 per cent will have no prodrome. Rash is uncommon, but eosinophilia is found in 70 per cent. It is important to recognize that jaundice may persist for extended periods after CPZ has been stopped. Only 30 per cent of patients are recovered at 4 weeks, 60 per cent at 8 weeks, 75 per cent at 12 weeks, and 93 per cent at 1 year. Ultimate resolution is the rule in the remaining 7 per cent.[3]

A syndrome mimicking primary biliary cirrhosis has been reported in 30 patients taking CPZ.[26] On clinical grounds, these patients cannot be separated from primary biliary cirrhosis, except for a higher frequency of males in the CPZ group. Biochemical and histologic findings may be identical. The frequency of occurrence of antimitochondrial antibodies, a marker for primary biliary cirrhosis, in CPZ-induced disease is not known. The eventual resolution of cholestasis in the majority of the patients taking CPZ, in contrast to the irreversibility of primary biliary cirrhosis, may be the only way to separate the groups.

ANDROGENS (17-ALKYLATED) AND ESTROGENS

If very sensitive tests of bile excretory function are used, the incidence of hepatic dysfunction with this group of steroids is almost universal. Clinical jaundice, however, is uncommon, indicating the importance of individual susceptibility. This is most clearly

TABLE 11–2. TYPES OF ACUTE HEPATIC INJURY CAUSED BY DRUGS*

Category of Drug	
Anesthetics	Halothane (H) Methoxyflurane (H)
Anticonvulsants	Carbamazepine (C) Phenytoin (HC)[g] Trimethadione (H) Valproic acid (H)
Antihypertensive Agents, Diuretics	Chlorthalidone (C) Methyldopa (HC) Metolazone (H)[g] Thiazides (C)
Antimicrobial Agents	Amoxicillin (H) Ampicillin (H) Carbenicillin (H) Cephalexin (H)[g] Chloramphenicol (HC) Clindamycin (H) Erythromycins (C) 5-Fluorocytosine (H) Griseofulvin (HC) Isoniazid (H) Nitrofurantoin (HC) Oxacillin (H)[g] Para-aminosalicylate (HC) Penicillin (HC)[g] Piperazines (C) Quinacrine (H) Rifampin (H) Sulfonamides (HC)[g] Tetracyclines (H)[f] Thiobendazole (C)
Antirheumatic Drugs, Analgesics, Muscle Relaxants	Acetaminophen (H) Allopurinol (H)[g] Carisoprodol (H) D-Penicillamine (C) Dantrolene (H) Diazepam (C) Gold (C) Ibuprofen (H) Indomethacin (H) Naproxen (C)[41] Oxyphenbutazone (H)[g] Phenylbutazone (H)[g] Probenecid (H) Propoxyphene (C) Salicylates (H) Sulindac (C)[39]
Cardiovascular	Aprindine (H) Papaverine (HC) Procainamide (HC)[g] Quinidine (HC)[g] Warfarin (C)
Chemotherapeutic Immunosuppressive Agents[14]	Azathioprine (HC) Busulfan (C) Corticosteroids[f] Cytosine arabinoside (H) L-Asparaginase (H)[f] 6-Mercaptopurine (HC) Methotrexate (H) Mithramycin (H) Mitomycin (H)[f] Nitrosoureas (H)
Hormonal Agents Drugs Used in Metabolic Disorders	Anabolic steroids (C) (C-17 alkylated) Bromocriptine (H) Chlorpropamide (C) Clofibrate (HC)[g] Contraceptives, oral (C) Estrogens (C) Methimazole (C) Nicotinic acid (HC) Propylthiouracil (HC) Tolazamide (C) Tolbutamide (C)
Psychotropic Drugs	Chlordiazepoxide (C) Diazepam (C) Flurazepam (C) Haloperidol (C) MAO-inhibitors (H) Phenothiazines (C) Tricyclic antidepressants (HC)
Miscellaneous	Cimetidine (HC)[42] Disulfiram (H) Danthron (H) Methoxsalen (H) Phenazopyridine (H)

H = Hepatocellular Necrosis: C = Cholestasis; HC = Necrosis and/or Cholestasis; g = Granulomas reported in some cases; f = Fatty change

*Table lists currently available therapeutic drugs that have been reported to cause hepatic injury; the predominant type of injury is shown in parentheses. The reader is urged to examine the original reports of these drug reactions; most are cited in references 11, 24, 25, and 26.

documented for birth control pills, in which the rare cases of overt jaundice are usually found in women with benign intrahepatic cholestasis of pregnancy.[10] This genetic disorder has a higher prevalence in Swedes and Chileans and commonly presents as pruritus alone in the second half of pregnancy.

The only anabolic steroids that cause cholestasis are alkylated at the C-17 position; thus, testosterone has never been reported to cause jaundice. Whether the anabolic steroids are administered orally or parenterally does not change the incidence of hepatotoxicity. In contrast to CPZ, however, the incidence of clinical jaundice increases with duration of exposure and higher doses of drug.[27] Biochemically it is a canalicular jaundice (Table 11–1), and symptoms abate quickly if the medication is stopped. The major long-term risk may be the development of hepatic adenomas and hepatocellular cancer,[20] but the true incidence of these complications is unknown.

Estrogens are the component of contraceptive steroids that leads to cholestasis. Jaundice usually occurs within the first two to three cycles, and pruritus is a common symptom that is seen in essentially all affected individuals. Since chronic estrogen use increases the incidence of gallstones,[28] there will be an initial concern of a partially obstructing common duct stone because of the canalicular biochemical profile. In addition to adenoma and hepatocellular cancer,[19] focal nodular hyperplasia and the Budd-Chiari syndrome (hepatic vein thrombosis) have been reported as sequelae of chronic estrogen use.

ANTIMICROBIALS

Erythromycin estolate has been the most commonly reported antimicrobial to cause cholestasis. Jaundice is rare in children (only 5 per cent of cases occur in children below 10 years of age) and almost always occur within three weeks of institution of drug therapy.[29] Clinical and biochemical features are identical to CPZ-induced jaundice, with jaundice subsiding within two to five weeks. Since the estolate is the only form of erythromycin that commonly causes jaundice and it offers no compensating therapeutic benefits, its use in adults is unwarranted. The FDA is currently considering removing erythromycin estolate from the market.[30]

Griseofulvin, nitrofurantoin, thiobendazole, and sulfonamides can cause cholestasis in addition to hepatocellular necrosis. The common presence of these agents in combination antimicrobials, emphasized by a case report of a patient who developed cholestasis after exposure to Tricofuron vaginal suppositories,[31] calls attention to the continued vigilance needed to uncover subtle drug exposures.

ANTIMETABOLITES

It has been suggested that several antineoplastic agents (busulfan, 6-mercaptopurine, azathioprine) cause cholestatic jaundice. If this occurs, it is a very rare event, and its pathogenesis must differ in some way from the more typical idiosyncratic drug reactions. In the majority of reports, patients have been taking the drug for more than a year, and jaundice has been associated with a worsening of their underlying disorder (i.e., transplant rejection, conversion of chronic to acute myelogenous leukemia).[32–34] Rechallenge studies have not been performed, and it is quite possible that the cholestasis was related to complications of the disease process (i.e., sepsis, leukemic infiltration of the liver) rather than to the treatment. Since these drugs are often irreplaceable and since specific diagnosis may be difficult, a carefully monitored rechallenge study may be warranted.

ANTICONVULSANTS

Although carbamazepine has been reported to cause cholestatic jaundice,[24] the more commonly used phenytoin causes hepatocellular necrosis and/or granulomatous hepatitis (see Chap. 10). However, chronic phenytoin therapy is associated with a high frequency of increases in both the alkaline phosphatase and GGT levels. The GGT level is abnormally elevated in more than 90 per cent of epileptics taking phenytoin alone or in combination with other drugs.[13] An elevated alkaline phosphatase level of both liver and bone origin can often be detected in patients on chronic phenytoin therapy.[35] The overall incidence of this combined biochemical abnormality is unknown. Whether the elevated liver alkaline phosphatase reflects cholestasis or nonspecific enzyme induction is not known, but these biochemical findings might lead to a costly diagnostic evaluation to rule out extrahepatic obstruction. At present, we recommend that a physical examination be performed and ultrasound be obtained in patients with increased GGT and/or alkaline phosphatase levels on chronic phenytoin therapy. If these evaluations are normal, no further evaluation need be considered in the asymptomatic patient.

DRUGS FOR RHEUMATIC DISEASES

Gold,[36] propoxyphene,[37] D-penicillamine,[38] and sulindac[39] have been reported to cause intrahepatic cholestasis that clinically mimics CPZ-induced jaundice. D-Penicillamine may present a particularly difficult diagnostic challenge, since it is also used to treat liver diseases (Wilson's disease, primary biliary cirrhosis) that have a significant degree of cholestasis as their primary manifestation. Differentiating an exacerbation of the underlying disease from drug toxicity can be difficult and often requires discontinuation of therapy.

HYDROCARBONS

All levels of society are exposed either accidentally or through industrial means to complex petrochemicals. In this regard, an epidemic of toxic hepatic injury that occurred in Epping, England, in 1965 is of interest.[40] *Epping jaundice*[40] refers to the cholestatic jaundice that occurred in 84 persons who ate bread accidentally contaminated by 4,4′-diaminodiphenylmethane, a hardener of epoxy resins. In 60 per cent of those affected, onset was abrupt with severe abdominal pain; initially, several patients had laparotomies before the clinical picture was formulated. Although clinically similar to CPZ-induced jaundice, liver histology tended to show more hepatocellular necrosis and neutrophilic infiltration of bile ducts that suggested extrahepatic obstruction with cholangitis. This epidemic emphasizes the importance of awareness of the possible role of environmental toxins in any form of unexplained liver injury.

DIFFERENTIAL DIAGNOSIS

It is important to keep in perspective that drugs are a relatively uncommon cause of jaundice. Chlorpromazine, perhaps the most frequently reported cause of drug-induced cholestasis, has a low (< 1 per cent) incidence of clinically significant hepatotoxicity. When Koff et al.[43] assessed the causes of jaundice among three Boston hospitals with diverse patient populations in 1969, drugs caused only 2 per cent of the cases. Alcohol (30 per cent), postoperative jaundice (18 per cent), hepatic disease (15 per cent), and extrahepatic biliary tract obstruction (15 per cent) were more commonly encountered. Thus, the clinician is faced with the statistical likelihood that drug-related cholestasis will be uncommon. However, concern about other lesions may lead to the performance of costly diagnostic tests and specific therapy (i.e., stopping the drug) not being initiated.

Although the differential diagnosis of cholestasis (Table 11–3) is broad, the history

TABLE 11–3. CAUSES OF CHOLESTASIS UNRELATED TO DRUGS*

MODE OF PRESENTATION	COMMENTS
Acute	
Extrahepatic obstruction	Choledocholithiasis Tumor → pancreas Inflammation → acute pancreatitis
Postoperative	Common, self-limiting, etiology?
Alcoholic liver disease	Hepatitis or steatosis
Hyperalimentation	See in adults and children
Severe sepsis	↑ ↑ Direct bilirubin with minimal ↑ alkaline phosphatase
Inspissated bile syndrome	Neonates only
Chronic	
Extrahepatic obstruction	Inflammation → stricture, chronic pancreatitis, sclerosing cholangitis Tumor → bile duct
Primary biliary cirrhosis	⊕ AMA; mainly women
Infiltrative disease of liver	Sarcoid, TB, tumor, etc.
Ulcerative colitis	Pericholangitis, sclerosing cholangitis, biliary cancer
Biliary atresia	Infants only
Genetic	
Dubin-Johnson syndrome	Melanin-like pigment in liver
Rotor syndrome	Autosomal dominant
Cholestasis of pregnancy	Will get contraceptive jaundice also

*Modified with permission from Zimmerman HJ: Intrahepatic cholestasis. Arch. Intern. Med. *139*:1038–1045, 1979.
AMA = antimitochondrial antibody.

TABLE 11–4. BILIARY TRACT IMAGING TO EXCLUDE EXTRAHEPATIC OBSTRUCTION

	Technique	Sensitivity/ Specificity	Morbidity	Cost*
Noninvasive	Ultrasound	95/95	0	$ 75–100
	CT Scan	95/95	Minimal radiation exposure	$225–300
Invasive	PTC	95/95	1% cholangitis 1% bile peritonitis	$140–180
	ERCP	95/95†	1% cholangitis	$450–600

*Denver, Colorado, 1980. Cost will vary depending on location.
†*If* duct is visualized after cannulation.

alone will suffice to exclude many of the causes. In fact, the rare genetic disorders are almost always historical diagnoses. Since drug-induced cholestasis may mimic both the clinical and biochemical features of acute or chronic extrahepatic obstruction, these remain the most important diagnostic considerations. Indeed, prior to 1970, many case reports of new drugs causing cholestasis included a laparotomy to exclude disease of the extrahepatic biliary tree. In the past decade, however, several noninvasive means of visualizing the biliary tree have largely replaced laparotomy in the jaundiced patient (Table 11–4). The sensitivity and specificity of *all* these tests approached 90 to 95 per cent when performed by experts using the most up-to-date equipment.[44-47] Selection of a test, therefore, will frequently depend on the availability of equipment and reliability of interpretation in the clinician's geographic location. If all are available, ultrasound (grey-scale with real-time) appears to be the ideal noninvasive screening modality on the basis of its being one-fourth to one-third the cost of a CT scan, while providing the same information.[44] At our institution, a normal ultrasound is accepted as strong evidence against extrahepatic obstruction. The invasive imaging techniques are currently reserved for preoperative assessment of the level of obstruction or for those few patients in whom the clinical course suggests obstruction in the face of a normal ultrasound (see the following section, Diagnostic Approach).

All lesions producing intrahepatic cholestasis (Table 11–3) are difficult to distinguish from drug-induced cholestasis by currently available criteria. However, evidence of "hypersensitivity" (i.e., fever, rash, eosinophilia) strongly suggests a drug-induced lesion.

Alcoholic liver disease may be the most common cause of jaundice seen in hospitals in the United States.[43] Cholestatic jaundice can be caused by the reversible lesion of steatosis or hepatitis and does not necessarily indicate the presence of cirrhosis. In general, the correct diagnosis is made on the basis of a careful history alone. However, a common error is the presumption that all jaundice in an alcoholic patient is related to alcohol ingestion. Thus, in a recent study of alcoholics, 25 per cent of liver disease could not be related to alcohol ingestion. The clinician must keep alert for the myriad of pharmaceuticals that may have been instituted for the neurologic, psychiatric, infectious, or other complications of alcoholism. Postoperative jaundice is seen frequently after major surgical procedures. The etiology of the cholestasis is unknown, but may be related in some way to voluminous blood transfusions that frequently accompany the syndrome. Sepsis, hepatitis, or drug toxicity are common diagnostic concerns, but ultimate complete clinical resolution is the rule.[48] The increasingly common use of total parenteral nutrition (TPN) has introduced a new source of intrahepatic cholestasis. Although initially felt to be seen only in infants,[49] more recent studies[50] have documented cholestatic jaundice in adults given TPN for 30 days, with 24 of 32 patients having an elevated alkaline phosphatase level and 19 of 32 becoming clinically jaundiced. The cholestasis was completely reversible on discontinuation of TPN and in three individuals by reducing the amount of fatty acids (Intralipid) in the infusion. Finally, bacterial sepsis secondary to either gram-positive or gram-negative bacteria can cause severe direct hyperbilirubinemia.[51] Frequently, the alkaline phosphatase level is minimally elevated compatible with a pure cholestatic lesion. Recent work suggests that this is a direct effect of endotoxin on the liver.[52]

Drugs are rarely involved in the etiology of chronic cholestasis, but the reasonably clear documentation of a "primary" biliary cirrhosis-like illness in approximately 30 patients who have used chlorpromazine and a few patients taking tolbutamide and thiobendazole emphasizes the need for continued reassessment of the possible role of drugs in any cholestatic lesion.[49] Although the clinical presentation of drug-induced chronic cholestasis is essentially indistinguishable from primary biliary cirrhosis, the prospect of ultimate recovery in a majority of the drug-related types separates them from the irreversible primary form.

DIAGNOSTIC APPROACH

An algorithm helpful in differentiating extrahepatic biliary tract obstruction from intrahepatic cholestasis in a patient taking drugs is depicted in Figure 11–3. Several presumptions underlie this approach.

First, although uncommon in a general population, drug-induced cholestasis is worth considering because it is treatable. Second, drug-induced cholestasis should be considered only if the duration of drug use is less than three months. Third, the presence of eosinophilia strongly supports a drug-related etiology, but the absence of eosinophilia is not helpful in the individual case. Fourth, although the initial historical, physical, and biochemical data base will allow the separation of cholestatic from hepatotoxic causes of jaundice in 90 per cent of cases, these factors will not differentiate cholestatic jaundice caused by drugs from extrahepatic obstruction. Finally, the algorithm is helpful only in the absence of cholangitis. The presence of cholangitis necessitates more rapid evaluation of the biliary tree.

Several branches of this algorithm require a more detailed explanation. About 95 per cent of patients who have cholestatic jaundice and an initially normal ultrasound do not have extrahepatic obstruction and will not require laparotomy to drain the biliary system. In fact, unless a drug or toxin (i.e., alcohol) can be stopped, most causes of intrahepatic cholesta-

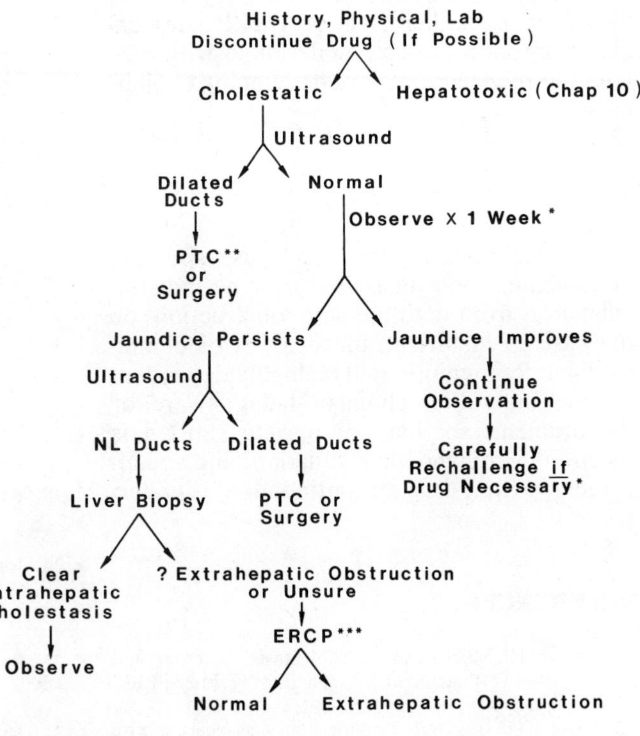

Figure 11–3. An algorithm for differentiating extrahepatic obstruction from intrahepatic cholestasis as the cause of jaundice in any patient using drugs.

sis have no specific therapy; thus, rapid diagnosis is unnecessary. With these considerations in mind, a period of observation after discontinuation of drug(s), without embarking on further tests, is warranted. In outpatients with minimal symptoms, this observation can be continued on an outpatient basis. In the few patients who actually have extrahepatic obstruction and do not improve, little has been lost, since permanent effects on the liver (i.e., biliary cirrhosis) are seen only after at least six weeks of complete obstruction.

In patients with persisting or worsening cholestasis, a repeat ultrasound examination is suggested. This will allow selection of patients with obstruction who have developed ductal system dilatation during the period of observation. In those with a normal ultrasound, a liver biopsy is most likely to provide specific diagnostic information. Since very few of these patients will have obstruction, the risk of bile peritonitis is minimal. Percutaneous transhepatic cholangiography (PTC) is the primary diagnostic modality in patients with evidence of bile duct dilatation. Endoscopic retrograde cholangiopancreatography (ERCP) is reserved for those individuals in whom extrahepatic obstruction is suggested on liver biopsy. If an obstructed biliary system is visualized by either PTC or ERCP, surgical decompression must be undertaken within 24 hours to reduce the risk of developing cholangitis.

SUMMARY

Pharmaceutical agents can cause sporadic intrahepatic cholestasis that may be indistinguishable from extrahepatic obstruction on the basis of historical, physical, or biochemical data. Recognition will be highly dependent on the individual clinician being aware of the problem, so that appropriate caution is taken in the diagnostic evaluation, and specific therapy (i.e., drug discontinuation) is undertaken.

REFERENCES

1. Popper H: Mechanism of cholestasis. *In* Liver and Bile (L'Bianchi, ed.). England: MTP Press, Ltd., Lancaster, 1977, pp. 189–201.
2. Ishak KG, Irey NS: Hepatic injury associated with the phenothiazines. Arch. Pathol. *93*:283–304, 1972.
3. Zimmerman HJ: Manifestations of hepatotoxicity. Ann. N.Y. Acad. Sci. *104*:954–987, 1963.
4. Kendler J, Bowry S, Seeff LB, et al.: Effect of chlorpromazine on the function of the perfused isolated liver. Biochem. Pharmacol. *20*:2439–2445, 1971.
5. Samuels AM, Carey MC: Effects of chlorpromazine hydrochloride and its metabolites on Mg^{2+}- and Na^+K^+-ATPase activities of canalicular-enriched rat liver plasma membranes. Gastroenterology *74*:1183–1190, 1978.
6. Elias E, Boyer JL: Chlorpromazine and its metabolites alter polymerization and gelation of actin. Science *206*:1404–1406, 1979.
7. Simon FR: Effects of estrogens on the liver. Gastroenterology *75*:512–514, 1978.
8. Adlercreutz H, Tenhunen R: Some aspects of the interaction between natural and synthetic female sex hormones and the liver. Am. J. Med. *49*:630–648, 1970.
9. Cohen L, Lewis C, Arias IM: Pregnancy, oral contraceptives and chronic familial jaundice with predominantly conjugated hyperbilirubinemia (Dubin-Johnson syndrome). Gastroenterology *62*:1182–1190, 1972.
10. Haemmerli VP: Recurrent intrahepatic cholestasis of pregnancy or pruritus gravidarum. Medicine *46*:299–321, 1967.
11. Zimmerman HJ: Hepatotoxicity — The Adverse Effects of Drugs and Other Chemicals on the Liver. 1st ed. New York: Appleton-Century-Crofts, 1978, p. 66.
12. Schenker S, Balint J, Schiff L: Differential diagnosis of jaundice: Report of a prospective study of 61 proved cases. Am. J. Dig. Dis. *7*:449–463, 1962.
13. Freer DE, Statland BE: Effects of ethanol on the activities of selected enzymes in sera of healthy young adults: 2. Interindividual variations in response of γ-glutamyltransferase to repeated ethanol challenges. Clin. Chem. *23*:2099–2102, 1977.
14. Heipertz R, Eickhoff K, Poser W: Anticonvulsant therapy and serum γ-glutamyltransferase. Klin. Wochenschr. *56*:921–928, 1978.
15. Scheuer PJ, Bianchi L: Guidelines for diagnosis of therapeutic drug-induced liver injury in liver biopsies. Lancet *1*:854–857, 1974.
16. Morris JS, Gallo GA, Scheuer PJ, et al.: Percutaneous liver biopsy in patients with large bile duct obstruction. Gastroenterology *68*:750–754, 1975.
17. Knauer CM: Percutaneous biopsy of the liver as a procedure for outpatients. Gastroenterology *74*:101–102, 1978.
18. Gall EA, Dobrogorski O: Hepatic alterations in obstructive jaundice. Am. J. Clin. Pathol. *41*:126–139, 1964.
19. Klatskin G: Hepatic tumors: Possible relationship to use of oral contraceptives. Gastroenterology *73*:386–394, 1977.
20. Johnson FL, Lerner KG, Siegel M, et al.: Association of androgenic-anabolic steroid therapy with development of hepatocellular carcinoma. Lancet *2*:1273–1276, 1972.
21. Berk PD, Martin JF, Young RS, et al.: Vinyl chloride-associated liver disease. Ann. Intern. Med. *84*:717–731, 1976.
22. Selinger M, Koff RS: Thorotrast and the liver: A reminder. Gastroenterology *68*:799–803, 1975.
23. Bloomer JR, Boyer JL: Phenobarbital effects in cho-

lestatic liver disease. Ann. Intern. Med. *82*:310–317, 1975.

24. Plaa GL, Priestly BG: Intrahepatic cholestasis induced by drugs and chemicals. Pharmacol. Rev. *28*:207–273, 1977.
25. Ludwig J: Drug effects on the liver. A tabular compilation of drugs and drug-related hepatic diseases. Dig. Dis. Sci. *24*:785–796, 1979.
26. Klatskin G: Toxic and drug-induced hepatitis. *In* Diseases of The Liver (L Schiff, ed.). 5th ed. Philadelphia: J.B. Lippincott, 1975, pp. 604–710.
27. Westaby D, Paradinas FJ, Ogle SJ, et al.: Liver damage from long-term methyltestosterone. Lancet *2*:261–263, 1977.
28. Bennion LJ, Ginsberg RL, Garnick MB, et al.: Effects of oral contraceptives on the gallbladder bile of normal women. N. Engl. J. Med. *294*:189–192, 1976.
29. Braun P: Hepatotoxicity of erythromycin. J. Infect. Dis. *119*:300–306, 1969.
30. FDA begins proceedings to remove erythromycin estolate from market. FDA Drug Bull. *9*:26–27, 1979.
31. Engel JJ, Vogt TR, Wilson DE: Cholestatic hepatitis after administration of furan derivatives. Arch. Intern. Med. *135*:733–735, 1975.
32. Underwood JCE, Shahani RT, Blackburn EK: Jaundice after treatment of leukemia with busulphan. Br. Med. J. *1*:556–557, 1971.
33. Hast R: Increase in serum alkaline phosphatase in chronic myelocytic leukemia — sign of drug-induced cholestasis. Acta Med. Scand. *203*:93–94, 1978.
34. Sparberg M, Simon N, del Greco F: Intrahepatic cholestasis due to azathioprine. Gastroenterology *57*:439–441, 1969.
35. Hahn TJ, Hendin BA, Sharp CR, et al.: Effect of chronic anticonvulsant therapy on serum 25-hydroxycalciferol levels in adults. N. Engl. J. Med. *287*:900–904, 1972.
36. Favreau M, Tannenbaum H, Lough J: Hepatic toxicity associated with gold therapy. Ann. Intern. Med. *87*:717–719, 1977.
37. Klein NC, Magida MG: Propoxyphene (Darvon) hepatotoxicity. Am. J. Dig. Dis. *16*:467–469, 1971.
38. Barzilai D, Dickstein G, Enat R, et al.: Cholestatic jaundice caused by D-penicillamine. Ann. Rheum. Dis. *37*:98–100, 1978.
39. Wolfe PB: Sulindac and jaundice. Ann. Intern. Med. *91*:656, 1979.
40. Kopelman H, Scheuer PJ, Williams R: The liver lesion in Epping jaundice. Q. J. Med. *35*:553–564, 1966.
41. Bass BH: Jaundice associated with Naproxen. Lancet *1*:998, 1974.
42. Lilly JR, Hitch DC, Javitz NB: Cimetidine cholestatic jaundice. J. Surg. Res. *24*:384, 1978.
43. Koff RS, Gardner R, Harinasuta U, et al.: Profile of hyperbilirubinemia in three hospital populations. Clin. Res. *18*:680, 1970.
44. Vallon AG, Lees WR, Cotton PB: Grey-scale ultrasonography in cholestatic jaundice. Gut *20*:51–54, 1979.
45. Levitt RG, Sagel SS, Stanley RJ, et al.: Accuracy of computed tomography of the liver and biliary tract. Radiology *124*:123–128, 1977.
46. Ferrucci JT, Wittenberg J: Refinements in Chiba needle transhepatic cholangiography. Am. J. Roentgenol. *129*:11–16, 1977.
47. Elias E, Hamlyn AN, Jain S, et al.: A randomized trial of percutaneous transhepatic cholangiography with the Chiba needle versus endoscopic retrograde cholangiography for bile duct visualization in jaundice. Gastroenterology *71*:439–443, 1976.
48. Kantrowitz PA, Jones WA, Greenberger NJ, et al.: Severe postoperative hyperbilirubinemia simulating obstructive jaundice. N. Engl. J. Med. *276*:591–598, 1967.
49. Zimmerman HJ: Intrahepatic cholestasis. Arch. Intern. Med. *139*:1038–1045, 1979.
50. Allardyce DB, Salvian AJ, Quenville NF: Cholestatic jaundice during total parenteral nutrition. Can. J. Surg. *21*:332–339, 1978.
51. Miller DJ, Keeton GR, Webber BL, et al.: Jaundice in severe bacterial infection. Gastroenterology *71*:94–97, 1976.
52. Utili R, Abernathy CO, Zimmerman HJ: Inhibition of Na^+,K^+-adenosinetriphosphatase by endotoxin: A possible mechanism for endotoxin-induced cholestasis. J. Infect. Dis. *136*:583–587, 1977.

Chapter 12

Drug Use in Patients With Liver Disease — An Overview

by

Rashmi V. Patwardhan,
and Steven Schenker

The aim of drug therapy is to administer an optimal dose of a drug to achieve an adequate blood concentration that provides the desired clinical and theraputic effect without toxicity. Owing to the large interpatient variability in disposition of drugs and pharmacologic response to them, this goal is not always achieved. Disease states of excretory organs further compound this variability, and it is essential for the physician to know normal pharmacokinetic and pharmacodynamic principles and how disease affects the fate of administered drugs. These variations in response are due to individual differences in the rate and extent of the processes of drug absorption, distribution, metabolism, and excretion. In addition, it is well recognized that age, sex, genetic constitution, environmental exposure to pollutants, and concomitantly administered drugs modify the disposition and elimination of a particular drug.

Since the liver is a major organ for metabolism and excretion of a number of drugs, liver disease significantly modifies the disposition and elimination of many therapeutic agents. It is, therefore, important to have knowledge of the metabolic fate of drugs that are prescribed for patients with liver disease. In addition to alterations in pharmacokinetics by liver disease there is evidence, albeit limited, that patients with liver disease have increased cerebral sensitivity for centrally acting drugs. There are limited experimental and clinical data regarding the effect of liver disease on drug disposition in humans. In recent years, progress has been made in the understanding of the pharmacokinetic principles of disposition of agents principally eliminated by the liver and the effect of liver diseases on disposition and elimination of some drugs.

This chapter is divided into two parts. Part I outlines the pharmacokinetic principles of drug disposition and elimination with emphasis on the liver as the organ of excretion, the importance and meaning of such pharmacokinetic parameters, and the difficulties encountered with the design and interpretation of clinical studies. Part II summarizes the present state of knowledge of some important drugs used in the diagnosis and/or treatment of patients with liver dysfunction.

PART I

PHARMACOKINETIC CONSIDERATIONS IN LIVER DISEASE

Pharmacokinetics is the quantitative study of the absorption, distribution, and elimination of drugs. To quantify these processes various derived pharmacokinetic terms and concepts have arisen.

HALF-LIFE

Most drug dispositional studies quantify drug removal from the body in terms of a first-order elimination rate constant or its equivalent, elimination half-life ($t1/2_{\beta}$), as estimated from the terminal portion of the blood concentration–time profile for the drug

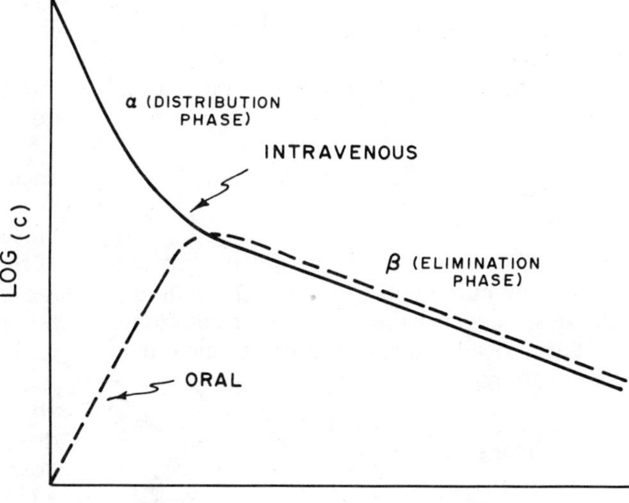

Figure 12–1. Blood (plasma) concentration/time profile after oral and intravenous administration of a drug.

(Fig. 12–1). There are considerable limitations to interpretation of half-life data *in vivo,* since the half-life is dependent on drug distribution and elimination. This dependency is described by the equation:

$$t1/2_{(\beta)} = \frac{V_d \times 0.694}{Cl_s} \qquad (1)$$

where V_d = volume into which the drug distributes and $C1_s$ = systemic clearance. Volume of distribution and systemic clearance are independent pharmacokinetic parameters and may separately influence the observed half-life. Thus, independent unidirectional changes in both could offset each other without altering the calculated half-life. This implies that the half-life *per se* is not a measure of the extraction capacity of the liver for the drug, and one requires knowledge of V_d, before the inverse relationship between $t1/2_{(\beta)}$ and Cl_s is assumed. Factors affecting half-life are shown in Table 12–1.

TABLE 12–1. POTENTIAL MECHANISMS INVOLVED IN PROLONGING THE ELIMINATION HALF-LIFE OF A DRUG ELIMINATED BY THE LIVER

Decreased hepatic blood flow and shunting through and around the liver
Decreased hepatic extraction
Reduced enzymatic activity
Altered uptake and/or binding to liver tissue
Increased binding to plasma,* i.e., restrictive versus nonrestrictive hepatic extraction (see text)
Increased volume of distribution
Decreased binding in plasma
Increased tissue binding (sequestration)

*Plasma drug binding is, however, generally unchanged or decreased in liver disease.

VOLUME OF DISTRIBUTION

Volume of distribution (V_d) refers to that volume into which the administered drug is distributed. The volume of distribution of a drug depends on the rate of drug elimination as well as the relative affinity for the drug binding in plasma and in the various tissue sites (i.e., lipid solubility). In general, drugs with high lipid solubility are extensively distributed (sequestered) in peripheral tissue depots (fat, bone) and tend to have a large V_d.[1] When drug elimination is visualized as a multicompartmental event, one can calculate the initial volume of distribution ($V_{d(\alpha)}$)(which is presumed to reflect drug equilibration during the initial rapid mixing of the drug in well-perfused tissue compartments) as well as drug distribution during the elimination phase, $V_{d(\beta)}$, and at steady state, $V_{d(ss)}$. A knowledge of these parameters indicates the extent to which the drug is distributed and how it would modify the value for a calculated elimination half-life.

CLEARANCE

A more useful approach would be the determination of total drug clearance from blood or plasma, since clearance is a measure of the efficiency with which a drug can be irreversibly removed from the body. Clearance does not depend on a particular compartmental model when calculated as:

$$Cl_s = \frac{FD}{AUC} \qquad (2)$$

where AUC = area under the plasma concentration/time curve and FD = the fraction of a drug dose reaching the systemic circulation.

Under steady-state conditions, clearance can be estimated as:

$$\text{Clearance} = \frac{I}{C_{B(ss)}} \qquad (3)$$

where I = infusion rate and $C_{B(ss)}$ = the steady-state drug concentration in blood. If individual organ blood flow is known and drug concentration in the arterial and venous systems (of the organ) can be estimated, then the individual organ clearance (liver for the purpose of this discussion) can be calculated as:

$$Cl_H = \frac{Q\,(C_a - C_v)}{C_a} = QE \qquad (4)$$

where Cl_H = hepatic clearance, Q = hepatic blood flow, C_a= arterial drug concentration, C_v = venous drug concentration, and E = the steady-state extraction ratio.

The sum of individual organ clearances will then equal total systemic clearance as:

$$Cl_s = Cl_H + Cl_{EH} \qquad (5)$$

where Cl_s = systemic clearance, Cl_H = hepatic clearance, and Cl_{EH} = extrahepatic clearance. For a drug solely eliminated by hepatic metabolism, plasma clearance would equal hepatic clearance. Despite the value of estimating alterations in systemic and hepatic drug clearance in the presence of liver disease as functions of overall drug metabolizing capacity, these determinations do not permit resolution of the relative contributions to this process of the controlling biologic factors — viz., hepatic blood flow, drug protein binding, etc.[2] The term *total intrinsic hepatic clearance,* $Cl_{(intrinsic)}$, has been used to indicate the maximum ability of the liver to irreversibly remove the drug by all pathways in the absence of any flow limitation.

$$Cl_H = QE = Q\,\frac{(Cl_{(intrinsic)})}{(Q + Cl_{(intrinsic)})} \qquad (6)$$

It then becomes apparent that hepatic clearance and extraction are influenced by two independent biologic factors: liver blood flow and $Cl_{(intrinsic)}$. A change in either will then affect plasma clearance and in turn the half-life of the drug.

LIVER BLOOD FLOW AND HEPATIC CLEARANCE

A number of physiologic and pathologic factors will influence liver blood flow; as hepatic flow increases, clearance of a drug will increase hyperbolically with an asymptote,

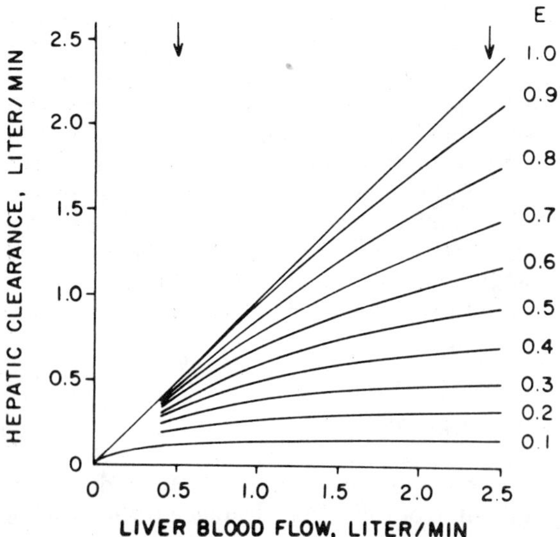

Figure 12–2. Effect of liver blood flow on hepatic clearance (E. = extraction ratio). (Reproduced with permission from Wilkinson, G. R., and Schand, D. G.: A physiological approach to hepatic drug clearance. Clin. Pharmacol. Ther. *18*:377–90, 1975.)

equivalent to $Cl_{(intrinsic)}$. Since there are physiologic limitations to the range of hepatic blood flow changes, the exact behavior of any drug will depend on the relative values of $Cl_{(intrinsic)}$ and liver flow (Fig. 12–2). Thus, when $Cl_{(intrinsic)}$ is very large compared to the flow, i.e., equivalent to an extraction ratio of > 0.8, the measured hepatic clearance does not reflect the activity of drug-metabolizing enzymes or other eliminating processes. The measured hepatic clearance does reflect the blood flow rate to the liver, and alterations in blood flow will produce proportional alterations in the measured clearance. The clearance of such drugs is, therefore, *flow-limited.* On the other hand, when hepatic blood flow is much greater than $Cl_{(intrinsic)}$, i.e., equivalent to an extraction ratio of < 0.2, clearance is approximately equal to this parameter and is essentially independent of flow. Clearance of such drugs is said to be *flow-independent* or *capacity-limited.* For intermediate extraction ratios, hepatic clearance is partly flow-dependent. Therefore, in *in vivo* studies of drug disposition and elimination, systemic clearance will estimate the efficiency of hepatic drug metabolizing enzymes only if the drug under consideration has a low extraction ratio of < 0.2 and its clearance is capacity-limited.

Patients with liver disease have varying degrees of abnormalities of portal circulation and total hepatic blood flow. Thus, in cirrhosis, the estimated total blood flow is reduced, while in viral hepatitis the hepatic blood flow is either normal or increased.[3] Patients with chronic liver disease may, in addition, have significant intra- or extrahepatic shunting of portal venous blood, possibly bypassing functional hepatocytes. Such shunting may have profound effects on orally administered drugs that would bypass the liver and reach high systemic concentrations. Thus, such changes in hepatic blood flow could significantly affect drug clearance and half-life, independent of any biochemical changes in hepatocyte function, and would either exaggerate or diminish the consequences of the functional impairment, depending on the direction of the flow change. Such changes would be most evident for drugs whose clearance is flow-dependent, e.g., lidocaine.[4]

INTRINSIC CLEARANCE

As mentioned earlier, hepatic clearance estimates the overall efficiency of the hepatic elimination process(es), which is dependent on several variables: (1) Rate of drug delivery, i.e., total hepatic blood flow (Q); (2) the extent of drug binding to blood constituents (usually expressed as the unbound [free] fraction of drug in plasma [f_B]; and (3) hepatic uptake from sinusoidal blood, intracellular transport and metabolism, and, in some instances, biliary secretion. This latter removal process is quantified as free intrinsic clearance ($Cl'_{(intrinsic)}$), which is the clearance of unbound drug from liver water.

If one assumes that the steady-state concentration of free drug in liver water is equal to the concentration of free drug in the hepatic vein ($f_B \bullet C_v$), then the rate of removal of free drug from water will be:

$$Cl'_{(intrinsic)} \times f_B C_v$$

The rate of removal is also given by:

$$Q\ (C_a - C_v)$$

Then:

$$Cl'_{(intrinsic)} \times f_B C_v = Q\ (C_a - C_v)$$

$$Cl_{(intrinsic)} = \frac{Q\ (C_a - C_v)}{f_B \times C_v}$$

Since:

$$\frac{C_a - C_v}{C_v} = E \qquad \text{from equation} \quad (4)$$

$$Cl'_{(intrinsic)} = \frac{QE}{f_B\ (1 - E)}$$

Therefore, rearranging:

$$E = \frac{f_B - Cl'_{(intrinsic)}}{Q + f_B Cl'_{(intrinsic)}}$$

Thus:

$$Cl_s = Cl_H = Q\ \frac{f_B Cl'_{(intrinsic)}}{Q + f_B Cl'_{(intrinsic)}} \qquad (7)$$

An advantage of the concept of intrinsic clearance is that it provides a way of relating changes in *in vivo* drug elimination to *in vitro* estimates of drug metabolism using Michaelis-Menton kinetics, whereby:

$$V = \frac{V_{max}\ S}{K_m + S} \qquad (8)$$

where V = initial velocity of the reaction at substrate concentration S, V_{max} = maximum velocity of reaction, and K_m is the Michaelis constant for the enzymatic reaction. When S $\ll K_m$, then the equation becomes:

$$V = \frac{V_{max}\,S}{K_m} \text{ or } \frac{V}{S} = \frac{V_{max}}{K_m}$$

as V/S is a measure of drug clearance from liver water, V_{max}/K_m is a measure of $Cl'_{(intrinsic)}$, provided the concentration of drug in liver water is much less than K_m.[5]

DRUG BINDING

Drugs circulate in the blood as the free moiety and as drug bound primarily to plasma proteins and other constituents of the blood. Binding of drugs to these substances and body tissues varies and depends on the chemical nature of the drug and its subsequent affinity to binding states. It is the free (unbound) drug that is available for distribution to the tissues which exerts pharmacologic effects and is metabolized prior to excretion. The process of drug binding to plasma proteins is a dynamic process whereby, as the free drug concentration falls secondary to metabolism and excretion, more free drug is released from binding sites to maintain a steady state between bound and unbound drug until the drug is completely eliminated from the body. Two types of drug binding to plasma constituents can be identified: (1) *Restrictive binding,* wherein only the circulating free drug is removed during its passage through the liver. In this situation, the extraction ratio, E, is less than or equal to the unbound fraction of drug in plasma, f_B. Hence, changes in drug binding will affect the elimination of such drugs, in addition to other factors that may affect drug disposition. (2) *Nonrestrictive binding,* wherein removal of both free (unbound) and bound drug occurs during its passage through the liver. In this situation, E $> f_B$. Changes in nonrestrictive drug binding will play an insignificant role in overall changes of drug disposition and elimination for this group of drugs.

To extend this concept of drug binding and its role in drug elimination, drugs may be classified according to elimination-extraction properties as shown in the following outline.[3]

I. Flow-dependent
II. Flow-independent (capacity-limited)
   A. Binding insensitive (nonrestrictive)
   B. Binding sensitive (restrictive)

The importance of this concept relates to drugs that are capacity-limited, binding sensitive (restrictive-binding). With such drugs, a decrease in binding (as may occur in liver disease) will increase the systemic clearance of the drug and, in addition, increase the amount of free drug available for pharmacologic action at the receptor sites in the effector organ(s). Such a change in binding, if not reflective of a further deterioration of hepatic function, may offset a fall in clearance secondary to hepatic disease.

DRUG ABSORPTION

After intravenous administration, all of the drug reaches the systemic circulation and estimation of elimination half-life, volumes of distribution, and clearance can be obtained by sequential measurement of circulating drug concentrations.

Since:

$$Cl_s = \frac{FD}{AUC} \qquad (2)$$

After intravenous administration:

$$Cl_s = \frac{D_{iv}}{AUC_{iv}}$$

where D_{iv} = the administered dose and AUC_{iv} = total area under the plasma concentration/-time curve after intravenous (IV) drug administration.

However, after oral administration, the amount of drug reaching the circulation will depend on the adequacy of the absorptive process under the experimental or disease conditions and on the first-pass extraction by the liver, since the drug has to pass through the liver prior to reaching the systemic circulation. This latter consideration is particularly relevant to high-clearance or flow-dependent drugs, since a large proportion of the drug would be extracted (metabolized) prior to reaching the systemic circulation; conversely, portal systemic shunting would enable the drug to bypass the liver leading to higher circulating drug concentrations.

In spite of these limitations, it has recently been demonstrated that after oral administration, providing that absorption is complete and all of the absorbed drug passes through the liver prior to reaching the systemic circulation, then[6]:

$$\frac{D_0}{AUC_0} = Cl_{(intrinsic)} + \frac{Cl_{EH}}{1 - E} \qquad (9)$$

where D_0 = fraction of the absorbed dose reaching the circulation and AUC_0 = the total area under the blood concentration–time curve after oral administration. If the drugs under question are essentially totally metabolized by the liver and there is little extrahepatic extraction, it follows that AUC_0 is a good indicator of hepatic metabolizing capacity, and estimation of systemic clearance after oral administration of such agents would be a reasonable indicator of hepatic clearance.

Since the various dispositional parameters are closely interrelated, it is important to have a fundamental knowledge of pharmacokinetics to understand the effects of various disease states on these parameters and the overall effect these changes would have on the disposition and elimination of drugs in the appropriate clinical setting. In spite of certain limitations, meaningful information can be obtained by conducting dispositional studies, and these can provide insight into the mechanisms of the changes observed. The problems in study design of drug disposition and elimination in patients with liver disease are briefly considered next.

PROBLEMS OF STUDY DESIGN AND INTERPRETATION

Human liver disease is an heterogeneous group of disease processes involving inflammatory, degenerative, and neoplastic changes of hepatic and biliary tissue, accompanied at times by alterations in hepatic blood flow. Most of these abnormalities are unique to the human; for example, adequate animal models of human cirrhosis and viral hepatitis are not available or are difficult to establish. As a result, dispositional studies are usually limited to patients, with the attendant clinical and ethical constraints.

Thus, a wide variety of diverse disease processes in various stages of evolution are examined when a group of patients with acute and/or chronic liver disease is studied. In such drug dispositional studies, it is important to subclassify adequately the patient population, as exemplified by studies with antipyrine.[7] There is a significant increase in the mean serum half-life of the drug in patients with liver disease generally, as compared to a normal control group (Fig. 12–3). Subclassification of patients according to their clinical diagnosis demonstrates, however, that pa-

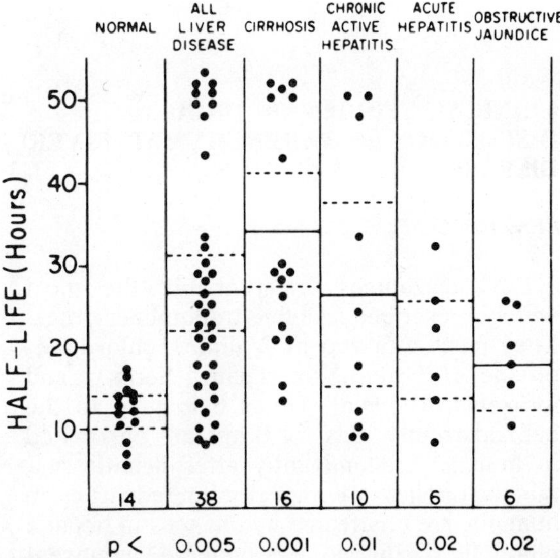

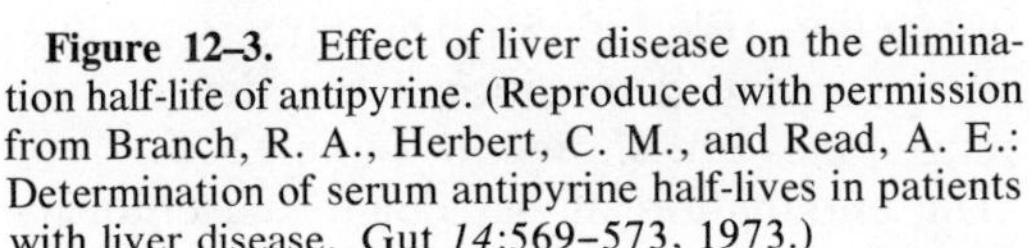
Figure 12–3. Effect of liver disease on the elimination half-life of antipyrine. (Reproduced with permission from Branch, R. A., Herbert, C. M., and Read, A. E.: Determination of serum antipyrine half-lives in patients with liver disease. Gut *14*:569–573, 1973.)

tients with obstructive jaundice and acute hepatitis have a much lesser degree of impairment than those with cirrhosis and chronic active hepatitis.[7] Many reported studies have neglected to provide such information, which is necessary to adequately relate changes to the type and severity of the disease state.

Similarly, patients under investigation are frequently receiving other drug therapy in addition to the drug under study. The influence of one drug on the disposition and elimination of another is well established; such interactions may modify the effect of liver disease *per se*. In the study by Levi et al.,[8] there was no significant difference in the mean half-life of phenylbutazone when a large group of patients with liver disease on drug therapy was compared to normal volunteers similarly tested. However, the half-life was significantly prolonged in the group of patients with hepatic damage not receiving other drugs as compared to controls (Fig. 12–4).

It is now well established that age and sex are also determinants of drug elimination and it is important that the patient group be compared to the appropriate age- and sex-matched control group.

In summary, it is vital to select a patient population that is as closely matched to controls as is possible. Alternatively, a carefully planned longitudinal study in a small group of patients throughout the evolution of the disease may be more informative than a large number of isolated observations in a heterogenous group of patients.

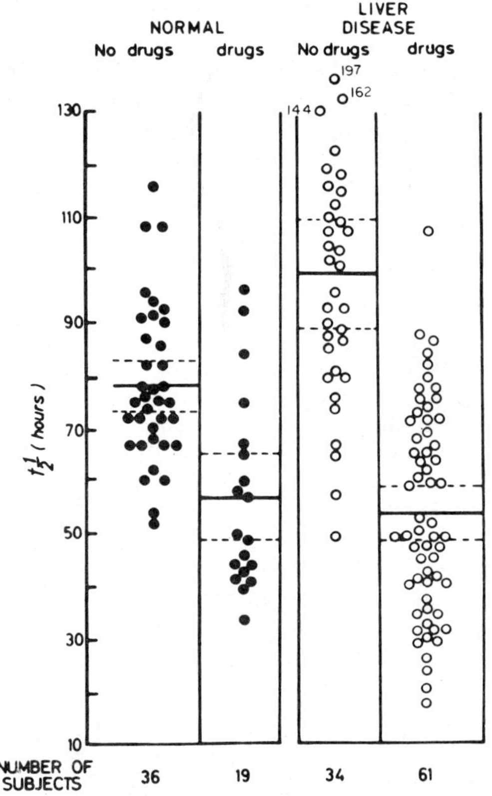

Figure 12–4. Effect of liver disease and concomitant drug therapy on the elimination half-life of phenylbutazone. (Reproduced with permission from Levi, A. J., Sherlock, S., and Walker, D.: Phenylbutazone and isoniazid metabolism in patients with liver disease in relation to previous drug therapy. Lancet 1:1275–1279, 1968.)

PART II

CLINICAL STUDIES OF DRUG DISPOSITION IN PARENCHYMAL LIVER DISEASE

BENZODIAZEPINES

Benzodiazepines are probably the most widely prescribed sedative-tranquilizer drugs. They include diazepam (Valium), chlordiazepoxide (Librium), oxazepam (Serax), and lorazepam (Ativan). Drugs belonging to the benzodiazepine class of drugs are eliminated in humans predominantly after hepatic metabolism. They are capacity-limited drugs in humans, are unaffected by changes in hepatic blood flow, and do not undergo significant first-pass extraction after oral administration. The metabolic pathways are interconnected and, for some drugs, there is generation of various metabolites that are pharmacologically active (Fig. 12–5). The effects of liver disease on the dispositional kinetics of benzodiazepines are shown in Table 12–2.

The elimination of diazepam and chlordiazepoxide is impaired by liver disease, while, in contrast, the removal from plasma of oxazepam and lorazepam is essentially unaffected. Inasmuch as the first two drugs are eliminated after oxidative metabolism while the latter two drugs are eliminated after conjugation as the glucuronide, this indicates that glucuronidating pathways of biotransforma-

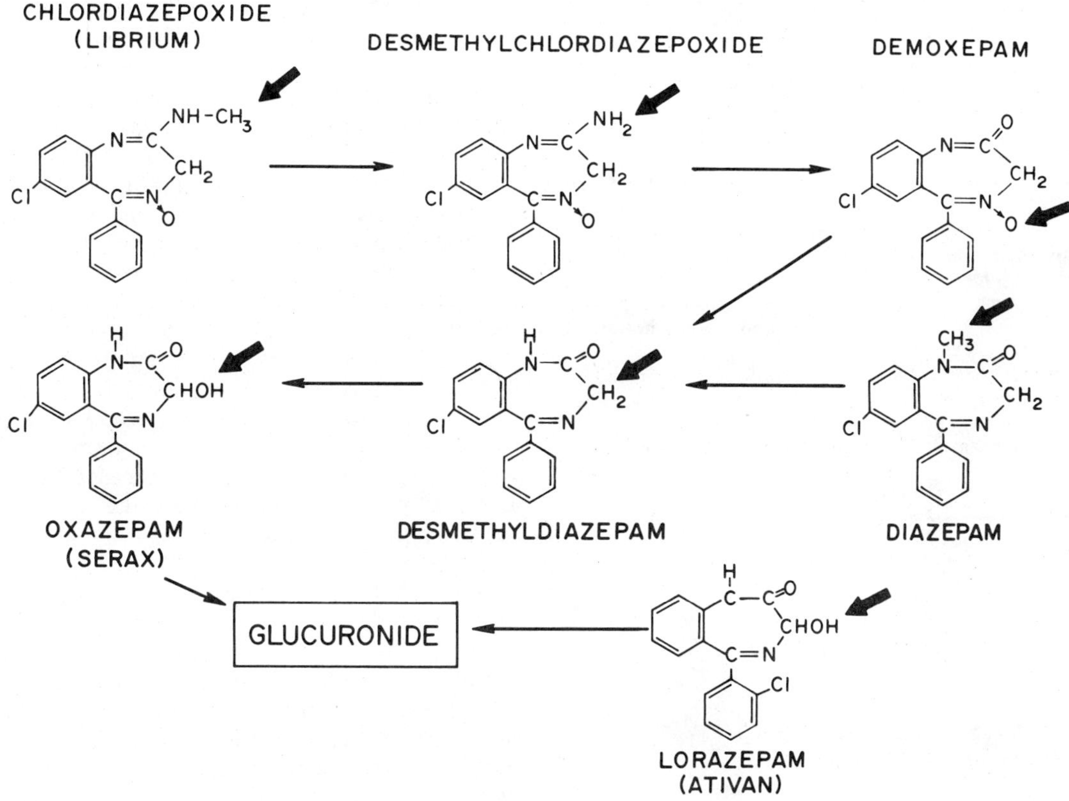

Figure 12–5. Metabolic pathway of commonly used benzodiazepines. (Broad arrows indicate sites of biotransformation.)

tion are resistant to acute and chronic liver disease and are relatively spared. This observation could be put to advantage when prolonged sedative therapy is required for patients with liver disease.

BARBITURATES AND OTHER SEDATIVE/TRANQUILIZERS

Until the appearance of the benzodiazepines, barbiturates were the commonest drugs used for their sedative, hypnotic, and antiepileptic properties. The duration of action of barbiturates is determined by the rate of hepatic elimination, with the longer-acting barbiturates being dependent predominantly on renal excretion. Intuitively, it was thought that elimination of long-acting barbiturates would be relatively unaffected by hepatic disease, since their elimination would be dependent on renal function. Studies with barbiturates in liver disease confirm this concept. The available data on the effects of liver disease on

TABLE 12–2. EFFECT OF LIVER DISEASE ON DISPOSITION AND ELIMINATION OF BENZODIAZEPINES

	Cirrhosis				Acute Viral Hepatitis			
	$t\frac{1}{2}_{\beta}$	Vd_{β}	*Cl's*	*Binding*	$t\frac{1}{2}_{\beta}$	Vd_{β}	*Cl's*	*Binding*
Diazepam[9]	↑	↑	↓*	↓	↑	↑	↓*	↓
Chlordiazepoxide[10]	↑	↑	↓*	↓	↑	↑	↓*	↓
Oxazepam[11]	0	0	0	0	0	0	0	0
Lorazepam[12]	↑	↑	0	↓	0	0	0	↓

↑ = Increase; ↓ = decrease; 0 = no change; * = delayed appearance and elimination of desmethylmetabolite.

TABLE 12–3. EFFECT OF LIVER DISEASE ON THE DISPOSITION OF BARBITURATES AND OTHER SEDATIVE/TRANQUILIZERS

DRUGS	EFFECTS
Hexobarbitone	Decreased clearance in cirrhosis and acute viral hepatitis. Reduced renal excretion of 3-keto hexobarbitone.[13]
Amylobarbitone Pentobarbitone	Impaired elimination in liver disease.[14-16]
Thiopentone	Increased cerebral sensitivity.[16] Data on V_d, $t^1/_{2\beta}$, and binding not available.
Phenobarbitone	Increase in half-life with cirrhosis.[17]
Meprobamate	Half-life prolonged in chronic liver disease.[14]
Chlorpromazine	No change with liver disease.[18] Plasma clearance greater in liver disease after reanalysis of data.[19]

barbiturates and other sedatives and tranquilizers are summarized in Table 12–3.

NARCOTICS, ANALGESICS, AND ANTI-INFLAMMATORY AGENTS

There is limited information regarding the effects of liver disease on the disposition and elimination of narcotics, analgesics, and anti-inflammatory agents. Although morphine, codeine, and methadone undergo hepatic metabolism, and increased cerebral sensitivity to morphine has been demonstrated in liver disease,[20] there are no detailed pharmacokinetic studies of these drugs in patients with liver disease. However, it has been shown that the elimination half-life of meperidine is prolonged in patients with viral hepatitis[21] and cirrhosis.[22] This was due to a fall in plasma clearance without changes in plasma drug binding and drug distribution. After recovery from viral hepatitis the dispositional parameters returned to normal. Among the nonnarcotic analgesic and anti-inflammatory drugs, aspirin disposition is unaffected by liver disease,[23] while the elimination of phenylbutazone,[8] acetanilide,[24] and acetaminophen[25] has been reported to be impaired.

Prednisone is being used with increasing frequency for the therapy of chronic hepatitis. The conversion of prednisone to its biologically active metabolite, prednisolone, is necessary for the pharmacologic effects of this steroid. In a detailed pharmacokinetic study, Schalm et al.[26] showed that serum prednisolone levels were significantly lower in patients with impaired liver function than in controls, but there was a greater percentage of pharmacologically active, unbound drug present in serum under such circumstances. In addition, the impairment of hepatic A ring reduction resulted in decreased elimination of the active metabolite.[27] Thus, impaired conversion of prednisone to prednisolone in severe liver disease may be compensated for by a decreased rate of elimination of the active metabolite, prednisolone, and by decreased protein binding leading to a higher level of unbound active drug in plasma. The higher unbound active drug level correlated well with decreased serum albumin. The increase in unbound prednisolone with decreased serum albumin may in part explain the reported increase in side effects of steroids in such patients. In a recent study, Madsbad et al.[28] indicate that mean serum prednisolone after oral prednisolone was independent of liver function, with better steady-state levels of prednisolone. Thus, though overall effects of liver disease on prednisone disposition may not affect the therapeutic effect of this drug, most authors accept that it is probably best to administer prednisolone rather than prednisone to patients with severe liver disease.

ANTIBIOTICS

Patients with cirrhosis are prone to repeated and often life-threatening infections and are subject to repeated therapy with numerous antibiotics. The use of antibiotics for treating infections is dictated by the sensitivity of the organisms to the therapeutic agent and knowledge of the effect of liver disease on the disposition of these drugs so that dosage schedules can be adjusted in order to avoid toxicity. The available data on the effect of liver disease on the disposition and elimination of antibiotics are summarized in Table 12–4. Since most antibiotics are eliminated by the kidneys essentially unchanged, modifications in dosage would be required in relatively few instances, as indicated in Table 12–4.

METHYLXANTHINES

Theophylline, caffeine, and theobromine are related methylated xanthines that share common pathways of hepatic drug elimination. Caffeine and theobromine are ingested in

TABLE 12-4. EFFECT OF LIVER DISEASE ON DISPOSITION AND ELIMINATION OF ANTIBIOTICS

Drugs	Effects
Penicillin G	Excretion primarily (~ 70%) renal.
Carbenicillin Methicillin Ampicillin	Severe liver disease prolongs $t^{1}/_{2\beta}$ of carbenicillin. Methicillin and Ampicillin unaffected by liver disease.[29]
Clindamycin	Impaired elimination in liver disease.[30]
Nafcillin	Predominant hepatic excretion. Cirrhosis and extrahepatic obstruction prolong $t^{1}/_{2\beta}$ and reduce plasma clearance.[31]
Chloramphenicol	Essentially normal disposition in liver disease; however, concomitant renal disease causes mild impairment in elimination.[32] Normal recovery of conjugate in urine of cirrhotic patients.[33]

large amounts in various drugs and in carbonated and noncarbonated beverages, while theophylline is the mainstay of therapy of acute and chronic pulmonary disease. Theophylline has a narrow therapeutic index and its elimination is reduced in infants,[34] with advancing age,[35] and by liver disease.[36] Nomograms are available[37] for the use of theophylline with respect to age and further modifications are required when theophylline is used in patients with liver disease. Blood drug levels during therapy should be monitored frequently to tailor the dosage schedule to the individual patient. Similarly, the elimination half-life of caffeine is significantly prolonged and the plasma clearance of bound and unbound caffeine is significantly reduced during pregnancy,[38] by oral contraceptive steroids,[39] and in patients with cirrhosis.[40] The metabolic or pharmacodynamic implications of this impaired caffeine elimination are not known at present.

CLINICAL CONSIDERATIONS IN THE USE OF DRUGS IN LIVER DISEASE

ACUTE VERSUS CHRONIC USE

Pharmacokinetic studies of drug disposition are usually conducted after a single intravenous dose and by following the circulating plasma–blood drug concentration/time profile over a sufficient time period. Usually, circulating drug concentrations are followed for at least three to five half-lives to obtain sufficient points on the drug elimination phase. Such data obtained after single-dose studies can be extrapolated to chronic drug administration by applying the pharmacokinetic concepts outlined earlier.

The rate of accumulation of a drug during chronic therapy depends on the elimination half-life. A longer half-life implies rapid drug accumulation. The plasma clearance dictates the steady-state drug concentration, with lower clearance giving a higher steady-state drug concentration. Patients with liver disease may, therefore, tend to accumulate some drugs more rapidly and achieve a higher circulating steady-state drug concentration. Such patients may be at a risk of exaggerated pharmacologic effects from routine doses of drugs. In some instances, as in the case of diazepam[9] and chlordiazepoxide,[10] metabolism of drugs leads to generation of pharmacologically active metabolites. Klotz et al. have shown that the elimination of desmethyldiazepam is depressed in chronic liver disease.[41] Thus, it is conceivable that accumulation of pharmacologically active metabolites may have pharmacologically additive effects. Though ideally dispositional studies should be performed during chronic dosing, meaningful information can be obtained from single-dose studies that are technically easier to perform.

ORAL VERSUS INTRAVENOUS ADMINISTRATION

As indicated earlier in the chapter, after oral administration the drug has to pass through the liver prior to reaching the systemic circulation. The extraction of drug by the liver during this passage through the liver is referred to as the first-pass effect, which is significant for flow-dependent (high-clearance) drugs. When such drugs are used orally, allowance is made for this first-pass extraction when dosage schedules are evolved. Occasionally, this first-pass extraction is so efficient that oral medication is virtually ineffective to obtain a pharmacologic response, e.g., morphine. Shunting of blood away from the liver as would occur by portal systemic shunting or by perfusion of nonfunctioning hepatocytes would lead to higher drug concentrations after oral drug administration. This could be a problem when treating patients with cirrhosis, especially after surgical shunting. Dosage adjustments may be necessary to avoid drug toxicity.

PHARMACODYNAMIC CONSIDERATIONS

The pharmacologic response(s) obtained after drug administration is referred to as the pharmacodynamics of the drug. This is dependent on the amount of free (unbound) concentration of the drug in circulation that is available for interaction with receptor sites in the effector organ. The effect of centrally acting drugs on cerebral receptor sites is especially important in patients with liver dysfunction, who are prone to altered cerebral function. The syndrome of altered cerebral function in the presence of acute or chronic liver disease has been referred to as hepatic encephalopathy. Various factors, such as ammonia, fatty acids, false neurotransmitters, and mercaptans, have been implicated in this metabolic encephalopathy. The precise mechanism for this metabolic encephalopathy has not been elucidated; however, the current belief is that a combination of the effects of various factors is probably responsible for altered cerebral function.[42]

In recent years, receptors have been identified in brain tissues of animals with high-affinity binding characteristics for benzodiazepines[43] and opiates[44] in addition to those for the naturally occurring neurotransmitters, i.e., gamma aminobutyric acid, acetylcholine, etc.[45, 46] It is conceivable that such cerebral receptors are altered in some way in patients with chronic liver disease prone to encephalopathy.

A clinical impression has existed for many years that patients with liver dysfunction have an altered sensitivity for drugs such as morphine and other sedatives. At the time of this writing, this hypothesis has not been substantiated with adequately designed studies or sufficient data. Quantification of cerebral function in response to centrally acting drugs is difficult. Conventionally, EEG changes have been used to quantify cerebral response to drugs. Laidlaw et al. were able to show that changes in derived EEG parameters (mean dominant frequency response to stimuli) following morphine administration were more prominent in patients with cirrhosis with a prior history of encephalopathy as compared to normal subjects and patients with cirrhosis without prior history of encephalopathy.[20] Similar findings were observed by Read et al. after small doses of chlorpromazine.[47] Interestingly, in this study, it was observed that while chlorpromazine had no effect on blood ammonia levels, clearance of an ammonia load was decreased when chlorpromazine was administered concomitantly. Tranylcypromine, a monoamine oxidase inhibitor, caused deterioration in the EEG while amitriptyline produced little change.[48] Two studies with diazepam have shown conflicting results. Murray-Lyon et al.[49] were unable to show an increased sensitivity to 5 mg of diazepam IV in patients with a history of prior encephalopathy, while Branch et al.[50] showed that patients with chronic liver disease required a significantly smaller dose of diazepam IV to achieve a predetermined end point of sedation as compared to control subjects. Also, in the latter study, EEG changes in patients with cirrhosis correlated with the degree of abnormality of baseline EEG and the level of serum albumin (lower albumin correlated with greater EEG change), and all EEG changes returned to baseline after 1 hour.

These investigations support the clinical impression of altered cerebral sensitivity, but more studies are required, using more quantitative EEG assessment and psychometric tests of cerebral function. Table 12–5 summarizes the potential mechanisms for altered cerebral sensitivity to centrally acting drugs. It is clear that there are multifactorial causes for altered cerebral sensitivity in patients with chronic liver disease, and much work is required in this field to elucidate the basic mechanisms involved.

TABLE 12–5. POTENTIAL MECHANISMS FOR ALTERED CEREBRAL SENSITIVITY IN PATIENTS WITH LIVER DISEASE

Decreased plasma drug binding (↑ unbound drug fraction in circulation)
Altered permeability of blood-brain barrier
Receptor interaction with sedatives and other exogenous substances Increased receptor sensitivity Competition for receptor binding between endogenous ligands and exogenous substances Alteration in endogenous ligands
Preexisting subclinical encephalopathy by circulating "toxins."

↑ = Increase.

CONCOMITANT DRUG THERAPY

Concomitant drug therapy can alter disposition and elimination of other therapeutic agents by a variety of mechanisms, and the net effect may cause either delayed or enhanced drug elimination. These effects of drug-drug interactions are independent of liver disease *per se*. The mechanism by which drug-drug interactions modify drug elimination are summarized in Table 12–6. In healthy individuals, chronic use of barbiturates, anticonvulsants, and glutethimide induces the hepatic microsomal mixed function oxidases and may accelerate the elimination of other coadministered drugs by these enzyme systems. Such an induction and acceleration of drug elimination has been observed in patients with liver disease,[8] and, as shown earlier, can complicate the interpretation of drug dispositional studies. Halogenated hydrocarbons inhaled in cigarette smoke have been shown to induce drug metabolism; however, their induction spectrum is narrower than that of the drugs mentioned. In contrast, drugs like disulfiram[51] and, more recently, cimetidine have been shown to inhibit some hepatic microsomal enzymes[52] and variably affect drug elimination in healthy subjects.[53, 54] Acute alcohol ingestion inhibits drug elimination, while chronic alcohol ingestion has been shown to induce drug metabolizing enzymes.[55] Thus, concomitant drug therapy modifies drug elimination in both normal subjects and in patients with liver disease. The potential for such drug-drug interaction should be kept in mind when multiple drugs are administered to patients with chronic liver disease.

TABLE 12-6. MECHANISMS BY WHICH CONCOMITANT DRUG THERAPY MODIFIES DRUG ELIMINATION

Alterations in absorption and distribution
Alterations in elimination
Induction of hepatic drug metabolizing enzymes
Inhibition of hepatic drug metabolizing enzymes
Competitive
Nonspecific (generalized)
Hepatotoxicity (parenchymal damage)
Nephrotoxicity (alteration in renal excretion of parent drug and metabolic degradation products)

CHOLESTASIS

In contrast to the many investigations of drug disposition in patients with parenchymal liver disease, there is little information available on the effects of hepatic cholestasis of either intra- or extrahepatic etiology on drug disposition. The mean half-life of antipyrine was significantly prolonged in six patients with obstructive jaundice[7]; however, the increase was modest. Patients with gallstones did not differ from control subjects and cholecystectomy did not influence antipyrine half-life.[56] Cholestasis theorectically would be expected to inhibit hepatic drug metabolism owing to the inhibitory action of bile acids, as has been demonstrated in the jaundiced rabbit.[57] However, obstructive jaundice is frequently associated with an increase in the hepatic smooth endoplasmic reticulum; it is possible that this, and the implied enhancement of drug metabolizing enzyme activity, largely offset any inhibitory action. In the absence of concomitant parenchymal liver disease, obstruction of biliary flow is usually a transient problem in clinical practice, and, therefore, does not require modification of drug therapy. However, more studies in this area are needed, particularly with drugs that are removed extensively from the body by biliary secretion.

HEPATIC MALIGNANCY

Primary and secondary (metastatic) liver cancer imply a grave prognosis, although newer radiographic and surgical techniques and cancer chemotherapy may have resulted in improved survival of patients with some hepatic tumors. Studies in laboratory animals with hepatoma indicate that drug metabolism occurs mainly in the healthy liver parenchyma and drug hydroxylation is negligible in the malignant tissue.[58] The effect of liver cancer on drug metabolism would appear to depend, therefore, on the volume of tumor-bearing tissue and accompanying hepatic parenchymal disease. Several endogenous peptides and/or hormones have been shown to alter variably drug metabolism[59]; production of such substances by hepatic and extrahepatic tumors could also alter drug disposition and elimination. Hepner and Vesell[60] and Sotaniemi et al.[61] have demonstrated marked variability in the metabolism of various drugs by patients with liver cancer. The important determinant, therefore, of drug metabolism in liver cancer is the functional reserve of normal hepatic parenchyma. In the absence of a reliable liver "function" test this functional reserve cannot be quantitated, and drug concentration should be monitored while treating patients with liver cancer, especially with those drugs with a narrow therapeutic index.

PREDICTIVE TESTS FOR HEPATIC FUNCTIONAL RESERVE

A prior knowledge of the clearance of each drug in the individual patient would be useful information for the clinician prescribing the drug. However, since this information is impossible to obtain in patients with liver disease, a practical alternative is needed. Unlike the creatinine clearance, which closely predicts renal functional reserve for most clinical situations, there is no single test readily available to predict hepatic functional reserve. Various laboratory tests have been conventionally called liver function tests, but none of these tests is a true measure of hepatic function. Liver disease is detected by abnormalities of all or some of the following tests: SGOT (serum glutamic-oxaloacetic transaminase), SGPT (serum glutamic-pyruvic transaminase), total bilirubin, gamma-glutamyl transpeptidase, albumin, BSP (Bromsulphalein) retention, and prothrombin time. Among these only serum albumin, serum bilirubin, BSP retention, and prothrombin time reflect hepatic function, but extrahepatic factors can also alter these tests. Correlations have been observed between serum albumin and/or prothrombin time and disposition of some drugs,[25] while no concordance could be obtained for other drugs.[9, 10]

Owing to the inadequacy of biochemical tests in assessment of hepatic function, clearance of model or marker drugs has been used to quantify hepatic functional reserve. Table 12–7 summarizes the data in such studies. The observations of studies on the clearance of these marker drugs suggest that (1) clearance of both high- and low-clearance drugs is mainly dependent on changes in intrinsic clearance and (2) changes in intrinsic clearance parallel the severity of the underlying liver disease. However, there are certain limitations to the applicability of such clearance measurements: (1) the present methods for determining intrinsic clearance do not account for intra- or extrahepatic shunting of blood through and around the liver, (2) results obtained cannot predict the rate of elimination of one drug from that of another in individual patients with liver disease, and (3) the present methods do not appear to be sensitive and specific enough for general applicability in clinical practice.

In more recent years, breath tests in man, using ^{14}C-aminopyrine,[64] ^{14}C-phenacetin,[65] ^{14}C-diazepam,[66] and ^{14}C-galactose or ^{13}C-galactose[67] are another attempt to quantitate hepatic function. Details of principles and methodology have been outlined elsewhere.[64] In brief, a substance labeled with ^{14}C, which is converted primarily in the liver to $^{14}CO_2$ as one metabolic product, is given orally or parenterally. The $^{14}CO_2$ exhaled in the breath is collected over a timed interval into an alkaline medium, such as a $^{14}CO_2$ trap. From the specific activity of the exhaled $^{14}CO_2$ over a given time interval one can semiquantitatively determine $^{14}CO_2$ output, and, therefore, the metabolism of a given labeled agent by the liver. The elimination profiles of unlabeled substrate from plasma after administration correlate well with the profile of $^{14}CO_2$ genera-

TABLE 12–7. MODEL OR MARKER DRUGS USED TO ESTIMATE HEPATIC FUNCTIONAL CAPACITY

COMPOUND	DISPOSTIONAL CHARACTERISTICS	RESULTS OBTAINED
Antipyrine[7]	Binding insensitive, reflects clearance from liver water. Flow-independent	Half-life prolonged in liver disease. Half-life normalized before that of SGOT, SGPT, and bilirubin.
Lignocaine[62]	High clearance, flow-limited	Did not reflect disease activity in acute viral hepatitis.
Indocyanine green[62]	High clearance, flow-limited	Reflected disease activity. Correlated with D-propranolol and antipyrine clearance.
D-Propranolol[63]	High clearance, flow-limited	Clearance decreased in both cirrhosis and hepatic fibrosis. Decreased clearance due to fall in intrinsic clearance. Correlated with albumin and prothrombin time.

tion after administration of labeled substrate. Thus, calculating the peak $^{14}CO_2$ production and elimination half-life of $^{14}CO_2$ gives a good measure of substrate metabolism and clearance, and, therefore, the hepatic metabolic capacity. The largest experience to date has been with the ^{14}C-aminopyrine breath test. In summary, the ^{14}C-aminopyrine breath test was positive in 72 per cent of patients with hepatic malignancy, as compared to 36 per cent positive liver scans. Though both tests were falsely negative with equal frequency, both tests were never false positive.[68] In one study,[69] the ^{14}C-aminopyrine breath test was as valuable as the SGOT in patients with parenchymal liver disease, while in another study,[70] the aminopyrine breath test correlated only with the one-stage prothrombin time among all conventional laboratory tests. The breath test in this study was more sensitive than SGOT. Studies conducted to establish the selectivity of the ^{14}C-aminopyrine breath test demonstrate that the ^{14}C-aminopyrine breath test does not discriminate between patients with cirrhosis, viral hepatitis, and hepatic malignancy. The ^{14}C-aminopyrine breath test correlates with BSP retention, galactose elimination, prothrombin time, and serum albumin,[60, 70] and in preliminary studies have been reported to predict the degree of hepatic damage better than conventional tests in patients with chronic viral hepatitis.[71] The other breath tests mentioned also differentiate between normal subjects and patients with chronic liver disease, but further evaluation is needed to determine their specificity, sensitivity, selectivity, and prognostic value.

Though considerable advance has been made in the last decade to develop a sensitive and predictable test of hepatic functional reserve, no one test has emerged that satisfies all the criteria for a function test. Further studies are required to validate these new tests and to develop newer probes of hepatic function.

SUMMARY AND CONCLUSIONS

The better understanding of the interrelationships of the independent biologic factors controlling and modifying drug disposition has provided some insights into the complex effects that human liver disease may have on these processes. It is now recognizable that liver dysfunction *a priori* does not lead to equal alterations in the hepatic handling of all drugs and that changes in other dispositional processes may occur. It appears that oxidative drug metabolism is affected to a greater degree in liver disease as compared to glucuronidating pathways of drug biotransformation. In spite of advances in development of tests to quantify hepatic functional reserve, the information necessary to predict quantitation of impairment in drug elimination is not yet available. The best advice to the clinician, at present, is to administer drugs carefully to patients with liver disease, especially drugs with a narrow therapeutic index and sedative-hypnotic agents. Careful titration of the dose to the observed and desired clinical response should be carried out. Whenever possible, serum levels of drugs with a low therapeutic index should be obtained. With further investigations in drug dispositional studies, more definitive guidelines for drug therapy in patients with liver disease are likely to become available.

REFERENCES

1. Blaschke, TF: Protein binding and kinetics of drugs in liver disease. Clin. Pharmacokinet. *2*:32–44, 1977.
2. Wilkinson, GR, Schenker, S: Drug disposition and liver disease. Drug Metab. Rev. *4*:139–175, 1975.
3. Preisig, R, Rankin, JG, Sweeting, J, Bradley, SE: Hepatic hemodynamics during viral hepatitis in man. Circulation *34*:188–197, 1966.
4. Thompson, PD, Melmon, KL, Richardson, JA, Cohn, K, Steinbrunn, W, Cudihee, R, Rowland, M: Lidocaine pharmacokinetics in advanced heart failure, liver disease and renal failure in humans. Ann. Intern. Med. *78*:499–508, 1973.
5. Winkler, K, Keiding, S, Tygstroup, N: Clearance as a quantitative measure of liver function. *In* The Liver: Quantitative Aspects of Stricture and Function (G Baumgartner and R Presig, eds.). Basel: Karger, pp. 144–155, 1973.
6. Wilkinson, GR, Schand, DG: A physiological approach to hepatic drug clearance. Clin. Pharmacol. Ther. *18*:377–390, 1975.
7. Branch, RA, Herbert, CM, Read, AE: Determination of serum antipyrine half-lives in patients with liver disease. Gut *14*:569–573, 1973.
8. Levi, AJ, Sherlock, S, Walker, D: Phenylbutazone and isoniazid metabolism in patients with liver disease in relation to previous drug therapy. Lancet *1*:1275–1279, 1968.
9. Klotz, U, Avant, GR, Hoyumpa, A, Schenker, S, Wilkinson, GR: The effects of age and liver disease on the disposition and elimination of diazepam in adult man. J. Clin. Invest. *55*:347–359, 1975.
10. Roberts, RK, Wilkinson, GR, Branch, RA, Schenker, S: The effect of age and parenchymal liver disease on the disposition and elimination of chlordiazepoxide (Librium®). Gastroenterology *75*: 479–485, 1979.

11. Shull, HJ, Wilkinson, GR, Johnson, R, Schenker, S: Normal disposition of oxazepam in acute viral hepatitis and cirrhosis. Ann. Intern. Med. *84*:420–425, 1976.
12. Krauss, JW, Desmond, PV, Marshall, JP, Johnson, RF, Schenker, S, Wilkinson, GR: The effects of aging and liver disease on the disposition of lorazepam in man. Clin. Pharmacol. Ther. *24*:411–419, 1978.
13. Breimer, DD: Pharmacokinetics of Hypnotic Drugs. Nijmegen, Netherlands: Drukkerij-Virgeverij Brakkenstein, 1974, pp. 291–307.
14. Held, HV, Olderhausen, HF, Remnier, H: Der abban von pentobarbitae bei leberschaden. Klin. Wochenschr. *48*:565–567, 1970.
15. Mawer, GE, Miller, NE, Turuberg, LA: Metabolism of amylobarbitone in patients with chronic liver disease. Br. J. Pharmacol. *44*:549–560, 1972.
16. Shideman, FE, Kelly, AR, Lee, LE, Lowell, VF, Adams, BJ: Role of the liver in detoxification of thiopental (Pentothal) in man. Anesthesiology *10*:421–428, 1949.
17. Alvin, J, McHorse, T, Hoyumpa, A, Bush, MT, Schenker, S: The effect of liver disease in man on the disposition of phenobarbital. J. Pharmacol. Exper. Ther. *192*:224–235, 1975.
18. Maxwell, GE, Carella, M, Parkes, JD, Williams, R, Mould, GP, Curry, SH: Plasma disappearance and clinical effects of chlorpromazine in cirrhosis. Clin. Sci. *43*:143–151, 1972.
19. Roberts, RK, Branch, RA, Desmond, PV, Schenker, S: The influence of liver disease on drug disposition. Clin. Gastroenterol. *8*:105–121, 1979.
20. Laidlaw, J, Read, AE, Sherlock, S: Morphine tolerance in hepatic cirrhosis. Gastroenterology *40*:380–396, 1961.
21. McHorse, TS, Wilkinson, GR, Johnson, RF, Schenker, S: Effect of acute viral hepatitis in man on the disposition and elimination of meperidine. Gastroenterology *68*:775–780, 1975.
22. Klotz, U, McHorse, TS, Wilkinson, GR, Schenker, S: The effect of cirrhosis on the disposition and elimination of meperidine in man. Clin. Pharmacol. Ther. *16*:667–675, 1974.
23. Brodie, BB, Burus, JJ, Weiner, M: Metabolism of drugs in subjects with Laennec's cirrhosis. Med. Exper. *1*:290–292, 1959.
24. Hammar, CH, Prellwitz, W: Die glucuronidbildung nach perorder belastung mit acetnilide bei chronischer hepatitis und lebercirrhose. Klin. Wochenschr. *44*:1010–1014, 1966.
25. Finlayson, NDC, Prescott, LF, Adjepon-Yamoiah, KK, Forrest, JAH: Antipyrine, lidocaine and parcetamol metabolism in chronic liver disease. Gastroenterology *67*:790, 1974.
26. Schalm, SW, Summerskill, WHJ, Go, VLW: Prednisone for chronic active liver disease: Pharmacokinetics, including conversion to prednisolone. Gastroenterology *72*:910–913, 1977.
27. Davis, M, Williams, R, Chakraborty, J, English, J, Marks, V, Ideo, G, Tempini, S: Prednisone or prednisolone for the treatment of chronic active hepatitis? A comparison of plasma availability. Br. J. Clin. Pharmacol. *5*:501–505, 1978.
28. Madsbad, S, Bjerregaard, B, Henriksen, JH, Juhl, E, Kehler, H: Impaired conversion of prednisone to prednisolone in patients with liver cirrhosis. Gut *21*:52–56, 1980.
29. Hoffman, TA, Cestero, R, Bullock, WE: Pharmacodynamics of carbenicillin in hepatic and renal failure. Ann. Intern. Med. *73*:173–178, 1970.
30. Avant, GR, Schenker, S, Alford, RH: The effect of cirrhosis on the disposition and elimination of clindamycin. Am. J. Dig. Dis. *20*:223, 1975.
31. Marshall, JP, Salt, WB, Elam, RO, Wilkinson, GR, Schenker, S: Disposition of nafcillin in patients with cirrhosis and extrahepatic biliary obstruction. Gastroenterology *73*:1388–1392, 1977.
32. Kumin, CM, Chazko, AJ, Finland, M: Persistence of antibiotics in the blood of patients with acute renal failure. II. Chloramphenicol and its metabolic products in the blood of patients with severe renal disease on hepatic cirrhosis. J. Clin. Invest. *38*:1498–1508, 1959.
33. Azzolini, F, Gazzaniga, A, Lodola, E, Natangelo, R: Elimination of chloramphenicol and thiamphenicol in subjects with cirrhosis of the liver. Int. J. Clin. Pharmacol. *6*:1059–1065, 1972.
34. Loughnan, PM, Sitar, DS, Ogilvie, RE, Eisen, A, Fox, Z, Neims, AH: Pharmacokinetic analysis of the disposition of intravenous theophylline in young children. J. Pediatr. *88*:874–879, 1976.
35. Nielsen-Kudsk, F, Magnussen, I, Jakobsen, P: Pharmacokinetics of theophylline in the elderly patients. Acta Pharmacol. Toxicol. *42*:226–234, 1978.
36. Mangione, A, Imhoff, TE, Lee, RV, Shum, LY, Jusko, WJ: Pharmacokinetics of theophylline in hepatic disease. Chest *73*:616–622, 1978.
37. Jusko, WJ, Koup, JR, Vance, JW, Schentag, JJ, Puritzky, P: Intravenous theophylline therapy: Nomogram guidelines. Ann. Intern. Med. *86*:400–404, 1977.
38. Neims, AH, Bailey, J, Aldridge, A: Disposition of caffeine during and after pregnancy. Clin. Res. *27*:236A, 1979.
39. Patwardhan, RV, Desmond, PV, Johnson, RF, Schenker, S: Impaired elimination of caffeine by oral contraceptive steroids. J. Lab. Clin. Med. *95*:603–608, 1980.
40. Desmond, PV, Patwardhan, RV, Johnson, RF, Schenker, S: Impaired elimination of caffeine in cirrhosis. Dig. Dis. Sci. *25*:93–197, 1980.
41. Klotz, U, Antonin, KH, Brügel, H, Breek, PR: Disposition of diazepam and its major metabolite desmethyldiazepam in patients with liver disease. Clin. Pharmacol. Ther. *21*:430–436, 1977.
42. Hoyumpa, AM, Desmond, PV, Avant, GR, Roberts, RK, Schenker, S: Clinical conferences: Hepatic encephalopathy. Gastroenterology *76*:184, 1979.
43. Squires, RF, Braestrup, C: Benzodiazepine receptors in rat brain. Nature *66*:732–734, 1977.
44. Pasternak, GW: Endogenous opioid systems in brain. (Editorial.) Am. J. Med. *68*:157–159, 1980.
45. Toffano, G, Guidotti, A, Costa, E: Purification of an endogenous protein inhibitor of the high-affinity binding of γ-aminobutyric acid to synaptic membrane of rat brain. Proc. Natl. Acad. Sci. USA *75*:4024–4028, 1978.
46. Yamamura, HI, Snyder, SH: Muscarinic cholinergic binding in rat brain. Proc. Natl. Acad. Sci. USA *71*:1725–1729, 1974.
47. Read, AE, Laidlow, J, McCarthy, CF: Effect of chlorpromazine in patients with hepatic disease. Br. Med. J. *1*:497–499, 1969.
48. Morgan, MH, Read, AE: Antidepressants and liver disease. Gut *13*:697–701, 1972.
49. Murray-Lyon, IM, Young, J, Parkes, JD, Knill-

Jones, RP, Williams, R: Clinical and electroencephalographic assessment of diazepam in liver disease. Br. Med. J. *2*:265–266, 1971.

50. Branch, RA, Morgan, MH, James, J, Read, AE: Intravenous administration of diazepam in patients with chronic liver disease. Gut *17*:975–983, 1976.
51. Lang, M, Marselos, M, Torroven, R: Modifications of drug metabolism by disulfiram and diethyldithiocarbamate. I. Mixed function oxidase. Chem. Biol. Inter. *15*:267–276, 1976.
52. Rendic, S, Sunjic, V, Toso, R, Kajfez, F, Ruff, HH: Interaction of cimetidine with liver microsomes. Xenobiotica *9*:555–564, 1979.
53. Desmond, PV, Patwardhan, RV, Schenker, S, Speeg, KV: Cimetidine impairs the elimination of chlordiazepoxide (Librium[R]) in man. Ann. Intern. Med. *93*:226–268, 1980.
54. Patwardhan, RV, Yarborough, G, Johnson, RF, Desmond, PV, Schenker, S, Speeg, KV, Jr.: Cimetidine spares the glucuronidation of lorazepam and oxazepam. Gastroenterology *79*:912–916, 1980.
55. Rubin, E, Lieber, CS: Hepatic microsomal enzymes in man and rat: Induction and inhibition by ethanol. Science *162*:690–691, 1968.
56. Hepner, GW, Vesell, ES: Normal antipyrine metabolism in patients with cholestrol cholelithiasis: Evidence that the disease is not due to generalized hepatic microsomal dysfunction. Am. J. Dig. Dis. *20*:9–12, 1975.
57. McLuen, EF, Fouts, JR: The effect of obstructive jaundice on drug metabolism in rabbits. J. Pharmacol. Exp. Ther. *131*:7–11, 1961.
58. Donelli, MG, Colombo, K, Garattini, S: Experiments aiming at demonstrating microsomal drug metabolism in the tumor tissue. Eur. J. Cancer *8*:181–183, 1972.
59. Kato, R: Sex related differences in drug metabolism. Drug Metab. Rev. *3*:1, 1974.
60. Hepner, GW, Vesell, ES: Quantitative assessment of hepatic function by breath analysis after oral administration of ^{14}C-aminopyrine. Ann. Intern. Med. *83*:632–638, 1975.
61. Sotaniemi, EA, Pelkonen, RO, Mokka, RE, Huttunen, R, Viyakaineu, E: Impairment of drug metabolism in patients with liver cancer. Eur. J. Clin. Invest. *1*:269–274, 1977.
62. Williams, RL, Blaschke, TF, Mettin, PJ, Melmon, KL, Rowland, M: Influence of acute viral hepatitis on the disposition of two compounds with high hepatic clearance. Lignocaine and indocyanine green. Clin. Pharmacol. Ther. *20*:290–229, 1976.
63. Pessayre, D, Lebree, D, Descatoire, V, Peignoux, M, Benhamon, JP: Mechanisms for reduced drug clearance in patients with cirrhosis. Gastroenterology *74*:566–571, 1978.
64. Hepner, GW, Vesell, ES: Assessment of aminopyrine metabolism in man by breath analysis after oral administration of ^{14}C-aminopyrine. Effects of phenobarbital, disulfiram and portal cirrhosis. N. Engl. J. Med. *291*:1384–1388, 1974.
65. Breen, KJ, Desmond, PV, Berry, R, Calder, I, Mushford, ML: A ^{14}C-phenacetin breath test in the assessment of hepatic function. Gastroenterology *72*:1033, 1977.
66. Hepner, GW, Vesell, EW, Lipon, A, Harvey, HA, Wilkinson, GR, Schenker, S: Disposition of aminopyrine, diazepam, and indocyanine green in patients with liver disease or an anticonvulsant drug therapy: Diazepam breath test and correlations in drug elimination. J. Lab. Clin. Med. *90*:440–456, 1977.
67. Shreeve, WW, Shoop, JD, Oh, DG, McInteer, BB: Test for alcoholic cirrhosis by conversion of (^{14}C) or (^{13}C) galactose to expire $^{14}CO_2$. Gastroenterology *71*:98–101, 1976.
68. Hepner, GW, Uhlin, SR, Lipton, A, Harvey, HA, Rohrer, CV: Abnormal aminopyrine metabolism in patients with hepatic neoplasm: Detection by breath test. J.A.M.A. *236*:1587–1590, 1976.
69. Galizzi, J, Long, RG, Billing, RH, Sherlock, S: Assessment of the (^{14}C) aminopyrine breath test in liver disease. Gut *19*:40–45, 1978.
70. Carlisle, R, Golambos, JT, Warren, WJ: The relationship between conventional liver tests, quantitative function tests and histopathology in cirrhosis. Dig. Dis. Sci. *24*:358–362, 1979.
71. Monroe, P, Baker, A, Krager, P, Schoeller, D, Klein, P: The aminopyrine breath test (CABT) predicts histology and correlates with course in patients with chronic hepatitis. Gastroenterology *78*:1314, 1980.

Chapter 13

Treatment of Infectious Complications

by

David M. Melikian

Antibiotic agents constitute a significant portion of drugs prescribed by physicians. Because of their widespread use and potential for toxicity, an understanding of their routes of elimination plays an important role in the success of therapy and potential toxicity. Guidelines for dosing modification (dosage or dosing interval) of antibiotics in patients with compromised renal or hepatic function are important in all clinical settings. Antibiotic dosing modification in patients with severe renal disease has been well established. However, guidelines for dosage adjustment in patients with significant hepatic dysfunction have not been given the same attention and, therefore, are not well established.

The purpose of this chapter is to help clinicians evaluate normal dosing guidelines and present accepted methods of altering dose or dosing interval when confronted with patients who have significant renal or hepatic disease. Data presented are based on specific pharmacokinetic parameters of each antibiotic agent as reported in the current literature.

PENICILLINS

GENERAL COMMENTS

Penicillin antibiotics are excreted mainly by the kidney; glomerular filtration and proximal tubular secretion may result in elimination of approximately 3 million units per hour of penicillin. Extrarenal mechanisms of penicillin elimination, such as hepatic metabolism and bile-fecal excretion, become important only as renal function deteriorates significantly.[1-4] The high therapeutic index of the penicillins makes dosage modification necessary only with severe renal insufficiency (glomerular filtration rate [GFR] $<$ 20 to 30 ml/min and serum creatinine $>$ 3 to 4 mg/dl). Penicillin G, ampicillin, amoxicillin, cyclacillin, carbenicillin, ticarcillin, and methicillin are excreted 75 to 95 per cent as unchanged drug in the urine. Dosage modification is usually necessary when GFR falls below 20 ml/min for penicillin G and below 30 ml/min for the other penicillins mentioned previously.[1-12] The isoxazolyl penicillins, cloxacillin and dicloxacillin, are excreted mainly through renal mechanisms, accounting for approximately 80 to 90 per cent of unchanged drug. Dosage modifications, however, for cloxacillin and dicloxacillin have not been shown to be necessary in severe renal insufficiency.[1,2,6] This must indicate compensation by nonrenal mechanisms. Approximately 50 to 70 per cent of oxacillin and nafcillin are eliminated through extrarenal mechanisms.[1,2,5-7] Dosage modification of these penicillins, therefore, may be necessary in patients with severe liver dysfunction.[5,6] Organic acids, such as probenecid, compete with penicillins for renal tubular secretion and, thus, may elevate penicillin blood levels. Unusually high and prolonged blood levels of penicillin may lead to complications in patients with renal insufficiency.[3] Patients receiving combinations of these drugs also should be monitored very closely for possible penicillin toxicity.

SPECIFIC DRUG MODIFICATIONS

PENICILLIN

Penicillin G is excreted approximately 80 per cent as unchanged drug in the urine. Dosage modification with liver dysfunction is not necessary. In patients with severe renal insufficiency (GFR < 20 ml/min), a dosage reduction is necessary. In this setting, doses in excess of 10 to 12 million units per day result in excessive penicillin blood levels and greater incidence of penicillin toxicity. Penicillin G doses in severe renal insufficiency, therefore, should be limited to 10 to 12 million units per day, at dosing intervals of 10 to 12 hours.[1-3] Hemodialysis may remove approximately 5 to 20 per cent of penicillin at a rate of 30 to 40 ml/min. The half-life of penicillin G may decrease by 45 per cent with hemodialysis.

AMPICILLIN, AMOXICILLIN, AND CYCLACILLIN

Ampicillin, amoxicillin, and *cyclacillin* are excreted 75 to 90 per cent as unchanged drug in the urine. Dosage modification of these penicillins in patients with liver dysfunction is unnecessary. Patients with moderate to severe renal insufficiency (GFR of 10 to 30 ml/min) require dosage modification. Dosing interval for these drugs should be extended from the normal of every 6 hours to every 9 to 12 hours in patients with GFR of 25 to 50 ml/min and every 12 to 18 hours in patients with GFR < 10 ml/min.[8-10] In a 6-hour hemodialysis period, 40 to 80 per cent of ampicillin may be removed and the half-life of ampicillin may be decreased by 75 per cent.[8, 14] Fifty per cent of amoxicillin may be removed in a 6-hour hemodialysis period. Approximately 70 to 80 per cent of cyclacillin may be removed and the half-life decreased by 75 per cent after a 6-hour hemodialysis period.

CARBENICILLIN AND TICARCILLIN

Carbenicillin and *ticarcillin* are excreted approximately 95 per cent unchanged in the urine.[11, 12] Dosage modification in patients with liver dysfunction is not necessary. Because significant quantities of carbenicillin and ticarcillin are excreted unchanged in the urine, significant dosage reduction in moderate and severe renal failure is indicated. GFR in the range of 10 to 50 ml/min may require a 25 to 50 per cent reduction in carbenicillin and ticarcillin dosage. GFR < 10 ml/min may require a reduction of ticarcillin and carbenicillin dosage by 50 to 75 per cent. With such advanced renal failure, the normal dosing interval of every 6 hours should be extended to every 12 to 24 hours.[1, 11, 12] A 4- to 6-gm daily dose may be sufficient to maintain adequate minimum inhibitory (or bactericidal) concentrations. A 6-hour hemodialysis period may remove 20 to 40 per cent of a carbenicillin or ticarcillin dose and the half-life of carbenicillin and ticarcillin may be decreased by 60 to 70 per cent. Additional maintenance doses, therefore, may be required after dialysis.[1, 11, 12]

METHICILLIN

Methicillin is excreted approximately 90 per cent unchanged in the urine. Ten per cent of methicillin is metabolized in the liver; therefore, modification of methicillin during severe liver dysfunction is unnecessary.[5] Patients with moderate renal insufficiency do not require dosage adjustments. Patients receiving methicillin with GFR < 10 ml/min require dosage and/or dosing interval changes. A 50 per cent reduction in methicillin dose may be required in patients with such severe renal insufficiency. The dosing interval should be increased from the normal of every 4 to 6 hours to a dosing interval of every 8 to 12 hours.[1] Unlike other penicillins, methicillin is not readily dialyzable; a 6-hour hemodialysis period removes very little methicillin.

ISOXAZOLYL PENICILLINS

The isoxazolyl penicillins, *cloxacillin* and *dicloxacillin,* are excreted 80 to 90 per cent unchanged in the urine.[1, 5, 6, 13] Because only 10 to 20 per cent of these penicillins is excreted as metabolized drug, dosage modification in liver disease is not necessary. It has been shown with these penicillins that renal disease does not affect tissue concentrations or half-life to a great extent. During severe renal insufficiency, extrarenal mechanisms of drug elimination become important. Dosage modifications for these drugs in the face of renal insufficiency, therefore, are not required.[1,5-7,13] Isoxazolyl penicillins are not readily dialyzable; a 6-hour hemodialysis period removes very little drug from the body.

Oxacillin and *nafcillin* are two isoxazolyl penicillins that are eliminated extensively through hepatic pathways. Approximately 50 per cent of oxacillin and 70 per cent of nafcillin are eliminated by hepatic metabolism.[5-7] Dosage modification, therefore, may be necessary in patients with moderate to severe liver dysfunction. Metabolites of these penicillins are microbiologically active, though their activity is very weak.[6] Accumulation of these active metabolites in patients with renal insufficiency has not proven to be significant enough to warrant dosage changes in renal failure. Nafcillin and oxacillin doses and dosing interval do not require modification in patients with renal insufficiency. Dialysis of these drugs is minimal and additional doses after dialysis are unnecessary.[1,7]

CEPHALOSPORINS

GENERAL COMMENTS

The majority of cephalosporins are eliminated by renal mechanisms; glomerular filtration and renal tubular secretion play a major role in elimination of these drugs.[15,16] Only cephalothin and cephapirin are eliminated to a significant extent through extrarenal (hepatic) mechanisms.[15-18] Because of their relatively high therapeutic/toxic index, dosage modification is needed only when GFR falls below 20 to 30 ml/min. Dosage changes for cephalothin, cephalexin, cephapirin, cephradine, and cephaloglycin are necessary in patients with renal insufficiency. Dosing interval may need to be increased when GFR falls below 20 ml/min.[15-26] Cefazolin, cefamandole, cefadroxil, cefoxitin, cefaclor, and cephaloridine also require dosage and dosing interval modifications in patients with renal insufficiency.[27-36]

SPECIFIC DRUG MODIFICATIONS

CEPHALOTHIN, CEPHALEXIN, CEPHAPIRIN, CEPHRADINE, AND CEPHALOGLYCIN

Cephalothin and *cephapirin* are two cephalosporins that undergo significant metabolism by the liver. Approximately 33 per cent of cephalothin is metabolized in the liver, and cephapirin is metabolized approximately 40 to 60 per cent by hepatic mechanisms. In patients with severe liver dysfunction, therefore, dosage adjustment of cephalothin and cephapirin may be necessary. These cephalosporins have desacetyl metabolites that are active, but the microbiologic activity of these compounds is very weak.[15,16,19] Accumulation of these active metabolites in patients with renal insufficiency has not proven to be of major significance.[19,21-23]

Cephalothin dosage and dosing interval need not be adjusted in patients with mild to moderate renal insufficiency (GFR $>$ 20 ml/min). In patients with GFR $<$ 20 ml/min, a normal loading dose may be initiated, but dosing interval should be increased from the normal of every 4 to 6 hours to every 8 to 24 hours.[1,22,23] All cephalosporins are significantly removed by hemodialysis and, to a lesser extent, by peritoneal dialysis. Supplementation of dosage following dialysis, therefore, may be needed to insure sustained therapeutic blood levels. A dosage of 1 gm after dialysis may be needed in patients with renal failure undergoing prolonged dialysis.

Cephalexin dosage need not be adjusted in patients with moderate renal insufficiency; however, dosage interval should be adjusted in patients with GFR $<$ 20 ml/min.[20,25] Dialysis may remove a significant portion of cephalexin; a 500-mg dose postdialysis may be appropriate to maintain therapeutic blood levels.[20,25] In this setting, the normal dosing interval of every 6 hours should be increased in these patients to a dosing interval of every 12 to 48 hours. Approximately 15 per cent of cephalexin is excreted through extrarenal mechanisms; therefore, dosage modification in patients with liver dysfunction is unnecessary.

Cephapirin dosage modification is unnecessary in patients with moderate renal insufficiency; however, dosage interval should be adjusted in patients with GFR $<$ 10 ml/min.[19,21] A normal dosing interval modification of every 6 hours should be increased to an every 12-hour regimen.

Cephapirin is significantly excreted through extrerenal mechanisms. Dosage adjustment in patients with severe hepatic dysfunction, therefore, may be necessary. Partial removal of cephapirin occurs after a 6-hour hemodialysis period. A dose of 18 mg/kg after hemodialysis is, therefore, recommended to maintain therapeutic concentrations.[1, 19, 21]

Cephradine requires no dosage modification in patients with moderate renal failure; however, a 50 per cent decreased dosage interval modification is necessary in patients with GFR less than 10 to 50 ml/min.[24-26] An increase in the normal dosage interval of every 6 hours should be modified to every 12 to 70 hours and dosage reduced by 25 to 75 per cent in these patients with GFR less than 10 ml/min. Extrarenal elimination of cephradine accounts for only 20 per cent of the total dosage; therefore, patients with severe liver dysfunction do not require dosage modification. Hemodialysis and peritoneal dialysis may remove significant portions of cephradine.[24, 26]

Cephaloglycin dosage modification in patients with moderate renal disease is unnecessary; however, in patients with severe renal insufficiency (GFR < 10 ml/min) a dosage interval modification is recommended.[16, 37] An increase over the normal 6-hour dosing interval to a 6- to 12-hour interval is suggested in patients with severe renal insufficiency. Peritoneal dialysis has been shown to remove approximately 40 per cent of cephaloglycin during a 6-hour dialysis treatment.[37, 128] Hemodialysis may remove only small amounts of cephaloglycin. Approximately 10 to 25 per cent of cephaloglycin is metabolized in the liver; therefore, dosage adjustment in patients with severe hepatic dysfunction is unnecessary.

CEFAZOLIN, CEFAMANDOLE, CEFOXITIN, CEFACLOR, AND CEFADROXIL

The dosage and dosage interval of these cephalosporins must be adjusted in patients with moderate to severe renal insufficiency.

Cefazolin dosage and dosage interval should be reduced in patients with moderate and severe renal insufficiency. A 50 per cent reduction of cefazolin dosage is needed in patients with GFR of 10 to 50 ml/min. The normal dosage interval of every 8 hours also should be increased to every 12 hours in these patients.[1, 16, 18, 27] GFR < 10 ml/min requires a dosage reduction to 25 per cent of normal and a dosing interval of every 24 to 48 hours. Hemodialysis and peritoneal dialysis remove significant amounts of cefazolin. An additional 250-mg dose of cefazolin after dialysis may be needed to maintain therapeutic levels. An insignificant proportion of cefazolin is metabolized by the liver; therefore, patients with severe liver dysfunction need not receive altered doses.[16, 18, 27]

Cefamandole doses should be decreased to 25 to 50 per cent of normal doses in patients with moderate renal insufficiency (GFR of 10 to 50 ml/min); the dosing interval should be increased from every 6 hours to 6 to 12 hours.[1, 17, 19, 28] Patients with severe renal insufficiency (GFR < 10 ml/min) should have cefamandole decreased to 10 to 25 per cent of normal doses and the dosing interval increased to every 8 to 12 hours. Cefamandole is an unusual cephalosporin in that dialysis removes very little drug from the body.[1, 19, 28] Approximately 15 to 25 per cent of cefamandole is metabolized by the liver. This amount is not sufficient to precipitate problems in patients with liver dysfunction. Patients with severe hepatic disease, therefore, will not need dosage modifications.

Cefoxitin doses and dosing interval may need reduction in patients with renal insufficiency.[27, 30, 31] A 25 per cent reduction in dose should be initiated in patients with GFR of 10 to 50 ml/min. The normal dosing interval of every 6 to 8 hours may need to be extended to every 8 to 12 hours. Patients with GFR < 10 ml/min may require a 50 per cent reduction in cefoxitin dose and an increase in dosing interval to every 24 to 48 hours.[1, 27, 30, 31] Peritoneal and hemodialysis may remove significant portions of cefoxitin from the serum. The total amount of cefoxitin metabolized by the liver is < 15 per cent; therefore, no dosage modification is necessary in patients with severe hepatic disease.

Cefaclor, an oral cephalosporin, may require dosage adjustment in patients with moderate or severe renal insufficiency.[32, 33] Dosing interval of cefaclor need not be adjusted in these patients. Patients with GFR of 10 to 50 ml/min require a cefaclor dosage reduction of 25 to 50 per cent of normal. GFR < 10 ml/min requires a 50 per cent or greater reduction of normal doses.[1, 32, 33] Hemodialysis may remove significant amounts of cefaclor. Hepatic elimination of cefaclor accounts for less than 10 per cent of total drug; therefore, dosage adjustment in patients with liver insufficiency is unnecessary.

Cefadroxil, another oral cephalosporin, may need dosage adjustment in patients with moderate renal insufficiency, but dosage interval does not require adjustment in these patients.[34, 35] A 50 per cent reduction in dosage may be necessary for patients with GFR < 10 to 15 ml/min. In patients with severe renal dysfunction (GFR < 10 ml/min), a dosage reduction of greater than 50 per cent may be necessary. A change in the every 12-hour dosage schedule to an every 24 to 48-hour dosage interval also may be necessary.[34, 35] Hemodialysis may remove significant portions of cefadroxil from the body. A 6-hour hemodialysis period may remove 75 per cent of total drug from the body. Only 12 per cent of cefadroxil is metabolized by the liver; therefore, no dosage modifications with hepatic failure are necessary for this drug.

Cephaloridine was one of the first injectable cephalosporins marketed. Because of its severe renal toxicity (renal tubular damage), cephaloridine should not be used in patients with any degree of renal insufficiency. Approximately 15 to 30 per cent of cephaloridine is metabolized by the liver, but dosage modification in patients with liver failure is not necessary.[1, 36]

AMINOGLYCOSIDES

Aminoglycoside antibiotics *(gentamicin, tobramycin, amikacin, kanamycin, neomycin,* and *streptomycin)* are extensively used in acute care facilities for treatment of serious gram-negative infections, bowel sterilization, and tuberculosis. Aminoglycosides are not significantly metabolized by the liver. They are eliminated almost entirely by the kidney in unchanged form, primarily through glomerular filtration.[37-46] Aminoglycosides have a relatively low therapeutic index; this coupled with their almost exclusive renal elimination may cause serious toxicities in patients with even mild renal insufficiency owing to accumulation of active drug.[37]

To effect rapid therapeutic blood levels in patients with renal failure, the usual aminoglycoside loading dose should always be administered. Subsequent maintenance therapy must be modified to avoid accumulation and toxicity in renal failure patients. Such maintenance therapy might involve either a reduced dosage administered at the usual interval or the usual dose given less frequently.[38] It must be remembered that considerable interindividual variation exists with drug kinetics in patients with renal failure. If possible, drug serum levels should be obtained in these patients to determine accurate dosage and dosing interval for the degree of renal failure.[37, 38]

The most widely used clinical method of dosing aminoglycosides in patients with renal failure involves an extension of the normal dosing interval.[1] The normal maintenance dose remains the same; however, the dosing interval may increase to an every second or third half-life. In most clinical settings, this regimen may be adequate; however, extremely large fluctuations in peak and trough aminoglycoside levels occur with this regimen. Aminoglycosides all have very similar half-lives, about three times the serum creatinine. When using the aforementioned dosing schedule, a serum creatinine of 3 mg/dl would result in maintenance doses being given every 18 to 27 hours. Simplification of this regimen would be to multiply the serum creatinine by a factor of 8 and 6 to determine the dosage interval in hours for gentamicin and tobramycin, respectively,[39-41] and to multiply the serum creatinine by a factor of 9 to determine the dosage interval for amikacin or kanamycin.[42-44] This extension of dosage interval assumes a 100 per cent normal maintenance dose. When the dosing interval falls at an unusual dosing period (e.g., 15, 27, 39 hours), an adjustment of this dosing interval to fit the needs of the acute care facility may be appropriate. Administration time may be either increased or decreased to coincide with the administration time of the facility. This increase or decrease must also be accompanied by a proportional increase or decrease of the maintenance dose. For example, if a patient were to receive 100 per cent of a maintenance dose every 18 hours, it might be more appropriate to decrease the dosage interval to every 12 hours and the maintenance dose to two-thirds of normal.

A more precise method of predicting serum aminoglycoside levels involves a method that reduces the normal maintenance dose but maintains the usual dosing interval. A simplified dosage reduction nomogram and an aminoglycoside dosing chart (Table 13–1) provide a more precise method of predicting desired serum aminoglycoside levels.[38]

Neomycin and streptomycin may accumulate in patients with renal dysfunction, requiring dosage and dosage interval modification in these patients.[1, 45, 56] Although less than 5 per cent of neomycin and streptomycin is metabolized in the liver, patients with concomitant renal and liver dysfunction are reported to

TABLE 13–1. AMINOGLYCOSIDE DOSING CHART

1. Select Loading Dose in mg/kg (ideal weight) to provide peak serum levels in range listed below for desired aminoglycoside.

AMINO-GLYCOSIDE	USUAL LOADING DOSE	EXPECTED PEAK SERUM LEVELS
Tobramycin Gentamicin	1.5 to 2.0 mg/kg	4 to 10 μg/ml
Amikacin Kanamycin	5.0 to 7.5 mg/kg	15 to 30 μg/ml

2. Select Maintenance Dose (as percentage of chosen loading dose) to continue peak serum levels indicated above according to desired dosing interval and the patient's corrected creatinine clearance.*

PERCENTAGE OF LOADING DOSE REQUIRED FOR DOSAGE INTERVAL SELECTED

C(c)cr (ml/min)	*Half-life*† *(hrs)*	*8 hrs*	*12 hrs*	*24 hrs*
90	3.1	84%	–	–
80	3.4	80	91%	–
70	3.9	76	88	–
60	4.5	71	84	–
50	5.3	65	79	–
40	6.5	57	72	92%
30	8.4	48	63	86
25	9.9	43	57	81
20	11.9	37	50	75
17	13.6	33	46	70
15	15.1	31	42	67
12	17.9	27	37	61
10‡	20.4	24	34	56
7	25.9	19	28	47
5	31.5	16	23	41
2	46.8	11	16	30
0	69.3	8	11	21

*Calculate corrected Creatinine Clearance C(c)cr as:
C(c)cr male = 140 − age/serum creatinine
C(c)cr female = 0.85 × C(c)cr male

†Alternatively, one-half of the chosen loading dose may be given at an interval approximately equal to the estimated half-life.

‡Dosing for patients with C(c)cr ≤ 10 ml/min should be assisted by measured serum levels.

(With permission from Hull, JH, Sarrubi FA: Gentamicin serum concentrations: Pharmakinetic predictions. Ann. Intern. Med. *85*:183–189, 1976.)

have prolonged half-lives that cannot be attributed to renal failure alone. Significant amounts of aminoglycosides may be removed by hemodialysis. Twenty to 60 ml/min of the aminoglycosides may be removed by hemodialysis.[1, 39, 40, 42] Peritoneal dialysis may remove on an average 5 to 15 ml/min of these drugs. Doses equivalent to the normal maintenance may be administered after each hemodialysis period. Removal of aminoglycosides after peritoneal dialysis is less complete and supplementary doses may not be necessary.

TETRACYCLINES

All tetracyclines, with the exception of minocycline and doxycycline, are relatively contraindicated in patients with mild to moderate renal insufficiency (GFR 10 to 50 ml/min). In patients with GFR < 10 to 30 ml/min, tetracyclines may promote a negative nitrogen balance by their antianabolic effect and precipitate metabolic acidosis and uremia in patients with preexisting renal insufficiency.[1, 47, 51] Tetracyclines also may produce renal sodium wasting and potentiate azotemia, especially in patients with concomitant diuretic therapy. Minocycline does have less antianabolic activity than tetracycline hydrochloride; however, its antianabolic activity is greater than doxycycline.[47, 51] Therefore, tetracyclines, with the exception of minocycline and doxycycline, should be avoided in patients with renal failure owing to their antianabolic effect on protein metabolism and their ability to worsen azotemia.

Approximately 70 per cent of tetracycline hydrochloride is eliminated as unchanged drug in the urine.[1, 50, 51] A 4-hour hemodialysis period decreases tetracycline levels by 14 to 27 per cent, but peritoneal dialysis removes very little tetracycline. Although only 30 per cent of tetracycline is metabolized in the liver, caution may be necessary in patients with hepatic insufficiency. These drugs may have direct nephrotoxic effects in patients with cirrhosis.[52] Dosing of tetracycline hydrochloride in patients with hepatic insufficiency, therefore, should be monitored closely; however, dosage modification may not be necessary.

Minocycline is metabolized approximately 90 per cent by the liver and its metabolites excreted in the urine are inactive. Dosage modification in patients with renal insufficiency, therefore, is not necessary.[47-49] Patients with hepatic failure should be monitored closely for minocycline accumulation; dosage modification may be necessary in these patients.

Doxycycline is excreted approximately 20 to 50 per cent as unchanged drug in the urine. Because doxycycline has insignificant antianabolic effects, it may be used at normal doses in patients with moderate to severe renal insufficiency.[47,48,50,51] Hemodialysis and peritoneal dialysis remove very small amounts of doxycycline. Doxycycline is eliminated 50 per cent by extrarenal mechanisms; liver metabolism and chelation in the intraluminal bowel wall account for this portion of administered drug.[47] Thus, patients with severe hepatic insufficiency must be monitored closely for accumulation of doxycycline serum levels and toxicity.

SULFONAMIDES AND TRIMETHOPRIM

Sulfonamides in general are eliminated through extrarenal mechanisms; however, in patients with severe renal failure, prolongation of sulfonamide half-lives is seen.[1,53-56]

Sulfisoxazole has 55 per cent of its total dose eliminated as unchanged drug by the kidney. In patients with moderate to severe renal insufficiency, sulfisoxazole dosage may remain unchanged, but dosage interval should be increased with severe renal dysfunction. Patients with GFR between 10 and 50 ml/min should have the dosing interval increased from every 6 hours to every 8 to 12 hours. Patients with GFR $<$ 10 ml/min should have dosing interval increased to an every 12 to 24 hour schedule.[1,53] Hemodialysis and peritoneal dialysis may remove significant amounts of sulfisoxazole from the serum. Forty-six per cent of sulfisoxazole is metabolized in the liver. Patients with severe liver insufficiency, therefore, should be monitored closely for sulfisoxazole accumulation.[53] Dosage modification in patients with hepatic insufficiency also may be necessary in certain instances.

Sulfamethoxazole is excreted 20 to 35 per cent as unchanged drug in the urine. Prolonged half-life may be seen in patients with renal insufficiency.[1,54,55,79] Normal dosages can be employed in patients with moderate to severe renal failure, but dosing interval should be increased to compensate for decreased clearance. The guidelines for changes in dosing intervals are similar to those of trimethoprim and sulfisoxazole. Hemodialysis may remove approximately 22 ml/min of sulfamethoxazole. Peritoneal dialysis may also remove sulfamethoxazole. Hepatic metabolism accounts for 65 to 80 per cent of sulfamethoxazole elimination.[54,55] Sulfonamide accumulation, therefore, may be seen in patients with severe hepatic insufficiency; thus, a dosage modification for these patients may be necessary.

Sulfasalazine may have a prolonged half-life in patients with severe renal insufficiency, although renal excretion accounts for less than 15 per cent of total drug elimination.[56] Patients with mild to moderate renal insufficiency, however, need no dosage modification. Guidelines for sulfasalazine dosage modification in patients with severe renal failure are not available. Eighty-five to 98 per cent of sulfasalazine is metabolized in the liver. Because the drug is almost totally metabolized by the liver, dosage modification in patients with severe renal insufficiency may not be necessary.[56] Liver metabolism results in several sulfonamide metabolites, which possess minor activity, and salicylic acid. Accumulation of sulfasalazine metabolites and salicylic acid has not been reported in patients with renal insufficiency and/or liver failure; however, dosage adjustment should be considered in patients with severe hepatic disease.[56] Five per cent of a sulfasalazine dose is excreted as unchanged drug in the feces.

Trimethoprim is eliminated largely through renal mechanisms; 65 to 80 per cent of trimethoprim is excreted as unchanged drug in the urine.[55,57] Dosage interval modifications, therefore, may be necessary in patients with moderate to severe renal disease. In patients with GFR of 10 to 50 ml/min, the normal dosage of trimethoprim should be administered; however, dosing interval should be increased from the normal of every 12 hours to every 18 hours. In patients with severe renal insufficiency (GFR $<$ 10 ml/min), the dosage interval should be increased to every 24 hours.[1,55-57] Hemodialysis may greatly reduce the prolonged trimethoprim serum half-lives; e.g., two-thirds decrease in half-life after 8 hours of dialysis. Hepatic metabolism of trimethoprim accounts for only 20 to 35 per cent of excreted drug. Thus, dosage adjustment in patients with severe liver failure would not seem necessary.[57]

ERYTHROMYCIN

The pharmacokinetics of erythromycin have not been well established; however, approximately 85 to 95 per cent of erythromycin is eliminated through nonrenal mechanisms.[58,59] Only 5 to 15 per cent of an administered erythromycin dose is recovered unchanged in the urine[58-60]; therefore, dosage modification in patients with severe renal insufficiency is not necessary.[1] Even though the metabolites of erythromycin are inactive, because of extensive hepatic metabolism, patients with impaired liver function should be monitored closely for accumulation of erythromycin in the serum. Dosage modification of erythromycin in patients with severe liver failure, therefore, may be necessary.[2, 58-60]

CLINDAMYCIN AND LINCOMYCIN

Clindamycin and lincomycin are excreted primarily through hepatic mechanisms.

Lincomycin has a greater dependency on renal excretion (10 to 30 per cent excreted unchanged in the urine) than clindamycin and may accumulate in patients with severe renal failure.[1, 61, 62] The half-lives of lincomycin may double or triple in patients with GFR < 10 ml/min. In these patients, a normal maintenance dose should be administered, but the dosing interval should be increased above the normal of every 6 hours to every 12 to 24 hours.[1, 61, 62] Lincomycin is not significantly removed by either hemodialysis or peritoneal dialysis. Four to forty per cent of lincomycin is recovered in the feces as active drug. Fifty to 70 per cent of lincomycin is metabolized to inactive compounds and excreted in the urine. Liver disease is reported to increase lincomycin half-life up to 11.8 hours (normal half-life 4 to 6 hours).[2, 61, 62] Dosage modification in patients with severe hepatic insufficiency, therefore, should be initiated for lincomycin.

Clindamycin is excreted approximately 10 to 15 per cent as unmetabolized drug in the urine and 5 per cent as active drug in the feces. The primary route of clindamycin elimination is through hepatic metabolism; therefore, patients with severe renal dysfunction do not require dosage adjustment.[1, 61, 63, 65, 66] Clindamycin is not significantly removed by either peritoneal dialysis or hemodialysis. Since 85 to 90 per cent of clindamycin is eliminated through hepatic metabolism, dosage adjustment in patients with liver disease is necessary. Liver dysfunction may increase the half-life of clindamycin to 7 to 14 hours (from the normal half-life of 2 to 4 hours).[63, 65, 66]

CHLORAMPHENICOL

The major route of excretion for chloramphenicol is by hepatic metabolism. Approximately 5 to 15 per cent of chloramphenicol is excreted unchanged in the urine.[67, 68] Anephric patients have a slight increase in chloramphenicol half-life; however, dosage adjustment in these patients is not necessary.[1] The hepatic metabolites of chloramphenicol are excreted in the urine. These microbiologically inactive chloramphenicol metabolites may accumulate in patients with advanced renal failure and cause depression of bone marrow erythrocytopoiesis.[1, 67, 68] Since 85 to 95 per cent of chloramphenicol is metabolized by the liver, dosage adjustment in patients with hepatic failure is necessary. Patients with combined liver and renal dysfunction may have a greatly prolonged half-life (12 hours).[2, 67, 68] Therefore, caution should be used and dosage adjustment initiated in patients with concomitant renal and liver dysfunction. Less than 5 per cent of chloramphenicol is eliminated in the feces. Peritoneal dialysis may remove small portions of chloramphenicol. Hemodialysis may significantly remove chloramphenicol from the serum; therefore, additional doses may be required after dialysis.[1, 67, 68]

METRONIDAZOLE

Metronidazole is eliminated primarily through hepatic mechanisms (45 to 55 per cent). Approximately 30 to 40 per cent of metronidazole is excreted as unchanged drug in the urine and 14 per cent unchanged drug and metabolites in the feces.[69, 70] Dosage modification in patients with moderate to severe renal insufficiency is not necessary; however, lengthening of the dosage interval in patients with GFR < 10 to 30 ml/min may be necessary. An increase from the normal every 8-hour dosage interval to 12 to 24 hours may be required in these patients.[1] The reason for this dosing interval modification is the activity of metronidazole metabolites. Metronidazole is metabolized to two active compounds. The acid metabolite is very weakly active with only 5 per cent of the parent compound activity. Metronidazole's hydroxy metabolite has approximately 30 per cent of the parent compound's microbiologic activity.[71] Accumulation of this hydroxy metabolite may result in prolonged metronidazole activity. Dosage modification in patients with severe liver insufficiency may be necessary with this drug.[1, 2, 69-71] Modification of dosage and cautious monitoring also would be prudent in patients with concomitant liver and renal failure. Peritoneal dialysis removes insignificant portions of metronidazole from the body, but the drug may be removed by hemodialysis.

VANCOMYCIN

Vancomycin is eliminated primarily through renal pathways. Eighty to 90 per cent is excreted as unchanged drug in the urine. The normal half-life of 4 to 8 hours may be greatly prolonged in patients with even mild renal insufficiency.[1, 72, 73] In patients with mild renal insufficiency (GFR 50 to 75 ml/min), a normal dose of vancomycin should be administered; however, the dosing interval should be increased to every 24 to 72 hours. Patients with GFR of 10 to 50 ml/min should have dosing intervals increased to every 72 to 144 hours. In patients with GFR < 10 ml/min, a dosing interval of 144 to 240 hours should be initiated.[1, 72-75] Neither peritoneal dialysis nor hemodialysis removes vancomycin from the serum. Because vancomycin is not removed by hemodialysis, it has proven to be very useful in treating arteriovenous shunt or fistula infections due to gram-positive organisms in patients with end-stage chronic renal failure.[75] A single dose of vancomycin may be given every 6 to 10 days with maintenance of therapeutic blood levels.[72, 74, 75] Accumulation of vancomycin in patients with renal insufficiency may result in serious oto- and nephrotoxicity; this results from blood levels in excess of 80 to 100 mg/ml.

URINARY TRACT ANTIMICROBIAL AGENTS

Drugs in this category (nitrofurantoin, nalidixic acid, oxolinic acid, and methenamine) are all used in the treatment of urinary tract infections.

Nitrofurantoin is eliminated mainly by extrarenal mechanisms; 50 to 80 per cent of nitrofurantoin is metabolized by the liver and/or inactivated by body tissues.[76] Renal excretion of unchanged drug is approximately 30 to 50 per cent. Nitrofurantoin may be used in patients with mild renal insufficiency, but as GFR becomes < 50 ml/min the efficacy of the drug decreases and toxicity may increase.[1, 76-79] Metabolites of nitrofurantoin accumulate in patients with severe renal insufficiency; these metabolites may induce a polyneuropathy.[1, 77, 78] Clinicians, therefore, should avoid this drug in patients with moderate to severe renal failure. Hemodialysis may remove 40 to 80 ml/min of nitrofurantoin. No data are available to assess modification of nitrofurantoin doses in patients with liver insufficiency. Because the liver inactivates a large portion of nitrofurantoin, patients with severe liver failure should be monitored closely for drug accumulation.[77, 79]

Nalidixic acid is eliminated mainly through extrarenal mechanisms; approximately 10 to 15 per cent of nalidixic acid is excreted unchanged in the urine.[72-82] This drug may be used in patients with mild renal insufficiency, but should be avoided in patients with moderate to severe renal failure.[1, 77-82] An active hydroxy metabolite and inactive monoglucuronide metabolites may accumulate in patients with renal failure. The half-life of nalidixic acid may increase from the normal of 1.0 to 2.5 hours to 21 hours when reported as inactive monoglucuronide metabolites.[80-82] Nalidixic acid should be avoided in patients with GFR < 50 ml/min owing to an increased incidence of dermatologic and gastrointestinal reactions in these patients.[81, 82] There are no data available on removal of nalidixic acid by peritoneal dialysis or hemodialysis. Eighty per cent of nalidixic acid is metabolized by the liver. Dosage modification of nalidixic acid in severe liver failure, therefore, should be considered, but precise dosage adjustments for these patients have not been established.

Oxolinic acid is almost exclusively metabolized by the liver; less than 2 per cent of oxolinic acid is excreted in the urine as unchanged drug.[82, 83] Sixteen per cent is excreted in the feces. Dosage modification in patients with moderate to severe renal disease has not been found to be necessary. Oxolinic acid is extensively metabolized (84 per cent) to eight metabolites. An oxolinic acid–glucuronide metabolite may have significant antimicrobial activity. Approximately 45 per cent of this metabolite is excreted in the urine.[82, 83] Accumulation of this metabolite with possible associated toxicity in patients with GFR < 50 ml/min warrants close monitoring.[83] There are no data available for removal of oxolinic acid by peritoneal dialysis or hemodialysis. Dosage modification in patients with liver disease has not been reported, but owing to its extensive hepatic metabolism, patients with severe liver failure should be monitored closely for drug accumulation.

Methenamine is eliminated primarily through renal mechanisms.[84-86] Seventy-five to 90 per cent of this drug is recovered in the urine.[84, 85] There are no data available on dosage modification in patients with renal failure, but methenamine should be avoided in patients with moderate to severe renal failure because of its ability to induce systemic acidosis in these patients.[1, 84, 85] Hemodialysis and peritoneal dialysis data are not available for removal of methenamine. A need for dosage modification of methenamine in patients with liver failure would not be anticipated, as only 10 to 25 per cent of the drug is metabolized by the liver.[84, 85]

ANTIFUNGAL AGENTS

Amphotericin B, flucytosine, and griseofulvin are the most common antifungal agents used for systemic mycoses. Miconazole is a systemic antifungal agent, but it is clinically used primarily as a topical agent.

Amphotericin B is eliminated mainly through extrarenal mechanisms; hepatic and bowel metabolism along with bile elimination account for the majority of amphotericin excreted.[87, 88] Only 3 to 5 per cent of amphotericin is excreted unchanged in the urine; dosage modification in patients with renal failure is not necessary.[1, 89] Peritoneal dialysis and hemodialysis do not remove significant portions of amphotericin from the plasma. Dosage adjustment in patients with severe liver failure may be necessary for patients receiving high doses of amphotericin. Amphotericin B does have intrinsic nephrotoxic activity; thus, possible accumulation of amphotericin in patients with liver disease requires close monitoring of both renal and liver function.

Flucytosine (5-fluorocytosine or 5-FU) is excreted 85 to 90 per cent unchanged in the urine. Fecal elimination of unchanged drug accounts for 10 per cent of 5-FU administered. Significant bone marrow toxicity and hepatic abnormalities may occur as accumulation of this drug develops in patients with renal failure.[90-92] Flucytosine's normal half-life of 2.5 to 4.0 hours may increase in severe renal failure to 75 to 250 hours. A dose of 12 to 35 mg/kg of 5-FU may be administered every 6 hours in patients with GFR $>$ 50 ml/min. Patients with moderate renal dysfunction (GFR of 10 to 50 ml/min) may require a dosage interval extension to every 12 to 36 hours. Patients with severe renal failure (GFR $<$ 10 ml/min) may require a dosage interval of 24 to 72 hours.[1, 90-92] Hemodialysis may clear significant portions of 5-FU (60 to 100 ml/min). Less than 5 per cent of 5-FU is metabolized by the liver; therefore, dosage adjustment is unnecessary in patients with severe hepatic failure.

Griseofulvin pharmacokinetics are not well established. The normal half-life of griseofulvin is reported to be 10 to 22 hours. The drug's half-life in anephric patients has not been determined[93]; however, less than 1 per cent of griseofulvin is excreted unchanged in the urine. Extensive liver metabolism (five metabolites) accounts for the majority of griseofulvin elimination.[93-95] Activity of these metabolites is unknown, and dosage modification based on accumulation of these metabolites in patients with renal failure has not been studied. No data are available on hemodialysis or peritoneal dialysis of griseofulvin. Owing to the extensive hepatic metabolism of griseofulvin, patients with severe liver impairment should be monitored closely for drug accumulation.[93] There are no data available for assessment of dosage modification in patients with liver failure, but adjustment of dosage in these patients may be indicated.

Miconazole is eliminated mainly through hepatic mechanisms. Less than 1 per cent is excreted in the urine as unchanged drug; 50 per cent is excreted in the feces unchanged.[96-98] Metabolism (hydrolysis and *N*-alkylation) accounts for 50 per cent of an administered dose. Activity of miconazole metabolites is unknown. Dosing and dosing interval changes would not seem necessary in patients with renal failure. Dosage modification in patients with severe hepatic disease has not been studied, but owing to its significant hepatic elimination, close monitoring and possible dose adjustment in these patients would be appropriate.[96, 98]

ANTITUBERCULOUS DRUGS

Isoniazid, rifampin, and ethambutol are the most common agents used for treatment of tuberculosis. The major route of isoniazid elimination is through hepatic metabolism.

Less than 20 per cent of *isoniazid* is excreted unchanged in the urine.[99, 101] Isoniazid metabolism is dependent on acetylator phenotype. Patients who are fast acetylators of isoniazid normally have a half-life of 1.5 hours; anephric fast acetylators will have half-lives in the range of 2.5 hours.[99, 100] Slow acetylators may have normal half-lives in the range of 5.0 hours; anephric slow acetylators may have prolonged half-lives of 10.7 hours. Since isoniazid is eliminated primarily through extrarenal mechanisms, no dosage modification in patients with mild or moderate renal failure is necessary.[1, 99] Patients with severe renal failure usually require no dosage modification, but small reductions of dose in anephric slow acetylators may be warranted (200 mg/day). Peritoneal dialysis removes less than 20 ml/min of isoniazid.[101-103] Hemodialysis may remove significant portions of isoniazid, and supplementation following dialysis may be necessary.[1, 102] Hepatic metabolism of isoniazid accounts for 65 to 95 per cent of a given dose (average 80 per cent); therefore, dosage modification in patients with severe hepatic failure may be indicated.[11, 100] Isoniazid half-life has been reported to increase in patients with severe liver dysfunction (up to 6.7 hours). Accumulation and toxicity of isoniazid may occur in these patients if dosage adjustment is not initiated.

Rifampin is eliminated primarily through extrarenal pathways; less than 15 per cent of rifampin is excreted unchanged in the urine.[104-106] Dosage modification of rifampin in patients with severe renal failure, therefore, is unnecessary.[1] Peritoneal dialysis and hemodialysis remove insignificant amounts of rifampin. Hepatic metabolism accounts for 85 to 95 per cent elimination of a rifampin dose. Since rifampin undergoes extensive intrahepatic circulation, severe hepatic failure or biliary obstruction may result in accumulation of rifampin in the serum.[104-106] Dosage adjustment in these patients may be necessary to avoid drug accumulation and toxicity.

Ethambutol is eliminated primarily through renal pathways; unchanged urinary ethambutol excretion accounts for 65 to 80 per cent of total drug administered.[107-109] Twenty per cent of ethambutol is excreted unchanged in the feces. Accumulation of ethambutol may occur in patients with moderate to severe renal failure; therefore, dosage adjustment is necessary in these patients. Patients with GFR of 10 to 50 ml/min should have a reduction in normal maintenance dose (15 to 25 mg/kg/day) by 50 per cent or dosage interval increased to every 36 hours. When GFR falls to < 10 ml/min, the normal maintenance dose should be decreased by 75 per cent or dosage interval increased to every 48 hours. Significant amounts of ethambutol are removed by hemodialysis (35 ml/min).[1, 108] Both peritoneal and hemodialysis remove approximately 35 per cent of administered ethambutol. Liver metabolism accounts for only 8 to 15 per cent of a given ethambutol dose. Dosage modification in patients with severe hepatic disease has not been necessary.

POLYMYXINS

Polymyxin B and colistimethate (polymyxin E) pharmacokinetics have not been studied extensively. The main route of elimination for polymyxins is through renal pathways. These drugs may be extremely ototoxic and nephrotoxic in patients with renal failure; therefore, avoidance of these drugs in patients with renal failure is generally recommended.[110-112]

Polymyxin B is predominantly handled by renal elimination, 60 per cent being excreted unchanged in the urine. The normal half-life of Polymyxin B (4.5 to 6.0 hours) may be increased in anephric patients to 36 hours. A dosage of 1 mg/kg every 3 days should be used in patients with GFR < 50 ml/min. In patients with GFR < 20 ml/min, a dosage of 1 mg/kg every 5 to 7 days should be used.[110] Peritoneal and hemodialysis remove insignificant portions of polymyxin B from the plasma. Patients with hepatic failure do not require dosage adjustment, as polymyxin B is almost exclusively eliminated via renal excretion.

Colistimethate is eliminated approximately 60 to 75 per cent as unchanged drug in the urine. Because of its marked nephro- and ototoxicity, colistimethate should be avoided in patients with severe renal failure.[111-113] Its administration in patients with decreased renal function requires dosage and dosing interval adjustment. The normal half-life of 1.5 to 8.0 hours may increase in anephric patients to 10 to 20 hours. Patients with GFR of 10 to 50 ml/min require a 25 to 50 per cent reduction in maintenance dose, and dosing interval should be increased to an every 3- to 5-day schedule. Severe renal failure requires a 75 per cent reduction in colistimethate doses with a dosing interval of 3 to 5 days.[111-113]

Hemodialysis does not remove significant amounts of colistimethate from the plasma. Peritoneal dialysis may remove small portions (10 ml/min). Peritoneal dialysis has been reported to remove 1 mg/hr of colistimethate. Hepatic metabolism and/or tissue inactivation account for only 25 to 50 per cent of drug elimination. The total contribution of liver inactivation is unknown. Dosage adjustment in patients with hepatic disease has not been studied, but modification of dosage schedules in these patients would not be anticipated.

ANTIVIRAL AGENTS

Amantadine and vidarabine (Vira-A) are the most widely used antiviral agents. Interferon is also included in this section for future reference.

Amantadine is eliminated predominantly through renal mechanisms. Ninety per cent of an administered dose is excreted unchanged in the urine.[114-116] Dosage modification in patients with moderate to severe renal failure, therefore, should be considered. Guidelines for amantadine use in patients with renal failure have not been established; however, accumulation and toxicity of amantadine in these patients would be anticipated and a reduced dosage or an increased dosage interval should be considered.[114-116] Hemodialysis removes very small amounts of amantadine from the serum (67 ml/min).[114] There is little evidence for significant hepatic metabolism of amatadine; thus, dosage adjustment in patients with severe liver dysfunction is not necessary.

Vidarabine (Vira-A) is deaminated in the peripheral tissues to arabinosylhypoxanthine, an active metabolite.[117] Forty-one to 53 per cent of this active metabolite is excreted in the urine. Vidarabine, as unchanged drug, accounts for only 1 to 3 per cent of total dose excreted in the urine.[117,118] Patients with renal disease should be monitored for accumulation of vidarabine's active metabolite. No guidelines have been established for dosage changes in patients with renal failure, but adjustment of dose or dosing interval should be considered in patients with severe kidney dysfunction.[117,118] Hepatic metabolism of vidarabine has not been established, but phosphorylation in the peripheral tissues has been shown to inactivate large amounts of vidarabine. Liver contribution to vidarabine inactivation is not expected to be significant; therefore, dosage modification in patients with severe liver failure would seem unnecessary.

Interferon is inactivated by many normal body fluids (saliva, serum, bile, urine, and stool).[119,120] Since these normal biologic fluids may inactivate interferon, little of the drug is excreted as the unchanged compound.[120,121] No data are available on dosage adjustment in patients with renal disease; however, based on interferon's extensive inactivation by physiologic fluids, dosage changes in renal failure would not be anticipated.[119-121] No data are available on removal of interferon by peritoneal dialysis or hemodialysis. Owing to its inactivation by normal body fluids, dosage modification of interferon in patients with hepatic disease is not necessary.

ANTIHELMINTICS

Few pharmacokinetic data are available on pyrvinum pamoate, mebendazole, thiobendazole, and quinacrine. However, these drugs do appear to be eliminated primarily through extrarenal mechanisms.

Pyrvinium pamoate is excreted less than 1 per cent as unchanged drug in the urine.[122] Dosage adjustment in patients with renal failure, therefore, would not be anticipated. Peritoneal dialysis and hemodialysis would not be expected to remove large portions of pyrvinium pamoate. The per cent of hepatic metabolism of pyrvinium pamoate has not been established, but a significant portion of the drug may be metabolized by the liver or eliminated through tissue inactivation.[122] Patients with severe liver dysfunction should be monitored closely for drug accumulation, and dosage modification of pyrvinium pamoate may be necessary in these patients.

Mebendazole is excreted less than 10 per cent as unchanged drug in the urine.[123] Dosage changes in patients with severe kidney disease, therefore, would not be anticipated. Hepatic metabolism accounts for 90 per cent of a given mebendizole dose. Twenty per cent of mebendazole metabolites are excreted as inactive decarbamated compounds and 75 per cent of a mebendazole dose is excreted as unidentified metabolites.[123] Hepatic dysfunction may lead to mebendazole accumulation, and dosage modification in these patients may be necessary. Guidelines for dosage modification, however, have not been established in patients with liver disease.

Thiobendazole is excreted less than 1 per cent as unchanged drug in the urine and 9 per cent is excreted unchanged in the feces.[124] Based on the small portion of thiobendazole excreted in the urine as unchanged drug, dosage modification in patients with severe renal insufficiency would not seem necessary. No data are available on thiobendazole's dialyzability. Approximately 90 per cent of thiobendazole is metabolized by hepatic mechanisms.[124] The metabolites do not possess significant antihelmintic activity. Accumulation of thiobendazole, therefore, may be anticipated in patients with severe liver dysfunction. Decreases in normal maintenance doses or an increase in the normal dosing interval thus may be necessary for patients with severe liver disease.

Quinacrine is rapidly metabolized by peripheral hydroxylase enzymes to hydroxyacridine.[125] No data are available on quinacrine's elimination in the urine. The metabolite hydroxyacridine is reported to be 88 per cent of a quinacrine dose in the serum.[125] The antihelmintic activity and toxicity of this metabolite are not known. Dosing guidelines in patients with renal failure have not been established, but dosage adjustment in patients with renal disease would not seem necessary. Guidelines for peritoneal and hemodialysis of quinacrine have not been reported. Dosage modification in patients with hepatic insufficiency has not been studied in patients receiving quinacrine. However, because of its peripheral inactivation, accumulation of quinacrine in patients with hepatic failure would seem unlikely, and dosage modification in severe hepatic disease would not seem necessary.

TABLE 13–2. RENAL EXCRETION OF ANTIBIOTIC AGENTS

Minimal Renal Excretion: No Dosage Adjustment Necessary (GFR 10 ml/min)		
Isoxazolyl Penicillins	Sulfasalazine	Vidarabine (Vira-A)
Oxacillin	Erythromycin	Interferon
Cloxacillin	Chloramphenicol	Thiobendazole
Dicloxacillin	Clindamycin	Mebendazole
Nafcillin	Griseofulvin	Pyrvinium pamoate
Minocycline	Miconazole	Quinacrine
Doxycycline	Rifampin	
Mild-Moderate Renal Excretion: Dosage or Dosage Interval Adjustment Necessary with Marked Decreases in Creatinine Clearance (GFR 10–30 ml/min)		
Penicillins	Cephalosporins	Sulfisoxazole
Penicillin G	Cephalothin	Sulfamethoxazole
Ampicillin	Cefazolin	Trimethoprim
Cyclacillin	Cefamandole	Lincomycin
Amoxicillin	Cephalexin	Metronidazole
Carbenicillin	Cephapirin	Amphotericin B
Tricarcillin	Cefaclor	Isoniazid
Methicillin	Cephradine	Ethambutol
	Cephaloglycin	Chloroquine
	Cephadroxil	
	Cefoxitin	
Substantial Renal Excretion: Dosage or Dosage Interval Adjustment Necessary with Moderate-Minimal Decreases in Creatinine Clearance (GFR 30–75 ml/min)		
Aminoglycosides	Cephaloridine	Oxolinic acid
Gentamicin	Tetracycline HCl	Methenamine
Tobramycin	Vancomycin	5-Fluorocytosine
Kanamycin	Colistimethate	Amantadine
Amikacin	Polymyxin B	
Neomycin	Nitrofurantoin	
Streptomycin	Nalidixic acid	

TABLE 13–3. HEPATIC METABOLISM OF ANTIBIOTIC AGENTS

Minimal Hepatic Metabolism: No Dosage Adjustment Necessary in Severe Hepatic Failure		
Penicillins (All except Oxacillin and Nafcillin)	Vancomycin	Amantadine
Cephalosporins (All except Cephalothin and Cephradine)	Colistimethate	Vidarabine (Vira-A)
Aminoglycosides (All except Streptomycin?)	Polymyxin B	Interferon
Trimethoprim	Methenamine	Quinacrine
	5-Fluorocytosine	Chloroquine?
	Ethambutol	
Moderate to Substantial Hepatic Metabolism: Dosage or Dosage Interval Adjustment Necessary with Moderate to Severe Liver Disease		
Oxacillin*	Metronidazole*	Oxolinic acid
Nafcillin*	Sulfisoxazole	Thiobendazole
Streptomycin	Sulfamethoxazole	Mebendazole
Cephalothin	Sulfasalazine	Pyrvinium pamoate
Cephapirin	Erythromycin*	
Tetracycline HCl	Chloramphenicol*	
Minocycline*	Clindamycin*	
Doxycycline*	Lincomycin	
Rifampin*	Nitrofurantoin	
Isoniazid*	Nalidixic acid	

*Drugs documented to have significantly prolonged $t^{1/2}$ and drug accumulation (increased toxicity) in patients with significant hepatic dysfunction.

ANTIMALARIAL AGENTS

Chloroquine is the most common antimalarial agent used today. The major route of chloroquine elimination is through renal mechanisms.[126, 127] Thirty-nine per cent of chloroquine is excreted unchanged in the urine and 10 per cent is excreted unchanged in the feces.[126] Accumulation of chloroquine in the serum is seen in patients with severe renal failure. Patients with GFR of 10 to 50 ml/min should have a decrease in the normal dosage to 150 mg/day. Patients with GFR < 10 ml/min should have a further decrease in dose to 50 to 100 mg/day.[1] Chloroquine does exhibit dose-dependent kinetics; i.e., as a dose increases the drug's half-life will also increase.[127] Patients receiving large single doses of chloroquine and having concomitant renal failure, therefore, may be at increased risk of developing chloroquine toxicity. Chloroquine is poorly hemodialyzed, with less than 5 per cent of chloroquine removed after a 6-hour hemodialysis treatment.[128] Chloroquine is concentrated in red blood cells (four times higher than serum) and has a large volume of distribution in the body. These two factors make hemodialysis ineffective in patients with chloroquine overdose.[128] Hepatic metabolism accounts for approximately 18 per cent of total dose eliminated. Activity of chloroquine's three metabolites is unknown.[126] No data on dosage modification in patients with hepatic failure are available; however, based on pharmacokinetic data, patients with severe hepatic failure would not require dosage modification. However, 33 per cent of the total chloroquine dose administered has an unknown fate.[126]

REFERENCES

1. Bennett WM, Muthers RS, Parker RA, et al.: Drug therapy in renal failure: dosing guidelines for adults. Ann. Intern. Med. *93*(Part I):62–83, 1980.
2. Pagliaro LA, Benet LZ: Critical compilation of terminal half-lives, percent excreted unchanged, and changes of half-life in renal and hepatic dysfunction for studies in humans with references. J. Pharmacokinet. and Biopharm. *3*:333–383, 1975.
3. Bryan CS, Stone WJ: Comparably massive penicillin G therapy in renal failure. Ann. Intern. Med. *82*:189–195, 1975.
4. Cole M, Kenig MD, Hewitt VA: Metabolism of penicillin to penicilloic acids and 6-aminopenicillanic acid in man and its significance in assessing penicillin absorption. Antimicrob. Agents Chemother. *3*:463–468, 1973.
5. Bulger RJ, Lindholm DD, Murray JS, et al.: Affect of uremia in methicillin and oxacillin blood levels. J.A.M.A. *187*:319–322, 1964.
6. Thijssen HW, Mattie H: Active metabolites of isoxazolylpenicillins in humans. Antimicrob. Agents Chemother. *10*:441–446, 1976.
7. Marshall JP, Salt WB, Elam RO: Disposition of nafcillin in patients with cirrhosis and extrahepatic biliary obstruction. Gastroenterology *73*:1388–1392, 1977.
8. Verbist L: Triple cross-over study on absorption and excretion of ampicillin, pivampicillin and amoxycillin. Antimicrob. Agents Chemother. *6*:588–593, 1974.
9. Lawson DH, Henderson AK, McGeachy RR: Amoxicillin: Pharmacokinetics study in normal subjects, patients with pernicious anemia and those with renal failure. Postgrad. Med. J. *50*:500–503, 1974.
10. Hertz CG: Serum and urinary concentrations of cyclacillin in humans. Antimicrob. Agents Chemother. *4*:361–365, 1973.
11. Parry MF, Neu HC: Pharmacokinetics of ticarcillin in patients with abnormal renal function. J. Infect Dis. *133*:46–49, 1976.
12. Hoffman TA, Cestero R, Bullick WE: Pharmacodynamics and carbenicillin in hepatic and renal failure. Ann. Intern. Med. *73*:173–178, 1970.
13. Bond JM, Lighbown JW, Barber M, et al.: A comparison of four phenoxypenicillins. Br. Med. J. *2*:956–961, 1963.
14. Whelton A, Sapir, DG, Carter CG, et al.: Intrarenal distribution of ampicillin in the normal and diseased human kidney. J. Infect. Dis. *125*:466–470, 1972.
15. Barza M, Miao PV: Antimicrobial spectrum, pharmacology and therapeutic use of antibiotics. Part 3: Chephalosporins. Am. J. Hosp. Pharm. *34*:621–629, 1977.
16. Nightingale CG, Greene DS, Quintiliani R: Pharmacokinetics and clinical use of cephalosporin antibiotics. J. Pharm. Sci. *64*:1899–1927, 1975.
17. Kirby WM, Demaine JB, Serrill WS: Pharmacokinetics of the cephalosporins in healthy volunteers and uremic patients. Postgrad. Med. J. *47*(Suppl.):41–46, 1971.
18. Andriole VT: Pharmacokinetics of cephalosporins in patients with normal or reduced renal function. J. Infect. Dis. *137*(Suppl):S88–S97, 1978.
19. Barza M, Melethil S, Berger S, et al.: Comparative pharmacokinetics of cefamandole, cephapirin, and cephalothin in healthy subjects and effect of repeated dosing. Antimicrob. Agents Chemother. *10*:421–425, 1976.
20. Reisberg BD, Mandelbaum J: Celphalexin: Absorption and excretion as related to renal function and hemodialysis. Infect. Immun. *3*:540–543, 1971.
21. McCloskey R, Terry E, McCracken A, et al.: Effect of hemodialysis in renal failure on serum and urine concentrations of cephapirin sodium. Antimicrob. Agents Chemother. *1*:90–93, 1972.
22. Kabins SA, Cohen S: Cephalothin serum concentrations in the azotemic patient. *In* Antimicrobial Agents and Chemotherapy. (JC Sylvester, ed.). Ann Arbor, Mich.: American Society of Microbiology, 1964, pp. 207–214.
23. Venuto RC, Plaut ME: Cephalothin handling in patients undergoing hemodialysis. *In* Antimicrobial Agents and Chemotherapy. (GL Hobby, ed.). Ann Arbor, Mich.: American Society of Microbiology, 1970, pp. 50–52.
24. Zaki A, Schreiber EC, Weliky I, et al.: Clinical pharmacology of oral cephradine. J. Clin. Pharmacol. *14*:118–126, 1974.
25. Finkelstein E, Quintiliani R, Lee R, et al.: Pharmacokinetics of oral cephalosporins: cephradine and cephalexin. J. Pharm. Sci. *67*:1447–1450, 1978.
26. Solomon AE, Buggs JD, McGleachy R, et al.: The administration of cephradine to patients in renal failure. Br. J. Clin. Pharmacol. *2*:443–448, 1975.

27. Welling PG, Craig WA, Amidon GL, et al.: Pharmacokinetics of cefazolin in normal and uremic subjects. Clin. Pharmacol. Ther. *15*:344–353, 1974.
28. Mellin HE, Welling PG, Madsen PO: Pharmcokinetics of cefamandole in patients with normal and impaired renal function. Antimicrob. Agents Chemother. *11*:262–266, 1977.
29. Fillastre JP, Leroy A, Godin M, et al.: Pharmacokinetics of cefoxitin sodium in normal subjects and uremic patients. J. Antimicrob. Chemother. *4*(Suppl. B):79–83, 1978.
30. Goodwin CS, Raftery EB, Goldberg AD, et al.: Effects of rate of infusion and probenecid on serum level, renal excretion, and tolerance of intravenous cefoxitin in humans: comparison with cephalothin. Antimicrob. Agents Chemother. *6*:338–346, 1974.
31. Sonneville PF, Kartodirdjo RR, Skeggs H, et al.: Comparative clinical pharmacology of intravenous cefoxitin and cephalothin. Eur. J. Clin. Pharmacol. *9*:397–403, 1976.
32. Levison ME, Santoro J, Agarwal BN: In vitro activity and pharmacokinetics of cefaclor in normal volunteers and patients with renal failure. Postgrad. Med. J. *55*(Suppl. 4):12–16, 1979.
33. Berman SJ, Boughton WH, Sugihara JG, Wong ECG: Pharmacokinetics of cefaclor in patients with end stage renal disease and during dialysis. Antimicrob. Agents Chemother. *14*:281–283, 1978.
34. Cutler, RE, Blair AD, Kelly MR: Cefadroxil kinetics in patients with renal insufficiency. Clin. Pharmacol. Ther. *25*:514–521, 1979.
35. Humbert G, Leroy A, Fillastre JP, et al.: Pharmacokinetics of cefadroxil in normal subjects and in patients with renal insufficiency. Chemotherapy *25*:189–195, 1979.
36. Pryor J, Joekes A, Foord R: Cephaloridine excretion in patients with normal and impaired renal function. Postgrad. Med. J. *43*(Suppl.):82–85, 1967.
37. Dahlgren JG, Anderson ET, Hewitt WL: Gentamicin blood levels: A guide to nephrotoxicity. Antimicrob. Agents Chemother. *8*:58–62, 1975.
38. Hull, JH, Sarubbi FA: Gentamicin serum concentrations: Pharmacokinetic predictions. Ann. Intern. Med. *85*:183–189, 1976.
39. Halpren BA, Axline SG, Coplon NS, et al.: Clearance of gentamicin during hemodialysis: comparison of four artificial kidneys. J. Infect. Dis. *133*:627–636, 1976.
40. Jaffee G, Meyers BR, Hirschman SZ: Pharmacokinetics of tobramycin in patients with stable renal impairment, patients undergoing peritoneal dialysis, and patients on chronic hemodialysis. Antimicrob. Agents Chemother. *5*:611–616, 1974.
41. Schentag JJ, Lasezkay G, Cumbo TJ, et al.: Accumulation pharmacokinetics of tobramycin. Antimicrob. Agents Chemother. *13*:649–656, 1978.
42. Reguer L, Colding H, Jensen H, et al.: Pharmacokinetics of amikacin during hemodialysis and peritoneal dialysis. Antimicrob. Agents Chemother. *11*:214–218, 1977.
43. McHenry MC, Wagner JG, Hall PM, et al.: Pharmacokinetics of amikacin in patients with impaired renal function. J. Infect. Dis. *135*(Suppl.):S343–S354, 1976.
44. Healy JK, Drum PJ, Elliot AJ: Kanamycin dosage in renal failure. Aust. N.Z. J. Med. *3*:474–479, 1973.
45. Edwards KOG, Whyte HM: Streptomycin poisoning in renal failure: an indication for treatment with an artificial kidney. Br. Med. J. *1*:752–754, 1959.
46. Last PM, Sherlock S: Systemic absorption of orally administered neomycin in liver disease. N. Engl. J. Med. *262*:385–389, 1960.
47. Whelton A: Tetracyclines in renal insufficiency: Resolution of a therapeutic dilemma. Bull. N.Y. Acad. Med. *54*:223–236, 1978.
48. Heaney D, Eknoyan G: Minocycline and doxycycline kinetics in chronic renal failure. Clin. Pharmacol. Ther. *24*:233–239, 1978.
49. McHenry TL, Gavan DG, Vidt S, et al.: Minocycline in renal failure. Clin. Pharmacol. Ther. *13*:146, 1972.
50. Kunin CM, Dornbush AC, Finland M: Distribution and excretion of four tetracycline analogues in normal young men. Clin. Invest. *38*:1950–1963, 1959.
51. Barza M, Schiefe T: Antimicrobial spectrum, pharmacology and therapeutic use of antibiotics. Part I: Tetracyclines. Am. J. Hosp. Pharm. *34*:49–57, 1977.
52. Lloyd-Still JD, Grand RJ, Vawter GF: Tetracycline hepatoxocity in the differential diagnosis of postoperative jaundice. J. Pediatr. *84*:366–370, 1974.
53. Kaplan SA, Weinfeld RE, Abruzzo CW, et al.: Pharmacokinetic profile of sulfisoxazole following intravenous, intramuscular, and oral administration to man. J. Pharm. Sci. *61*:773–778, 1972.
54. Bourgault A, Van Scoy RE, Brewer NS, et al.: Trimethoprim and sulfamethoxazole for treatment of infection with pneumocystis carinii in renal insufficiency. Chest *74*:91–92, 1978.
55. Craig, WA, Kunin CM: Trimethoprim-sulfamethoxazole: Pharmacodynamic effects of urinary pH and impaired renal function. Ann. Intern. Med. *78*:491–497, 1973.
56. Peppercorn MA, Goldman P: Distribution studies of salicylazosulfapyridine and its metabolite. Gastroenterology *64*:240–245, 1973.
57. Sigel CPW, Grace ME, Nichol CA: Metabolism of trimethoprim in man and measurement of a new metabolite: A new fluorescence assay. J. Infect. Dis. *128*(Suppl.):S580–S583, 1973.
58. Sabath, LD, Gerstein DA, Loder PB, et al.: Excretion of erythromycin and its enhanced activity in urine against gram negative bacilli with alkalinization. J. Lab. Clin. Med. *72*:916–923, 1968.
59. Lee CC, Anderson RC, Chen KK: Renal clearance of erythromycin. Proc. Soc. Exp. Biol. Med. *88*:584–586, 1955.
60. Knothe H, Dette GA: Pharmacokinetics of erythromycin. Scott. Med. J. *22*:397–400, 1977.
61. McGehee RF, Smith CB, Wilcox C, et al.: Comparative studies of antimicrobial activity in vitro and absorption and excretion of lincomycin and clinimycin. Am. J. Med. Sci. *256*:279–292, 1968.
62. Malacoff RF, Finkelstein FO, Andriole VT: Affect of peritoneal dialysis on serum levels of tobramycin and lincomycin. Antimicrob. Agents Chemother. *8*:574–580, 1975.
63. Keusch GT, Present DH: Summary of a workshop

on clindamycin colitis. J. Infect. Dis. *133*:578–587, 1976.
64. Williams DN, Crossley K, Hoffman C, et al.: Parenteral clindamycin phosphate: Pharmacology with normal and abnormal liver function and effect of nasal staphylococci. Antimicrob. Agents Chemother. *7*:153–158, 1975.
65. Peddie DA, Dann E, Bailey RR: The effect of impairment of renal function and dialysis on the serum and urine levels of clindamycin. Aust. N.Z. J. Med. *5*:198–202, 1975.
66. Joshi AM, Stein RM: Altered serum clearance of intravenously administered clindamycin phosphate in patients with uremia. J. Clin. Pharmacol. *14*:140–144, 1974.
67. Kunin CM, Glazko AJ, Finland M: Persistance of antibiotics in blood of patients with acute renal failure. Part 2: Chloramphenicol and its metabolic products in blood of patients with severe renal disease or hepatic cirrhosis. J. Clin. Invest. *38*:1498–1508, 1959.
68. Lindberg AA, Nilsson LH, Bucht H, et al.: Concentration of chloramphenicol in the urine and blood in relation to renal function. Br. Med. J. *2*:724–728, 1966.
69. Wheller LA, Demeo M, Halula M, et al.: Use of high pressure liquid chemotography to determine plasma levels of metronidazole and metabolites after IV administration. Antimicrob. Agents Chemotherapy *13*:205–209, 1978.
70. Ralph ED, Clarke JT, Libke RD, et al.: Pharmacokinetics of metronidazole as determined by bioassay. Antimicrob. Agents Chemother. *6*:691–696, 1974.
71. Ralph ED, Kirby WM: Bioassay of metronidazole with either anaerobic or aerobic incubation. J. Infect. Dis. *132*:587–591, 1975.
72. Lindholm DD, Murray JS: Persistance of vancomycin in the blood during renal failure and its treatment by hemodialysis. N. Engl. J. Med. *274*:1047–1051, 1966.
73. Krogstad DJ, Moellering RC, Greenblatt DJ: Single dose kinetics of intravenous vancomycin. J. Clin. Pharmacol. *74*:197–201, 1980.
74. Gambertoglio J: Dosage of vancomycin. (Letter.) Mayo Clin. Proc. *53*:197–198, 1978.
75. Eykyn S, Phillips I, Evans J: Vancomycin for staphylococcal shunt site infections in patients on regular hemodialysis. Br. Med. J. *3*:80–86, 1970.
76. Reckendorf HK, Castringius RG, Spingler HK: Comparative pharmacodynamics, urinary excretion and half-life determinations of nitrofurantoin sodium. *In* Antimicrobial Agents and Chemotherapy (JC Sylvester, ed.). Ann Arbor, Mich.: American Society of Microbiology, 1964, pp. 531–537.
77. Felts JH, Hayes DM, Gergen JA, et al.: Neurohematologic and bacteriologic effects of nitrofurantoin in renal insufficiency. Am. J. Med. *51*:331–339, 1971.
78. Loughridge LW: Peripheral neuropathy due to nitrofurantoin. Lancet *2*:1133–1135, 1962.
79. Goff JB, Schleger JU, O'Dell RM: Urinary excretion of nalidixic acid, sulfamethoxazole, and nitrofurantoin with reduced renal function. J. Urol. *99*:371–375, 1968.
80. Portmann GA, McChesney EW, More WE: Pharmacokinetic model for nalidixic acid in man. Part I: Kinetic pathway for hydroxynalidixic acid. Part II: Parameters for absorption, metabolism and excretion. J. Pharm. Sci. *55*:59–62, 72–78, 1966.
81. Adams WR, Dawborn JK: Plasma levels and urinary excretion of nalidixic acid in patients with renal failure. Aust. N.Z. J. Med. *17*:126–131, 1971.
82. Mannisto PT: Pharmacokinetics of nalidixic acid and oxolinic acid in healthy women. Clin. Pharmacol. Ther. *19*:37–46, 1976.
83. Dicarlo RJ, Crew MC, Melgar MD, et al.: Oxolinic acid metabolism by man. Arch. Int. Pharmacodyn. Ther. *174*:413–427, 1968.
84. Scudi JB, Reinhard JF: Absorption, distribution and renal excretion of mandelamine. J. Lab. Clin. Med. *33*:1304–1310, 1948.
85. Knight V, Draper JW, Brady EA, et al.: Methenamine mandelate: Antimicrobial activity, absorption and excretion. Antimicrob. Agents Chemother. *2*:615–635, 1952.
86. Musher DM, Griffith DP: Generation of formaldehyde from methenamine: effect of pH and concentration, and antibacterial effect. Antimicrob. Agents Chemother. *6*:708–711, 1974.
87. Bindschandler DD, Bnnett JE: A pharmacologic guide to the clinical use of amphotericin B. J. Infect. Dis. *120*:427–436, 1969.
88. Feldman HA, Hamilton JD, Gutman RA: Amphotericin B therapy in an anephric patient. Antimicrob. Agents Chemother. *4*:302–305, 1973.
89. Block ER, Bennett JE, Livoti LG, et al.: Flucytosine and amphotericin B: hemodialysis effects on the plasma concentrations and clearance. Ann. Intern. Med. *80*:613–617, 1974.
90. Koechlin BA, Rubio F, Palmer S, et al.: The metabolism of 5-fluorocytosine-2-14-C in the rat and the disposition of 5-fluorocytosine in man. Biochem. Pharmacol. *15*:435–446, 1966.
91. Wade D, Sudlow G: The kinetics of 5-fluorocytosine elimination in man. Aust. N.Z. J. Med. *2*:153–158, 1972.
92. Dawborn JK, Page MD, Schiavone DJ: Use of 5-fluorocytosine in patients with impaired renal function. Br. Med. J. *4*:382–384, 1973.
93. Lin C, Magat J, Chang R, et al.: Absorption, metabolism and excretion of 14C-griseofulvin in man. J. Pharmacol. Exp. Ther. *187*:415–422, 1973.
94. Roth FJ, Jr.: Griseofulvin. Ann. N.Y. Acad. Sci. *89*:247–253, 1960–1961.
95. Busfield D, Child KJ, Atkinson RM, et al.: An effect of phenobarbitone on blood levels on griseofulvin in man. Lancet *2*:1042–1043, 1963.
96. Brugmans G, Van Cutsem J, Heykants J, et al.: Systemic antifungal potential, safety, biotransport and transformation and miconazole nitrate. Eur. J. Clin. Pharmacol. *5*:93–99, 1972.
97. Hoeprich PD, Goldstein E: Miconazole therapy for coccidioidomycosis. J.A.M.A. *230*:1153–1157, 1974.
98. Lewi PJ, Boelaert J, Daneels R, et al.: Pharmacokinetic profile of intravenous miconazole in man: Comparison of normal subjects and patients with renal insufficiency. Eur. J. Clin. Pharmacol. *10*:49–54, 1976.
99. Hughes HB: On the metabolic fate of isoniazid. J. Pharmacol. Exper. Ther. *109*:444–452, 1953.
100. Mitchell JR, Zimmerman HF, Ishak KG, et al.: Isoniazid liver injury: Clinical spectrum, pathol-

ogy, and probable pathogenesis. Ann. Intern. Med. *84*:181–192, 1976.

101. Bowersox DW, Winterbauer RH, Stewart GS, et al.: Isoniazid dosage in patient with renal failure. N. Engl. J. Med. *289*:84–87, 1973.
102. Sitprija V, Holmes JH: Isoniazid intoxication. Am. Rev. Resp. Dis. *90*:248–254, 1964.
103. Reidenberg MM, Shear L, Cohen RV: Elimination of isoniazid in patients with impaired renal function. Am. Rev. Resp. Dis. *108*:1426–1428, 1973.
104. Maggi N, Furesz S, Pallanza R, et al.: Rifampicin deacetylation in the human organism. Arzneim. Forsch. *19*:651–654, 1969.
105. Proust AJ: The Australian rifampicin trial. Med. J. Aust. *2*:85–94, 1971.
106. Dickinson JM, Aber VR, Allen BW, et al.: Assay of rifampicin in serum. J. Clin. Pathol. *27*:457–462, 1974.
107. Strauss I, Erhardt F: Ethambutol absorption, excretion and dosage in patients with renal tuberculosis. Chemotherapy *15*:148–157, 1970.
108. Christopher TG, Blair AD, Forrey AW, et al.: Kinetics of ethambutol elimination in renal disease. Proc. Clin. Dial. Transplant. Forum *3*:96–101, 1973.
109. Lee CS, Gambertoglio JG, Brater DC, et al.: Kinetics of oral ethambutol in normal subjects. Clin. Pharmacol. Ther. *22*:615–621, 1977.
110. Hoeprich PD: The polymyxins. Med. Clin. North Am. *54*:1257–1276, 1970.
111. Goodman NJ, Friedman EA: The effects of renal impairment, peritoneal dialysis and hemodialysis on serum colistimethate levels. Ann. Intern. Med. *68*:984–994, 1968.
112. Swick HM, Maxwell E, Charache P, et al.: Peritoneal dialysis in colistin intoxication. J. Pediatr. *74*:976–980, 1969.
113. MacKay DN, Kaye D: Serum concentrations of colistin in patients with normal and impaired renal function. N. Engl. J. Med. *270*:394–397, 1964.
114. Soung L, Ing S, Dugirdas JT, et al.: Amantadine hydrochloride pharmacokinetics in hemodialysis patients. Ann. Intern. Med. *93*(Part I):46–49, 1980.
115. Armbruster KFW, Rahn AC, Ing TS, et al.: Amantadine toxicity in a patient with renal insufficiency. Nephron *13*:183–186, 1974.
116. Ing TS, Dugirdas JT, Soung LS, et al.: Toxic effects of amantadine in patients with renal failure. Can. Med. Assoc. J. *120*:695–698, 1979.
117. Kinkel AW, Buchanan RA: Human Pharmacology. *In* Adenine Arabinoside: An Antiviral Agent (D Pavan-Langstone, RAP Buchanan, and CA Alford, eds). New York: Raven Press, 1975.
118. Glazko AJ, Change T, Drach JC, et al: Species differences in the metabolic disposition of adenine arabinoside. *In* Adenine Arabinoside: An Antiviral Agent (D Pavan-Langston, RA Buchanan, CA Alford, eds.). New York: Raven Press, 1975.
119. Hirsch MS, Swritz MN: Antiviral agents. N. Engl. J. Med. *302*:903–907; 949–953, 1980.
120. Merigan TC: Pharmacokinetics and side effects of interferon in man. Tex. Rep. Biol. Med. *35*:541–547, 1977.
121. Pollard RB, Merigan TC: Experience with clinical applications of interferon and interferon inducers. Pharmacol. Ther. *2*:783–811, 1978.
122. Buchanan RA, Barrow WB, Heffelfinger JC, et al.: Pyrvinium pamoate. Clin. Pharmacol. Ther. *16*:716–719, 1974.
123. Brugmans JP, Thienpont DC, Wijngaarden ID, et al.: Mebendazole in enterobiasis: Radiochemical and pilot clinical study in 1,278 subjects. J.A.M.A. *217*:313–316, 1971.
124. Tocco DJ, Rosenblum D, Martin CM, et al.: Absorption, metabolism, and excretion of thiobendazole in man and laboratory animals. Toxicol. Appl. Pharmacol. *9*:31–39, 1966.
125. Tsou KC, Ledis S, Steiger E, et al.: Facile preparation of 6-chloro-9-amino-2-hydroxyacridine, a urinary metabolite of quinacrine and quinacrine mustard. J. Pharm. Sci. *64*:1418–1419, 1975.
126. Frish-Holmberg M, Bergkvist Y, Domeij-Nyberg B, et al.: Chloroquine serum concentrations and side effects: Evidence for dose-dependent kinetics. Clin. Pharmacol. Ther. *25*:345–350, 1979.
127. VanStone JC: Hemodialysis and chloroquine poisoning. J. Lab. Clin. Med. *88*:87–90, 1976.
128. Johnson WD, Appelstein JM, Kaye J: Cephaloglycin. J.A.M.A. *206*:2698–2702, 1968.

Chapter 14

Analgesics, Sedatives, and Sedative-Hypnotics

by

Melton B. Affrime
and David T. Lowenthal

Renal and hepatic disease both present complex situations that modify pharmacokinetic responses to drugs. Thus, the incidence of adverse drug reactions is increased in patients with renal and hepatic disease.[1-4] In many instances, these adverse drug reactions are related to diminished metabolism, altered elimination of the parent compound, and retention of toxic metabolites. Many of the adverse responses that occur when drugs are administered to patients with kidney and liver disease involve analgesics and sedative-hypnotic agents.[5-7] This chapter will, therefore, provide a comprehensive review of the clinical pharmacology of these agents.

When the kidney serves as the major pathway of drug elimination, any alteration of renal function results in parallel changes in creatinine clearance and drug kinetic parameters. Several of the drugs cited in this chapter require modification of the dosage, and careful monitoring for toxic effects when used in renal failure. This is particularly important for drugs with a low therapeutic ratio that are eliminated mainly unchanged by the kidneys or those that are metabolized to polar moieties that are pharmacologically active. As mentioned in Chapter 2, this dosage alteration should take into account changes in renal function as well as the effects of dialysis. Those agents eliminated by a compensatory route (e.g., bile) or those that have a large therapeutic ratio can generally be used without dosage modification. However, in many cases, unexplained symptoms in the seriously ill patient with renal failure may still be due to unrecognized or unexpected drug toxicity.[8] Therefore, it must be stressed that drugs should be used only if there is a definite indication and therapy is monitored appropriately.

While an accurate assessment of the severity of the liver disease is essential, unlike renal disease, there is no simple test of hepatic function that enables the therapeutic regimen to be easily adjusted for all drugs predominantly metabolized by the liver. It is thought that the liver has a great reserve capacity and it is only in severe liver disease, particularly cirrhosis, that problems in therapy may occur owing to decreases in rate of biotransformation or increases in oral bioavailability. However, it is important to recognize that even mild degrees of liver abnormalities may occasionally alter pharmacologic response to a drug.[8-14] As a general rule, adverse reactions are most likely to occur when drugs with either a low therapeutic ratio or with potential for enhancement of effect are administered to patients with advanced liver disease.

James[12] described sound guidelines for the use of drugs in patients with liver disease:

1. As in all therapeutic decisions, evaluate the possible benefit-to-risk ratio. If risk outweighs benefits, do not prescribe the drug.

2. If possible, select drugs that have no potential for hepatotoxicity.

3. If possible, select drugs that are mainly eliminated unchanged by the kidney.

4. Avoid drugs that have an effect on the central nervous system.
5. Start treatment with small doses.
6. Clinical and laboratory observations, including estimations of the plasma drug concentrations when feasible, provide the best means for adjusting dosing regimens in patients with impaired or fluctuating liver function.

Since this chapter deals with agents that have central nervous system depression as either an intended or a predictable pharmacologic effect, further nervous system depression often arises when these agents are administered to patients with severe liver disease. Thus, patients in hepatic coma or precoma are known to be extremely sensitive to drugs such as morphine and barbiturates, contraindicating their use under such circumstances.[13, 14]

ANALGESICS

SALICYLATES

The complex pharmacokinetics of salicylate elimination involve two saturable pathways and three linear, parallel pathways. The nonlinearity of the saturable pathways makes it difficult to predict the pharmacokinetic implications of changes in the dosing regimen of salicylate without direct clinical trials. There are also nonlinear relationships between salicylate dose and steady-state salicylate level, as well as dose-dependent changes in the time required to attain steady state and in percentage of protein binding.[16] However, with careful monitoring of serum salicylate concentration, and careful attention to dosage interval and body weight, salicylates can be used with great versatility.[17]

Individuals with normal hepatic and renal function have been observed to attain plateau serum salicylate concentrations that correlate better with urinary excretion of the capacity-limited biotransformation product, salicylurate, than with the total urinary excretion of salicylates.[18] Brodie and his group studied the metabolism of salicylates in patients with Laennec's cirrhosis diagnosed on clinical grounds and found the half-life of acetylsalicylic acid to be unaltered.[19]

Lowenthal et al. studied the kinetics of salicylate elimination in six anephric patients following intravenous 500 mg sodium salicylate per 1.73 sq mm of body surface area.[20] Detailed pharmacokinetic analysis revealed no significant differences in apparent volume of distribution and elimination rate constants between the anephric patients and normal adult subjects. Metabolism of salicylate in the anephric patients, determined by the rate of formation of salicyluric acid from salicylate, was unchanged in the anephric patients. Thus, there is no pharmacokinetic basis for altering the dosage in chronic renal or hepatic disease. However, the irritative effects of salicylate on the gastric mucosa in combination with the effect of salicylate on platelet function serve as strong relative contraindications to the use of salicylates in patients with chronic renal and hepatic disease.

Salicylic acid excretion by the kidney involves glomerular filtration, active tubular secretion, and passive tubular reabsorption.[21] The latter process is dependent on the quantity of nonionized salicylate present, which is in turn dependent on the pH of the tubular fluid. When the pH of the urine is less than 6.0, clearance of salicylic acid approximates only 5 to 15 per cent of the creatinine clearance, but at a urine pH greater than 7.4 the clearance of salicylic acid is greater than the creatinine clearance.[22]

Hemodialysis readily removes salicylate with clearances of 35 to 100 ml/min reported.[23] Peritoneal dialysis removes some salicylates; in infants intoxicated with salicylate, salicylate clearances of 45 to 90 ml/hr have been reported.[24] Forced alkaline diuresis is also an efficient method of salicylate removal.[25, 26]

PROPOXYPHENE

Propoxyphene, a widely described oral analgesic agent, is metabolized entirely by hepatic biotransformation.[26] The major metabolite of D-propoxyphene, D-norpropoxyphene, has a longer biologic half-life than its precursor.[27] Elimination of propoxyphene occurs by both biliary excretion and renal excretion of drug metabolites. Consequently, norpropoxyphene accumulation is more pronounced in anephric patients.[28] Recent studies in propoxyphene-intoxicated patients suggested that the elimination kinetics are directly related to dose.[29]

In normal individuals, propoxyphene half-life values range from 6 to 18 hours. A large fraction of orally administered D-propoxyphene is biotransformed by first-pass metabolism. Thus, oral doses of propoxyphene in patients with liver disease will be associated with increased bioavailability and pharmacologic effect. Recent pharmacokinetic analyses of D-propoxyphene following both oral and intravenous administration show two- to threefold interindividual variations in systemic clearance, apparent volume of distribution, and D-propoxyphene and norpropoxyphene half-lives.[30] Because of this variability, interpretation of data in renal or hepatic disease is difficult.

Plasma protein binding of D-propoxyphene and D-norpropoxyphene is 76 per cent in normal subjects and 80 per cent in anephric patients.[31] Also, there is no correlation between the free fraction propoxyphene level and serum albumin concentrations.[31] D-Norpropoxyphene concentrations did not affect the propoxyphene plasma protein binding.[31] Very low hemodialysis clearances of D-propoxyphene and D-norpropoxyphene have been obtained.[32]

Although D-propoxyphene is extensively metabolized by the liver, this drug has not been studied in either acute or chronic hepatic insufficiency. However, it is suggested that extreme caution be exercised along with dosage modification for use in patients with hepatic disease owing to the high first-pass extraction of this agent. In addition, the central nervous system toxicity of D-propoxyphene and D-norpropoxyphene at high serum concentrations[33, 34] demands extreme care in the use of this agent in patients with kidney and liver dysfunction.

ACETAMINOPHEN

Acetaminophen (paracetamol, *N*-acetyl-para-aminophenol) is a commonly used mild analgesic and antipyretic. Alone or in combination with other drugs, it is found in the United States in more than 200 formulations promoted for symptomatic relief of pain, cough, and colds. Its popular use is partly due to low incidence of adverse effects relative to salicylates.[35]

In subjects with normal renal and hepatic function, acetaminophen is rapidly absorbed from the gastrointestinal tract, reaching peak plasma concentrations within 40 to 60 minutes of ingestion.[36] Its binding to plasma proteins is less than that of salicylates.[37] Biotransformation takes place mainly in the liver. The polar metabolites are excreted by the kidneys and elimination half-life has been found to range from 2 to 4 hours.[38-40]

Studies have indicated that following acetaminophen overdosage[41] with hepatic dysfunction,[42] the apparent elimination half-life is prolonged. Furthermore, there have been suggestions in the literature that modest dosages of acetaminophen can cause liver damage in individuals with preexistent hepatic dysfunction.[43, 44]

Lowenthal et al. studied the pharmacokinetics of acetaminophen elimination in five surgically anephric and five physiologically anephric patients on an intermittent dialysis day.[45] There were no significant differences in the biologic half-life and volume of distribution of acetaminophen when patients were compared with normal controls. However, the anephric patients, unlike the normal subjects, showed pronounced accumulation of acetaminophen glucuronide and sulfate in plasma. The authors concluded that the kidneys do not contribute significantly to the elimination of unchanged acetaminophen in humans, but do play a role in elimination of drug metabolites.

In order to determine the effect of hemodialysis on the biologic half-life of acetaminophen in anephric patients and to assess the relative efficacy of hemodialysis for the removal of acetaminophen and its glucuronide and sulfate conjugates from plasma, four anephric patients were studied during hemodialysis and on nondialysis days.[46] There was a strong correlation between the dialyzer extraction ratios of acetaminophen and urea nitrogen. Hemodialysis was the major route of elimination of acetaminophen sulfate in the anephric patients. These observations suggest that acetaminophen is substantially removed by hemodialysis.

Because acetaminophen is a known hepatotoxin[47] and because patients with hepatic disease may be more likely to develop acetaminophen hepatotoxicity, this drug should be avoided in patients with compromised hepatic function. However, there seems to be no reason to alter the dosage or to avoid the use of acetaminophen in patients with chronic renal disease. Since this drug may also be nephrotoxic (see Chap. 8), chronic use of large amounts of acetaminophen is contraindicated in patients with renal disease. Phenacetin (acetophenetidin) is an established antipyretic-analgesic that, in combination with other analgesics and caffeine, was very popular in the past. At present, it is available in only about 10 products.[48] Phenacetin is a predictable nephrotoxic agent that is metabolized to acetaminophen by the liver.[49] Thus, it should be utilized with extreme caution in patients with renal and hepatic disease.

NARCOTIC ANALGESICS

Morphine, codeine, and methadone are metabolized by the liver. The sedative effects of morphine are prolonged in animals with experimentally induced liver damage and in patients with liver disease.[50] Generally, the effects of narcotic analgesics have been shown to be prolonged in anuric patients.[51] Patients with chronic or acute renal failure receiving morphine[52] or meperidine[51] have been shown to have increased sensitivity to these narcotic analgesics, as indicated by a response to naloxone antagonism at a time when no naloxone response would be predicted. The narcotic analgesics are not removed by hemodialysis.

MORPHINE

Although detailed pharmacokinetic studies of morphine have not been done in patients with either hepatic or renal dysfunction, Olsen et al. have undertaken a study of the plasma protein binding in patients with uremia, jaundice, and hypoalbuminemia.[53] These patients were found to be very sensitive to usual clinical doses of morphine. This increased sensitivity correlated with decreased morphine binding to plasma proteins. However, until detailed pharmacokinetic studies are done in these patients precise dosage recommendations cannot be suggested.

MEPERIDINE (Demerol)

In vitro and *in vivo* animal experiments have demonstrated that the liver plays a major role in the biotransformation of meperidine.[54] These studies underscore the need for cautious use of the meperidine in patients with hepatic dysfunction.[54]

Normeperidine, one of the metabolites of meperidine biotransformation, accumulates in patients with chronic renal disease, and it has been shown to possess significant central nervous system pharmacologic activity.[55] Studies in animals have shown that this *N*-demethylated metabolite is half as potent as meperidine as an analgesic, but twice as potent as a convulsant.[56, 57]

Klotz and his group[58] studied the effects of cirrhosis on the disposition and elimination of meperidine in humans. Ten male patients with biopsy-proven cirrhosis of the liver were studied. The cirrhosis was presumed to be due to alcoholism in nine patients and the result of viral hepatitis in one patient. The patients received 0.8 mg/kg of meperidine hydrochloride by rapid intravenous injection over 1 min into an antecubital vein. Appropriate blood samples were drawn for meperidine and normeperidine assay. There were no significant correlations between the prolonged plasma half-life and decreased plasma clearance of the drug and biochemical hepatic function tests in patients with liver disease. The metabolite, normeperidine, was not detected in the plasma of either group (normal or cirrhotics). This study suggests that the prolonged elimination of meperidine in cirrhosis is due to impaired hepatic biotransformation.[57, 58]

Szeto and her group paid special attention to the *N*-demethylated metabolite of meperidine in a drug kinetic study in patients with renal failure or cancer.[59] After a dose of meperidine, meperidine blood concentration in cancer patients was 0.1 to 0.5 μg/ml 1 hour after administration and was 0.05 to 0.14 μg/ml in patients during the oliguric period after renal transplantation. Normeperidine concentrations were 0.05 to 0.29 μg/ml in these cancer patients and 0.13 to 0.36 μg/ml in the patients with renal failure. Higher normeperidine concentrations and very high normeperidine:meperidine ratios were observed in two patients receiving multiple doses of meperidine. These high ratios were associated with signs of central nervous system excitation, suggesting that normeperidine can contribute to the excitatory effects seen after multiple doses of meperidine. Thus, patients with renal failure treated with many doses of meperidine are particularly susceptible to this problem.

The disposition of parenteral meperidine in patients with hepatitis B acute viral hepatitis and in normal volunteers has been studied.[60] The terminal plasma half-life of meperidine was significantly prolonged ($p < 0.001$) in patients with acute viral hepatitis compared to the age-matched control subjects: 6.99 ± 2.74

hr versus 3.37 ± 0.82 hr, respectively (mean ± standard deviation). A similar twofold change in the total plasma clearance of the drug was observed. No significant differences occurred in either the volume of distribution of meperidine or its plasma protein binding. Normeperidine was not detected in the plasma of either group, and only small amounts of normeperidine were found in the urine. Thus, it is clear that a significant proportion of the patients with acute viral hepatitis will accumulate meperidine if this agent is administered in the standard fashion over a prolonged period.

The central role of the liver in the biotransformation of meperidine and the increasing evidence that this drug's sedative properties may precipitate hepatic encephalopathy limit the use of meperidine in patients with liver disease.

CODEINE, METHADONE, AND PENTAZOCINE

Codeine, methadone, and pentazocine are more than 80 per cent metabolized by the liver. These drugs also undergo substantial first-pass metabolism by the liver. Thus, use of these agents in patients with acute or chronic hepatic disease will be associated with increased bioavailability and can precipitate central nervous system depression and hepatic encephalopathy. Therefore, cautious use is suggested.

Codeine, pentazocine, and methadone can be used without dosage modification in renal failure, although the sedative effects may be enhanced.[61] Although methadone is partially eliminated as unchanged drug in the urine (in some cases, up to 58 per cent of the dose), accumulation may not occur in renal failure owing to increased elimination by the fecal route.[62] The major metabolites of methadone are not pharmacologically active. Methadone is not significantly removed by hemodialysis.

SEDATIVE-HYPNOTICS

BARBITURATES

PHENOBARBITAL

The clinical pharmacokinetics of phenobarbital have been studied extensively in patients with normal renal and hepatic function. However, few studies are available in patients with liver or renal disease. Lous has described elevated serum concentrations of phenobarbital in patients with liver disease.[63] The same author has also observed increased toxicity to phenobarbital in patients with renal disease.[64] Moreover, in usual circumstances, up to 50 per cent of phenobarbital is excreted unchanged in the urine.[65] Thus, patients with kidney and liver disease need dosage modification when phenobarbital is utilized.

Essentially all of the information available on dialysis of the barbiturates is derived from overdose cases. Forced alkaline diuresis can result in enhanced elimination of long-acting barbiturates. Alkalinization of the urine to a pH of greater than 7.5 has caused only a small increase in excretion of secobarbital and pentobarbital, while the excretion of phenobarbital is increased significantly. The reason for this is the greater ionization of phenobarbital at higher pH values in which the ionized form of the drug becomes unreabsorbable by the renal tubule. With a urine pH less than 7.5 and a urinary flow rate of 1 ml/min, the clearance of phenobarbital is only 2 ml/min. This clearance can be increased to greater than 15 ml/min with a urine flow of 5 to 10 ml/min and urine pH greater than 7.5.[66, 67] Clearance of pentobarbital during peritoneal dialysis has been measured at 12 ml/min and that of phenobarbital at 13 ml/min.[66] Hemodialysis is an efficient method of removal of barbiturates. Again, the short-acting barbiturates are less well removed than the long-acting compounds.[68] Clearance values during hemodialysis for various barbiturates have been reported as: pentobarbital, 42 to 55 ml/min; amobarbital, 25 ml/min; and phenobarbital, 48 to 72 ml/min.[69]

Interestingly, phenobarbital, a classic inducer of hepatic microsomal enzyme systems, has been shown to improve liver function tests in patients with cholestatic liver disease.[70] Alvin et al. studied the effect of liver disease on the disposition of phenobarbital.[71] Three groups of male individuals were studied, one group with normal hepatic function, a second group of patients with cirrhosis, and a third group of patients with acute viral hepatitis. In cirrhotic patients, plasma half-life was prolonged from 86 to 130 hr ($p < 0.0001$). In patients with acute viral hepatitis, phenobarbital half-life was not significantly prolonged and urinary excretion of phenobarbital and its metabolites was within the normal range. Thus, phenobarbital will exert a cumulative effect when administered to patients with chronic liver disease.

HEXOBARBITAL

Hexobarbital has a shorter half-life (4 hours) than phenobarbital (50 to 140 hours). The half-life of hexobarbital has been studied in patients with acute hepatitis and following apparent clinical recovery.[72] The elimination half-life was 8 hours in the hepatitis patients and 4 hours in the control group. Clearance was significantly reduced in the hepatitis group, whereas the volume of distribution at steady state was not significantly altered. In six of the patients, following recovery (as judged by normal serum transaminase and bilirubin levels), the half-life of hexobarbital was shorter and the clearance value was higher than during the acute illness. However, the values did not return to normal. This suggests that clinical recovery from liver disease is not accompanied by corresponding complete recovery of drug metabolizing capability. Based on these observations, hexobarbital should be used cautiously in patients with hepatic dysfunction. No data are available on hexobarbital use in renal disease.

THIOPENTAL

Shideman et al. demonstrated the significantly longer duration of action of a standard induction dose of thiopental (4 mg/kg) in patients with hepatic dysfunction compared with normal controls.[73] A few years later, Dundee and Richards observed that only half of the normal intravenous dose of thiopental was necessary to induce anesthesia in patients with chronic renal failure.[74] Such findings[74] caused Ghoneim and Pandya to study the plasma protein binding of thiopental in patients with impaired renal and hepatic function.[75] Following 24 hours of equilibrium dialysis, the plasma from healthy volunteers bound 72 per cent of thiopental. In plasma from patients with hepatic disease, 47 per cent of thiopental was bound, while in patients with renal disease, 46 per cent was bound. The decreased binding in uremia could not be explained completely by competitive displacement by nitrogenous end products or by hypoalbuminemia, but hypoalbuminemia appeared to account for the decreased binding in patients with cirrhosis. These data indicate that it is necessary to decrease the dose of thiopental in patients with impaired renal or hepatic dysfunction. Some of the enhanced effect of thiopental may be due to more free (unbound) active drug.

PENTOBARBITAL

The sedative-hypnotic agent pentobarbital has not been studied in patients with hepatic disease. However, it has been studied in patients with poor renal function.[76] Reidenberg et al.[76] concluded that pentobarbital elimination is normal in patients with renal failure. Moreover, some uremic patients have shortened pentobarbital plasma half-life values. These more likely result from low apparent volume of distribution with normal metabolic clearance rates rather than from accelerated metabolism of pentobarbital.

BENZODIAZEPINES

CHLORDIAZEPOXIDE (Librium)

Chlordiazepoxide has been used widely as a sedative and antianxiety agent for 20 years. It is extensively metabolized with less than 1 per cent of an administered dose appearing in the urine as the parent drug.[77] After a single dose, the major circulating metabolite is *N*-desmethylchlordiazepoxide;[78] much lower levels of a subsequent hydroxylated metabolite, demoxepam,[79] are also seen. Both of these metabolites are active in animals.[4] Additional metabolites have also been identified.[77, 80]

Greenblatt and coworkers found the apparent elimination half-life of chlordiazepoxide (17.8 ± 2.2 hr) following acute intravenous (IV) administration to be the same for males and females with normal renal and hepatic function.[81]

Roberts et al. studied the effect of age and parenchymal liver disease on the disposition and elimination of chlordiazepoxide.[82] Eight male patients, ages 40 to 61 with biopsy-proven alcoholic cirrhosis, and five patients (4 female, 1 male), ages 20 to 29, were studied during HB_sAg–positive acute viral hepatitis. Over the age range 20 to 80 years, decreases in plasma clearance from 30 ml/min to 10 ml/min (r^2, 0.71; $p < 0.01$) and increases in volume of distribution from 0.26 to 0.38 L/kg (r^2, 0.60; $p < 0.05$) were seen. Similarly, a decrease in plasma clearance in cirrhosis (7.7 ± 2.1 compared to 15.3 ± 4.4 ml/min in normals; $p < 0.01$) and an increase in the volume of distribution resulted in the prolongation of the elimination half-life in both forms of liver disease (cirrhosis and viral hepatitis). There was borderline significance in the decrease in plasma protein binding in those patients with hepatic disease (94.6 ± 2.0) and normals (96.5 ± 1.8; $p = 0.056$).

Thus, cirrhosis and acute viral hepatitis produce significantly altered disposition of chlordiazepoxide. The absence of the close correlation between the standard liver function tests and the disposition parameters of chlordiazepoxide is consistent with the observation of many investigators with most, but not all, drugs and emphasizes the difficulty of individualizing drug therapy patients with liver disease.[82, 83]

Sellers and his group also studied chlordiazepoxide disposition in 14 normal subjects and 11 patients with biopsy-proven cirrhosis following a 50-mg IV infusion over 10 min. In the cirrhotics, half-lives of chlordiazepoxide were 20 to 90 per cent longer and plasma clearance 33 to 87 per cent lower than in normals.[84] However, the extent of drug accumulation does not necessarily predict the intensity of clinical sedation, and adaptation or tolerance to central depressant effects may develop. Taken together, these observations suggest care in the use of chlordiazepoxide in patients with liver disease.

The kinetics of chlordiazepoxide have not been studied in patients with renal disease. However, little dosage modification would be anticipated. Chlordiazepoxide is not substantially removed by hemodialysis (see Chap. 20).

DIAZEPAM (Valium)

Diazepam is one of the most widely used of the benzodiazepine group of drugs. The clinical pharmacokinetics have been extensively studied.[85] In normal individuals, there is up to thirtyfold interindividual variation in dose:blood level ratios, especially following acute diazepam administration. There is accumulation of the active *N*-desmethyldiazepam during chronic treatment.[86]

In patients with liver disease, significant alterations of kinetic properties of diazepam have been observed. Diazepam is extensively metabolized by hepatic microsomal enzymes. It also exhibits capacity-limited, protein binding–sensitive hepatic clearance. Thus, it is understandable why liver disease may be associated with alterations of kinetic properties. Most of the studies of diazepam in liver disease are following acute dosage, rather than chronic dosing in which steady-state concentrations are examined. These acute studies suggest that there is a lower peak plasma concentration in patients with liver disease.[87] A possible explanation for this lower plasma concentration is a larger volume of distribution in patients with cirrhosis[88, 89] and in patients with biliary disease.[90] Klotz et al. observed that the elimination half-life increased about twofold in acute viral hepatitis but returned to normal on recovery from the illness.[88] However, both Klotz et al.[88] and Andreasen et al.[89] noted that patients with alcoholic cirrhosis have a two- to fivefold increase in the elimination half-life of diazepam. Thus, there is a definite need to decrease the dose and to lengthen the dosage interval in patients with hepatic dysfunction.[90]

The plasma protein binding of diazepam has been observed to be decreased from 98 to 92 per cent in patients with renal insufficiency.[91-93] The clinical implications of these findings are unclear at this time. Diazepam elimination is unaffected in patients with chronic renal disease; thus, there is no need to modify diazepam dosage in these patients. Diazepam is not substantially removed by dialysis.

OXAZEPAM (Serax)

Oxazepam pharmacokinetics are unaltered in patients with hepatic dysfunction.[94, 95] The kinetics of oxazepam also have been found to be unaltered in patients with chronic renal disease.[96]

LORAZEPAM (Ativan)

Lorazepam, a benzodiazepine that undergoes a metabolic pathway similar to that of oxazepam (i.e., glucuronidation or oxidation), has a lesser degree of impairment in systemic plasma clearance in patients with liver disease than would be expected for the benzodiazepines in general.[97] Lorazepam kinetics have been found to be unchanged in patients with chronic renal disease.[98]

FLURAZEPAM (Dalmane)

Flurazepam is one of the most commonly prescribed hypnotic agents in hospitalized medical patients in the United States and Canada, but it has not been studied extensively in patients with hepatic and renal disease. The desalkylated metabolite of flurazepam has been shown to have pharmacologic activity in animals.[99] Kales et al. have suggested that this metabolite and others may intensify the hypnotic effect of flurazepam because peak hypnotic effectiveness occurs only after the third dose of the drug.[100]

In summary, oxazepam is probably the safest drug for sedation in patients with liver disease. Unlike diazepam and chlordiazepoxide, oxazepam does not form active metabolites and is not likely to accumulate with repeat doses in patients with liver disease. However, it should be given with care and in smaller doses because of possible increased cerebral sensitivity. Patients with chronic renal disease have been observed to have decreased plasma protein binding of diazepam. However, the therapeutic ratio of the drug is large and no major toxicity is likely even in overdosage. Therefore, no modification of dose regimen is required in patients with renal failure. Finally, the rates of elimination of oxazepam and flurazepam do not change in patients with impaired renal function.

MISCELLANEOUS SEDATIVES AND HYPNOTIC AGENTS

MEPROBAMATE

Meprobamate is about 80 per cent metabolized by the liver, with 8 to 19 per cent eliminated unchanged in the urine. Its half-life of 6 hours has been observed to double in patients with acute hepatitis and in several patients with cirrhosis.[101] This agent should be avoided in patients with compromised hepatic function. Slightly reduced doses can be utilized on a short-term basis in patients with kidney disease. Relatively low clearance rates of meprobamate occur during hemodialysis (10 to 20 ml/min).[102]

CHLORAL HYDRATE (Noctec) AND ETHCHLORVYNOL (Placidyl)

Choral hydrate, one of the first hypnotic agents, is administered as a liquid or in a solid form as a prodrug (e.g., chloral betaine, dichloralphenazone, triclofos). Marshall and Owens and Owens et al. studied the metabolism of chloral hydrate in humans and found that its metabolite, trichloroethanol, is responsible for its hypnotic effects.[103, 104] There are no data regarding chloral hydrate pharmacokinetics in patients with hepatic and renal dysfunction. Trichloracetic acid, the toxic acidic end product of trichloroethanol metabolism, is avidly bound to serum albumin and has been shown to displace other organic acids from binding sites.[105] There is also evidence that organic acids are abnormally bound to plasma proteins of patients with chronic renal disease.[106] Therefore, it is conceivable that patients with renal disease would have more active trichloracetic acid available for pharmacologic effect. Chloral hydrate is rapidly removed by hemodialysis.

Ethchlorvynol is a noncyclic tertiary alcohol that in doses of 0.5 to 1.0 gm is a potent short-acting hypnotic. There are no data available regarding the pharmacokinetics about the need for dosage modification of this drug in patients with hepatic and renal disease. However, the drug is metabolized by the liver and increased half-life would be anticipated in patients with hepatic disease. Ethchlorvynol is not removed by dialysis (see Chap. 20).

GLUTETHIMIDE (Doriden), METHAQUALONE (Quaalude), AND METHYPRYLON (Noludar)

Glutethimide, methaqualone, and methyprylon are structurally related piperidinedione derivatives. Pharmacokinetically, glutethimide[108] and methaqualone[109-111] have been studied in subjects with normal renal and hepatic function. Glutethimide half-life following oral administration ranges from 5 to 22 hours. It is metabolized via the liver with less than 2 per cent excreted unchanged in the urine. It has an active metabolite, 4-hydroxyglutethimide, which has a longer half-life than the parent compound. Methaqualone has an apparent plasma half-life ranging from 20 to 60 hours. Only 2 per cent of the parent compound is eliminated unchanged in the urine. The safety and efficacy of these "miscellaneous" agents in patients with renal and hepatic disease have not been established. These agents do not undergo significant removal with hemodialysis. However, the pharmacokinetics and favorable therapeutic ratio of the benzodiazepines in these patients have been discussed at length in this chapter. Therefore, it is strongly suggested that a benzodiazepine be used if a sedative or sedative hypnotic is required.

In summary, for the treatment of pain in patients with renal failure, short courses of standard doses of acetaminophen, propoxyphene, pentazocine, codeine, meperidine, morphine, or methadone can be used. Close monitoring of patients is necessary, since uremic patients may be unusually susceptible to the analgesic and sedative effects of these drugs. Normeperidine, a metabolite of meperidine with convulsant properties, may accumulate in patients with renal failure and lead to central nervous system excitation and seizures. Anephric patients eliminate small doses of salicylate as rapidly as normal subjects. However, the long-term administration of phenacetin and acetaminophen should be avoided in patients with renal failure due to these drugs.

The treatment of pain in patients with liver disease is more difficult, since most analgesics are metabolized by the liver. Mild analgesia can best be obtained with acetaminophen. For severe pain, none of the parenterally administered analgesics appears superior. Marked dosage reduction and close clinical monitoring of the patient are required for all of these agents in patients with severe liver disease.

CONCLUSIONS

For sedation in patients with uremia, satisfactory results without significant toxic reaction can be obtained in using standard short-term doses of diazepam, flurazepam, chlordiazepoxide, meprobamate, chloral hydrate, short-acting barbiturates, ethchlorvynol, and diphenhydramine. Because of significant renal elimination and potential drug accumulation, the use of long-acting barbiturates should be avoided in patients with renal failure. Glutethimide, methaqualone, and methyprylon should probably be avoided in patients with renal failure owing to a lack of pharmacokinetic data in renal failure and because of their abuse potential. Oxazepam and lorazepam are suggested for sedation in patients with hepatic dysfunction. Flurazepam is the hypnotic agent of choice in patients with both renal and hepatic dysfunction.

Fessel and Conn found that sedatives and analgesics were a common precipitant of coma in individuals with severe liver disease.[7] Similar data are available for patients with renal disease.[5] Furthermore, the information presented in this chapter points out that the elimination of many sedatives and analgesics is impaired in patients with even mild hepatic dysfunction. Until a test is elaborated that can predict hepatic drug metabolism, it is necessary to make dosage adjustments based on clinical guidelines plus appropriate plasma drug concentration determinations.

REFERENCES

1. Smith JW, Seidl LG, Cluff LE: Studies on the epidemology of adverse drug reactions. V. Clinical factors influencing susceptibility. Ann. Intern. Med. *65*:629, 1966.
2. Reidenberg MM: Renal Function and Drug Action. Philadelphia: W. B. Saunders, 1971.
3. Jick H: Adverse drug effects in relation to renal function. Amer. J. Med. *62*:514, 1977.
4. Drayer DE: Pharmacologically active drug metabolites: Therapeutic and toxic activities, plasma and urine data in man, accumulation in renal failure. Clin. Pharm. *1*:426, 1976.
5. Ricket, G, deNovales EL, Verroast P: Drug intoxication and neurological episodes in chronic renal failure. Br. Med. J. *2*:394–396, 1970.
6. Taclob L, Needle M: Drug-induced encephalopathy in patients on maintenance dialysis. Lancet *2*:704–705, 1976.
7. Fessel JM, Conn HO: An analysis of causes and prevention of hepatic coma. Gastroenterology *62*:191, 1972.
8. Brater DC, Morelli HF: Rational drug therapy in patients with renal disease. West. J. Med. *123*:393, 1975.
9. Farrell GC, Cooksley WGE, Powell LW: Drug metabolism in liver disease: Activity of hepatic microsomal metabolizing enzymes. Clin. Pharmacol. Ther. *26*:483, 1979.
10. Hefner WG, Vasell ES, Lipton A, Harvey HA, Wilkinson GR, Schenker S: Disposition of aminopyrine, antipyrine, diazepam and indocyanine green in patients with liver disease or on anticonvulsant drug therapy: diazepam breath test and correlations in drug elimination. J. Lab. Clin. Med. *90*:440, 1977.
11. Klotz U, Fischer C, Muller-Seydlitz P, Schulty J, Muller WA: Alterations in the disposition of differently cleared drugs in patients with cirrhosis. Clin. Pharmacol. Ther. *26*:221, 1979.
12. James I: Prescribing in patients with liver disease. Br. J. Hosp. Med. *3*(Suppl. 1):67, 1975.
13. Laidlaw J, Read AE, Sherlock S: Morphine toler-

ance in hepatic cirrhosis. Gastroenterology *40*:389, 1961.
14. Sessions JT, Minkel HP, Bullard JC, Ingelfinger FJ: The effect of barbiturates in patients with liver disease. J. Clin. Invest. *33*:1116, 1954.
15. Levy G, Tsuchiya T, Amsel LP: Limited capacity for salicylphenolic glucuronide formation and its effect on the kinetics of salicylate elimination in man. Clin. Pharmacol. Ther. *13*:258, 1972.
16. Levy G, Tsuchiya T: Salicylate accumulation kinetics in man. N. Engl. J. Med. *287*:430, 1972.
17. Levy G, Giacomini KM: Commentary: rational aspirin dosage. Clin. Pharmacol Ther. *23*:247, 1978.
18. Gupta W, Sarkissian E, Paulus HE: Correlation of plateau serum salicylate level with rate of salicylate metabolism. Clin. Pharmacol. Ther. *18*:350, 1975.
19. Brodie BB, Burns JJ, Weiner M: Metabolism of drugs in subjects with Laennec's cirrhosis. Med. Exp. *1*:290, 1959.
20. Lowenthal DT, Briggs WA, Levy G: Kinetics of salicylate elimination by anephric patients. J. Clin. Invest. *54*:1221, 1974.
21. Levy G: Pharmacokinetics of salicylate elimination in man. J. Pharmacol. Sci. *54*:959, 1965.
22. Davison C: Salicylate metabolism in man. Ann. N.Y. Acad. Sci. *179*:249, 1971.
23. Kallen RJ, Zaltzman S, Coe FL, Metcoff J: Hemodialysis in children: technique, kinetic aspects related to varying body size and application to salicylate intoxication, acute renal failure and some other disorders. Medicine *45*:1, 1966.
24. Fischer RL: Intermittent peritoneal dialysis using 5 per cent albumin in the treatment of salicylate intoxication in children. J. Pediatr. *56*:226, 1961.
25. Prowse K, Pain M, Marston AD: The treatment of salicylate poisoning using mannitol and forced alkaline diuresis. Clin. Sci. *38*:327, 1970.
26. Verebely K, Inturrisi CE: Disposition of propoxyphene and norpropoxyphene in man after single oral dose. Clin. Pharmacol. Ther. *15*:320, 1974.
27. Verebely K, Inturrisi CE: The simultaneous determination of propoxyphene and norpropoxyphene in human body fluids using gas–liquid chromatography. J. Chromatog. *75*:195, 1973.
28. Giacomini KM, Gibson TP, Levy G: Effect of hemodialysis on propoxyphene and norpropoxyphene concentrations in blood of anephric patients. Clin. Pharmacol. Ther. *27*:508, 1980.
29. Schaw J, Dam AH, Christensen JM: Pharmacokinetics of dextropropoxyphene in acute poisoning. Arch. Toxicol. *1*(Suppl.):343, 1978.
30. Gram LF, Schou J, Way WL, Heltberg J, Bodin NO: D-Propoxyphene kinetics after single oral and intravenous doses in man. Clin. Pharmacol. Ther. *26*:473–482, 1979.
31. Giacomini KL, Gibson TP, Levy G: Plasma protein binding of D-propoxyphene in normal subjects and anephric patients. J. Clin. Pharmacol. *18*:106, 1978.
32. Giacomini KM, Gibson TP, Levy G: Effect of hemodialysis on propoxyphene and norpropoxyphene concentrations in blood of anephric patients. Clin. Pharmacol. Ther. *27*:508–514, 1980.
33. Holland DR, Steinberg MI: Electrophysiologic properties of propoxyphene and norpropoxyphene in canine cardiac conducting tissues in vitro and in vivo. Toxicol. Appl. Pharmacol. *47*:123, 1979.
34. Nickarder R, Smitz SE, Steinberg MI: Propoxyphene and norpropoxyphene: pharmacologic and toxic effects in animals. J. Pharmacol. Exp. Ther. *200*:245, 1977.
35. Miller RR: Analgesics in Drug Effects in Hospitalized Patients: Experiences of the Boston Collaborative Drug Surveillance Program, 1966–1975, (RR Miller and DG Greenblatt, eds.). New York: John Wiley & Sons, 1976.
36. Dordini B, Wilson RA, Thompson RPH, Williams R: Reduction of absorption of paracetamol by activated charcoal and cholestyramine: a possible therapeutic measure. Br. Med. J. *3*:86, 1973.
37. Gazzard BG, Ford-Hutchinson AW, Smith MJH, Williams R: The binding of paracetamol to plasma proteins of man and pig. J. Pharmacol. *25*:964, 1973.
38. Albert KS, Sedman AJ, Wagner JG: Pharmacokinetics of orally administered acetaminophen in man. J. Pharmacokinet. Biopharm. *2*:381, 1974.
39. Miller RP, Roberts RJ, Fischer J: Acetaminophen elimination kinetics in neonates, children and adults. Clin. Pharmacol. Ther. *19*:284, 1976.
40. Prescott LF, Sansur M, Levin W, Conney AH: The comparative metabolism of phenacetin and N-acetyl-p-aminophenol in man with particular reference to effects on the kidney. Clin. Pharmacol Ther. *9*:605, 1968.
41. Slattery JT, Levy G: Acetaminophen kinetics in acutely poisoned patients. Clin. Pharmacol. Ther. *25*:184, 1979.
42. Finlayson HDC, Prescott LF, Adiepon-Yamoah KK, Forrest JAH: Antipyrine, lidocaine and paracetamol metabolism in chronic liver disease. Gastroenterology *67*:790, 1974.
43. Varker JD, Vecarle DG, Anuras S: Chronic excessive acetaminophen use and liver damage. Ann. Intern. Med. *87*:299, 1977.
44. Johnson GK, Tolman KG: Chronic liver disease and acetaminophen. Ann. Intern. Med. *87*:302, 1977.
45. Lowenthal DT, Øie S, Vanstone JC, Briggs WA, Levy G: Pharmacokinetics of acetaminophen elimination by anephric patients. J. Pharmacol. Exp. Ther. *196*:570, 1976.
46. Øie S, Lowenthal DT, Briggs WA, Levy G: Effect of hemodialysis on kinetics of acetaminophen elimination by anephric patients. Clin. Pharmacol. Ther. *18*:680, 1975.
47. Mitchell JR, Jollow DJ, Potter WZ, et al.: Acetaminophen-induced hepatic necrosis. I. Role of drug metabolism. J. Pharmacol. Exp. Ther. *187*:185, 1973.
48. Van Tyle WK: Internal analgesic products. *In* Handbook of Non-Prescription Drugs (LL Corrigan, ed.). 6th ed. Washington, D.C.: American Pharmaceutical Association, 1979.
49. Prescott LS: Effects of acetylsalicylate acid, phenacetin, paracetamol and caffeine on renal tubular epithelium. Lancet *2*:91, 1965.
50. Hoyumpa A: Diagnosis and management of hepatic encephalopathy. *In* Hepatic Support in Acute Liver Failure (GGR Kuster, ed.). Springfield, Illinois: Charles C Thomas, 1976, pp. 88–124.

51. Don HG, Dieppa RA, Taylor P: Narcotic analgesics in anuric patients. Anesthesiology *42*:745, 1975.
52. Mostert JR, Evers JL, Hobika GH, et al.: Cardiorespiratory effects of anaesthesia with morphine or fentanyl in chronic renal failure and cerebral toxicity after morphine. Br. J. Anesthesiol. *43*:1053–1060, 1971.
53. Olsen GD, Bennett WM, Porter GA: Morphine and phenytoin binding to plasma proteins in renal and hepatic failure. Clin. Pharmacol. Ther. *17*:677, 1976.
54. Way EL, Swanson R, Gimble AI: Studies in vitro and in vivo on the influence of the liver on isonipecaine (Demerol) activity. J. Pharmacol. Exp. Ther. *91*:178–184, 1947.
55. MacDonald AD, Woolfe G, Bergel F, et al.: Analgesic action of pethidine derivates and related compounds. Br. J. Pharmacol. *1*:4–14, 1946.
56. Miller JW, Anderson HH: The effect of *N*-demethylation on certain pharmacologic actions of morphine, codeine and meperidine in the mouse. J. Pharmacol. Exp. Ther. *112*:191–196, 1954.
57. Deneau GA, Nakai K: The toxicity of meperidine in the monkey as influenced by its rate of absorption. Bulletin, Drug Addiction and Narcotics App. *6*:2460–2469, 1961.
58. Klotz U, McHorse TS, Wilkinson GR, et al.: The effect of cirrhosis on the disposition and elimination of meperidine in man. Clin. Pharmacol. Ther. *16*:667–675, 1974.
59. Szeto HH, Inturrisi CE, Houde R, Saal S, Cheigh J, Reidenberg MM: Accumulation of normeperidine, an active metabolite of meperidine, in patients with renal failure or cancer. Ann. Intern. Med. *86*:738–741, 1977.
60. McHorse TS, Wilkinson GR, Johnson RF, et al.: Effect of acute viral hepatitis in man on the disposition and elimination of meperidine. Gastroenterology *68*:775–780, 1975.
61. Wright N, Roleson JS: Renal Diseases in Drug Treatment (GS Avery, ed.). 2nd ed. Sydney and New York: Adis Press, 1980, pp. 800–845.
62. Inturrisi CE: Disposition of narcotics in patients with renal disease. Am. J. Med. *62*:528, 1977.
63. Lous P: Plasma levels and urinary excretion of three barbituric acids after oral administration to man. Acta Pharmacol. Toxicol. *10*:147–165, 1954.
64. Lous P: Elimination of barbiturates. *In* Barbiturate Poisoning and Tetanus (SH Johansen, ed.). Boston: Little, Brown, 1966, pp. 341–350.
65. Kallberg N, Agurell S, Ericsson O, Bucht E, Jalling B, Boreus LO: Quantitation of phenobarbital and its main metabolites in human urine. Eur. J. Clin. Pharmacol. *9*:161–168, 1975.
66. Bloomer HA, Maddock RK, Jr.: An assessment of diuresis and dialysis for treating acute barbiturate poisoning. *In* Acute Barbiturate Poisoning (H Mathew, ed.). Amsterdam: Excerpta Medica, 1971, p. 223.
67. Bloomer, HA: A critical evaluation of diuresis in the treatment of barbiturate intoxication. J. Lab. Clin. Med. *64*:898, 1966.
68. Butler TC, Mabaffee C, Waddell WJ: Phenobarbital: studies of elimination, accumulation. tolerance and dosage schedules. J. Pharmacol. Exp. Ther. *111*:425, 1954.
69. Henderson LW, Merrill JP: Treatment of barbiturate intoxication. Ann. Intern. Med. *64*:876, 1966.
70. Bloomer JR, Boyer JL: Phenobarbital effects in cholestatic liver disease. Ann. Intern. Med. *82*:310–317, 1975.
71. Alvin J, McHorse T, Hoyumpa A, Bush MT, Schenker S: The effect of liver disease in man on the disposition of phenobarbital. J. Pharmacol. Exp. Ther. *192*:224–235, 1975.
72. Breimer DD, Zilly W, Richter E: Pharmacokinetics of hexobarbital in acute hepatitis and after apparent recovery. Clin. Pharmacol Ther. *18*:433–440, 1975.
73. Shideman FE, Kelly AR, Lee LE, et al.: The role of the liver in the detoxification of thiopental (Pentothal) by man. Anesthesiology *10*:421–428, 1949.
74. Dundee JW, Richards RK: Effect of azotemia upon the action of intravenous barbiturate anesthesia. Anesthesiology *15*:333–346, 1954.
75. Ghoneim MM, Pandya H: Plasma protein binding of thiopental in patients with impaired renal or hepatic function. Anesthesiology *42*:545, 1975.
76. Reidenberg MM, Lowenthal DT, Briggs W, Gasparo M: Pentobarbital elimination in patients with poor renal function. Clin. Pharmacol. Ther. *20*:67–71, 1976.
77. Koechlin BA, Schwarz MA, Krol G, Oberhansli W: The metabolic fate of C^{14}-labelled chlordiazepoxide in man, in the dog and in the rat. J. Pharmacol. Exp. Ther. *148*:399–411, 1965.
78. Schwartz MA, Postma E: Metabolic N-demethylation of chlordiazepoxide, J. Pharm. Soc. *55*:1358–1362, 1966.
79. Schwartz MA, Postma E, Gout A: Biological half-life of chlordiazepoxide and its metabolite, demoxepam in man. J. Pharm. Sci. *60*:1500–1503, 1971.
80. Dixon R, Brooks MA, Postma M, Hackman A, Spector S, et al.: *N*-Desmethyldiazepam: A metabolite of chlordiazepoxide in man. Clin. Pharmacol. Ther. *20*:450–457, 1976.
81. Greenblatt DJ, Shader RI, Franke K, MacLaughlin DS, Ransil BJ, Koch-Weser J: Kinetics of intravenous chlordiazepoxide: sex differences in drug distribution. Clin. Pharmacol. Ther. *22*:893, 1977.
82. Roberts RK, Wilkinson GR, Branch RA, Schenker S: Effect of age and parenchymal liver disease on the disposition and elimination of chlordiazepoxide (Librium). Gastroenterology *75*: 479–485, 1978.
83. Wilkinson GR, Schenker S: Effects of liver disease on drug disposition in man. Biochem. Pharmacol. *25*:2675, 1976.
84. Sellers EM, Greenblatt DJ, Giles HG, et al.: Chlordiazepoxide and oxazepam disposition in cirrhosis. Clin. Pharmacol. Ther. *26*:240, 1979.
85. Mandelli M, Tognoni G, Garattini S: Clinical pharmacokinetics of diazepam. Clin. Pharmacokinet. *3*:72–91, 1978.
86. Dasberg HH, Van der Kleijn E, Guelen PJR, Van-Praag HM: Plasma concentrations of diazepam and of its metabolite N-desmethyldiazepam in relation to anxiolytic effect. Clin. Pharmacol. Ther. *15*:473, 1974.
87. Sellman R, Kanto J, Pekkarinen J: Biliary excretion of diazepam and its metabolites in man. Acta Pharmacol Toxicol. *37*:242–249, 1975.

88. Klotz U, Avant GR, Hoyumpa A, et al.: The effects of age and liver disease on the disposition and elimination of diazepam in adult man. J. Clin. Invest. *55*:347–359, 1975.
89. Andreasen PB, Hendel J, Greisen G, Hvidberg EF: Pharmacokinetics of diazepam in disordered liver function. Eur. J. Clin. Pharmacol. *10*:115–120, 1976.
90. Mahon WA, Inaba T, Umeda T, et al.: Biliary elimination of diazepam in man. Clin. Pharmacol. Ther. *19*:443–450, 1976.
91. Kangas L, Kanto J, Forsström J, Iisalo E: The protein binding of diazepam and N-demethyldiazepam in patients with poor renal function. Clin. Nephrol. *5*:114–118, 1976.
92. Andreassen F: The effect of dialysis on the protein binding of drugs in patients with acute renal failure. Acta Pharmacol. Toxicol. *34*:284–294, 1974.
93. Kober A, Sjoholm I, Borga O, Odar-Cederlof I: Protein binding of diazepam and digitoxin in uremic and normal serum. Biochem. Pharmacol. *28*:1037–1042, 1978.
94. Wilkinson GR: The effects of liver disease and aging on the disposition of diazepam, chlordiazepoxide, oxazepam and lorazepam in man. Acta Psychiatr. Scand. *274*(Suppl.):561, 1978.
95. Shull, HJ, Jr, Wilkinson GR, Johnson R, Schenker S: Normal disposition of oxazepam in acute viral hepatitis and cirrhosis. Ann. Intern. Med. *84*:420–425, 1976.
96. Odar-Cederlof I, Vessman J, Alvan G, Sjoqvist F: Oxazepam disposition in uraemic patients. Acta Pharmacol. Toxicol. *40*(Suppl. 1):52, 1977.
97. Kraus JW, Desmond PV, Marshall JP, et al.: Effects of aging and liver disease on disposition of lorazepam. Clin. Pharmacol. Ther. *24*:411, 1978.
98. Verbeeck R, Tjandramaga TB, Verberckmoes R, DeSchepper PJ: Biotransformation and excretion of lorazepam in patients with chronic renal failure. Br. J. Clin. Pharmacol. *3*:1033, 1976.
99. Randall LO, Kappell B: Pharmacological activity of some benzodiazepines and their metabolites: *In* The Benzodiazepines (Garattini S, Mussini E, and Randall LO, (eds.). New York: Raven Press, 1973, pp. 27–51.
100. Kales A, Bixler EO, Scharf M, Kales J: Sleep laboratory studies of flurazepam: A model for evaluating hypnotic drugs. Clin. Pharmacol. Ther. *19*:576, 1976.
101. Weld H, Von Oldershausen HF: Zur Pharmakokinetik von Meprobamat bei chronischen Hepatopathien und Arzneimittelsucht. Klin. Wochenschr. *47*:78–80, 1969.
102. Maher JF, Schriener GE: The clinical dialysis of poisons. Trans. Am. Soc. Artif. Intern. Organs *9*:385, 1963.
103. Marshall EK, Owens AH: Absorption, excretion and metabolic fate of chloral hydrate and trichloroethanol. Bull. Johns Hopkins Hosp. *94*:1–18, 1954.
104. Owens AH, Marshall EK, Broun GO, Zubrod CG, Lasagna L: Comparative evaluation of the hypnotic potency of chloral hydrate and trichloroethanol. Bull. Johns Hopkins Hosp. *96*:71, 1955.
105. Sellers EM, Koch-Weser J: Kinetics and clinical importance of displacement of warfarin from albumin by acidic drugs. Ann. N.Y. Acad. Sci. *179*:213–225, 1971.
106. Reidenberg MM, Affrime MB: Influence of disease on binding of drugs to plasma proteins. Ann. N.Y. Acad. Sci. *226*:115–126, 1973.
107. Curry SH, Riddall D, Gordon JS, Simpson P, et al.: Disposition of glutethimide in man. Clin. Pharmacol. Ther. *12*:849–857, 1971.
108. Kadar D, Inaba T, Endrenyi L, et al.: Comparative drug elimination capacity in man — glutethimide, amobarbital, antipyrine and sulfinpyrazone. Clin. Pharmacol Ther. *14*:552–560, 1974.
109. Morris RN, Gunderson GA, Babcock SW, Zarostinski JF: Plasma levels and absorption of methaqualone after oral administration to man. Clin. Pharmacol. Ther. *13*:710–723, 1972.
110. Alvan G, Ericsson O, Levander S, Lindgren JE: Plasma concentrations and effects of methaqualone after single and multiple oral doses in man. Eur. J. Clin. Pharmacol *7*:449–454, 1974.
111. Nayak RK, Smyth RD, Chamberlain JH, et al.: Methaqualone pharmacokinetics after single and multiple dose administration in man. J. Pharmacokinet. Biopharm. *2*:107–121, 1974.

Chapter 15

Antihypertensive Agents and Diuretics

by

John G. Gerber

Antihypertensive and diuretic agents are among the most frequently prescribed drugs in current use. Moreover, these drugs are frequently utilized in the treatment of patients with kidney and liver disease. For example, hypertension and edema often complicate the course of patients with kidney disease. Current estimates suggest that 20 to 50 per cent of the 45,000 patients in chronic dialysis programs are on antihypertensive medications. In patients with liver disease, the presence of ascites and edema often results in diuretic use. The widespread use of antihypertensive and diuretic agents in general practice as well as in patients with kidney and liver disease demands maximal understanding of these complex agents by the clinician. This chapter will develop a background to aid the clinician in his use of antihypertensive and diuretic drugs in the general population and in patients with hepatic and kidney disease.

THE USE OF ANTIHYPERTENSIVE AGENTS IN PATIENTS WITH KIDNEY AND LIVER DISEASE

The pharmacology of antihypertensive drugs differs from that of many other drug groups. For example, blood levels of these drugs do not correlate with the hypotensive effect. Moreover, antihypertensive drug half-lives do not correlate with duration of hypotension. This dissociation between pharmacodynamic (hypotensive) effect and pharmacokinetic (blood levels, $T_{1/2}$) parameters does not necessarily mean that these drugs behave irregularly. Rather, this dissociation suggests that there may be sequestered pools for these drugs, resulting in slow turnover at the site of action. Methyldopa is a classic example. This drug has a plasma half-life of 2 hours, but its duration of action can be as long as 24 hours. Since methyldopa requires metabolism to methylnorepinephrine in the brain to exert its antihypertensive activity, the duration of action of the drug correlates best with the turnover of methylnorepinephrine in the brain, and not with plasma methyldopa concentration. Hydralazine also has a short plasma half-life, but its duration of action can be as long as 12 hours. It has been suggested that hydralazine accumulates in the vascular smooth muscle where the drug turnover is slower than measurable blood levels could indicate. Thus, only by understanding the distribution and metabolism of antihypertensive drugs can we explain the apparent pharmacokinetic and pharmacodynamic dissociation.

Fortunately, antihypertensive drugs as a group are quite safe; excessive hypotension is the first sign that too much drug has been administered. This easily measurable response makes empiric adjustments of doses of these drugs, without obtaining drug blood levels, justifiable. Nonetheless, only by knowing both the pharmacokinetics and pharmacodynamics of these drugs can intelligent dosage intervals be established.

METHYLDOPA (Aldomet)

Since its introduction in 1963, methyldopa (Fig. 15–1) has been an extremely useful antihypertensive agent. Although initially it was thought that the drug caused hypotension by inhibiting dopa decarboxylase, thus depleting norepinephrine peripherally, the present evidence indicates that methyldopa has to penetrate the central nervous system and be metabolized to methylnorepinephrine to be active.[1] In the central nervous system, methylnorepinephrine decreases sympathetic traffic to peripheral vessels.

The drug is indicated for moderate to severe hypertension. Although methyldopa is not considered a first-line drug for the treatment of hypertension, many hypertensive patients do very well when methyldopa is combined with a diuretic.[2] The use of a diuretic is necessary when a patient is treated with methyldopa because salt and water retention gradually occurs and "overrides" the hypotensive effect of the drug. Since a decrease in perfusion pressure to the kidneys is a very potent signal to enhance tubular sodium and water reabsorption, the use of diuretics is always necessary when treating patients with antihypertensive agents.

Mild toxicity associated with the use of methyldopa is common, but life-threatening toxicity is rare. Somnolence and fatigue occur in as many as 28 per cent of the patients using the drug. This central depressant effect is the most common reason for stopping the medication in practice. Generally, young and active people have low tolerance to methyldopa. Because of the drug's central nervous system effects, many consultants avoid the use of methyldopa in patients who have occupations requiring mental alertness and manual dexterity. Other common effects that occur with the use of methyldopa include dry mouth, headaches, impotence, diarrhea, nasal congestion, and mental depression.

Although these adverse effects have profound influence on patient compliance, they are not life-threatening. This is not the case with the development of methyldopa-related hemolytic anemia and hepatitis. The development of a positive Coombs' test is seen in at least 20 per cent of the patients on chronic methyldopa therapy. Usually, this laboratory finding is of no consequence except for the difficulty in crossmatching the patient for blood transfusions. The antibody to the red cells is an IgG warm antibody aimed at the Rh locus. Actual hemolysis develops in less than 1 per cent of patients taking methyldopa. The development of a positive Coombs' test is not sufficient reason to discontinue methyldopa therapy because only a small fraction of patients who do so develop actual hemolysis. However, the drug must be discontinued when hemolysis develops. Although the Coombs' test can remain positive for as long as a year after the discontinuation of methyldopa, the hemolysis resolves in less than a week. In a few resistant cases, short-term corticosteroid therapy has been used successfully to treat severe methyldopa-induced hemolysis.

The exact incidence of hepatic abnormalities with the use of methyldopa is not known. Less than 5 per cent of patients taking methyldopa develop transient rises in transaminases, and the incidence of severe hepatitis must be much less. Patients who develop methyldopa hepatitis frequently develop prodromal symptoms of fatigue and anorexia followed by

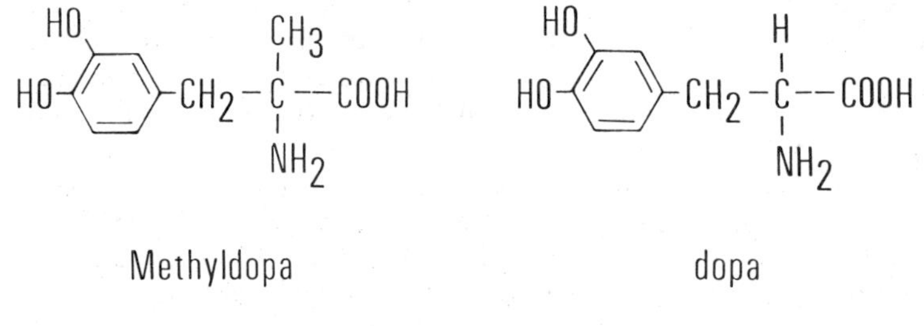

Figure 15–1. The structure of methyldopa as compared to the endogenous catecholamine dopa.

clinical jaundice. These symptoms usually occur in the first 2 to 3 months after methyldopa therapy. The liver biopsy shows a picture very similar to that of viral hepatitis. However, occasionally a biopsy may show a picture compatible with chronic active hepatitis or granulomatous hepatitis.

In the majority of the reported cases of methyldopa hepatitis, the outcome is very good when the medication is discontinued. There are a few reported cases of severe hepatic necrosis and death with continued administration of the drug in the face of liver function derangements. The mechanism by which methyldopa can induce liver disease is not known, but a hypersensitivity-type reaction has been proposed.[3]

In addition to hemolysis and hepatitis, chronic methyldopa therapy can result in a drug-induced lupus syndrome and hyperpyrexia. Both of these conditions require the immediate cessation of the drug therapy.

The pharmacokinetic parameters of methyldopa have been studied in humans, but the understanding of the peripheral kinetics of the drug does not help to explain the duration of action of the drug in the treatment of hypertension. Rather, a thorough understanding of the kinetics of the metabolism of methyldopa to methylnorepinephrine, as well as the kinetics of methylnorepinephrine and norepinephrine in the central nervous system, is necessary to understand the drug's duration of action.

Methyldopa is only 50 per cent absorbed from the gastrointestinal tract. There is evidence that the absorption may rely on an active amino acid transport process that is stereoselective. Once methyldopa is absorbed, it is distributed into a small apparent volume and excreted mostly as methyldopa or conjugated methyldopa in the urine with a half-life of about 1 to 2 hours. Some of the methyldopa is metabolized to methyldopamine and further metabolized to 3-*O*-methyl-α-methyldopamine in the liver. In renal failure, the plasma half-life of methyldopa is prolonged to 3 to 4 hours. However, the significance of the prolonged half-life in renal insufficiency is questionable, since the duration of action of methyldopa is about 24 hours. Human studies have demonstrated that patients in renal failure are more sensitive to the hypotensive action of methyldopa. However, plasma levels of methyldopa in patients with renal failure were not elevated above those of patients with normal renal function, suggesting that accumulation of the drug is not the mechanism of this increased sensitivity. The possibility that more methyldopa can diffuse into the brain in renal failure needs to be explored. Whatever the mechanism of increased sensitivity, the dose of methyldopa should be reduced in patients with renal failure.[4]

The use of methyldopa in acute liver disease is contraindicated because of methyldopa's potential for hepatotoxicity. In chronic liver disease, methyldopa probably should not be used because of its depressant effect on the central nervous system. Since the major portion of ingested methyldopa is excreted in the urine unchanged, the plasma clearance of methyldopa in liver disease is probably altered very little. However, the effect of liver disease on the integrity of the blood-brain barrier could potentially increase methyldopa's accessibility to its site of action. Although general information is lacking in the use of methyldopa in liver disease, the drug should probably be reserved for hypertensives with normal hepatic function.

In summary, methyldopa is an efficacious drug in the treatment of hypertension. The drug should be used carefully in renal disease because of the heightened sensitivity such patients exhibit for the drug. However, methyldopa does not affect renal function and renal hemodynamics, thus making it a good drug for treatment of hypertension with renal failure. Methyldopa should be avoided in acute or chronic hepatic insufficiency.

GUANETHIDINE (Ismelin)

Guanethidine was introduced in 1959 as an antihypertensive agent. Before the availability of potent arteriolar vasodilators, guanethidine was the drug of choice in the treatment of severe hypertension. The popularity of guanethidine is on the decline, mainly because of the development of severe orthostatic hypotension and sexual dysfunction with the use of the drug. Guanethidine's advantages over other antihypertensive agents in use today are that it need be administered only once a day and no central nervous system side effects have been associated with its use.[5]

Guanethidine lowers blood pressure by causing peripheral sympathetic denervation, thus decreasing both the cardiac output and peripheral vascular resistance (Table 15–1).

Guanethidine enters the postganglionic sympathetic nerve endings through the norepinephrine reuptake pump. Once inside the neurovesicles, it inhibits norepinephrine accumulation and release. Because guanethidine has to penetrate sympathetic nerve endings to be active, any drugs that interfere with the norepinephrine pump will inactivate the sympatholytic effect of the drug. Thus, tricyclic antidepressants, phenothiazines, cocaine, and ephedrine are a few of the drugs that interfere with guanethidine's antihypertensive activity through the inhibition of the norepinephrine pump.[6]

Guanethidine is indicated in the treatment of moderate to severe hypertension. The concomitant use of a diuretic is mandatory because salt and water retention can blunt the antihypertensive effect of the drug. Major side effects of guanethidine are secondary to the drug's sympatholytic property. Orthostatic hypotension to some degree is seen with all patients on guanethidine. This orthostatic hypotension poses a problem in maintaining both supine and upright blood pressures in the normal range. Other side effects of the drug are diarrhea, nasal stuffiness, ejaculatory impairment, and bradycardia, all related to the sympatholytic action of guanethidine. Rarely, patients on guanethidine develop congestive heart failure as a consequence of cardiac sympathetic blockade and salt retention.

Guanethidine's bioavailability is variable among individual patients and ranges from 3 to 50 per cent. Once absorbed, the drug is both metabolized by the liver at a clearance rate of about 300 ml/min and excreted unchanged in the urine at a renal clearance rate of 300 ml/min. The drug is widely distributed into sympathetic neurons and is felt to have a very large volume of distribution. Once distributed, guanethidine is eliminated with a half-life of 5 days. Because of its long half-life, the drug can be given once a day. Since it takes three half-lives to reach 87.5 per cent of steady-state drug levels, adjustments in daily maintenance dose are usually made at 2- to 3-week intervals.[7]

Data on alterations of guanethidine kinetics in renal and hepatic diseases are not available. Acutely, patients with low endogenous creatinine clearances respond to guanethidine similarly to patients with normal renal function. However, when the drug is given chronically, a decrease in renal function should increase the steady-state blood level of the drug. Whether or not this increased blood level is of clinical importance is unknown. The interindividual variation in bioavailability for guanethidine is much greater than the variation in total body clearance of the drug that is expected in renal failure.[8] Because of these variables in patients with renal or hepatic dysfunction, guanethidine dosage should be adjusted according to clinical response. In patients with renal or hepatic dysfunction, the time required

TABLE 15–1. PHYSIOLOGIC EFFECTS OF ANTIHYPERTENSIVE AGENTS

	Effect on		
	Cardiac Output	*Vascular Resistance*	Major Side Effect
Peripheral Sympatholytic Agents			
Guanethidine	↓	↓	Orthostasis
Reserpine	↓	↓	Sedation
Prazosin	↓	↓	Orthostasis
Central Sympatholytic Agents			
α-Methyldopa	↓	↓	Sedation
Clonidine	↓	↓	Sedation
Arteriolar Vasodilators			
Hydralazine	↑	↓	Tachycardia
Minoxidil	↑	↓	Tachycardia
Diazoxide	↑	↓	Tachycardia
Arteriolar and Venular Vasodilator			
Nitroprusside	↑	↓	Slight tachycardia

↑ = Increase.
↓ = Decrease.

to reach a steady-state blood concentration of guanethidine is prolonged because of the drug's longer elimination half-life. Thus, in patients with significant renal and hepatic diseases with lower than normal plasma clearance of guanethidine, small initial doses with adjustments of the daily maintenance dose at 3- to 4-week intervals (instead of 2- or 3-week intervals) should avoid excessive hypotension and adverse effects.

CLONIDINE (Catapres)

Clonidine was introduced in the United States in 1974.[9] The drug was originally developed in the early 1960's as a nasal decongestant, and lowering of blood pressure was noted as a side effect. The mechanism of action of clonidine is incompletely understood. It is clear that the drug has to penetrate the central nervous system to be active.[10] The drug is then thought to interact with an α-receptor in the brain to decrease sympathetic traffic to the peripheral vasculature. The drug works by a mechanism similar to that of α-methyldopa, except that clonidine does not have to be metabolized to be active.

Clonidine is indicated for the treatment of moderate hypertension. Clonidine remains an effective antihypertensive agent only if used together with a diuretic, because salt and water retention will blunt the hypotensive effect of the drug. Clonidine is probably not considered a first-line drug for the treatment of hypertension because of the severe sedation that a substantial percentage of patients taking this drug experience. In addition to the sedation, xerostomia is a common side effect of the drug. As with methyldopa, orthostatic hypotension is rarely experienced with clonidine unless the patient is dehydrated. Impotence occurs in about 5 per cent of males taking the drug. Major gastrointestinal symptoms also occur in 5 per cent of patients using clonidine. The most consistent reason why patients stop taking clonidine is severe sedation experienced with its use. Logically, patients who have jobs necessitating mental alertness should not be started on clonidine because of the predictable somnolence the drug will cause. On abrupt cessation of clonidine, a small fraction of patients will experience a blood pressure overshoot phenomenon associated with excessive catecholamine excretion in the urine.[11] There are reports of the development of hypertensive encephalopathy when clonidine is abruptly withdrawn, particularly in patients on high doses (> 1 to 2 mg) of the drug. These patients are best treated with α-adrenergic blocking agents like phentolamine to control the blood pressure. The onset of severe hypertension after cessation of clonidine usually occurs between 12 and 48 hours after the last dose. Since there is no way to predict which patients will develop this drug withdrawal phenomenon, a tapering regimen of clonidine over 4 to 7 days may be the safest means of discontinuing the drug.

The pharmacokinetics of clonidine have been well studied in humans. The drug is 80 per cent absorbed after oral administration and distributed extensively with an apparent volume of distribution of about 3 L/kg. At least 50 per cent of the drug is excreted unchanged in the urine and some fraction is metabolized by the liver. The drug has a plasma half-life of 7 to 12 hours. Peak concentration of the drug is achieved 2 hours after oral administration. The hypotensive effect of the drug is only slightly correlated with plasma concentration. However, both the sedative effect of clonidine and the decrease in saliva flow correlate with plasma drug levels.[12] Some investigators have observed that at very high plasma clonidine concentrations, the decrease in blood pressure is attenuated. This observation is consistent with the peripheral α-adrenergic agonist activity of clonidine in higher concentrations.

Clonidine can be used safely in renal failure, but the dose generally has to be less. However, interindividual requirements for clonidine are quite variable, and the best parameter to follow in treating hypertensive patients with renal disease is the blood pressure response. Also, fluid status plays an important role in drug responsiveness in the hypertensive patient. Patients who are salt and water overloaded may respond very poorly to clonidine, but after vigorous diuresis may actually develop hypotension while using the drug. Thus, there are factors other than pharmacokinetics that determine antihypertensive drug requirement.

Clonidine is probably a safer drug to use in liver disease than methyldopa because no documented case reports of clonidine-induced hepatitis have been reported. However, in patients with chronic liver disease and borderline encephalopathy, the central depressive actions of clonidine may be deleterious. The actual pharmacokinetics of clonidine in liver disease have not been examined. Since 50 per cent of clonidine's metabolism occurs in the liver, the plasma clearance of clonidine must be somewhat impaired in liver disease. Thus, as a safety measure, clonidine should be started at a low dose in hypertensive patients with liver disease and slowly titrated to a desired hypotensive response.

RESERPINE

Reserpine is one of many chemicals derived from the root of the plant *Rauwolfia serpentina*. Although the whole root has been used in primitive medicine for many centuries, the extract and the more purified reserpine have been in clinical use in the United States only in the last three decades.

The drug is indicated in mild to moderate hypertension. Reserpine as a sole drug for the treatment of hypertension is not very effective, because the consequent salt and water retention limits the antihypertensive effect of the drug. However, a combination of a diuretic plus reserpine has additive antihypertensive effects. Reserpine should not be used in the treatment of hypertensive emergencies because even when given parenterally, the onset of action is variable (30 minutes to several hours). Also, the sedation that accompanies parenteral reserpine can render mental status evaluation difficult in patients with hypertensive encephalopathy.

The mechanism of action of reserpine has been studied extensively. The drug appears to bind to neurotransmitter storage vesicles in both the central and peripheral nervous systems. In the sympathetic neuron, the binding of reserpine to storage vesicles results in catecholamine depletion; however, the drug depletes serotonin storage sites as well. Most researchers believe that the main mechanism of reserpine's hypotensive action is through peripheral, rather than central, catecholamine depletion.[13]

The toxicity of reserpine is dose related. At a relatively low dose of 0.25 mg/day, reserpine has no more side effects than other antihypertensive drugs like methyldopa or propranolol. But at doses greater than 0.50 mg/day, the toxicity of reserpine is substantial. By far the most dangerous side effect is the development of severe psychotic depression with suicidal ideation.[14] This side effect occurs usually after several months of reserpine administration. Drowsiness, sedation, and lethargy are observed in nearly all patients on high doses of reserpine. Nasal congestion is also seen frequently after higher doses of reserpine. Reserpine can increase gastric acid production and cause symptoms of peptic ulcer disease; therefore, patients with peptic ulcer disease should not be given reserpine. Bronchospasm also has been described in patients on reserpine; thus, reserpine should be used very cautiously in patients with asthma. The purported association between reserpine use and breast cancer has not been confirmed.

Although reserpine was quite a popular antihypertensive drug in the 1960's, its use is presently declining. The drug's major advantage over other antihypertensive drugs is its long duration of action and, therefore, the convenience of once-a-day administration. The pharmacokinetics of reserpine have not been studied extensively because of the difficulty in measuring plasma reserpine levels, which are usually less than one nanogram per milliliter. Moreover, the pharmacokinetic studies involving radioactive reserpine fail to distinguish between the native drug and its metabolites. In one study in which such separation was made, only two patients were studied after a 1-mg oral dose and then restudied several weeks later after a 1-mg intramuscular dose of reserpine. Although no numbers were reported in that study, the area under the curve after the oral dose of reserpine appeared much lower than after the intramuscular dose of reserpine, thus suggesting low bioavailability of the drug after oral administration. The apparent volume of distribution was quite high, in the range of 5 to 7 L/kg, and the $t_{1/2}$ was at least 48 hours.[15] Reserpine is extensively metabolized by the liver, and the native drug itself is not excreted unchanged in the urine. Therefore, it is unlikely that renal dysfunction will affect the pharmacokinetics of reserpine. The metabolism of reserpine has not been studied in patients with hepatic disease. However, since reserpine is extensively metabolized by the liver, it would be wise to reduce the dose of reserpine in patients with liver disease and carefully titrate dosage according to blood pressure response. Since reserpine has marked central depressive effects, the drug should not be used in patients who may develop hepatic encephalopathy. The basic problem in using reserpine in the treatment of hypertension is that it is not a versatile drug. If a 0.25 mg/day dose does not bring a patient's blood pressure under control, increasing the dose will usually be accompanied by some serious drug toxicity.

PRAZOSIN (Minipres)

Prazosin has been recently introduced as an antihypertensive agent in the United States. Prazosin was initially marketed as a peripheral vasodilator because of its ability to inhibit phosphodiesterase, thereby increasing vessel cyclic AMP content. More recently, a potent postsynaptic α-adrenergic receptor inhibition of prazosin has been recognized. Since the concentration *in vitro* necessary to inhibit phosphodiesterase is almost 1000 times that required to inhibit α-adrenergic receptors, it is more likely that the drug's antihypertensive effect is through its adrenergic blocking actions.[16]

As with other α-adrenergic blockers, the use of prazosin is associated with orthostatic hypotension. However, unlike other α-adrenergic blockers, prazosin-induced hypotension is not associated with a large compensatory increase in heart rate and renal renin release. Because prazosin blocks both venous and arterial postsynaptic α-receptors, the drug decreases both cardiac afterload and cardiac preload (Table 15–1). It is exactly these properties of the drug that have made it useful for the treatment of chronic congestive heart failure.

Prazosin is indicated for use in mild to moderate hypertension. However, the drug has been used successfully for severe hypertension when combined with both a β-adrenergic blocker and a diuretic agent. Prazosin should always be used together with a diuretic drug to prevent the salt and water retention associated with prazosin-induced hypotension.

The incidence of toxicity for patients taking prazosin is similar to what is described for drugs like methyldopa and propranolol. By far the most common side effect observed is orthostatic hypotension. This effect is most prominent following the first few doses of the drug. Reports of syncope after the first dose of prazosin have been described; therefore, many physicians prescribe the first dose of the drug at bedtime to prevent the development of orthostasis. Other side effects of prazosin are more nonspecific and include headache, drowsiness, weakness, dry mouth, and nausea and other gastrointestinal disturbances. Overall, however, the drug is well tolerated.[17]

The pharmacokinetic parameters of prazosin have not been well delineated. The bioavailability of prazosin, however, is good but varies with food intake. Some studies suggest that food increases prazosin's absorption, while other studies report the opposite. In fact, the intake of food probably makes very little overall difference in the treatment of hypertension with prazosin. Once absorbed, prazosin is extensively metabolized by the liver to less active compounds by *O*-dealkylation and conjugation. Only a very small percentage of the total drug is excreted unchanged in the urine. Prazosin has a plasma half-life of about 2.5 to 4.0 hours and a volume of distribution of 1.2 to 1.5 L/kg. The drug is about 97 per cent protein bound. The usual dose of the drug is 1 to 10 mg twice a day. Even though the drug's plasma half-life is 2.5 to 4.0 hours, its duration of action is as long as 12 hours. The reason for this pharmacokinetic and pharmacodynamic dissociation is not known. However, the relationship between drug effect and plasma drug concentration is generally not linear for most antihypertensive drugs.

The use of prazosin in renal disease has not been well studied. Since the drug is mainly excreted through extrarenal routes, the dosage schedule probably does not need to be altered in renal failure. However, Curtis[18] reported that patients with renal failure responded with a fall in blood pressure after very low doses of prazosin, thus suggesting that patients with renal failure are more sensitive to the drug. Since no blood levels of the drug were obtained and the volume status of these patients was not investigated, it is difficult to define the exact cause of this increased drug sensitivity in renal failure. There is no doubt that patients with extracellular volume depletion are exquisitely sensitive to the antihypertensive effects of drugs that interfere with sympathetic function and that volume-expanded patients tend to be resistant. Thus, a patient with renal failure taking prazosin who is hypertensive prior to dialysis may become hypotensive after ultrafiltration and removal of fluid after or during dialysis.

The use of prazosin in liver disease has not been examined. However, since prazosin is almost exclusively metabolized by the liver, significant liver disease probably will affect the drug's plasma clearance. The practicing physician, therefore, should probably initiate prazosin at a low dose in hypertensive patients with liver disease, and titrate the maintenance dose according to blood pressure response.

HYDRALAZINE (Apresoline)

Hydralazine lowers blood pressure by having a direct effect on arterioles to decrease peripheral vascular resistance. Since the pathophysiology of essential hypertension is an increase in peripheral vascular resistance, hydralazine is theoretically an excellent drug in the treatment of hypertension. Hydralazine was introduced as an antihypertensive agent almost two decades ago, but the drug lost its popularity early because of the frequent occurrence of toxic side effects. However, there has been a resurgence of the use of hydralazine recently because hydralazine has been found to be quite effective when used together with a β-adrenergic blocking agent and a diuretic.[19] It is now clear that much of the toxicity associated with the use of hydralazine was secondary to the reflex sympathetic activation, an effect abolished by β-blockers. In addition, the frequently encountered resistance in the treatment of hypertension with hydralazine alone was secondary to salt and water retention, an effect blocked by diuretics.

Hydralazine is indicated in mild to severe hypertension. However, as stated previously, the drug has to be used together with a β-adrenergic blocker and a diuretic to prevent reflex tachycardia and salt and water retention associated with a hydralazine-induced decrease in blood pressure. The big advantage in using hydralazine over the sympatholytic drugs is that hydralazine has no effect on venous tone; thus, orthostatic hypotension does not occur. Although, theoretically, there is no maximal dose of hydralazine in lowering blood pressure, drug toxicity does develop frequently when the oral dosage of the drug exceeds 200 mg/day.

The most common side effects of the drug are headache, heart palpitations, nausea, and lethargy. The headache limits use of hydralazine in patients with vascular headaches. The palpitations and tachycardia both can be inhibited by use of β-adrenergic blocking agents. The physician should avoid using hydralazine in patients with coronary artery disease because precipitation of myocardial infarction can occur. If hydralazine use is necessary in such patients, the physician must be certain that the patient has undergone adequate β-adrenergic blockade.

Chronic administration of hydralazine can lead to an acute rheumatoid state resembling systemic lupus erythematosus. If this occurs, the drug should be discontinued immediately and the syndrome will then regress.[20] Both the total dosage used and the rate of acetylation play a role in the development of drug-induced lupus syndrome. The syndrome eventually appears in 10 to 20 per cent of patients treated with doses of 400 mg/day or more. However, several cases of lupus-like syndrome have developed in patients on low doses of the drug. Patients that are slow acetylators may be especially prone to develop hydralazine-induced lupus. The safest way to follow patients on hydralazine is to obtain plasma antinuclear antibody levels twice a year. With the appearance of a high antinuclear antibody titer, another antihypertensive agent should be substituted for hydralazine.

Patients on chronic hydralazine therapy occasionally develop a pyridoxine-responsive neuropathy. This neuropathy is very similar to that observed with isoniazid. Other side effects are rare with hydralazine.

The understanding of the metabolism of hydralazine is complex and is currently undergoing some revision owing to use of better analytic techniques. Clearly, some of the oral drug undergoes *N*-acetylation prior to reaching the systemic circulation. Thus, patients who are rapid acetylators have lower bioavailability of the drug than slow acetylators. The bioavailability difference is the major reason why rapid acetylators require more drug both to achieve a hypotensive response and to develop the drug-induced lupus syndrome. Once in the systemic circulation, the total plasma clearance of hydralazine in slow and rapid acetylators is comparable. This suggests that most of the drug metabolism is neither by transacetylation nor by liver metabolism. Indeed, the plasma clearance of hydralazine is severalfold greater than liver blood flow. It has been suggested that the high plasma clearance of the drug is secondary to intravascular conversion of hydralazine to hydralazine pyruvic acid hydrazone. The actual half-life of hydralazine itself is less than an hour in the plasma, but several conjugated metabolites have longer half-lives.[21] The duration of action of hydralazine is frequently as long as 12 hours. The explanation for this pharmacokinetic and pharmacodynamic dissociation is not readily apparent. It has been suggested that hydralazine is concentrated and bound in the vascular smooth muscle and released slowly into the circulation to explain the drug's long duration of action.[22] However, with the more recent evidence that many of hydralazine's metabolites have vascular activity equal to that of hydralazine, it is quite possible that the persistence of a metabolite in the plasma is responsible for the duration of the antihypertensive activity of hydralazine.[23]

The exact alteration of hydralazine dosage in patients with renal and hepatic insufficiency has not been well established. Earlier studies have shown that the half-life of hydralazine is prolonged in renal failure. However, in these investigations, both the parent drug and the metabolites were probably measured in the plasma. Since the major route of elimination of the hydralazine conjugates is in the urine (and these metabolites are vasoactive), hydralazine should be used carefully in renal failure. Since the interindividual dose requirement for hydralazine is variable, it is difficult to recommend a precise dosage for renal failure. As a general rule, therefore, starting hydralazine at a low dose and carefully titrating the drug dose to the desired level of blood pressure response should avoid excessive hypotension.

A similar approach also is recommended with use of hydralazine in patients with hepatic disease. Severe hepatic cellular structural disease (e.g., cirrhosis) could limit acetylation and, thus, increase the bioavailability of hydralazine. Since the bioavailability of hydralazine is 10 per cent in fast acetylators and 25 per cent in slow acetylators, the drug's bioavailability could be increased severalfold. In addition, since hydralazine elimination is partially through liver metabolism, liver disease could prolong the half-life of the native drug.

Overall, however, hydralazine can be used safely and effectively in patients with either liver or renal disease if the prescribing physician starts with a low dose and titrates the dose gradually until the desired blood pressure is achieved.

MINOXIDIL (Loniten)

Minoxidil has only recently been marketed in the United States, although the drug has been studied for over a decade. Minoxidil is a very useful addition to the antihypertensive armamentarium, especially in the treatment of otherwise severe drug-resistant hypertension. The hypotensive action of minoxidil is by decreasing peripheral vascular resistance through dilating arterioles. Thus, it has a mechanism similar to hydralazine. In contrast, however, minoxidil is more potent and may have an antihypertensive effect in patients that do not respond to hydralazine.[24]

As with hydralazine, the lowering of blood pressure with minoxidil is associated with reflex sympathetic activation and salt and water retention. Consequently, the drug has to be used together with a β-adrenergic blocker and a diuretic to prevent tachycardia and salt and water retention, respectively. Since the drug decreases arteriolar but not venous tone, orthostasis is not a symptom associated with the use of minoxidil. The combination of minoxidil, furosemide, and propranolol is often effective even in the most difficult of hypertensive patients.

The drug has been reported to cause pulmonary hypertension when used chronically. Most likely, the pulmonary hypertension is a result of salt and water retention with subsequent congestive heart failure. Minoxidil use will result in excess hair growth in places where there are hair follicles. This cosmetic problem is usually well tolerated, but some patients have stopped taking minoxidil because of this side effect. Unlike hydralazine, minoxidil use is not associated with drug-induced lupus syndrome. The usual dosage can be anywhere from 2 mg/day to as high as 80 mg/day. Until wider experience is available, minoxidil is indicated only in severe hypertension, or in hypertension not responsive to the usual agents.

The pharmacokinetic parameters of minoxidil have been well studied. The drug is well absorbed, but its bioavailability is probably less than unity because of first-pass liver metabolism. The drug is not protein bound, and 90 per cent is metabolized in the liver to various conjugates. Total body clearance of the drug is 600 ml/min, but only 70 ml/min represents renal clearance. Volume of distribution is 2 to 3 L/kg, and the reported half-life is 4.2 hours.[25] Although the half-life of minoxidil is short, the duration of action of the drug is as long as 24 hours. Some researchers have suggested that minoxidil is sequestered by the arteriolar smooth muscles where it exerts a persistent effect on receptor sites.[26] In addition, the possibility of persistence of active metabolites has not been thoroughly examined.

Since the renal clearance of minoxidil represents only a small fraction of the total clearance of the drug, renal insufficiency will not cause much accumulation of the drug. In fact, in patients with renal failure who have been unresponsive to other antihypertensive drugs, minoxidil has been widely and successfully utilized. The effect of liver disease on minoxidil pharmacokinetics has not been studied. Since most of the drug is cleared by the liver, drug accumulation would be expected to occur with significant liver disease. However, the interindividual variability in the dose requirement is quite high for minoxidil. Thus, it is impossible to predict what the dosage requirement for a particular patient with liver disease might be. As a rule, the higher the blood pressure, the more minoxidil is required to return blood pressure to the normotensive range. In patients with significant liver disease, it would be reasonable to start minoxidil at lower doses and titrate the dose to the desired blood pressure.

SODIUM NITROPRUSSIDE (Nipride)

Sodium nitroprusside has been approved in the United States for treatment of severe hypertension since 1974. This agent has also been utilized in the management of aortic dissection, severe congestive heart failure, and in the setting of acute myocardial infarction.[27-30] Nitroprusside causes relaxation of arterial and venous smooth muscle. This relaxation is not mediated through any known receptor system and the cellular mechanism of action of nitroprusside remains uncertain. The chemical responsible for the vascular smooth muscle relaxation properties of nitroprusside is also unknown. Thus, neither cyanide nor thiocyanate, metabolites of nitroprusside, can be implicated as sole mediators of the hypotensive effect.

Nitroprusside is rapidly decomposed by nonenzymatic conversion to cyanide. This conversion to cyanide probably occurs by a direct interaction of nitroprusside with sulfhydryl groups in red blood cells and tissues. The cyanide formed is rapidly converted to thiocyanate, which has a half-life of 7 to 10 days and is excreted by the kidneys. The conversion of cyanide to thiocyanate requires the mitochondrial enzyme rhodanase, a sulfhydryl transferase located in hepatic and renal tissue. The rhodanase system is dependent on an adequate supply of sulfur in order to form thiocyanate.

When utilizing nitroprusside therapy, prevention of cyanide and thiocyanate toxicity is mandatory. Such toxicity is more likely to occur in patients with renal and hepatic disease who may lack rhodanase and in patients receiving high doses (> 3 μg/kg/min) for longer than 72 hours.[27-30] Cyanide combines with cytochrome *c* of the respiratory chain, thereby inhibiting aerobic metabolism and increasing lactate production. Thus, metabolic acidosis is often an early indication of cyanide toxicity.[28-30] Some observers feel that significant tachyphylaxis to the hypotensive effect of nitroprusside may also be an early indication of cyanide accumulation.[29] Thiocyanate toxicity is usually neurologic in nature, with seizures, confusion, and hyperreflexia occurring. Thiocyanate levels less than 10 mg/dl are usually well tolerated, while levels greater than 20 mg/dl may be associated with toxicity.

Therapy of suspected or confirmed cyanide toxicity includes infusions of thiosulfate (to serve as a sulfur donor, thereby facilitating conversion of cyanide to cyanate), and sodium nitrate (to induce methemoglobinemia, which combines with cyanide to form cyanomethemoglobinemia). In addition, vitamin B_{12} combines with cyanide to form cyanocobalamin. The prophylactic infusion of hydroxycobalamin (25 mg/hr) can decrease red blood cell cyanide and tissue hypoxia during nitroprusside infusion.[28] Thiocyanate toxicity is best managed by discontinuation of nitroprusside and the use of dialysis.

Nitroprusside can be administered only parenterally. The hypotensive half-life of the drug is very short. Additional pharmacokinetic parameters for nitroprusside are not available. Both hepatic and renal disease may be expected to enhance the likelihood of development of cyanide and thiocyanate accumulation. Thus, in these circumstances, utilization of low dosage with careful clinical, blood gas, and cyanide and thiocyanate level monitoring (when available) should be considered if prolonged (> 72 hrs) therapy is needed.

DIAZOXIDE (Hyperstat)

Diazoxide, a nondiuretic thiazide derivative, effectively lowers arterial pressure by directly decreasing peripheral vascular resistance.[31-39] The ability of diazoxide to diminish muscle tone is not limited to the vascular tree. For example, diazoxide also diminishes uterine contractile response to oxytocin.[33] Oral absorption is dependent on the physical properties of the drug, with suspensions of the drug being better absorbed than capsules or tablets. Only the parenteral form is available in the United States. In adult volunteers with normal renal function, the oral administration of 200 to 300 mg gives peak plasma levels of 15 to 25 μg/ml at 2 to 6 hours, which persist for several hours. For hypertensive emergencies, maximal blood pressure–lowering effect is seen immediately following rapid (3 to 5 mg/kg) intravenous administration. Following 3 to 5 mg/kg rapid intravenous pulses of diazoxide, immediate peak blood levels of 15 to 25 μg/ml occur, while blood levels greater than 5 μg/ml occur up to 36 hours. However, the hypotensive activity of diazoxide does not correlate well with plasma levels of the drug. Greater hypotensive effect is usually seen after the rapid intravenous administration of the drug, as opposed to oral administration; although oral administration does result in decreases in blood pressure. The hypotensive effect of diazoxide is only one-third as long as its half-life. Diazoxide is 90 per cent protein bound and crosses the placenta. The protein binding of diazoxide diminishes with increasing blood levels and is also decreased in renal failure. No data on distribution of diazoxide are availabile for humans. In dogs and rats, diazoxide is widely distributed in tissues with kidneys, adrenals, liver, lungs, pancreas, and heart all demonstrating tissue:plasma ratios greater than 1. Diazoxide likely undergoes some metabolism in humans; recent studies suggest that 20 per cent of the diazoxide excreted by the kidneys is a polar metabolite. The metabolites of diazoxide are not protein bound and are devoid of vasodilator activity. Variable reports suggest that from 10 to 90 per cent of diazoxide or its metabolites are excreted by the kidneys and that the renal clearance of diazoxide is 4 to 5 ml/min. The half-life of diazoxide in patients with normal renal function is 20 to 36 hours. In patients with impaired renal function, the half-life of diazoxide has been reported to increase with decreasing renal function. Although diazoxide accumulation likely occurs in patients with impaired renal function, both parenteral and oral therapy is efficacious in these cases without excess secondary effects.

Among the untoward effects are hypotension, seizures, arrhythmias, gastrointestinal symptoms, hypersensitivity reactions, pain at injection site, bone marrow suppression, pancreatitis, and hirsutism.[31, 33, 34] At hypotensive doses, diazoxide will result in transient decreases in renal blood flow, glomerular filtration rate, and sodium and water excretion. Prolonged oral administration has also resulted in increases in plasma volume and body weight. Increases in serum uric acid due to decreases in renal uric acid excretion are frequent. Diazoxide has a pronounced hyperglycemic effect following both oral and intravenous therapy that appears to be due to insulin suppression. Nonketotic and ketotic hyperglycemia and coma can result. Diazoxide may stop labor and, by displacing coumadin from albumin, can be synergistic with the effect of coumarin derivatives. Recently, extrapyramidal symptoms occurred in 15 per cent of diazoxide-treated patients in one series.

The dialysance of diazoxide during hemodialysis is 23 to 28 ml/min.[39] In a single patient undergoing peritoneal dialysis, 18 hours of dialysis lowered plasma diazoxide concentrations from 45 mg/L to 15 mg/L.[10] The high degree of protein binding substantially limits dialyzability.

Since the half-life of diazoxide increases with decreasing renal function, it may be anticipated that smaller doses or longer dosage intervals of diazoxide would be required in patients with impaired renal function. However, diazoxide responsiveness does not appear to correlate well with serum levels. To date, standard rapid intravenous doses (3 to 5 mg/kg) and oral doses (100 to 400 mg/day) of diazoxide have been observed to be effective in some patients with impaired renal function. It should be noted that extensive experience with chronic oral diazoxide in patients with renal failure is not available, and some reports suggest that patients with renal failure are susceptible to untoward secondary effects of the drug.[32, 36] As with other antihypertensives, titration of dose and frequency of administration should be monitored by blood pressure responses and observation for secondary effects. Since diazoxide induces sodium retention, the concomitant administration of a potent diuretic, such as furosemide, may often potentiate the effect of diazoxide. No information is available on the use of diazoxide in patients with liver disease. The low albumin levels seen in patients with liver disease will decrease protein binding and enhance the hypotensive effect of diazoxide.

THE USE OF DIURETIC DRUGS IN PATIENTS WITH KIDNEY AND LIVER DISEASE

The diuretic drugs are unusual in that the magnitude of the diuresis in an individual can be titrated by altering the dose administered without resorting to blood levels. This readily observable dose-response relationship is unfortunately not available for most drugs used clinically. Nevertheless, in order to estimate the frequency of administration of the diuretic agent and how to alter diuretic administration in renal and hepatic diseases, a knowledge of their pharmacokinetics and their mode of action is of utmost importance. The diuretic furosemide illustrates the importance of the understanding of the pharmacokinetics and pharmacodynamics in the rational use of a drug. Drugs that are removed by the kidneys accumulate in the body in renal failure; thus, a decrease in dosage is necessary to avoid toxic accumulation and excessive response. However, with a drug like furosemide, whose action is dependent on the drug reaching the luminal surface of the nephron, an actual increase in dosage is necessary in renal failure. In patients with renal disease, diuretic agents are often utilized to maintain sodium and water balance. In general, once the glomerular filtration rate declines below 30 ml/min, only the "loop" diuretics, and possibly metolazone, continue to be effective natriuretic agents.

The use of potassium-sparing diuretics should be limited in patients with renal disease, since these agents can result in severe hyperkalemia, even with mild renal failure. This hyperkalemia is most pronounced in diabetic patients who are deficient in humoral factors important in transcellular potassium transport (i.e., insulin, aldosterone, catecholamines).

With regard to liver disease, several studies suggest that diuretic therapy in the cirrhotic patient may be associated with a substantial risk of adverse effects. The results of Sherlock's survey of diuretic-related complications occurring in cirrhotics treated from 1962 to 1965 suggest that 10 to 40 per cent of patients develop drug-related encephalopathy, hypokalemia, or azotemia.[40, 41]

A dangerous complication in the cirrhotic patient is the induction of azotemia by the overzealous use of diuretic. Shear and associates[42] have demonstrated that the maximum rate of mobilization of ascites from the peritoneum is 300 ml/day and with peripheral edema, 600 ml/day.[35] Thus, a more rapid rate of diuresis (i.e., > 1 L/day of negative fluid balance) occurs only at the expense of diminishing plasma volume and deterioration in renal function.[43] Fortunately, such diuretic-induced azotemia is often reversible. Diuretics, however, have been demonstrated to precipitate nonreversible renal failure in patients with cirrhosis.

General principles in the treatment of ascites include:

1. Exclusion of specific, treatable causes of ascites.
2. Daily weights and careful clinical and biochemical monitoring.
3. Ascertainment of stability of liver and renal function before institution of diuretic therapy.
4. An initial trial of bedrest and restriction of dietary sodium before diuretic therapy, since this therapy may result in a diuresis in 10 to 25 per cent of cirrhotic patients.
5. A daily weight loss of 1 to 2 pounds in patients with ascites and peripheral edema and 0.3 pound in patients with ascites without peripheral edema should be considered optimal.
6. The end point of therapy is maximum patient comfort with a minimum of drug-induced complications. This may require slight liberalization of sodium intake at the expense of increased dosage of diuretics and the maintenance of some residual ascites in selected patients.

A suggested regimen for diuretic therapy of ascites includes:

1. Sodium restriction (10 to 40 mEq/day).
2. If no diuresis occurs in 3 to 4 days, add spironolactone (100 mg/day); increase spironolactone by 100 mg every 3 to 5 days to a maximal dose of 400 mg/day. This results in a diuresis in 40 to 60 per cent of patients.
3. If no diuresis results with 400 mg of spironolactone, add hydrochlorothiazide (50 to 200 mg/day) or furosemide (20 to 80 mg/day).
4. If no diuresis is observed on this regimen after reassessment of dietary intake, and hepatic and renal function show no deterioration, increasing doses of furosemide may be used.

Utilizing a similar protocol, Gregory and co-workers[44] demonstrated effectiveness and relative lack of adverse effects in the treatment of ascites complicating cirrhosis.

Under usual circumstances, restriction of water is not necessary unless the patient has evidence of impaired renal water excretion (hyponatremia < 130 mEq/L). In cirrhotic patients with ascites and hyponatremia, modest water restriction to allow a negative water balance results in improvement of the hyponatremia. In rare instances, ascites not responsive to the above regimen may be treated by portacaval shunting or mechanical diversion procedures (peritoneal-venous [LeVeen] shunt). Whether or not the surgical mortality and morbidity of such procedures (e.g., hepatic encephalopathy, peritonitis, intravascular coagulation) outweigh the advantages remains to be shown.

BENZOTHIADIAZINES

The diuretic agent chlorothiazide was discovered in 1956 and was marketed shortly afterward.[45] Since then, hydrochlorothiazide has become the most popular agent in the treatment of hypertension and edema. Both chlorthalidone and metolazone are heterocyclic variants of thiazide diuretics (benzothiadiazines) (Fig. 15–2) and act in the same area of the nephron as the more classic benzothiadiazines; these agents, therefore, will also be considered in this section.

The diuretic effects of the benzothiadiazine compounds are due to inhibition of the sodium reabsorption in the early part of the distal convoluted tubule. Although some researchers have suggested a proximal tubular effect of these drugs, this action is unimportant relative to the more distal effect. Because of their effect on the early part of the distal tubule, these drugs impair maximal urinary dilution. This distal effect, as well as the diminished distal fluid delivery that occurs secondary to volume depletion, makes them useful drugs in the treatment of diabetes insipidus.[46] The drug's main indication is in the treatment of hypertension. In fact, benzothiadiazines are the mainstay of therapy for the majority of patients with mild to moderate hypertension. No benzothiadiazine compound has a particular advantage over another in the treatment of hypertension. Since hydrochlorothiazide is the least expensive in the group, it has been preferred by the majority of practitioners. One requirement of the diuretic in the treatment of hypertension is that diuresis has to be achieved.[47] Since renal failure has been shown to significantly blunt the diuretic effect of the benzothiadiazines, these drugs are not that useful in hypertensive with significant renal failure (glomerular filtration rate < 25 ml/min). One exception may be the use of metolazone, which retains a significant diuretic effect even when the glomerular filtration rate is below 25 ml/min.[48]

Benzothiadiazines are also useful in the treatment of chronic congestive heart failure with normal renal function. However, the drugs should not be used in acute pulmonary edema, in which a faster-acting drug like furosemide, which also has venodilator properties, is more useful.

The toxicity of benzothiadiazines is usually an extension of their effect to induce a diuresis. Thus, salt and water depletion is a frequently encountered problem with the use of any of the diuretic agents. In these patients, blood urea nitrogen and serum creatinine will rise and postural hypotension will develop. Hyponatremia can occur after benzothiadiazine therapy if the patient has access to free water, since volume depletion stimulates vasopressin release, thereby preventing free water clearance.

Potassium deficiency is a common problem with benzothiadiazine therapy. Although usually mild, occasionally potassium deficien-

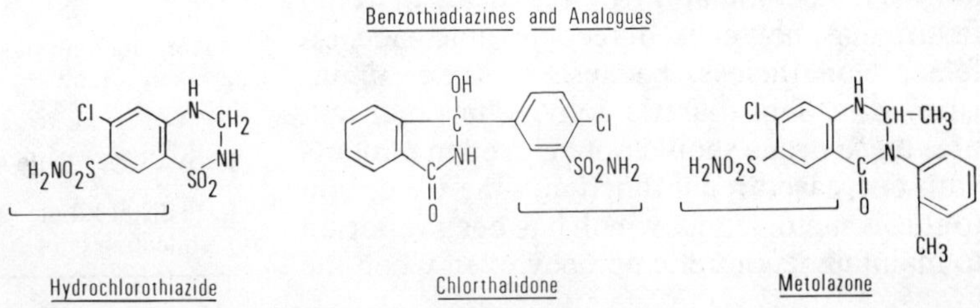

Benzothiadiazines and Analogues

Hydrochlorothiazide — Chlorthalidone — Metolazone

Figure 15–2. The structure of hydrochlorothiazide as compared to the benzodiathiazine analogues metolazone and chlorthalidone.

cy can be severe enough to cause muscle weakness. Patients who are on a digitalis preparation are especially prone to develop cardiac arrhythmias if hypokalemia is also present. Metabolic alkalosis is seen along with hypokalemia, mainly because of secondary aldosteronism. Carbohydrate intolerance is frequently found with chronic use of benzothiadiazine therapy and is likely related, at least partially, to the hypokalemia, since hypokalemia is known to impair insulin release. A few cases of hyperosmolar nonketotic coma have been described in older maturity-onset diabetics treated with any of these drugs. Hyperuricemia and hypertriglyceridemia are regular findings with the use of benzothiadiazines. In addition, allergic reactions have been ascribed to these drugs; thiazide diuretics have also been rarely reported to induce an allergic interstitial nephritis.[49]

Although the benzothiadiazines have been discussed together, they do differ in one important respect; namely, their duration of action. Both chlorothiazide and hydrochlorothiazide have plasma half-lives in the 8- to 10-hour range, while chlorthalidone has a plasma half-life well over 24 hours.[50, 51] Metolazone's plasma half-life has been reported to be only 8 hours. All of the benzothiadiazines are excreted unchanged by the kidney through both filtration and tubular secretion. The principal differences in these drugs' half-lives are secondary to variability in plasma protein binding and volume of distribution. Chlorthalidone is more lipid soluble than hydrochlorothiazide and, consequently, has a higher volume of distribution, which partially accounts for its longer half-life.

Since the benzothiadiazines are exclusively eliminated through the kidney, liver disease does not influence the clearance of these drugs. However, in severe liver disease, hypokalemic alkalosis can precipitate hepatic coma, therefore cautioning against injudicious use of these diuretics in patients with liver disease. In renal disease, benzothiadiazines will accumulate; however, since most side effects of these drugs are related to their diuresis, accumulation of the drug in renal failure has not caused recognizable side effects. Nonetheless, because of their diminished or absent diuretic activity in renal failure, these drugs should not be used in patients with decreased renal function. One exception to this is metolazone, which has been reported to maintain its diuretic potency even when the glomerular filtration rate falls below 25 ml/min. To summarize, benzothiadiazines are very useful drugs in the treatment of both hypertension and chronic congestive heart failure. Since hydrochlorothiazide is the least expensive of the group of drugs, it should be the one selected most frequently for treatment. In renal failure, metolazone may be more effective. If a long duration of action is desired, as in the treatment of diabetes insipidus, chlorthalidone is preferred.

FUROSEMIDE

Furosemide is an extremely potent diuretic agent that was introduced in 1966, almost 10 years after the benzothiadiazines. However, at present, furosemide has become the most frequently prescribed diuretic agent.

Furosemide is structurally different from the benzothiadiazines in that it contains an anthranilic acid derivative of the thiadiazine group. Furosemide acts on the ascending limb of the loop of Henle to inhibit active chloride transport. Since the ascending limb of the loop of Henle reabsorbs a greater fraction of the total solute load than the distal tubule (Table 15–2), furosemide is a more potent diuretic than the benzothiadiazines. Furosemide has to reach the luminal side of the loop of Henle to inhibit chloride transport.[52] The drug gains entrance into tubular lumen mainly through active secretion in the straight portion of the proximal tubule via the organic acid pump.

Furosemide may be used in both acute and chronic congestive heart failure. In acute pul-

TABLE 15–2. DIURETICS AND THEIR SITE OF ACTION

Segment of Nephron	Per Cent of Filtrate Reabsorbed	Diuretics Interfering with the Function of Segment
Proximal tubule	~70%	Carbonic anhydrase inhibitors
Ascending limb of Henle's loop	~20%	Furosemide Ethacrynic acid Mercurials
Early distal tubule	~5%	Benzothiadiazines
Late distal tubule collecting duct	~1–2%	Spironolactone Triamterene

monary edema, furosemide not only produces a rapid diuresis, thereby reducing intravascular volume, but also has a direct effect to decrease venous tone, thereby reducing cardiac preload. In chronic congestive heart failure, furosemide administration may prevent salt and water accumulation associated with decreased cardiac function. Although also used in the treatment of hypertension, furosemide offers no advantage over the benzothiadiazines when the renal function is adequate. However, in renal insufficiency, furosemide will cause diuresis in patients resistant to benzothiadiazines.

The side effects of furosemide are mostly related to its potent diuretic properties. Consequently, salt and water depletion is common. Hypokalemia, hyperuricemia, and hyperglycemia are observed as frequently with furosemide as with the benzothiadiazines. Ototoxicity has been reported occasionally after large doses of intravenous furosemide.[53] This ototoxicity may be especially common when large doses of furosemide are administered to patients with renal failure. However, ototoxicity has also been observed with small doses in patients with normal renal function.[54] The ototoxicity is usually reversible, although some patients fail to recover auditory function. The mechanism for this ototoxicity is incompletely understood.

The pharmacokinetic parameters of furosemide have been extensively studied.[55, 56] The drug is well absorbed after oral administration and has minimal first-pass metabolism. In the systemic circulation, it distributes into a volume of 0.15 L/kg. The drug is highly protein bound (~ 95 per cent). Furosemide is cleared from the plasma by both renal and hepatic routes, with renal routes predominating in patients with normal renal function. The drug has a half-life of about 90 to 100 minutes. The drug is secreted into the renal tubular lumen via the organic acid transport pump. Thus, drugs like probenecid will interfere with the tubular secretion of furosemide, but probably not with its diuretic potency, since higher plasma drug concentrations compensate for this inhibition. In patients with renal failure, furosemide is metabolized by the liver; then the half-life of the drug can be as long as 10 to 12 hours. There is evidence that the hepatic uptake of furosemide is via an organic acid transport pump as well. Thus, both in renal failure, because naturally occurring organic acids accumulate, and after probenecid administration, the hepatic clearance of the drug is decreased because of competitive inhibitor at the organic transport site.[55, 56]

In renal failure, furosemide is still active when a higher plasma drug concentration is achieved. Thus, the actual dose of the drug has to be increased in patients with renal failure. The main danger of these high doses is the development of ototoxicity. However, ototoxicity is usually reversible and relatively uncommon.

In severe hepatic disease, the renal function is frequently affected as well, making it difficult to evaluate the role of hepatic disease alone on furosemide pharmacokinetics. Since a significant part of the total plasma clearance of the drug is hepatic in origin, severe liver disease with normal renal function results in some drug accumulation and intensification of the diuretic effect of a given dose of furosemide. Another important consideration is the effect of chronic furosemide administration to produce hypokalemic alkalosis, which may lead to the development of hepatic encephalopathy.

Overall, the popularity of furosemide is justified. The drug is a very safe and efficacious drug over a wide range of renal function. In renal failure, the dosage of furosemide should be adjusted upward to elevate plasma furosemide concentrations so as to compete effectively for organic acid secretory pumps in the proximal tubule.

ETHACRYNIC ACID (Edecrin)

Ethacrynic acid was discovered as a result of a search for a nonmercurial inhibitor of sulfhydryl-catalyzed enzyme system in the kidney. Although ethacrynic acid is frequently used interchangeably with furosemide, their mechanisms of action are different. Both ethacrynic acid and furosemide exert their major effect on the ascending limb of the loop of Henle to inhibit chloride transport. Ethacrynic acid, however, competes for the same excretory carrier and diuretic receptor as the mercurials, while furosemide does not.[57] Ethacrynic acid by itself is inactive to inhibit chloride transport and has to form an ethacrynic-cysteine complex to be active.

The indications for ethacrynic acid are the same as for furosemide. Ethacrynic acid exhibits no therapeutic advantages over furosemide and possible disadvantages in terms of toxicity. The alleged efficacy of ethacrynic acid in cases of furosemide resistance is more anecdotal than factual. In fact, a controlled study comparing the diuretic efficacy of furosemide 80 mg, ethacrynic acid 100 mg, and mercaptomerin 125 mg, revealed that furosemide was slightly better than ethacrynic acid, and much better than mercaptomerin.[49] Volume depletion, potassium deficiency, metabolic alkalosis, hyperuricemia, and hyperglycemia are all seen with the use of ethacrynic acid at the same frequency as with the use of furosemide. However, gastrointestinal symptoms, including upper gastrointestinal bleeding, as well as ototoxicity are more commonly observed with the use of ethacrynic acid than with furosemide.[59] There are reported instances of ototoxicity after standard intravenous doses of ethacrynic acid in patients without renal failure.

The pharmacokinetic parameters of ethacrynic acid have not been extensively studied in humans. The drug is well absorbed after oral administration and appears to distribute into a small volume of distribution (~ 0.1 L/kg). The drug is highly protein bound and has a half-life of about 60 minutes. The drug is cleared through both renal and hepatic routes. The renal excretion occurs via tubular secretion in the proximal tubule by the active organic acid pump. The pharmacokinetics of ethacrynic acid have not been extensively studied in either renal failure or hepatic disease, which is reason enough to avoid the use of the drug in these disease states. The only clear-cut circumstance in which ethacrynic acid is superior to furosemide for diuresis is if the patient has demonstrated an allergic reaction to furosemide.

MERCURIAL DIURETICS

Mercurial diuretics are of historic importance but have no practical use in clinical medicine today. Inorganic mercury has been used as a diuretic since the sixteenth century. Organic mercurial compounds used in the early twentieth century for the treatment of syphilis were found to have diuretic activity as well. Various organic mercurial compounds were developed between 1920 and 1960 as diuretic agents for the treatment of edematous states. Some older physicians still prefer to use mercurials for the treatment of congestive heart failure even though the more versatile orally active diuretics are more efficacious.

Not all organic mercurials have diuretic activity. Only organic mercurials that are acid labile and release inorganic mercury in renal tissues are active.[60] It is the inorganic mercury that interacts with the sulfhydryl-containing enzymes in the renal tissue to poison tubular reabsorptive sites. Mercurials most likely work in the ascending limb of the loop of Henle to inhibit chloride reabsorption. The drug is ineffective during hypochloremic metabolic alkalosis.

Organic mercurials are excreted almost exclusively by the renal route. The drug should not be used in patients with renal failure because accumulation of the drug can precipitate organic mercurial poisoning. Fatal cardiac arrhythmias have occurred from high organic mercurial plasma concentrations when the drug has been given intravenously. These drugs can probably be given safely in patients with liver disease if the renal function is normal. However, chronic use of mercurials will result in the development of hypokalemic alkalosis that could precipitate hepatic encephalopathy.

SPIRONOLACTONE (Aldactone)

Spironolactone was introduced as a diuretic agent in 1960. The drug is a direct aldosterone antagonist and, consequently, appears to be most effective in disease states associated with high aldosterone levels. Since the fraction of the total glomerular filtrate reaching the distal tubular sites is small, the drug is a weak diuretic as compared to the loop diuretics or even to the benzothiadiazines. Since the drug indirectly interferes with potassium secretion, the use of this diuretic is associated with potassium retention rather than potassium depletion. Spironolactone is frequently used together with another diuretic to avoid potassium depletion or the necessity for potassium supplementation.

Spironolactone may be used in the treatment of hypertension (particularly secondary to primary hyperaldosteronism), congestive heart failure, and nephrotic syndrome, especially when used together with one of the benzothiadiazines. The drug has been used alone in high doses (100 to 400 mg/day) to treat the ascites and edema associated with hepatic cirrhosis.

There are several potential toxicities associated with spironolactone use.[61] Hyperkalemia is a frequent occurrence and can be especially dangerous if the patient is on a high potassium diet as well. The concomitant use of spironolactone and salt substitute (which is mostly KCl) is an especially dangerous situation. Gastrointestinal irritation consisting of nausea, vomiting, and diarrhea can occur in 10 per cent of patients using the drug. A most annoying side effect of the drug is gynecomastia in males; this may also be accompanied by impotence. This effect is dose related and is more commonly observed when the daily dose of the drug exceeds 200 mg/day. Amenorrhea and rarely menorrhagia are seen in some women taking spironolactone. These latter side effects are related to the steroid-like structure of spironolactone (Fig. 15–3). Volume depletion is rarely a significant problem with the use of spironolactone alone.

The pharmacokinetic parameters of spironolactone have not been extensively studied, since measurement of plasma levels of spironolactone is difficult. After oral administration of spironolactone, the bioavailability is greater than 90 per cent. Spironolactone is very rapidly metabolized to canrenone, which is as active as spironolactone in inhibiting aldosterone activity. Canrenone is 90 to 98 per cent bound to plasma proteins and after its distribution phase the plasma levels decline with a half-life of about 16 hours.[62] Canrenone is eliminated by both liver metabolism and renal excretion. The drug would be expected to accumulate if used in renal or hepatic failure. Moreover, because of the high probability of the development of hyperkalemia, spironolactone should not be used in patients with renal failure.

Since spironolactone's transformation to canrenone occurs in the liver, and at least 50 per cent of the circulating canrenone is further metabolized by the liver, one would expect both of these drugs to accumulate in patients with liver disease. Nonetheless, high doses of spironolactone have been used in patients with cirrhosis of the liver without important side effects. Hyperchloremic, hyperkalemic, metabolic acidosis, however, has been observed to occur.[63] Since cirrhotic patients may have very high circulating concentrations of aldosterone, a very high spironolactone concentration is required to induce a natriuretic effect.

TRIAMTERENE (Dyrenium)

Triamterene, like spironolactone, is a most useful diuretic when utilized together with either a "loop" diuretic or benzothiadiazine to prevent potassium wasting. The drug was introduced in the early 1960's. Triamterene acts in the distal tubule to prevent sodium reabsorption and potassium secretion. However, unlike spironolactone, the action of triamterene is not dependent of the presence of aldosterone.

There are only a few indications for triamterene use. The drug is less potent than spironolactone in lowering blood pressure in hypertensives. The diuresis attained from the use of triamterene alone is small; consequently, the drug cannot be used alone for edematous states. Used together with another diuretic, triamterene will potentiate the natriuresis and inhibit potassium wasting.

The most common side effect associated with the use of triamterene is the development of hyperkalemia. Mild hyperuricemia and gastrointestinal symptoms occur in 10 to 20 per cent of patients using triamterene. Since the drug is a weak inhibitor of dihydrofolate reductase, patients with borderline folic acid deficiency can develop a megaloblastic anemia.[64]

The pharmacokinetics of triamterene have been examined in humans.[65] The absorption of the drug after oral administration ranges from 40 to 70 per cent. In addition, the drug under-

Figure 15–3. The steroid-like structure of the aldosterone antagonist spironolactone as compared to triamterene.

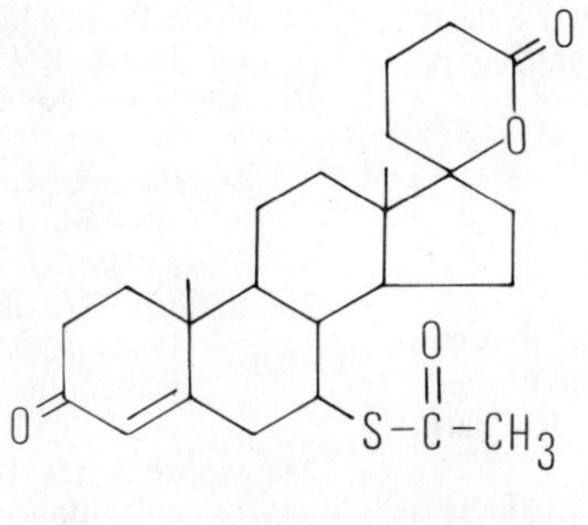

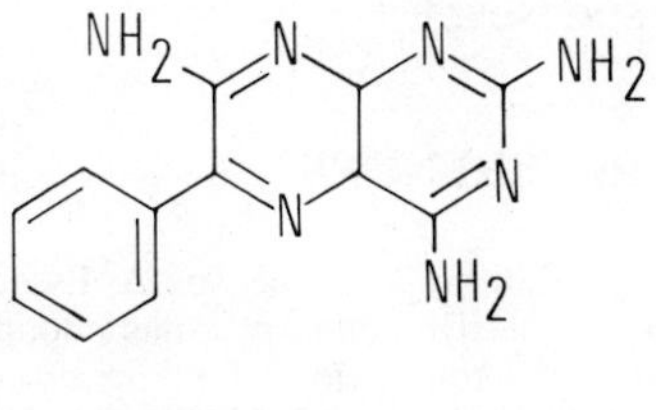

goes significant first-pass liver metabolism, making the total bioavailability of the drug quite low. Once in the systemic circulation, the drug distributes into a volume of 2 to 3 L/kg and has an elimination half-life of 2 hours. Total body clearance of the drug is somewhere in the 800 to 1000 ml/min range. Renal clearance represents only 15 per cent of this, while the hepatic clearance accounts for the remainder. The drug is only 50 per cent protein bound and is metabolized to an inactive compound.

Triamterene should not be used in patients with significant renal dysfunction because of the danger of developing hyperkalemia. In mild renal disease, the overall plasma clearance of the drug should be unaltered. In contrast, in severe liver disease, not only is the plasma clearance of the drug decreased, but the drug's bioavailability is enhanced; therefore, development of toxic drug levels is likely. It is wise to reduce triamterene dosage in patients with significant functional or structural liver disease.

CONCLUSIONS

Both the antihypertensive drugs and the diuretic drugs used in clinical practice alter physiologic functions in humans (e.g., blood pressure, renal excretion) that can be monitored easily. Such a luxury does not exist for many other drugs used in clinical practice. The pharmacologic properties needed to assess dosage interval are detailed in the Appendix.

The common adverse side effects of these drugs are generally extensions of their pharmacologic actions and can be minimized by dosage adjustment or by administration of other drugs to counteract the untoward effects. By understanding the pharmacokinetics and pharmacodynamics of these drugs, dosages can be adjusted rationally in patients with either renal or hepatic insufficiency, thus avoiding drug accumulation and excessive responses.

REFERENCES

1. Henring M, Rubenson A: Evidence that the hypotensive action of α-methyldopa is mediated by central action of methylnoradrenaline. J. Pharm. Pharmacol. *23*:407–411, 1971.
2. Horwitz D, Pettinger WA, Orvis H, et al.: Effects of methyldopa in fifty hypertensive patients. Clin. Pharmacol. Ther. *8*:224–234, 1967.
3. Rodman JS, Deutsch DJ, Gutman SI: Methyldopa hepatitis. Amer. J. Med. *60*:941–948, 1976.
4. Stenback O. Myhre E, Brodwall EK, Hansen T: Hypotensive effect of methyldopa in renal failure associated with hypertension. Acta Med. Scand. *191*:333–337, 1971.
5. Woosley RL, Nies AS: Guanethidine. N. Engl. J. Med. *295*:1053–1057, 1976.
6. Mitchell JR, Cavanaugh JH, Arias L, Oates JA: Guanethidine and related agents. III. Antagonism by drugs which inhibit norepinephrine pump in man. J. Clin. Invest. *49*:1596–1604, 1970.
7. Lukas G: Metabolism and biochemical pharmacology of guanethidine and related compounds. Drug Metab. Rev. *2*:101–116, 1973.
8. Leishman AWD, Sandler G: Guanethidine and hypertension after five years. Angiology *18*:705–716, 1967.
9. Pettinger WA: Clonidine, a new antihypertensive drug. N. Engl. J. Med. *293*:1179–1180, 1975.
10. Reid JL, Wing LM, Mathias CJ, Frankel HL, Neill E: The central hypotensive effect of clonidine. Studies in tetraplegic subjects. Clin. Pharmacol. Ther. *21*:375–381, 1977.
11. Hansson L, Hunyor JN, Julius S, Hobbler SW: Blood pressure crisis following withdrawal of clonidine, with special reference to arterial and urinary catecholamine levels, and suggestions for acute management. Am. Heart J. *85*:605–610, 1973.
12. Davies DS, Wing LMH, Reid JL, et al.: Pharmacokinetics and concentration-effect relationships of intravenous and oral clonidine. Clin. Pharmacol. Ther. *21*:593–601, 1977.
13. Stitzel RE: The biological fate of reserpine. Pharmacol. Rev. *28*:179–205, 1977.
14. Quetsch RN, Achor RWP, Litin EM, Faucett RL: Depressive reactions in hypertensive patients: a comparison of those treated with rauwolfia and those receiving no specific antihypertensive treatment. Circulation *19*:366–375, 1959.
15. Tripp SL, Williams E, Wagner WE, Lukas G: A specific assay for subnanogram concentrations of reserpine in human plasma. Life Sci. *16*:1167–1178, 1975.
16. Hess HJ: Biochemistry and structure activity studies with prazosin. *In* Prazosin: Evaluation of a New Antihypertensive Agent (DWK Cotton, ed.). Amsterdam: Excerpta Medica, 1974, pp. 3–15.
17. Brogden RN, Heel RC, Speight TM, Avery GS: Prazosin: A review of its pharmacological properties and therapeutic efficacy in hypertension. Drugs *14*:163–197, 1977.
18. Curtis JR: Prazosin in patients with chronic renal failure. Br. Med. J. *3*:742–743, 1974.
19. Koch-Weser J: The comeback of hydralazine. Am. Heart. J. *95*:1–3, 1978.
20. Alarcon-Segovia D, Wakim KG, Worthington JW, Ward LE: Clinical and experimental studies on the hydralazine syndrome and its relationship to systemic lupus erythematosus. Medicine *46*:1–33, 1967.
21. Ludden TN, Shepherd AMM, Lin MS, McNay JL: Pharmacokinetics of hydralazine following intravenous administration of hypertensive patients. Clin. Pharmacol. Ther. *27*:268, 1980.
22. Moore-Jones D, Perry HM: Radioautographic localization of hydralazine-1-C^{14} in arterial walls. Proc. Soc. Exp. Biol. Med. *122*:576–579, 1966.
23. Haegele KD, McLean AJ, duSouich P, et al.: Identifi-

cation of hydralazine and hydralazine hydrazone metabolites in human body fluids and quantitative *in vitro* comparisons of their smooth muscle relaxant activity. Br. J. Clin. Pharmacol. *5*:489–494, 1978.

24. Dormois JC, Young JL, Nies AS: Minoxidil in severe hypertension: value when conventional drugs have failed. Amer. Heart. J. *90*:360–368, 1975.
25. Gottlieb TB, Thomas RC, Chidsey CA: Pharmacokinetic studies of minoxidil. Clin. Pharmacol. Ther. *13*:436–441, 1971.
26. Pluss RG, Orcutt J, Chidsey CA: Tissue distribution and hypotension effects of minoxidil in normotensive rats. J. Lab. Clin. Med. *79*:639–647, 1972.
27. Cohn JN, Burke LP: Nitroprusside. Ann. Intern. Med. *91*:752–757, 1979.
28. Cottrell JE, Casthely P, Brodie JO, et al.: Prevention of nitroprusside-induced cyanide toxicity with hydroxy cobalamin. N. Engl. J. Med. *298*:808–811, 1978.
29. Cottrell JE, Patel K, Casthely, et al.: Nitroprusside tachyphylaxis without acidosis. Anesthesiology *49*:141–142, 1978.
30. Tinker JH, Michenfelder JD: Sodium nitroprusside. Anesthesiology *45*:340–354, 1976.
31. Pearson RM: Pharmacokinetics and response to diazoxide in renal failure. Clin. Pharmacokinet. *2*:198–204, 1977.
32. Pearson RM, Breckenridge AM: Renal function, protein binding and pharmacologic response to diazoxide. Br. J. Clin. Pharmacol. *3*:169–175, 1976.
33. Paulissian R: Diazoxide. Int. Anesthesiol. Clin. *16*:201–237, 1978.
34. Pruitt AW, Dayton PG, Patterson JH: Disposition of diazoxide in children. Clin. Pharmacol. Ther. *14*:73–82, 1973.
35. Sellers EM, Koch-Weser J: Protein binding and vascular activity of diazoxide. N. Engl. J. Med. *281*:1141–1145, 1969.
36. Pohl JE, Thurston H: Use of diazoxide in hypertension with renal failure. Br. Med. J. *4*:142–145, 1971.
37. Mroczek WJ, Davidov M, Gavrilovich L, Finnerty F: The value of aggressive therapy in the hypertensive patient with azotemia. Circulation *40*:893–904, 1969.
38. Pruitt AW, Faraj BA, Dayton PG: Metabolism of diazoxide in man and experimental animals, J. Pharmacol. Exp. Ther. *188*:248–256, 1974.
39. DeBrae M, Mussche M, Ringoir S, Bosteels V: Oral diazoxide for malignant hypertension. Lancet *1*:1397, 1972.
40. Sherlock S: Ascites formation in cirrhosis and its management. Scand. J. Gastroenterol. *7* (Suppl.):9–15, 1970.
41. Senewiratne B, Sherlock S: Amiloride (MK870) in patients with ascites due to cirrhosis of the liver. Lancet *1*:120–122, 1968.
42. Shear L, Ching S, Gabuzda GJ: Compartmentalization of ascites and edema in patients with hepatic cirrhosis. N. Engl. J. Med. *282*:1391–1396, 1970.
43. Lieberman FL, Reynolds TB: Renal failure with cirrhosis. Observations on the role of diuretics. Ann. Intern. Med. *64*:1221–1228, 1966.
44. Gregory PB, Broedelschen DH, Hill MD: Complications of diuresis in the alcoholic with ascites: a controlled trial. Gastroenterology *73*:534, 1977.
45. Novello FC, Sprague JM: Benzothiadiazine dioxides as novel diuretics. J. Am. Chem. Soc. *79*:2028–2029, 1957.
46. Lant AF, Wilson GM: Long-term therapy of diabetes insipidus with oral benzothiadiazine and phthalimidine diuretics. Clin. Sci. *40*:497–511, 1971.
47. Coleman TG, Bower JD, Langford HG, Guyton AC: Regulation of arterial pressure in the anephric state. Circulation *42*:509–514, 1970.
48. Bennett WM, Porter GA: Efficacy and safety of metolazone in renal failure and the nephrotic syndrome. J. Clin. Pharmacol. *13*:357–364, 1973.
49. Fuller TJ, Barcenas CG, White MJ: Diuretic-induced interstitial nephritis. J.A.M.A. *235*:1998–1999, 1976.
50. Beerman B, Groschinsky-Grund M, Rosen A: Absorption, metabolism and excretion of hydrochlorothiazide. Clin. Pharmacol. Ther. *19*:531–537, 1976.
51. Riess W, Dubach UC, Burckhardt D, et al.: Pharmacokinetic studies with chlorthalidone in man. Europ. J. Clin. Pharmacol. *12*:375–382, 1977.
52. Bing M, Stoner L, Cardinal J, Green N: Furosemide effect on isolated perfused tubules. Am. J. Physiol. *225*:119–124, 1973.
53. Gallagher KL, Jones JK: Furosemide-induced ototoxicity. Ann. Intern. Med. *91*:744–745, 1979.
54. Quick CA, Hoppe W: Permanent deafness associated with furosemide administration. Ann. Otol. Rhinol. Laryngol. *84*:94–101, 1975.
55. Cutler RE, Blair AD: Clinical pharmacokinetics of furosemide. Clin. Pharmacokinet. *4*:279–296, 1979.
56. Huang CM, Atkinson AJ, Levin M, Levin NW, Quintanilla A: Pharmacokinetics of furosemide in advanced renal failure. Clin. Pharmacol. Ther. *16*:659–666, 1974.
57. Nigrovic V, Koechel DA, Cafruny EJ: Renal interaction between ethacrynic acid and mercurial diuretics. J. Pharmacol. Exp. Ther. *186*:331–344, 1973.
58. Olesen KH: A comparison of the diuretic action of mercaptomerin, ethacrynic acid and furosemide in congestive heart failure. Acta Med. Scand. *187*:391–399, 1970.
59. Pillay VKG, Schwartz FD, Aimi K, Kark RM: Transient and permanent deafness following treatment with ethacrynic acid in renal failure. Lancet *1*:77–79, 1969.
60. Clarkson TW, Rothstein A, Sutherland R: The mechanism of action of mercurial diuretics in rats: The metabolism of ^{203}Hg-labelled chlormerodrin. Br. J. Pharmacol. Chemother. *24*:1–13, 1965.
61. Greenblatt DJ, Koch-Weser J: Adverse reactions to spironolactone. J.A.M.A. *225*:40–43, 1973.
62. Karim A, Zagarella J, Hribar J, Dooley M: Spironolactone I. Disposition and metabolism. Clin. Pharmacol. Ther. *19*:158–169, 1976.
63. Gabow PA, Moore WS, Schrier RW: Spironolactone induced hyperchloremic acidosis. Ann. Intern. Med. *90*:338–340, 1979.
64. Lieberman FL, Bateman JR: Megaloblastic anemia possibly induced by triamterene in patients with alcoholic cirrhosis. Ann. Intern. Med. *68*:168–173, 1968.
65. Pruitt AW, Winkel JS, Dayton PG: Variations in the fate of triamterene. Clin. Pharmacol. Ther. *21*:610–619, 1977.

Chapter 16

Cardiac Glycosides and Antiarrhythmic Drugs

by

David T. Lowenthal
and Melton B. Affrime

Drugs that are administered to patients with renal and hepatic failure undergo the conventional processes of biotransformation, which include absorption, distribution, metabolism, and elimination. Abnormalities in any of these processes may predispose these patients to adverse drug reactions. Smith et al. reported that the incidence of adverse drug reactions was increased when blood urea nitrogen was greater than 40 mg/dl and when there was an increase in hepatic enzymes.[1] These observations opened the horizons to clinical research in which causes for such adverse drug reactions were identified. It is now appreciated that the causes of drug toxicity in renal and hepatic failure[2-4] are impaired renal or biliary excretion of parent drug or active metabolite(s), impaired hepatic metabolism (increased or decreased), increased drug sensitivity (due to altered protein binding and abnormal blood-brain barrier) and drug interactions (see Chap. 3). An understanding of the ways in which these patients differ from normal can enable one to individualize therapy for this group of patients and achieve better therapeutic results. Cardiovascular disease may occur with high frequency in end-stage renal disease.[5] Thus, hypertension, irregularities in rate and rhythm conduction, and heart failure are commonly observed in this population. Moreover, cardiac disease often leads to impaired renal and hepatic function. Thus, a clear understanding of the clinical pharmacology of cardiovascular drugs is needed for the clinician dealing with patients with renal, hepatic, and cardiac disease.

The pharmacokinetics of the cardiovascular drugs that have been studied in patients with renal and hepatic insufficiency will be discussed individually. The data are summarized in tabular form in the Appendix of this book.

DIGITALIS PREPARATIONS

Digoxin and digitoxin are the two most commonly used digitalis glycosides. They find wide clinical usage for both their inotropic and antiarrhythmic effects. However, wide usage has been accompanied by widespread toxicity. Up to 23 per cent of inpatients receiving digoxin demonstrate evidence of digitalis toxicity.[6, 7] Even more significantly, these digitalis toxic patients had twice the mortality of nontoxic patients. Familiarity with the details of the clinical pharmacology and pharmacokinetics of these two glycosides is necessary to avoid untoward effects. Indeed, a decrease in the incidence of digitalis toxicity has been noted when glycoside therapy is guided by appropriate pharmacokinetic models and digitalis plasma concentration measurements.[8-10]

PHARMACOKINETICS OF DIGOXIN AND DIGITOXIN IN RENAL DISEASE

Clinical pharmacologic studies of digoxin and digitoxin in normal individuals have demonstrated that digoxin is more dependent on renal excretion. Thus, its elimination will be significantly hindered in patients with renal failure. In general, digoxin clearance is directly proportional to creatinine clearance.[11-13] As renal impairment progresses, there is an increase in the fecal excretion of digoxin.[12] However, this alternate pathway of digoxin elimination cannot completely compensate for the loss of the renal excretory route, and overall elimination of digoxin is impaired.[14-16] Digoxin half-life can be prolonged up to 4 to 10 days in patients with renal failure.[17] Nomogram methods utilizing serum creatinine to judge digoxin dosage are available.[20]

Recently, the formulas used to assess digoxin dosage in uremic patients based on serum creatinine alone have been challenged along several lines. The correlation of digoxin half-life and creatinine clearance was shown to be poor ($r = 0.4$).[21] Furthermore, the volume of distribution of digoxin is very variable and often decreased in patients with renal failure.[22] Thus, serum creatinine alone does not predict digoxin half-life in a simple fashion.[23, 24] Others, reporting that digoxin is handled by tubular as well as glomerular mechanisms, suggest that the blood urea nitrogen (BUN) concentration might better be used to adjust digoxin dosage.[25] This approach has not found wide clinical application. Still others suggest measuring digoxin urinary output to circumvent the problem of variability of digoxin volume of distribution.[26] Digoxin clearance (ml/min) may be calculated by obtaining a timed urinary digoxin concentration (mg/min) and drawing a digoxin serum level (mg/ml) at the midpoint of the urinary collection. This latter method also has not been found to be practical for widespread clinical usage.

As a general rule, serum digoxin half-life in patients with severe renal failure can be estimated to be 4 days.[11, 27, 28] This means that 14 per cent per day of the digoxin in the body is excreted by nonurinary routes. Thus, replacement of 14 per cent of body digoxin stores is necessary to maintain steady-state body stores. Of interest, if one neglects to discontinue digoxin for 2 days in the face of an absolute decrease in renal function, there is only a 21 per cent increase in the total body digoxin stores. Thus, although renal function is of great clinical importance in judging digoxin dosage, other factors are involved.[15] In general, no significant change in digoxin dosage is advised until the creatinine clearance is less than 50 ml/min.[18] Thus, no change is needed for patients who have undergone a unilateral nephrectomy. A decrease in digoxin dose of 50 per cent with a serum creatinine of 3 to 5 mg/dl and a decrease in digoxin dose of 75 per cent in patients without renal function is advised.[11, 13, 19]

Although it has been stated that only the maintenance dose of digoxin needs to be changed in patients with uremia,[28] the decrease in volume of distribution of digoxin in uremic patients suggests that a decrease in initial dosage may also be warranted in some cases. In addition, the binding of digoxin to serum proteins was shown to be significantly decreased in the face of uremia (25 ± 4 per cent in controls vs. 18 ± 6 per cent in uremic plasma, $p < 0.01$).[29] However, such a change amounts to only a 10 per cent increase in the free fraction of digoxin and is usually not of clinical importance.

There is some disagreement about the effect of uremia on digitoxin metabolism, binding, and excretion. Some authors[30] have reasoned that renal elimination of digitoxin can amount to as much as 30 per cent of digitoxin elimination in normals. These observations suggest that alterations in digitoxin pharmacokinetics must occur in patients with renal failure. Moreover, good estimates suggest that uremic patients eliminate 7.6 per cent of their digitoxin stores per day, as opposed to the normal 11 per cent elimination per day. This would result in only a slight prolongation of digitoxin half-life to 8.8 days. A digitoxin dosage formula was derived from this information: $7.7 + (0.035 \times \text{creatinine clearance}) = \text{dose of digitoxin in milligrams}$.

Total digitoxin protein binding may be slightly decreased in uremic patients because of lower plasma protein levels. In addition, there seems to be a shift in the metabolism of digitoxin to more cardioactive metabolites with lower affinity for protein binding sites in patients with renal failure. Therefore, in uremic patients with decreased plasma proteins, serum concentrations of digitoxin tend to be lower, but the total active, unbound drug concentration is near normal.[29, 31, 32] The time needed to reach steady-state plateau levels when digitoxin is given in only maintenance dose form is 1 month in both uremic and normal patients. This implies that digitoxin half-life is not substantially prolonged in severe renal failure.[32-34]

In patients with the nephrotic syndrome, digitoxin binding to albumin is slightly decreased, with resultant increases in the volume of distribution. However, decreases in half-life of digitoxin due to increased availability of free drug for renal excretion are present. The decreased half-life and increased volume of distribution imply that greater drug doses may be needed in individual patients; however, the decrease in binding dictates that for any given drug level there is an increased amount of free pharmacologically active drug present.[35] The pharmacokinetics of digitoxin in uremic patients are complex. However, the net result is that little alteration in digitoxin dosage is necessary.

Dialysis does not significantly decrease the total body stores of digoxin or digitoxin in that digoxin is sparingly distributed in the plasma space and digitoxin is highly protein bound.[34, 36, 37] It is suggested that digoxin be given to uremic patients undergoing dialysis at 0.125 mg/day, 5 days per week and digitoxin at 0.1 mg/day, 5 days per week. The serum half-life of digoxin and digitoxin approximate each other in renal failure, and 30 days are needed to reach a plateau concentration when these drugs are started in maintenance form or a change in drug dosage occurs. These dose levels will result in a low therapeutic, nontoxic serum concentration for digoxin of 0.84 ± 0.05 ng/ml and 19 ± 1 ng/ml for digitoxin. No glycoside should be given on the day of dialysis to avoid increasing body glycoside stores in the face of the electrolyte (potassium) shifts that occur during dialysis. Heparin used with dialysis also alters the binding of glycosides to serum proteins. Following renal transplantation, digoxin clearance parallels the overall renal function of the patient.[38] In patients with renal and hepatic failure, determinations of digoxin or digitoxin blood levels may aid in dosage adjustments. However, the conventional radioimmunoassay method for digoxin assay may overestimate digoxin concentrations in dialysis patients.[39]

One of the therapeutic debates in literature has been whether digoxin or digitoxin is the preferred glycoside in renal failure. Obviously, digitoxin is less altered by renal failure; however, digoxin is altered in a reasonably predictable manner. Thus, there is no definite preference if these agents are used cautiously.[34]

PHARMACOKINETICS OF DIGOXIN AND DIGITOXIN IN LIVER DISEASE

In acute hepatitis, there is no impairment in digoxin elimination. However, if a precursor, β-methyldigoxin, is administered, there is a significantly retarded elimination of the drug.[40] For this drug, there is an increase in plasma concentration and in pharmacologic activity related to decrease in the hepatic process of demethylation. In chronic liver disease, such as cirrhosis, the metabolism of digoxin as studied by analysis of blood, feces, and urine is unimpaired.[41] Since digitoxin appears to be eliminated primarily by hepatic metabolism, it might be anticipated that hepatic impairment would influence the elimination of this drug. However, there are no clinical data to substantiate this hypothesis. Digitoxin is 50 to 75 per cent metabolized via the liver in normal individuals. In one patient with hepatocellular disease, 55 per cent of a given dose of digitoxin was excreted in the urine and 33 per cent was found in the feces as unchanged digitoxin. Only 12 per cent of the dose was metabolized. However, this finding is from only one particular case; therefore, large-scale conclusions cannot be drawn.[42]

An enterohepatic circulation is thought to be responsible for the long elimination half-life of digitoxin in humans.[43] Cholestyramine will reduce the enterohepatic circulation of digitoxin and shorten its half life.[44] Storstein and Amlie[45] have studied the biliary excretion of digitoxin in two patients with biliary fistulas and have found the excretion via this route to be 1.5 per cent in 24 hours. The elimination half-life of digitoxin was shorter in patients with biliary T-tubes than in controls with an intact enterohepatic circulation, but still longer than for other glycosides, indicating that factors other than enterohepatic circulation are important in the slow elimination of this drug.[46] Digitoxin is a capacity-limited, binding-sensitive glycoside (97 per cent protein bound) with a correspondingly very low hepatic extraction ratio (0.005).[47] Biliary excretion and enterohepatic circulation do not play a role in digoxin elimination.[48] In summary, there is no apparent need to alter digitalis glycoside dosing in patients with acute or chronic liver disease. Chronic renal disease requires dosage adjustments for digoxin.

ANTIARRHYTHMIC DRUGS

PROPRANOLOL

Propranolol, a nonselective β-adrenergic antagonist, is used primarily in the treatment of hypertension, angina pectoris, and cardiac arrhythmias. When administered orally, propranolol undergoes first-pass hepatic extraction with a high extraction ratio of 0.6 to 0.8. Propranolol is metabolized (hydroxylation) by the hepatic oxidative pathway to 4-hydroxypropranolol.[49] The hepatic clearance of propranolol is proportional to hepatic blood flow and, therefore, sensitive to factors that alter this flow.[50] In subjects with normal renal function, propranolol is well absorbed when taken orally. Owing to the avid hepatic uptake, oral doses result in lower plasma concentrations than equivalent intravenous doses. In addition, long-term administration of propranolol to normal individuals results in saturating hepatic uptake and metabolic processes that may result in higher plasma concentrations and a prolongation of the biologic half-life.[51] There is significant interindividual variability[52] in the plasma concentration–dose relationship as well as significant intraindividual[53] variability in plasma propranolol concentration. Technical interference by Vacutainer-type tubes[54] as well as by heparin[55] may contribute to the variability in propranolol plasma levels that often results in reported low plasma concentrations.

Previous studies[56] in our laboratory have not demonstrated an impairment of propranolol absorption in patients with chronic renal disease. However, significantly higher plasma concentrations of propranolol 1.5 hours after the administration of 80 mg occurs when patients with renal failure are compared with normal controls[56] (Fig. 16–1). In patients with renal failure, the dose per kilogram was significantly greater, yet the metabolic clearance was lower when compared with the control group. Elimination half-life and the elimination rate constant (Table 16–1) of propranolol were not significantly altered by renal failure.[56] Yet, because of the significantly higher plasma concentrations of propranolol, the area under the curve (AUC) was threefold greater in renal failure (Table 16–2). These observations suggest an impairment in the first-pass effect of propranolol in renal insufficiency.[56, 57] We have also recently found a decrease in volume of distribution of propranolol in two patients with end-stage renal disease[58] (Table 16–2). Since propranolol is largely extracted by the liver, severe hepatic disease with diminished hepatic blood flow and drug extraction efficiency would also be expected to result in higher blood levels.

In contrast to normal individuals, when propranolol is given in long-term maintenance doses (that is, 40 to 80 mg every 8 hours) to patients with renal failure, the elimination half-life is shorter than when the drug is given in single doses[59] (Fig. 16–2). There is evidence that some drugs, such as antipyrine,[60] phenytoin,[61] and pentobarbital,[62] which, like propranolol, are metabolized by oxidation processes, have accelerated rates of metabolism and shortened biologic half-lives in patients with end-stage renal disease. It is likely that the chronic administration of propranolol may also be associated with increased metabolism when the drug is given over a long period. This may reflect an increase in the activity of the microsomal oxidation system in chronic renal failure.

In summary, propranolol dosage should be carefully monitored in patients with kidney

TABLE 16–1. SINGLE DOSE PHARMACOKINETICS OF ORAL ANTIARRHYTHMICS

	PROPRANOLOL*	PROCAINAMIDE*	QUINIDINE*	PHENYTOIN†	DISOPYRAMIDE*
			Normal Subjects		
T ½ (hr)	4.4	3.5	7.2	0.7	4.4
Elimination rate constant, Ke (hr^{-1})	0.157	0.198	0.096	0.05	0.16
			Patients with End-Stage Renal Disease		
T½	3.2	12.8 (N)‡	6.6	1.4	8.3
Ke	0.216	19.3 (A)§	0.105	0.1	0.08

*Active metabolite. See text.
†T½ is shorter when drug is given in multiple doses.
‡Physiologic anephric.
§Anatomic anephric.

TABLE 16–2. COMPARISON OF MEAN PHARMACOKINETIC PARAMETERS: NORMAL VOLUNTEERS AND PATIENTS WITH END-STAGE RENAL DISEASE RECEIVING PROPRANOLOL, 80 MG.

Dose/kg	Peak Concentration (ng/ml)	AUC (ng/ml × hr)	Metabolic Clearance* (L/min)	fs†	F‡
		Control Group			
1.05 ± 0.5	51.6 ± 1.0	274 ± 49	0.817 ± 0.039	0.254 ± 0.04	0.158 ± 0.02
		Patients with End-Stage Renal Disease			
1.44 ±0.2	155 ± 40	716 ± 149	0.637 ± 0.04	0.440 ± 0.05	0.275 ± 0.03
P <0.01	P <0.05	P <0.05	P <0.05	P <0.05	P <0.05

*Metabolic clearance $= \frac{F \cdot D}{AUC}$

†fs $= \frac{Q}{Q + \frac{D-T}{AUC}}$ where Q = hepatic blood flow of 1.1 L/min
T = 30 mg. threshold dose
D = 80 mg dose

‡F $= fs \frac{(D-T)}{D}$

disease. Careful attention must be paid to blood pressure and pulse rate change as a result of the early elevated plasma concentrations. However, the increased plasma propranolol level is transient and, generally, when long-term dosing is prescribed no accumulation of propranolol occurs. Although 4-hydroxypropranolol, naphthoxylactic acid, and naphthoxyacetic acid accumulation may occur, these substances do not result in ad-

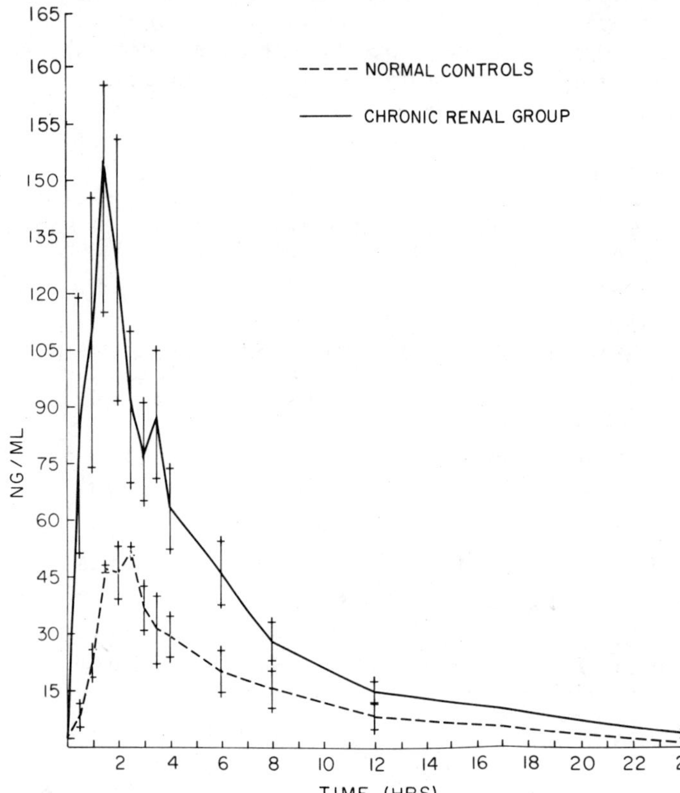

Figure 16–1. Propranolol concentrations in normal subjects (broken line) and in patients with end-stage renal failure (solid line) after the administration of a single dose of 80 ng.

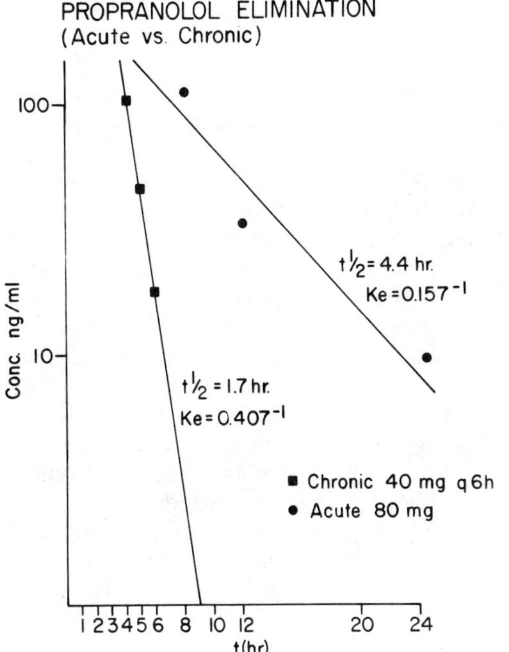

Figure 16–2. Propranolol elimination in patients with end-stage renal disease receiving long-term therapy, 40 mg every 6 hours (solid box), versus those receiving a single dose of 80 ng (solid circles).

verse or overt hemodynamic alterations.[63, 64] Therefore, dosage alteration is unnecessary for chronic propranolol therapy in patients with advanced renal disease.

Protein binding studies in our laboratory with radioactive carbon (^{14}C)–labeled propranolol or unlabeled drug, by means of ultracentrifugation and equilibrium dialysis, demonstrate that the binding of propranolol is not impaired in patients with renal insufficiency. However, when patients are treated with long-term peritoneal dialysis, the binding of propranolol is significantly less; this is probably due to the loss of albumin during the peritoneal dialysis procedure. Because of its avid protein binding of 90 per cent or greater, it can be predicted that the dialyzability of propranolol is small. Previous work has demonstrated that this is the case with propranolol.[56]

Changes have been reported in the distribution and disposition of intravenous propranolol in patients with cirrhosis and chronic active hepatitis compared with normal subjects.[3, 4, 65] The clearance of propranolol decreases as the severity and derangement of hepatic function increases, as documented by hypoalbuminemia, hyperbilirubinemia, and a prolongation of the prothrombin time.[3, 4, 65] The average clearance and volume of distribution of propranolol are 0.44 L/min and 448 L, respectively, in patients with hepatic disease as compared with 0.92 L/min and 220 L in normal subjects. There is an increase in free propranolol concentration in patients with chronic liver disease. It is difficult to extrapolate these data generated by the intravenous administration of propranolol to chronic oral dosing because of the unknown effect of chronic liver disease on hepatic enzyme activity (intrinsic hepatic clearance), hepatic blood flow, and volume of distribution. However, because of the increase in the free fraction of propranolol in patients with impaired hepatic function, increasing oral doses should be given with caution. Interestingly, in patients with portacaval shunt, high plasma concentrations occur because the oral dose circumvents the avid hepatic extraction process. Branch et al.[65] have found an eightfold increase in propranolol half-life in cirrhotics with hypoalbuminemia even though hepatic clearance is reduced to only one third of normal. This is probably related to the fact that there is a significant increase in the volume of distribution of propranolol as noted previously.

QUINIDINE

Quinidine undergoes oxidation in the liver to several hydroxy derivatives. With normal renal function, renal excretion is rapid and 10 to 50 per cent of a given dose is found unchanged in the urine within 24 hours of administration. Since quinidine is a weak base, the urinary excretion of quinidine is enhanced by acidification and delayed by alkalinization of the urine.[66] The half-life of quinidine has been shown to be equivalent in normal subjects, in patients with impaired renal function, and in patients with congestive heart failure. Mean half-life is 7 hours after a single dose of quinidine.[67] Previous studies [68] have contended that higher plasma levels of quinidine occur in patients with impaired renal function. However, the nonspecificity of the assay techniques resulted in the measurement of quinidine plus its polar metabolites. More recently, improved assay methodology has resulted in the measurement of the parent quinidine as well as the metabolites. Studies by Drayer et al.[69] have demonstrated in animal models that the quinidine metabolites 3-

hydroxyquinidine, 2-oxoquinidinone, and O-desmethylquinidine exert antiarrhythmic effects.

Figure 16–3 shows plasma quinidine concentrations measured by a double extraction method in steady-state studies. The concentrations of the drug are within the normal therapeutic range in patients in renal insufficiency, in patients with congestive heart failure, and in control subjects being treated for arrhythmias. The biologic half-life of quinidine following its long-term use appears longer than that following a single dose.[69] This may be a reflection of rapid tissue uptake, avid tissue binding, and slow release following long-term quinidine administration. At equilibrium, tissue to serum concentration ratios may be as large as 20.

Quinidine is 80 per cent protein bound. This binding is not altered in patients with impaired renal function but is diminished in patients with liver disease. There is a 300 per cent increase in the free fraction of quinidine in patients with cirrhosis, probably due to hypoalbuminemia.[70, 71] It is unlikely that the drug is dialyzable because of high protein binding. Since the therapeutic concentrations of standard doses of quinidine in end-stage renal failure do not exceed the normal range, this antiarrhythmic may be safer to administer than procainamide. Dosage adjustments are advised during maintenance therapy because of potential accumulation of metabolites. The initial dose of quinidine should remain unchanged once the GFR (glomerular filtration rate) is less than 50 ml/min, and maintenance dosages of 100 mg every 8 hours are often therapeutic.

The effect of hepatic disease on quinidine metabolism has not been thoroughly studied. Patients with both chronic liver and renal disease may have seizure activity requiring the administration of phenytoin. When phenytoin is given simultaneously with quinidine, it may accelerate the metabolism of quinidine, yielding a lower plasma concentration and a decrease in therapeutic effect.[72] Recently, another significant drug interaction involving quinidine and digoxin has been demonstrated.[73] When quinidine is added to a regimen including digoxin, plasma digoxin levels increase. The pharmacokinetic basis of this interaction has not been clarified. However, a decrease in digoxin volume of distribution and renal elimination may occur.

PROCAINAMIDE

Fifty to 60 per cent of a dose of procainamide is excreted by the kidney unchanged and 7 to 24 per cent is acetylated to *N*-acetylprocainamide (NAPA), an active metabolite. Contrary to previous data, urinary

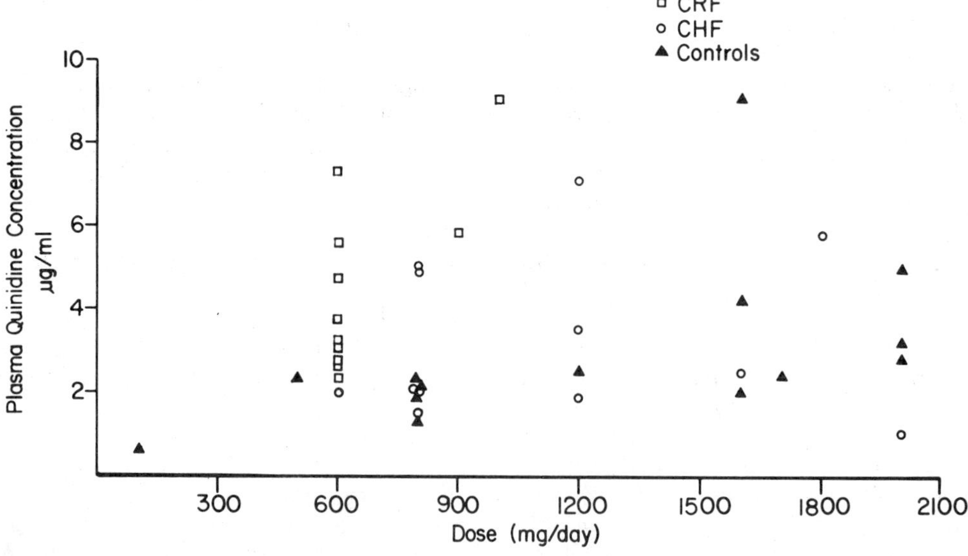

Figure 16–3. Plasma quinidine concentrations measured by the double-extraction method under steady state conditions. CRF = chronic renal failure; CHF = congestive heart failure.

acidification does not increase the renal excretion of procainamide and, consequently, does not lower the half-life of the drug.[74] In patients with renal disease, urinary excretion of procainamide decreases proportionately as creatinine clearance diminishes. In renal failure, elimination of the parent compound decreases, while the major metabolite, NAPA, a potent active antiarrhythmic,[75, 76] often accumulates. There are no data on procainamide biotransformation or acetylation in acute or chronic hepatic disease.

There is no impairment of procainamide absorption in chronic renal insufficiency, and the plasma concentration peaks within 1.5 to 2.0 hours after a single dose of 500 mg.[77] The normal half-life of the drug is 3.5 to 4.0 hours, and this can be prolonged three to fourfold in patients with impaired renal function (Table 16–1). Normally, the drug is only 15 per cent protein bound and is readily dialyzable. With long-term administration, there is slight prolongation of the half-life (9 to 19 hours). The biologic half-life of the NAPA metabolite is very long.[75] NAPA is present in significant concentration in the plasma of patients taking procainamide for more than 1 to 2 days.[75] It has an antiarrhythmic activity similar to that of procainamide in animal models and in humans.[78, 79] Over 85 per cent of a dose of NAPA in man is excreted unchanged in the urine.

Measurements of plasma concentrations of procainamide by the usual fluorometric or colorimetric methods do not detect the pharmacologically active metabolite. In patients with high NAPA levels (patients that rapidly acetylate drugs or patients with renal failure who are receiving long-term procainamide therapy), determination of procainamide blood levels alone by these methods can be misleading. The acetylator phenotype can be determined by using the NAPA to procainamide concentration ratio in plasma. Assuming that the procainamide has been given for 3 or more days and that the plasma is obtained 3 hours after the administration of a dose of procainamide, the ratio is below 0.85 in slow acetylators and above 1.0 in rapid acetylators. A slow acetylator would have a higher concentration of procainamide than of NAPA, and the reverse would be true in patients who are rapid acetylators. In patients with renal failure, the prolonged half-life of NAPA in plasma is due to synthesis from procainamide as well as the impaired renal excretion of NAPA. Since the NAPA accumulates in patients with poor renal function, both NAPA and procainamide concentrations should be monitored in these patients.[75] The maintenance dosage of procainamide should be lowered and the dosing interval extended to a dose every 12 rather than 8 hours; this should be commensurate with maintenance of good arrhythmia control as the NAPA accumulates. In patients with renal failure, the acetylator phenotype cannot be determined on the basis of measuring NAPA and procainamide plasma ratios as is done for nonazotemic patients because of the accumulation of NAPA.

LIDOCAINE

The parenteral use of lidocaine is confined primarily to patients with ventricular arrhythmias. It is used often as a local anesthetic for minor surgical procedures and in customary doses has not created or been associated with any adverse reactions. Lidocaine is metabolized by the liver via an oxidative pathway through *N*-dealkylation to monoethyglycinexylidide (MEGX) and glycinexylidide (GX), both of which are active metabolites.[80] Lidocaine has a biphasic elimination process with both a short and a long half-life. In subjects with chronic renal insufficiency, the half-lives of 9.3 minutes and 77 minutes, respectively, are comparable to those of normal control subjects.[81] MEGX and GX are active metabolites with local anesthetic, antiarrhythmic, hypotensive, and central nervous system toxic properties, but only GX accumulates in patients with chronic renal insufficiency and, rarely, creates adverse pharmacologic responses.[82] Normally, lidocaine is 60 per cent protein bound; this binding is directly dependent on drug concentration.[81] Protein binding and dialyzability of lidocaine and its metabolites in patients with renal insufficiency have not been studied.

Lidocaine is normally metabolized by the liver with 65 per cent of the drug extracted on the first pass, leaving 35 per cent free (of which 40 per cent is unbound to protein) to act pharmacologically in the system.[85] If the first-pass extraction by the liver is deranged because of liver disease (acute viral hepatitis, chronic alcoholic liver disease)[81, 82] or disorders that diminish hepatic blood flow (congestive heart failure), biotransformation of lidocaine might be slowed and cumulative effects of the drug might occur. Lidocaine clearance is reduced by approximately 50 per cent with resulting threefold prolongation of elimination half-life and twofold increase in the plasma lidocaine concentrations in patients with severe hepatic dysfunction. The usual loading dose of lidocaine may be given, but the infusion rate should be reduced by approximately one-half. Subsequently, lidocaine blood concentrations may be of value in the management of such patients.

DISOPYRAMIDE (NORPACE)[86]

Oral administration of disopyramide as the phosphate salt or free base results in rapid and complete absorption. The relative systemic availability of these two oral forms has varied between studies, but appears to be approximately 70 to 85 per cent compared with intravenous administration. Disopyramide undergoes limited hepatic first-pass metabolism of approximately 10 to 20 per cent.[86] The extent of protein binding of disopyramide shows wide interpatient variability and is concentration dependent. The fraction not bound to plasma proteins increases with total plasma concentrations, and plasma clearance is independent of the concentration of the free drug. This results in the concentration of free or unbound drug increasing proportionally with dose, but total drug concentration shows a less than proportionate increase.

Peak plasma concentrations 2 hours after oral administration[86] are lower in patients with acute myocardial infarction; i.e., less than 1 μg/ml as compared to 2 to 3 μg/ml in healthy subjects receiving the same dose. The intravenous administration of 1.5 to 2.0 mg/kg results in a rapid peak in disopyramide plasma concentrations, declining immediately after injection to about 4 μg/ml at 5 minutes. The distribution half-life if disopyramide is approximately 3 minutes in healthy subjects and is five times prolonged in patients with recent myocardial infarction. The steady-state volume of distribution after intravenous administration is greater in healthy subjects (40 to 89 L) than in patients with acute myocardial infarction (33 to 60 L) and is slightly reduced in patients with impaired renal function.

Approximately 50 to 60 per cent of an administered dose of disopyramide is excreted unchanged, with the majority eliminated in the urine. A small amount is eliminated in feces. Disopyramide undergoes *N*-dealkylation as the primary metabolic pathway and the major metabolite is excreted by the kidney. In animals, the *N*-dealkylated metabolite has some antiarrhythmic activity, but less than disopyramide. The elimination half-life after intravenous administration is longer in patients with recent myocardial infarction (7.0 to 11.8 hr) and severe renal dysfunction (8.3 to 43.0 hr, the value increasing as renal function worsens) and shortest in healthy subjects (4.4 to 8.2 hr). Similarly, an oral dose of 200 to 300 mg is excreted more slowly in patients with ventricular arrhythmias (half-life of 9.3 to 33.8 hs) than in healthy volunteers (8.2 to 8.9 hr). There are no data on disopyramide biotransformation in acute or chronic liver disease.

Previous studies of disopyramide kinetics in normal subjects have shown total clearance varying from 6 to 200 ml/min.[87] It has been demonstrated that disopyramide clearance falls significantly when the creatinine clearance has dropped to 20 to 25 ml/min. The half-life then becomes prolonged and may be up to five times that found under normal circumstances. Dosage modification is, therefore, necessary when serum creatinine exceeds 3 mg/dl to avoid excessive plasma concentrations.[88] It appears prudent to alter the dosage of disopyramide in patients with impaired renal function and to increase this reduction in dosage and/or prolong the dosage interval when the combined disease entities of acute myocardial infarction and chronic renal failure coincide. Studies correlating plasma levels of disopyramide with clinical effects are limited, but it appears that a plasma concentration of approximately 3 to 6 μg/ml represents a desirable therapeutic range.

If one assumes an average plasma concentration of 4μg/ml, with patients with normal renal function showing a half-life of 7 to 8 hours, the disopyramide dose should be 150 to 200 mg every 6 hours. Whiting and Elliott[88] have suggested that in patients whose creatinine clearance is less than 8 ml/min, the dose would be 150 mg every 24 hours or 75 mg every 12 hours or 50 mg every 8 hours. For patients with less severe renal impairment, the dosage might be 150 mg every 12 hours or 100 mg every 8 hours.[88] Disopyramide dialyzability has been demonstrated *in vitro* using human blood containing an initial plasma concentration of 22 mg/L, which was then dialyzed at body temperature in a Cordis-Dow number 4 artificial kidney at a blood flow rate of 250 ml/min and the disopyramide plasma concentration fell to 3 mg/L within 2 hours. Karim[89] concluded that, based on the *in vitro* data, hemodialysis may be of potential use in enhancing the elimination of toxic concentrations of disopyramide from the body.

Disopyramide has anticholinergic activity that may result in dryness of the mouth and difficulty in urination. Patients with impaired renal function receiving disopyramide may alter their fluid intake as a consequence of dryness of the mouth and those that are still able to produce urine may have difficulty in doing so if there is urinary retention. The drug may also cause pruritus. Rarely, peripheral neuropathy may develop in patients receiving disopyramide; this drug may also complicate existing peripheral neuropathy. No information is available on the use of disopyramide in patients with hepatic disease. Based on the pharmacokinetic parameters of the drug, little dosage modification would be anticipated.

PHENYTOIN (DILANTIN)

Phenytoin absorption in renal failure is normal and plasma concentrations are adequate for anticonvulsant and antiarrhythmic activity, even when reduced dosages of the drug are administered. Phenytoin kinetics are dose dependent. Increasing the amount of phenytoin administered results in more hepatic saturation and increased half-life. These kinetics are substantially different in patients with impaired renal function. Early observations demonstrated that plasma concentrations as low as 2 μg/ml, which ordinarily is subtherapeutic (10 to 20 μg/ml is the normal therapeutic range), were effective in reducing seizure activity in patients with impaired renal function. This, in fact, was also sufficient to produce symptoms of phenytoin toxicity; namely, nystagmus and ataxia. Reidenberg and colleagues[62] demonstrated that advancing renal impairment decreases total plasma concentration of phenytoin and more of the drug is in the free form. It has also been demonstrated that phenytoin is extensively metabolized to a hydroxy metabolite that is conjugated to glucuronide and excreted by the kidney in normal individuals. This metabolite has little, if any, pharmacologic activity. However, this metabolite accumulates in patients with renal insufficiency. In patients with impaired renal function, the plasma half-life of phenytoin is shortened, most likely because there is more free drug to be metabolized by the liver.

Patients with impaired renal function have abnormalities in carbohydrate metabolism regardless of whether or not they are diabetic. In this regard, phenytoin also has been demonstrated to impair insulin release.[96] Phenytoin, likewise, interacts with vitamin D, an effect which may result in hypocalcemia, hypophosphatemia, and clinical manifestations of rickets in children.[96] In patients with renal disease, the latter metabolic effect of phenytoin may worsen the existing renal osteodystrophy and secondary hyperparathyroidism. When given with digitoxin, phenytoin can induce the metabolism of this glycoside. This results in more digoxin being produced and a shortening of the digitoxin half-life. The increase in free phenytoin in uremia can certainly explain such an interaction.[97] There appears to be no need to alter the dosage of phenytoin in patients with renal impairment, although the therapeutic and toxic effects may be seen at lower plasma concentrations owing to the protein binding abnormalities.

The dialyzability of phenytoin is insignificant. This is probably related to the fact that of the total amount of phenytoin ingested, small amounts (less than 10 per cent) of unchanged phenytoin are excreted in the urine and feces, while 60 to 80 per cent is excreted in the urine as the parahydroxy derivative or glucuronide conjugate.[98, 99]

Phenytoin has low hepatic extraction (0.03) and is 90 per cent protein bound.[100] In patients with cirrhosis and with acute and viral hepatitis,[70, 100] there is a marked increase in the percentage of free phenytoin. There is no influence of acute viral hepatitis on the volume of distribution or clearance of phenytoin as compared with values found in patients on recovery. However, these studies were performed in the setting of subtherapeutic plasma concentrations in the range of linear phenytoin kinetics. Hyperbilirubinemia can displace phenytoin from plasma protein and elevate the free phenytoin level. Therefore, dosage reduction, broadening of the dosage interval, and plasma level monitoring are recommended for patients with both renal and hepatic disease.

OTHER β-ADRENORECEPTOR BLOCKING AGENTS

Timolol[101] is six times as potent with regard to β-adrenergic blocking activity as propranolol and has no cardiac selectivity and membrane-stabilizing activity. Timolol is only 10 per cent protein bound. The elimination half-life of timolol in patients with renal disease is four hours, which is similar to the half-life in patients with normal renal function.[101] Following 20 mg of timolol given in single dose, there does seem to be a prolongation of the blood pressure response as well as heart rate response, with the systolic and diastolic pressure and heart rate very gradually returning to predosing levels by 24 hours. When given prior to hemodialysis, there are significant hemodynamic effects leading to hypotention, bradycardia, nausea, and sweating. These effects contraindicate the use of timolol prior to dialysis.[101] Timolol does not give rise to active metabolites, in contrast to propranolol. No data exist concerning the pharmacodynamics or biotransformation of timolol in patients with acute or chronic liver disease.

Labetolol is an investigational antihypertensive agent with both α- and β-adrenoreceptor blocking properties. It is extensively metabolized in the liver with less than 5 per cent being excreted unchanged in the urine. Based on this fact, it would be safe to give to the patient with chronic renal disease. However, in patients with chronic liver disease, bioavailability studies with labetolol demonstrate increased bioavailability owing to a reduction in first-pass metabolism.[102] This effect correlated negatively with serum albumin concentrations. In addition, the decrease in heart rate and blood pressure was greater after oral administration, suggesting an exaggerated response due to the increased bioavailability. Similar results have been reported with increased bioavailability for propranolol. Oxyprenolol, alprenolol, and metoprolol, which also have high hepatic extraction, have not yet been studied in this setting of chronic hepatic disease, but similar results must be anticipated.

Pindolol is six times as potent as propranolol as a β-adrenergic antagonist. Another major difference is that it has significant partial agonist activity. Its half-life in normal renal function is 3 to 4 hours, and 40 per cent of a single dose of pindolol is recovered unchanged in the urine.[103, 104] Nevertheless, there has not been any correlation found between the overall elimination rate constant of pindolol and endogenous creatinine clearance. Ohnhaus et al.[103] concluded that the extrarenal elimination rate constant was increased in chronic renal failure. However, Øie and Levy[104] found a statistically significant positive correlation between the renal clearance of pindolol and creatinine.

Sotalol is approximately one tenth as potent as propranolol and has no cardioselectivity, agonist activity, or membrane-stabilizing activity. Sotalol is excreted mainly by the kidneys as unchanged drug. In patients with end-stage renal disease, the plasma half-life is approximately 42 hours, as compared with 5 hours in normal subjects.[105] Thus, significant dosage reduction and widening of dosage interval is suggested in patients with renal failure.

Nadolol is a noncardioselective β-adrenergic blocking agent, which has the longest plasma half-life of any known β-blocking drug and, thus, can be administered once daily. It is two to four times as potent as propranolol as a β-adrenergic antagonist. Nadolol is only about 30 per cent protein bound, and more than 90 per cent is recovered in the urine and feces unchanged.[106, 107] No active metabolites have been identified. Nadolol has a half-life in patients with normal renal function of 17 to 24 hours following a single oral dose. The renal clearance of nadolol has been found to correlate directly with creatinine clearance. As a consequence, the plasma half-life is prolonged in patients with impaired renal function. Therefore, dosage intervals in patients with decreased renal function receiving nadolol should be lengthened. Hemodialysis can effectively reduce serum concentrations of the drug and, thus, be useful as a means of treating nadolol intoxication. When creatinine clearance is below 50 ml/min, the dosage can be reduced by 50 per cent and the dosage interval can be widened to every other day.

Metoprolol is a cardioselective β-adrenergic blocking agent at lower doses ($<$ 150 mg/day). It is 12 per cent protein bound, and primarily undergoes hepatic biotransformation with some first-pass effect. The half-life of oral metoprolol in normal persons is 3 to 4 hours, and about 3 per cent of a dose is recovered unchanged in the urine. There are no known active metabolites. There is no need to alter the dosage in patients with impaired renal function.[108] Interestingly, about 95 per cent of an oral or intravenous dose of metoprolol is recovered in the urine over a period of 72 hours. Whereas the elimination half-life of the total metabolites after oral administration is about 3 hours, after an intravenous dose it is about 5 hours. This indicates that the route of administration might influence the metabolic pathways of metoprolol. This phenomenon might reflect the first-pass elimination of metoprolol that results in 50 per cent of administered dose reaching the systemic circulation. The first-pass process may be impaired in chronic hepatic disease, resulting in an enhanced bioavailability and pharmacodynamic effect of metaprolol.

When compared to propranolol, alprenolol has less bioavailability (10 per cent) and is avidly protein bound with an elimination half-life similar to that of propranolol. Less than 1 per cent of the drug is excreted unchanged, and like propranolol, it too has active metabolites. Alprenolol is nonselective and equipotent to propranolol, but it does have greater partial agonist activity. Although the pharmacokinetics of alprenolol have not been delineated in patients with impaired renal function, the fact that hepatic biotransformation gives rise to an active metabolite would suggest that a dosage reduction be recommended in order to avoid significant accumulation of the active metabolite. This recommendation would apply in advanced renal failure and careful observation of pharmacodynamic activity would be necessary. In patients with chronic liver disease, a decreased first-pass effect may result in increased bioavailability and enhanced pharmacologic effect.

Atenolol has an elimination half-life in subjects with normal renal function of 6 to 9 hours.[109] It is equipotent to propranolol, it is cardioselective, and it may be the only adrenoreceptor blocker that may not cross the blood-brain barrier. There are no active metabolites, and approximately 40 per cent of atenolol is recovered unchanged in the urine following a single dose. It would seem, therefore, that some dosage reduction be employed if given to patients with impaired renal function.

ANGIOTENSIN II ANTAGONIST (SARALASIN) AND CONVERTING ENZYME INHIBITOR (CAPTOPRIL)

The elimination half-life of saralasin in hypertensive patients is 3.2 minutes.[109] The pharmacologic half-life is approximately 8 minutes, as determined by the rate of return of blood pressure after saralasin-induced reduction in blood pressure.[110] There is a brief time required to reach steady-state plasma concentrations with saralasin and a plateau is achieved in a 15-minute period.[110] There are no data on the elimination kinetics of saralasin in patients with impaired renal function. In view of its brief duration of action in subjects with normal renal function, the angiotensin II antagonist probably does not accumulate to any significant degree in impaired renal function. The effect of saralasin on blood pressure in patients with terminal renal failure has been studied. The observed fall in blood pressure in some of these patients demonstrated that high renin and angiotensin levels may be involved in the pathogenesis of hypertension in some patients with terminal renal failure.[111]

Although pharmacokinetic data are not available for captopril, its clinical effect has been studied in the hypertension of chronic renal failure.[112] In those patients studied, the drug was effective but adverse side effects and dosage reduction were necessary. Patients with impaired renal function have received maintenance doses of 200 mg two times a day in the setting of as much as 250 mg of furosemide.[112] Adverse effects, e.g., agranulocytosis, leukopenia, ageusia, fever, maculopapular skin eruption, and proteinuria have been observed at high doses of captopril.

SUMMARY AND CONCLUSIONS

In patients with renal failure, cardiovascular drugs that require significant dosage modifications include digoxin, procainamide, disopyramide, sotolol, naldolol, and atenolol. In contrast, digitoxin, propranolol, quinidine, lidocaine, phenytoin, labetolol, and metoprolol can be cautiously utilized in more standard doses. A large number of cardiovascular drugs, including propranolol, lidocaine, phenytoin, labetolol, oxyprenolol, and metoprolol, require significant reduction of dosage and/or drug interval in patients with liver disease, heart failure, or portacaval shunts. Digoxin and disopyramide can be utilized in standard doses in patients with liver disease and normal renal function.

Patients with kidney and liver disease may be especially prone to some of the potentially adverse hemodynamic-cardiovascular effects of the drugs discussed in this chapter. Thus, in addition to careful dosage alterations, close clinical, electrocardiographic, and plasma drug level monitoring are often essential adjuncts to therapy.

REFERENCES

1. Smith, JW, Seidl LG, Cluff LE: Studies on the epidemiology of adverse drug reactions. V. Clinical factors influencing susceptibility. Ann. Intern. Med. *65*:629, 1966.
2. Reidenberg MM: Renal function and drug action. Philadelphia: W. B. Saunders Co., 1971.
3. Wilkinson GR, Schenker S: Drug disposition and liver disease. Drug Metabol. Rev. *4*(2):139–175, 1975.
4. Blaschke TF: Protein binding and kinetics of drugs in liver disease. Clin. Pharmacokinet. *2*:32–44, 1977.
5. Lindner A, Charra B, Sherrard DJ, et al.: Accelerated atherosclerosis in prolonged maintenance hemodialysis. N. Engl. J. Med. *290*:697, 1974.
6. Beller GA, Smith TW, Abelmann WH, et al.: Digitalis intoxication. A prospective clinical study with serum level correlations. N. Engl. J. Med. *284*:989, 1971.
7. Lasagna L: How useful are serum digitalis measurements? N. Engl. J. Med. *294*:898, 1976.
8. Koch-Weser J, Duhme DW, Greenblatt DJ: Influence of serum digoxin concentration measurements on frequency of digitoxicity. Clin. Pharmacol. Ther. *16*:284, 1973.
9. Duhme DW, Greenblatt DJ, Koch-Weser J: Reduction of digoxin toxicity associated with measurement of serum levels. Ann. Intern. Med. *80*:516, 1974.
10. Jelliffe RW, Buell J, Kalaba R: Reduction of digitalis toxicity by computer-assisted glycoside dosage regimens. Ann. Intern. Med. *77*:891, 1972.
11. Doherty JE, Flanigan WJ, Perkins WH, et al.: Studies with tritiated digoxin in anephric human subjects. Circulation *35*:298, 1967.
12. Maloney C, Ahmed M, Tweeddale M, et al.: Biotransformation and elimination of digoxin with normal and minimal renal function. Clin. Res. *24*:651A, 1976.
13. Doherty JE, Kane JJ: Clinical pharmacology of digitalis glycosides. Ann. Rev. Med. *26*:159, 1975.
14. Doherty JE, Perkins WH, Wilson MC: Studies with tritiated digoxin in renal failure. Am. J. Med. *37*:536, 1964.
15. Marcus FI, Peterson A, Salel A, et al.: The metabolism of tritiated digoxin in renal insufficiency in dogs and man. J. Pharmacol. Exp. Ther. *152*:372, 1966.
16. Doherty JE, Bissett JK, Kane JJ, et al.: Tritiated digoxin: Studies in renal disease in human subjects. Int. J. Clin. Pharmacol. *12*:89, 1975.
17. Gault MH, Jeffrey JR, Chirito E, et al.: Studies of digoxin dosage, kinetics and serum concentrations in renal failure and review of the literature. Nephron *17*:161, 1976.
18. Doherty JE, Flanigan WJ, Patterson RM, et al.: The excretion of tritiated digoxin in normal human volunteers before and after unilateral nephrectomy. Circulation *40*:555, 1969.
19. Blood PM, Nelp WB, Truell SH: Relationship of the excretion of tritiated digoxin to renal function. Am. J. Med. Sci. *251*:133, 1966.
20. Paulson MJ, Welling PG: Calculation of serum digoxin levels in patients with normal and impaired renal function. J. Clin. Pharmacol. *16*:660, 1976.
21. Marcus FI: Current concepts of digoxin therapy. Mod. Concepts Cardiovasc. Dis. *45*:77, 1976.
22. Reuning RH, Sams RA, Notari RE: Role of pharmacokinetics in drug dosage adjustment. I. Pharmacologic effect kinetics and apparent volume of distribution of digoxin. J. Clin. Pharmacol. *13*:127, 1973.
23. Jusko WJ, Szefler SJ, Goldfarb AL: Pharmacokinetic design of digoxin dosage regimens in relation to renal function. J. Clin. Pharmacol. *14*:525, 1974.
24. Wagner JG, Yates JD, Willis PW, 3rd, et al.: Correlation of plasma levels of digoxin in cardiac patients with dose and measures of renal function. Clin. Pharmacol. Ther. *15*:291, 1974.
25. Halkin H, Sheiner LB, Melmon KL: Determinants of the renal clearance of digoxin. Clin. Pharmacol. Ther. *17*:385, 1975.
26. Koup JR, Jusko WJ, Elwood CM, et al.: Digoxin pharmacokinetics: Role of renal failure in dosage regimen design. Clin. Pharmacol. Ther. *18*:9, 1975.
27. Jelliffe RW: A mathematical analysis of digitalis kinetics in patients with normal and reduced renal function. Math. Biosci. *1*:305, 1965.
28. Jelliffe RW: An improved method of digoxin therapy. Ann. Intern. Med. *69*:703, 1968.
29. Storstein L: Studies on digitalis. V. The influence of impaired renal function, hemodialysis and drug interaction on serum protein binding of digitoxin and digoxin. Clin. Pharmacol. Ther. *20*:6, 1976.
30. Jelliffe RW, Buell J, Kalaba R, et al.: An improved method of digitoxin therapy. Ann. Intern. Med. *72*:453, 1970.
31. Sheiner LB: The use of serum concentrations on digitalis for quantitative therapeutic decisions. Cardiovasc. Clin. *6*:141, 1974.
32. Rasmussen K, Jervell J, Storstein L, et al.: Digitoxin kinetics in patients with impaired renal function. Clin. Pharmacol. Ther. *13*:6, 1972.
33. Vohringer HF, Reitbrock N, Spurny P: Disposition of digitoxin in renal failure. Clin. Pharmacol. Ther. *19*:387, 1976.
34. Finkelstein FO, Foffinet JA, Hendler EO, et al.: Pharmacokinetics of digoxin and digitoxin in patients undergoing hemodialysis. Am. J. Med. *58*:525, 1975.
35. Storstein L: Studies on digitalis. VII. Influence of nephrotic syndrome on protein binding, pharmacokinetics and renal excretion of digitoxin and cardioactive metabolites. Clin. Pharmacol. Ther. *20*:158, 1976.
36. Ackerman GL, Doherty JE, Flanigan WJ: Peritoneal dialysis and hemodialysis of tritiated digoxin. Ann. Intern. Med. *67*:718, 1967.
37. Lukas DS, DeMartino AG: Binding of digoxin and some related cardenolides to human plasma proteins. J. Clin. Invest. *48*:1041, 1969.
38. Doherty JE, Flanigan WJ, Perkins WH: Tritiated digoxin excretion of patients following renal transplantation. Circulation *37*:865, 1968.
39. Gibson TP, Nelson HA: Evidence for accumulation of digoxin metabolites in renal failure. Clin. Pharmacol. Ther. *27*:219, 1980.

40. Zilly W, Richter E, Rietbrock N: Pharmacokinetics and metabolism of digoxin- and beta-methyl-digoxin-12 alpha-[3] H in patients with acute hepatitis. Clin. Pharmacol. Ther. *17*:302–309, 1975.
41. Marcus FI, Kapadia GG: Metabolism of tritiated digoxin in cirrhotic patients. Gastroenterology *47*:517–524, 1964.
42. Lukas DS: Changing concepts of digitalis therapy and toxicity. *In* Cardiovascular Problems (H Russek, ed.) Baltimore: University Park Press, 1976, pp. 295–319.
43. Okita GI: Species differences in duration of action of cardiac glycosides. Fed. Proc. *26*:1125–1129, 1967.
44. Caldwell JH, Greenberger NJ: Interruption of the enterohepatic circulation of digitoxin by cholestyramine. I. Protection against lethal digitoxin intoxication. J. Clin. Invest. *50*:2626–2637, 1971.
45. Storstein L, Amlie J: Studies on digitalis XII. Kinetic pattern of digitoxin metabolism in patients with biliary fistulas. Clin. Pharmacol. Ther. *21*:659–674, 1977.
46. Rollins DE, Klaassen CD: Biliary excretion of drugs in man. Clin. Pharmacokinet. *4*:368–379, 1979.
47. Lukas DS, DeMartino AG: Binding of digitoxin and some related cardenolides to human plasma proteins. J. Clin. Invest. *48*:1041–1053, 1969.
48. Storstein L: Studies on digitalis. III. Biliary excretion and enterohepatic circulation of digitoxin and its cardio-active metabolites. Clin. Pharmacol. Ther. *17*:313–320, 1975.
49. Evans GH, Nies AS, Shand DG: The disposition of propranolol. III. Decreased half-life and volume of distribution as a result of plasma binding in man, monkey, dog and rat. J. Pharmacol. Exp. Ther. *186*:114–122, 1973.
50. Nies AS, Shand DG, Wilkinson GR: Altered hepatic blood flow and drug disposition. Clin. Pharmacokinet. *1*:135–155, 1976.
51. Evans GH, Shand DG: Disposition of propranolol. V. Drug accumulation and steady-state concentrations during chronic oral administration in man. Clin. Pharmacol. Ther. *14*:487, 1973.
52. Shand DG, Nukolls EM, Oates JA: Plasma propranolol levels in adults. Clin. Pharmacol. Ther. *11*:112, 1970.
53. Briggs WA, Lowenthal DT, Cirksena W, et al.: Propranolol in hypertensive dialysis patients: efficacy and compliance. Clin. Pharmacol. Ther. *18*:606, 1975.
54. Cotham RH, Shand D: Spuriously low plasma propranolol concentrations resulting from blood collection methods. Clin. Pharmacol. Ther. *18*:535, 1975.
55. Wood M, Shand DG, Wood AJJ: Altered drug binding due to sampling through heparin locks. Clin. Pharmacol. Ther. *25*:255, 1979.
56. Lowenthal DT, Briggs WA, Gibson TP, et al.: Pharmacokinetics of oral propranolol in chronic renal disease. Clin. Pharmacol. Ther. *16*:761, 1974.
57. Bianchetti G, Graziani G, Brancaccio D, et al.: Pharmacokinetics and effects of propranolol in terminal uraemic patients and in patients undergoing regular dialysis treatment. Clin. Pharmacokinet. *1*:373, 1976.
58. Affrime MB, Ruch E, Pirano AJ, DiGregorio GJ, Lowenthal DT: Apparent volume of distribution of propranolol in patients with normal and abnormal renal function. Clin. Res. *28*:233A, 1980.
59. Lowenthal DT: Pharmacokinetics of antiarrhythmics: propranolol, quinidine, procainamide, lidocaine. Am. J. Med. *62*:532, 1977.
60. Lichter M, Black M, Arias IM: The metabolism of antipyrine in patients with chronic renal failure. J. Pharmacol. Exp. Ther. *187*:612, 1973.
61. Reidenberg MM, Odar-Cederlof I, von Bahr C, et al.: Protein binding of diphenylhydantoin and desmethylimipramine in plasma from patients with poor renal function. N. Engl. J. Med. *285*:264, 1971.
62. Reidenberg MM, Lowenthal DT, Briggs WA, et al.: Pentobarbital elimination in patients with poor renal function. Clin. Pharmacol. Ther. *20*:67, 1976.
63. Walle T, Conradi E, Walle K, et al.: 4-Hydroxypropranolol and its glucuronide after single and long-term doses of propranolol. Clin. Pharmacol. Ther. *27*:22, 1980.
64. Schneck DW, Gibson TP, Pritchard JF, Hayes AF, Jr.: The plasma concentrations of napthoxylactic acid and napthoxyacetic acid in uremic patients receiving chronic propranolol. Clin. Res. *27*:602A, 1979.
65. Branch RA, James J, Read AE: A study of factors influencing drug disposition in chronic liver disease using the model drug (+)-propranolol. Br. J. Clin. Pharmacol. *3*:243–249, 1976.
66. Gerhardt RE, Knouss FR, Thyrum PT, et al.: Quinidine excretion in aciduria and alkaluria. Ann. Intern. Med. *71*:927, 1969.
67. Kessler KM, Lowenthal DT, Warner H, et al.: Unimpaired quinidine elimination in patients with poor renal function or congestive heart failure. N. Engl. J. Med. *290*:706, 1974.
68. Bellett S, Roman LR, Boza A: Relation between serum quinidine levels and renal function: studies in normal subjects and patients with congestive failure and renal insufficiency. Am. J. Cardiol. *27*:368, 1971.
69. Drayer DE, Lowenthal DT, Restivo KM, Schwartz A, Cook CE: Steady-state serum levels of quinidine and active metabolites in cardiac patients with varying degrees of renal function. Clin. Pharmacol. Ther. *24*:31–39, 1978.
70. Affrime MB, Reidenberg MM: The protein binding of some drugs in plasma from patients with alcoholic liver disease. J. Clin. Pharmacol. *8*:267–269, 1975.
71. Ueda CT, Williamson BJ, Dzinkzio BS: Absolute quinidine bioavailability. Clin. Pharmacol. Ther. *20*:260–265, 1976.
72. Data JL, Wilkinson J, Nies N: Interactions of quinidine with the anticonvulsant drugs. N. Engl. J. Med. *294*:699, 1976.
73. Bigger JT: The quinidine-digoxin interaction. What do we know about it? N. Engl. J. Med. *301*:799–781, 1979.
74. Galeazzi RL, Sheiner LB, Lockwood T, et al.: The renal elimination of procainamide. Clin. Pharmacol. Ther. *19*:55, 1976.

75. Drayer DE, Lowenthal DT, Woosley RL, et al.: Cumulation of *N*-acetylprocainamide, an active metabolite of procainamide in patients with impaired renal function. Clin. Pharmacol. Ther. *22*:63, 1977.
76. Gibson TP, Matusik EJ, Briggs WA: *N*-Acetylprocainamide levels in patients with end-stage renal failure. Clin. Pharmacol. Ther. *19*:206, 1976.
77. Gibson TP, Lowenthal DT, Nelson HA, et al.: Elimination of procainamide in end-stage renal failure. Clin. Pharmacol. Ther. *17*:321, 1975.
78. Drayer D, Reidenberg MM, Sevy RW: *N*-Acetylprocainamide: an active metabolite of procainamide. Proc. Soc. Exp. Biol. *146*:358, 1974.
79. Elson J, Strong JM, Lee WK, et al.: Antiarrhythmic potency of N-acetylprocainamide. Clin. Pharmacol. Ther. *17*:134, 1975.
80. Collinsworth KA, Kalman SM, Harrison DC: The clinical pharmacology of lidocaine as an antiarrhythmic drug. Circulation *50*:1217, 1974.
81. Thomson PD, Melmon KL, Richardson JA, et al.: Lidocaine pharmacokinetics in advanced heart failure, liver disease and renal failure in humans. Ann. Intern. Med. *78*:499, 1973.
82. Collingsworth KA, Strong JM, Atkinson AJ, Jr.: Pharmacokinetics and metabolism of lidocaine in patients with renal failure. Clin. Pharmacol. Ther. *18*:59, 1975.
83. Williams RL, Blaschke TF, Mefflin PJ, et al.: Influence of viral hepatitis on the disposition of two compounds with high hepatic clearance: lidocaine and indocyanine green. Clin. Pharmacol. Ther. *20*:290, 1976.
84. Boyes RN, Scott DB, Jebson PJ, et al.: Pharmacokinetics of lidocaine in man. Clin. Pharmacol. Ther. *12*:105, 1971.
85. Boyes RN, Adams HJ, Duce BR: Oral absorption and disposition kinetics of lidocaine hydrochloride in dogs. J. Pharmacol. Exp. Ther. *174*:1, 1970.
86. Mason DT: Disopyramide: a new agent for effective therapy of ventricular dsyrhythmias. Drugs *15*:329, 1978.
87. Hinderling PH, Garrett ER: Pharmacokinetics of the antiarrhythmic disopyramide in healthy humans. J. Pharmacokinet. Biopharm. *4*:199, 1976.
88. Whiting B, Elliott HL: Disopyramide in renal impairment. Lancet *2*:1363, 1977.
89. Karim A: Disopyramide dialyzability. Lancet *2*:214, 1978.
90. Reidenberg MM, Affrime MB: Influence of disease on binding of drugs to plasma proteins. Ann. N.Y. Acad. Sci. *226*:115–126, 1973.
91. Reidenberg MM: The biotransformation of drugs in renal failure. Amer. J. Med. *62*:482–485, 1977.
92. Letteri JM, Mellk H, Louis S, et al.: Diphenylhydantoin metabolism in uremia. N. Engl. J. Med. *285*:648–652, 1971.
93. Odar-Cederlof I, Borga O: Kinetics of diphenylhydantoin in uraemic patients: consequences of decreased protein binding. Eur. J. Clin. Pharmacol. *7*:31–37, 1974.
94. Odar-Cederlof I: Studies of the plasma protein binding of drugs in patients with renal failure. (Thesis.) Stockholm: Karolinska Institutet, Sweden, 1975.
95. Reynolds F, Ziroyanis PN, Jones NF, et al.: Salivary phenytoin concentrations in epilepsy and in chronic renal failure. Lancet *2*:384–386, 1976.
96. Boston Collaborative Drug Program. Diphenylhydantoin side effects and serum albumin levels. Clin. Pharmacol. Ther. *14*:529, 1973.
97. Solomon HM, Reuh SD, Spirt N: Interactions between digitoxin and other drugs *in vitro* and *in vivo*. Ann. N.Y. Acad. Sci. *17*:362, 1971.
98. Butler TC: The metabolic conversion of 5,5′diphenylhydantoin to 5-*p*-hydroxyphenyl-5-phenylhydantoin. J. Pharm. Exp. Ther. *119*:1, 1957.
99. Manard FW: The metabolic state of diphenylhydantoin in the dog, rat and man. J. Pharm. Exp. Ther. *130*:275, 1960.
100. Blaschke TF, Mefflin PJ, Melmon KL, Rowland M: Influence of acute viral hepatitis on phenytoin kinetics and protein binding. Clin. Pharmacol. Ther. *17*:685–691, 1975.
101. Lowenthal DT, Pitone JM, Affrime MB, et al.: Timolol kinetics in chronic renal insufficiency. Clin. Pharmacol. Ther. *23*:606, 1978.
102. Homeida M, Jackson L, Roberts CJD: Decreased first-pass metabolism of labetolol in chronic liver disease. Br. Med. J. *2*:1048–1050, 1978.
103. Ohnhaus EE, Nuesch E, Meier J, Kalberer F: Pharmacokinetics of unlabelled and C^{14}-labelled pindolol in uremia. Eur. J. Clin. Pharmacol. *7*:25, 1974.
104. Øie S, Levy G: Relationship between renal function and elimination kinetics of pindolol in man. Eur. J. Clin. Pharmacol. *9*:115, 1975.
105. Tjandramaga TB, Thomas J, Verbeeck R, et al.: The effect of end-stage renal failure and hemodialysis on the elimination kinetics of sotalol. Br. J. Clin. Pharmacol. *3*:259, 1976.
106. Frishman W: Clinical pharmacology of the new beta-adrenergic blocking drugs. Part 9 — Nadolol — A new long acting beta-adrenoreceptor blocking drug. Am. Heart J. *99*:124, 1980.
107. Herrere J, Vukovich RA, Griffith DJ: Elimination of nadolol by patients with renal impairment. Br. J. Clin. Pharmacol. *7*:227S, 1979.
108. Brogden RN, Heel RC, Speight TM, Avery GS: Metoprolol: A review of its pharmacological properties and therapeutic efficacy in hypertension. Drugs *14*:321, 1977.
109. Johnsson G, Regàrdh CG: Clinical pharmacokinetics of beta-adrenoreceptor blocking drugs. Clin. Pharmacol. *1*:233, 1976.
110. Pettinger WA, Mitchell HC: Clinical pharmacology of angiotensin antagonists. Fed. Proc. *35*:2521, 1976.
111. Tuma J: Effect of saralasin on blood pressure and on hemodynamics in patients with terminal renal failure. Schweiz. Med. Wochenschr. *107*:704, 1977.
112. Brunner HR, Wauters JP, McKinstry D, et al.: Inappropriate renin secretion unmasked by captopril (SQ 14225) in hypertension in chronic renal failure. Lancet *2*:704, 1978.

Chapter 17

Treatment of Musculoskeletal Disorders

by

James C. Steigerwald

In a 1976 report published by the Arthritis Foundation,[1] it was estimated that over 20,000,000 persons in the United States suffer from some form of arthritis or related disease. Some of these diseases, such as systemic lupus erythematosus, progressive systemic sclerosis, and polyarteritis nodosa, may have severe renal disease as one of their primary organ involvements. Others, such as osteoarthritis, occur so commonly that many people with kidney or liver disease will suffer from both conditions. There are also a few musculoskeletal conditions that occur more commonly in patients with preexisting liver or kidney disease. An example of this is the increased incidence of hyperuricemia and, occasionally, gout in patients with chronic renal disease. Finally, there are a number of diseases in which patients appear to be more at risk of developing renal or liver problems after use of drugs used to treat musculoskeletal disorders. An example of this is the aspirin-induced hepatotoxicity seen in some patients with systemic lupus erythematosus.

In an attempt to cover the multiple issues involved in the treatment of musculoskeletal disorders in patients with kidney and liver disease, this chapter will be divided into four sections: (1) acute musculoskeletal disorders associated with renal and hepatic disease; (2) chronic musculoskeletal disorders associated with renal and hepatic disease; (3) drugs that may cause renal and hepatic toxicity in musculoskeletal diseases; and (4) the specific use of antirheumatic drugs in renal and hepatic disease.

ACUTE MUSCULOSKELETAL DISORDERS ASSOCIATED WITH RENAL AND HEPATIC DISEASE

SEPTIC ARTHRITIS

Patients with chronic renal disease — especially those receiving immunosuppressive therapy following renal transplantation — are particularly susceptible to bacteremia. Moreover, loss of the bacterial filtering ability of the hepatic reticuloendothelial system, as occurs in patients with advanced liver disease, also predisposes to septicemia; thus, acute septic arthritis will be encountered in patients with kidney and liver disease. In patients on chronic maintenance dialysis programs, septic arthritis due to staphylococcal organisms will be especially prevalent. However, any bacterial organism can cause an acute arthritis, while mycobacterial or fungal infections may result in a more chronic synovitis.

In all patients in whom synovitis develops, it is mandatory to perform a joint aspiration. The following examination should be performed on the synovial fluid:

1. *White blood cell and differential count.* If the white blood cell count is over 30,000 cells/mm^3 with a predominance of polymorphonuclear cells and no crystals are seen, it should be assumed that a bacterial infection is present and antibiotic coverage instituted. The most likely organisms are gram-positive cocci (70 to 80 per cent) or gram-negative bacilli (20 to 30 per cent). If no organisms are identified on Gram stain and no other cause of acute

arthritis can be found, empirical treatment should be started with an isoxazolyl penicillin plus an aminoglycoside antimicrobial while cultures are pending. Careful dosage adjustment of the aminoglycoside will be required (see Chap. 13).

2. *Gram stain.* The cells present should be spun down and Gram stained. If organisms are seen, appropriate antibiotic coverage should be begun.

3. *Polarized light microscopy.* The procedure should be performed with careful examination for uric acid or calcium pyrophosphate dihydrate crystals.

4. *Aerobic and anerobic cultures.* Unless there is a high index of suspicion, cultures for mycobacteria or fungi are not done routinely on an effusion that has developed acutely. If, however, the synovitis is of a chronic nature, these organisms should be looked for in synovial fluid. If synovial fluid smears and cultures are negative but one still suspects mycobacterial or fungal infection, a synovial biopsy is then indicated.

In addition to bacterial or fungal infections, viral infections are frequently associated with arthritis. One infection in particular, hepatitis B, is particularly prevalent in patients on a chronic dialysis program. Joint manifestations occur in approximately 25 per cent of patients with hepatitis B infection, usually beginning a few days to several weeks before other manifestations of the disease are present. The joint manifestations rarely persist after clinical evidence of liver disease is manifest, although elevations of serum liver enzymes will often be present while the arthritis is still present. Joint manifestations vary from arthralgias to a symmetrical polyarthritis. The most commonly involved joints are the small finger joints, knees, shoulders, and ankles, although any synovial joint may, at times, be affected. About one-half of the patients who have arthritis associated with hepatitis also develop a rash that is most commonly urticarial. It has been suggested that the presence of circulating immune complexes, hepatitis B surface antigen, and antibody to hepatitis B surface antigen (HB_sAg and anti-HB) correlates with the presence of joint and skin disease in hepatitis B infection.[2] Not until antibody excess occurs do the complexes disappear, and the joint and skin symptoms resolve.

Since the joint disease is self-limited, aggressive therapy is not indicated. Salicylates or one of the nonsteroidal anti-inflammatory drugs (NSAIDs) (ibuprofen, fenoprofen, naproxen, or indomethacin) are generally satisfactory and can all be used at full dosage schedules in patients on hemodialysis.

CRYSTALLINE-INDUCED DISORDERS IN RENAL AND HEPATIC DISEASE (Table 17–1)

HYPERURICEMIA AND GOUT

Hyperuricemia, a consistent elevation of the serum uric acid level to greater than 8 mg/dl, develops late in the course of chronic renal disease. Most patients are able to maintain a normal serum uric acid level until their creatinine clearance drops below 15 ml/min. This appears to be at least partially explicable on the basis of a marked increase in urate excretion per nephron.[3] When the creatinine clearance falls below 10 ml/min, the ability of the nephron to secrete urate falls markedly and hyperuricemia results. Although hyperuricemia does develop late in chronic renal failure, the occurrence of clinical gout in these patients is quite uncommon. In a study of 496

TABLE 17–1. CRYSTALLINE-INDUCED DISORDERS IN CHRONIC RENAL AND HEPATIC DISEASE

Description of Arthritis	Type of Crystal
Gout—acute inflammatory arthritis responds well to colchicine or the NSAIDs	Monosodium urate
Pseudogout—acute inflammatory arthritis seen in association with chondrocalcinosis responds to treatment with NSAIDs	Calcium pyrophosphate dihydrate
Apatite Deposition Disease—acute or chronic periarticular inflammation and/or chronic synovitis responds to colchicine or the NSAIDs	Calcium hydroxyapatite

patients with chronic renal insufficiency, Sarre found six cases with clinical gout. In only two of these did the gout develop following the onset of chronic renal disease.[4]

There are a number of reasons why gouty arthritis may be uncommon in chronic renal insufficiency. First, it is well known that arthritis develops in primary gout only after 20 to 30 years of sustained hyperuricemia at a time when the uric acid pool has increased by two- to threefold. Since most patients with chronic renal disease do not survive that long, they would not be expected to develop a similar elevation in their total uric acid pools that leads to the development of gouty arthritis. Second, uremic patients show a significantly diminished inflammatory response to urate crystals injected either subcutaneously or intradermally.[5] If a similar response to the presence of urate crystals occurs within joints, a typical attack of gout seems less likely to occur.

If significant hyperuricemia does develop in patients with kidney and liver disease, allopurinol is the therapeutic agent of choice. Once creatinine clearance declines below 40 ml/min, uricosuric agents are ineffective. Moreover, these agents can markedly further increase uric acid excretion per nephron, further predisposing the kidney to additional damage. If the creatinine clearance is under 50 ml/min, the daily dose of allopurinol should be reduced to 200 mg/day. Occasionally, higher doses will be needed to maintain the uric acid at a normal level. If an acute gouty arthritis attack develops in a patient with chronic renal disease, colchicine or one of the NSAIDs, such as indomethacin, can be used at full dosage for brief courses of therapy. These NSAIDs can also be utilized in patients with liver disease. It should be recalled that these agents may cause gastrointestinal irritation, sodium and water retention, and diminution in renal function when administered to patients with renal and hepatic disease; thus, close clinical observation is necessary.

In the absence of any specific enzyme deficiency (for example, glycogen storage disease type I and glucose-6-phosphatase deficiency), there is no increased incidence of hyperuricemia and gout in patients with liver disease. Indeed, liver disease, because of an associated decreased rate of uric acid production, is frequently associated with hypouricemia, and serum uric acid levels of 2 mg/dl may be encountered.

PSEUDOGOUT

Deposition of calcium pyrophosphate may occur in hyaline and fibrocartilage in a syndrome referred to as chondrocalcinosis. When the calcium pyrophosphate crystals shed into a joint, they induce an inflammatory reaction that has been termed pseudogout because of its clinical similarity to an acute gouty attack. Although chondrocalcinosis and pseudogout are usually thought to be idiopathic, they are particularly prone to occur in patients with primary hyperparathyroidism. Since almost all patients with chronic renal disease have persistently elevated levels of parathyroid hormone (secondary hyperparathyroidism), acute pseudogout can and does occur in patients with chronic renal disease. Moreover, the high plasma pyrophosphate levels in renal failure can also predispose to calcium pyrophosphate dihydrate deposition. In a recent study, the presence of chondrocalcinosis, considered a radiographic "marker" of pseudogout, was found in 4 per cent of patients on chronic dialysis.[6] This percentage is similar to age-matched patients without renal failure.

Two chronic liver diseases, hemochromatosis and Wilson's disease, are reported to be associated with chondrocalcinosis and pseudogout. Thus, the occurrence of pseudogout in association with significant liver disease should raise the suspicion of underlying hemochromatosis or Wilson's disease. The acute arthritis is treated with any of the NSAIDs; like acute gouty attacks, however, it is not common.

APATITE DEPOSITION DISEASE

In 1964, Caner and Decker[7] reported on five patients who developed acute attacks of arthritis or periarthritis in association with chronic hemodialysis. Two patients had typical podagra and most likely had acute gouty arthritis. In contrast, the other three patients developed chronic, recurrent attacks of arthritis after having been on hemodialysis for from 8 to 16 months. These attacks usually lasted from 3 to 7 days and occurred one to three times each month. They involved a single area of inflammation of synovia, tendons, tendon sheaths, bursae, or other periarticular soft tissue. The adjacent synovium, when involved, was nontender but did contain an effusion. The involvement was seen predominantly in the upper extremity with the dorsa of the hands and wrists the most common areas affected. When synovial fluid was examined, it demonstrated a good mucin clot, few white blood cells, and no crystals by polarized light microscopy. The authors were unsure of the specific cause of these inflammatory episodes but thought they could be related to the soft tissue calcification frequently found in the areas of inflammation.

In 1969, Moskowitz et al.[8] described in detail a patient with crystal-induced inflammation associated with chronic renal failure who was being treated with periodic hemodialysis. In this patient, like the patients of Caner and Decker,[7] the acute inflammatory episodes appeared to develop in association with periarticular metastatic calcifications. Analysis of this soft tissue crystalline material revealed calcium apatite but neither urates nor pyrophosphates. The acute attacks responded well to colchicine therapy. The frequency of attacks appeared to decrease after treatment with aluminum hydroxide gel, which led to a decrease in serum phosphorus levels. The authors felt that the syndrome had a direct relationship to hyperphosphatemia with resultant high calcium × phosphorus product.

In 1976, Dieppe et al.[9] first clearly described an arthritis that appeared to be caused by the presence of apatite crystals in synovial fluid or synovial tissue. These patients all had chronic degenerative arthritis (osteoarthritis) with a superimposed acute episode of joint swelling and effusions. All patients had involvement of knee joints, and three of six had affected distal interphalangeal joints. Although no crystals were seen on light microscopy of the synovial fluid or synovial tissue, hydroxyapatite crystals were identified by their characteristic morphology under scanning electron microscopy and by their ratios of phosphorus:calcium calculated by energy-dispersive microanalysis. The authors thus suggested that a third type of crystal-deposition disease had been identified — calcium–hydroxyapatite crystal deposition disease.

A short time after Dieppe's suggestion, Schumacher et al.[10] reported the similar finding of needle-shaped crystals, 75 to 250 Å in diameter, in a variety of joint diseases. In 4 of their 11 cases, the crystals were seen in synovial effusion cells in patients with otherwise unexplained acute arthritis. Three of these four patients did have osteoarthritis, while the other developed an acute effusion while on dialysis for chronic renal failure. These authors were able to confirm a calcium:phosphate ratio in these crystals consistent with apatite. They further were able to induce synovitis in dogs by intra-articular injections of hydroxyapatite. We have recently seen three patients on hemodialysis who developed chronic effusions of the knees.[11] Roentgenograms of the knees were normal in all patients. Synovial fluid analysis demonstrated low white blood cell counts (<200 cells/mm^3), and no crystals were seen on polarized light microscopy. Synovial biopsies, however, demonstrated weakly positive and negative birefringent crystals on polarized light microscopy in two patients. Electron microscopy examination in all three patients demonstrated an amorphous material present, along with microcrystal-like structures resembling previously described calcium hydroxyapatite.[10] It would thus seem that calcium hydroxyapatite can be the cause of acute periarticular inflammation as well as acute or chronic synovitis in patients on dialysis for renal failure.

MISCELLANEOUS

Acute arthritis or arthralgias often occur as part of the spectrum of chronic liver disease. These joint problems are seen most commonly in chronic active hepatitis. Mackay[12] has reported an incidence of 50 to 60 per cent, while Golding et al.[13] report an incidence of 27 per cent joint involvement in their patients. Both large and small joints can be affected, with activity tending to coincide with episodes of activity of the liver disease. The synovial fluid is mildly inflammatory and only rarely leads to any erosive changes on radiographic examination. Arthritis and/or arthralgias have also been reported in primary biliary cirrhosis, cryptogenic cirrhosis, or alcoholic cirrhosis, but the incidence in these conditions is much lower. As previously discussed, joint manifestations also occur in approximately 25 per cent of patients with hepatitis B infection.

CHRONIC MUSCULOSKELETAL DISORDERS ASSOCIATED WITH RENAL AND HEPATIC DISEASE

ASEPTIC NECROSIS OF BONE

Aseptic necrosis (also called osteonecrosis, avascular necrosis, and ischemic necrosis) of subchondral bone with subsequent collapse of the articular surface was first associated with corticosteroid therapy in 1957.[14] Since that time, ample clinical evidence has suggested that aseptic necrosis of bone is related to corticosteroid therapy. Patients treated with high-dose corticosteroid therapy for prolonged periods of time are most at risk. Renal transplant patients, patients with severe renal disease, and patients with systemic lupus erythematosus are, thus, commonly affected with aseptic necrosis. Bravo et al.,[15] in reviewing musculoskeletal disorders after renal homotransplantation, observed 5 of 60 patients, who were followed a mean duration of 105 to 232 days, developed avascular necrosis of the hips (4 patients) and knee (1 patient). Four of the 5 patients had been administered prednisone, 3 to 5 mg/kg/day, while the other patient was taking 2 mg/kg/day. All 5 patients were also receiving azathioprine, 1.5 to 4.0 mg/kg/day. In another study,[16] 6 per cent of patients surviving longer than 3 months after renal transplantation developed aseptic necrosis in one or more bones. Although weight-bearing areas are most commonly affected (femoral head, femoral condyles, and talus), about 20 to 25 per cent of cases will be seen in non–weight-bearing areas, with the humeral head most frequently involved.

The pathophysiology of aseptic bone necrosis in patients on long-term corticosteroid therapy has not been clearly delineated. The most prevalent hypothesis suggests that corticosteroid therapy alters fat metabolism and transport, especially in the liver. Fat microemboli then result, occluding terminal vessels in bone and causing subchondral bone infarction.

The clinical diagnosis of this condition can be very difficult in the early stages when routine roentgenographic findings are absent despite the fact that the patients complain of pain. If tomography or radionuclide imaging of the painful areas is done, however, focal changes may be seen. At this stage, there is still a chance that nonsurgical treatment may be useful. Patients should avoid any mechanical stress to the areas involved, and if it is a weight-bearing surface, crutches should be utilized. If revascularization does not occur, and necrosis progresses, surgical intervention, particularly total joint replacement, may be required.

METABOLIC BONE DISEASES

Essentially all patients with chronic renal disease will have a combination of osteoporosis, osteomalacia, and osteitis fibrosa when bone biopsy specimens are examined.[17, 18] The clinical significance of these findings varies greatly in individuals. In patients on chronic hemodialysis, excess parathyroid hormone secretion and abnormalities in vitamin D metabolism may lead to symptomatic osteitis fibrosa and/or osteomalacia, while renal transplant recipients frequently suffer the complications of corticosteroid-induced osteoporosis. In the following paragraphs, each of these metabolic bone diseases will be discussed in some detail. It is important to reemphasize, however, that in any given patient, elements of all three states often coexist.

OSTEOPOROSIS

Osteoporosis is defined as a reduction in bone mass below the normal level. A parallel loss of both bone mineral and bone protein matrix occurs. In patients with chronic renal and, occasionally, chronic hepatic disease, a number of factors, alone or in combination, predispose to the development of osteoporosis. These factors include:

1. *Physical inactivity*. Physical activity essential to maintain a normal bone mass is often greatly diminished in patients with chronic renal and liver disease.
2. *Decreased calcium absorption*. In order to maintain a positive calcium balance, all individuals must have 1.0 to 1.5 gm of calcium in their diets. With age, the gut is less able to absorb calcium, so higher dietary calcium is often required. Patients with chronic renal and hepatic disease often do not have substantial quantities of calcium or protein in their diet. Moreover, diminished production of 1,25-dihydroxyvitamin D_3 in renal failure and diminished absorption of this vitamin in some liver diseases can diminish gastrointestinal calcium absorption.
3. *Hormonal deficiency*. After the age of 30 to 35 years, all individuals have a decrease in bone mass that is accentuated in women at menopause. Menopausal loss of bone is thought to be due to estrogen deficiency. Individuals whose maximum bone mass is low (Caucasian women) are most at risk for accentuation of bone loss at menopause.
4. *Corticosteroids*. Patients receiving long-term high-dose corticosteroids (e.g., renal transplant recipients, patients treated with corticosteroids for chronic active hepatitis), develop a decreased bone mass as determined

radiologically and histologically. Since the vertebrae are particularly susceptible to these changes, vertebral compression occurs commonly in this disorder.

The mechanisms by which corticosteroids cause these changes appear to be twofold: First, corticosteroids exert a direct effect on bone to decrease bone formation and increase bone resorption. The decrease in bone formation seems related to a direct inhibition of osteoblast function, while the increase in bone resorption may be mediated by parathyroid hormone. It is known that serum parathyroid hormone (PTH) levels are often elevated in patients on long-term corticosteroid therapy. Also, parathyroidectomy abolishes the osteoclastic response to corticosteroids in animals. Secondly, corticosteroids result in inhibition of intestinal calcium absorption. The mechanism by which intestinal calcium absorption is decreased by corticosteroids is not clear but may be due to competition with the effect of 1,25-dihydroxyvitamin D to promote intestinal calcium absorption. Any decrease in calcium absorption results in an increase in PTH secretion that further stimulates bone resorption.

OSTEITIS FIBROSA AND OSTEOMALACIA

Secondary hyperparathyroidism complicating chronic renal failure is believed to start early in the course of the disease.[17-21] A decrease in ionized calcium in the blood is probably the major factor that leads to parathyroid hyperplasia. Several factors in turn interact to lower ionized calcium. Among these factors, hyperphosphatemia has been felt by many to be important. According to this view, transient and undetectable increases in serum phosphorus occur as glomerular filtration rate falls early in renal failure. Such transient hyperphosphatemia lowers blood calcium, thereby inducing PTH secretion. Increased levels of PTH induce phosphaturia, returning serum calcium and phosphorus levels toward normal. When renal function falls to less than 25 per cent of normal, overt persistent hyperphosphatemia develops. The resultant decrease in ionized calcium serves as a constant stimulus to PTH secretion. Considerable evidence, derived largely from studies in uremic dogs, supports this view.

Much evidence also suggests an important role for abnormalities in vitamin D metabolism to lower ionized calcium and induce increased secretion of parathyroid hormone in renal insufficiency. Thus, the active form of vitamin D, 1,25-dihydroxyvitamin D, is synthesized in the kidney. Synthesis is stimulated by hypocalcemia, increased levels of PTH, and hypophosphatemia. Conversely, synthesis of 1,25-dihydroxyvitamin D is impaired with significant destruction of renal mass and hyperphosphatemia. Any decrease in 1,25-dihydroxyvitamin D early in the course of renal failure would diminish gastrointestinal calcium absorption and the effect of parathyroid hormone to mobilize skeletal calcium. Hypocalcemia with increased secretion of parathyroid hormone would then occur in an attempt to restore serum calcium levels to normal. While conflicting data are available on 1,25-dihydroxyvitamin D levels early in the course of chronic renal failure, uniformally low levels have been found in severe chronic renal failure.

Finally, skeletal resistance to the calcemic action of parathyroid hormone occurs with renal failure and accentuates hypocalcemia and, therefore, parathyroid hyperplasia. Both hyperphosphatemia and diminished active vitamin D levels appear to be factors underlying this skeletal resistance.

The factors causing osteomalacic bone disease seen in patients with chronic renal failure have not been so clearly elucidated.[18, 19] In this regard, the lack of mineralization of osteoid seen in this disorder may be due to abnormal bone collagen synthesis, abnormalities in crystal growth and maturation, accumulation of inhibitors of bone crystallization (such as magnesium and pyrophosphate), and reduction in bone carbonate content due to metabolic acidosis. Finally, a defect in production of a vitamin D metabolite may also be operative.

In some patients, congenital and acquired renal tubular syndromes (e.g., vitamin D–resistant rickets and proximal Fanconi syndrome) result in hyperphosphaturia; secondary hypophosphatemia and eventually osteomalacia can occur. Similarly, either a proximal (Type II, Fanconi's) or a distal (Type I, classic) renal tubular defect may result in renal tubular acidosis. Metabolic acidosis in itself mobilizes calcium from the skeleton in the form of calcium carbonate.

Bone pain felt primarily in the axial skeleton — back, hips, and ribs — is the most common complaint of patients with renal osteodystrophy. Pain can also involve other areas, such as knees, heels, shoulders, and elbows. Movement tends to aggravate the pains. Proximal muscle weakness may be a striking feature of the disease. Otherwise, physical examination is often unrevealing.

The diagnosis of renal osteodystrophy is based on clinical findings, laboratory abnormalities, bone x-rays, and bone histology. Occasionally, measurements of serum parathyroid hormone assays will be helpful. Mild abnormalities of serum calcium and phosphorus are usually present. The bone component of alkaline phosphatase is usually high, but normal levels do not preclude this diagnosis. Muscle enzymes are normal. Bone x-rays may be helpful, especially when special techniques and a radiologist with expertise in metabolic bone disease are available. In general, x-ray techniques may suggest osteitis fibrosa (subperiostial bone reabsorption) but are less helpful when predominantly osteomalacia is present; often, a definitive diagnosis can be established only with bone biopsy.

Management of renal osteodystrophy includes:

1. Maintenance of blood calcium and phosphorus as normal as possible in patients with renal failure by appropriate phosphate-binding antacids and calcium supplementation if necessary.

2. Vitamin D therapy should be considered when (a) There is clinical, radiographic, and bone biopsy evidence of overt hyperparathyroidism and serum calcium is less than 10 mg/dl; (b) There is significant hypocalcemia unresponsive to oral calcium supplementation present; (c) There is osteomalacia, particularly when osteitis fibrosa and osteomalacia coexist.

In some patients with significant hyperparathyroidism, manifest by high parathyroid hormone levels, bone disease, metastatic calcification, and/or hypercalcemia, parathyroidectomy may be indicated. Some patients with osteomalacia may respond to other vitamin D analogues.[19]

The liver is essential for the conversion of vitamin D to 25-hydroxyvitamin D. When measured, 25-hydroxyvitamin D levels are low in cirrhosis. Nevertheless, except for primary biliary cirrhosis in which there is also malabsorption secondary to an obstructive jaundice, clinical signs and symptoms of osteomalacia are not common in liver disease. Vitamin D supplementation should be considered in patients with chronic cholestasis.

MISCELLANEOUS

Metastatic calcification frequently occurs in patients with chronic renal failure. The metastatic calcification that occurs in periarticular tissue can result in chronic musculoskeletal pains. This form of calcification is made up of hydroxyapatite and correlates well with a prolonged increase in the calcium × phosphorus product. Often, severe secondary hyperparathyroidism is present. This form of metastatic calcification is potentially reversible with restoration of a normal calcium × phosphorus product by use of phosphate-binding antacids.

DRUGS THAT MAY CAUSE RENAL AND HEPATIC TOXICITY IN MUSCULOSKELETAL DISEASES

SALICYLATES AND THE NONSTEROIDAL ANTI-INFLAMMATORY DRUGS (Table 17–2)

SALICYLATES

It has been known for many years that salicylates cause some minor alteration in glomerular and tubular function in the kidney. These changes, however, rarely affect the clinical course or management of patients. In a recent report, however, Kimberly and Plotz[22] observed elevations of serum creatinine and blood urea nitrogen and a decrease in creatinine clearance in patients taking anti-inflammatory doses of aspirin. These changes were most marked in patients with systemic lupus erythematosus, occurring in 13 of 25 patients studied. The decrease in renal function began after 2 to 3 days of aspirin therapy. The peak decrease in renal function was observed at about 7 days. The changes seemed

TABLE 17–2. DRUGS THAT MAY CAUSE A DECREASE IN RENAL FUNCTION IN SYSTEMIC LUPUS ERYTHEMATOSUS AND/OR RHEUMATOID ARTHRITIS

Salicylates
Nonsteroidal anti-inflammatory drugs
Phenylbutazone
Indomethacin
Ibuprofen
Naproxen
Fenoprofen
Gold salts
Penicillamine

to correlate with the serum salicylate level because, at and below levels of 10 mg/dl, there was no decline in function. When serum salicylate levels reached about 25 mg/dl the changes were apparent. In this study, the maximum changes noted at 7 to 8 days persisted but did not worsen as long as aspirin was continued. The maximum follow-up of patients on high doses of salicylates, however, was only 2 to 3 weeks. Once salicylates were discontinued, renal function returned to baseline values over a period of about 5 days.

Further work by this same group,[23] again studying a group of patients with systemic lupus erythematosus, noted a mean decrease of 47 per cent in urinary prostaglandin E–like material accompanying the decline in renal function during aspirin therapy. They suggest from these observations that the mechanism for these salicylate-induced changes in renal function may be the inhibition of renal prostaglandin synthesis.

The liver as well as the kidney seems to be particularly susceptible to damage by salicylates. Salicylates have been reported to cause abnormalities of liver function in rheumatic fever, juvenile rheumatoid arthritis, and systemic lupus erythematosus. Liver function abnormalities are manifested primarily by an elevation of transaminase levels, but mild increases in alkaline phosphatase, bilirubin, and prothrombin time can also be seen. In most cases, the patients are asymptomatic, although a few patients with juvenile rheumatoid arthritis and systemic lupus erythematosus have developed clinical signs of hepatitis. In these symptomatic patients, liver biopsies all demonstrated evidence of chronic hepatitis. In 1976, Seaman and Plotz reported a prospective study of the effect of aspirin (serum salicylate levels of 25 to 30 mg/dl) on liver tests in patients with systemic lupus erythematosus and rheumatoid arthritis and in normal individuals.[24] One of three normal individuals developed a mild increase in his serum glutamic-pyruvic transaminase (SGPT), while four of 20 patients with rheumatoid arthritis increased their SGPT levels to twice normal after 2 weeks of salicylate therapy. In the patients with systemic lupus erythematosus, 7 of the 16 patients developed a rapid rise in SGPT after 1 week of therapy, and in 6 of these patients, the rise was higher than any seen in patients with rheumatoid arthritis or normal subjects. Four of these patients also developed symptoms. All of the patients with lupus, except one who developed signs of hepatotoxicity while using salicylates, were considered to have active disease. When the salicylates were discontinued, evidence of hepatotoxicity disappeared in all patients.

NONSTEROIDAL ANTI-INFLAMMATORY DRUGS

The observation that salicylates may decrease renal blood flow and glomerular filtration in some patients and that this decrease in function appeared to be related to inhibition of prostaglandin E synthesis prompted further studies of the nonsteroidal anti-inflammatory drugs (NSAIDs) that also inhibit prostaglandin synthesis. Kimberly et al.[25] studied three patients with systemic lupus erythematosus taking one of the propionic acid derivatives: ibuprofen, naproxen, or fenoprofen. In a manner similar to aspirin, each of these drugs reduced renal function associated with reduced excretion of urinary prostaglandin E–like material. Two of the three patients did show attenuation or reduction of the changes in renal function within a few days, even though the drugs were continued. Of importance was their observation that the effects of different NSAIDs or salicylates on renal function was not necessarily identical in any one patient. For example, a patient may be able to tolerate salicylates but not necessarily ibuprofen, or conversely, ibuprofen but not salicylates.

In addition to this decline in renal function with the NSAIDs (it has also been reported with indomethacin and phenylbutazone), there are now a number of case reports of reversible renal failure and/or the nephrotic syndrome associated with this group of drugs. Ibuprofen,[26] fenoprofen, or naproxen[27] and indomethacin and phenylbutazone[28] have all been implicated. In contrast to the studies in patients with systemic lupus erythematosus, all of these patients had essentially normal renal function prior to the onset of their renal failure and were given the medication for treatment of osteoarthritis, rheumatoid arthritis, or crystalline-induced arthritis. Renal biopsies done in two of the patients displayed an interstitial nephritis as the predominant pathologic finding. After the medications were discontinued, the renal function of all patients returned to baseline values (see Chap. 6).

In contrast to salicylates, hepatotoxicity from the NSAIDs is quite rare. There are isolated reports of indomethacin, phenylbutazone, and ibuprofen causing hepatotoxicity, but at least for the present, these have not been clinically important problems.

GOLD SALTS

Since the 1920's, when it was first used to treat rheumatoid arthritis, gold has remained one of the most effective forms of treatment of chronic rheumatoid arthritis. Approximately 80 per cent of patients who are begun on a course of gold therapy will derive a significant benefit from the course of gold. Unfortunately, however, about 15 to 20 per cent of those who have noted improvement will be forced to discontinue the gold because of toxic reactions. Although dermatitis is by far the most common side effect of gold therapy, proteinuria develops at some time during treatment in about 10 per cent of patients and generally requires discontinuation of therapy. Nephritis and/or the nephrotic syndrome may develop in a few individuals, particularly if the gold is continued after proteinuria develops. The major lesion on renal biopsy is a membranous glomerulonephritis with deposition of immunoglobulins and complement in the glomeruli. These lesions almost always resolve after discontinuation of treatment. This disorder is discussed in detail in Chapter 7.

PENICILLAMINE

Penicillamine, a structural analogue of the naturally occurring amino acid cysteine, has been used in the treatment of rheumatoid arthritis for the past 15 to 20 years, but has become widely accepted only in the past few years. It has been shown in clinical trials to be superior to placebo and at least as efficacious as gold therapy. Like gold salts, however, side effects from penicillamine therapy are common. The most common of the late toxic manifestations is proteinuria, occurring in about 20 per cent of patients. Even though the lesion responsible for the proteinuria (determined by renal biopsy) may be stable and the urine protein excretion is less than 2 gm/24 hr,[29] most physicians would stop therapy, since continued treatment can result in the development of a chronic glomerulonephritis and renal insufficiency (see Chap. 7).

ANALGESIC NEPHROPATHY (see Chap. 8)

Since 1953,[30] it has been observed that overuse or misuse of certain analgesic drugs or drug combinations can be associated with interstitial nephritis and/or renal papillary necrosis. The drugs implicated (salicylates, acetaminophen, and phenacetin) are ones commonly used in the treatment of musculoskeletal disorders. Although these drugs have, occasionally, been reported to cause renal damage when given alone and in high dosage, most workers now feel that it is the combination of two of these drugs that has the greatest potential for damaging the kidneys. Indeed, in a study of 763 patients with rheumatoid arthritis and 145 patients with osteoarthritis, there was no association between the chronic use of salicylates alone and analgesic nephropathy.

There are a number of mechanisms proposed to explain why these drug combinations may cause renal damage. As discussed by Mitchell et al.,[32] salicylates, acetaminophen, and phenacetin are all converted by microsomal enzymes to chemically reactive intermediates that concentrate in the medullae and papillae of the kidneys. This concentration may then cause a primary lesion, leading to papillary necrosis and eventually to cortical damage. Molland,[33] using mixtures containing salicylates, suggests that early papillary changes might be a result of the salicylates acting as an inhibitor of prostaglandins. This could cause ischemia because of reduced blood flow to the medulla and render the kidney more susceptible to the salicylates themselves or, more likely, to other drugs in the combination (phenacetin or acetaminophen). Whatever the mechanism, if the analgesic overuse continues, permanent and severe damage to the kidney results. Discontinuation of the offending medication, however, generally prevents further damage to the kidneys.

It is well known that acetaminophen overdosage may cause an acute centrilobular hepatic necrosis that may be fatal (see Chap. 11). In 1977, however, a report appeared in which a patient with arthritis developed liver function abnormalities while taking therapeutic doses of acetaminophen for 1 year.[34] A liver biopsy showed both acute and chronic inflammatory cell infiltration. Rechallenge with acetaminophen again induced marked elevations of serum glutamic-oxalacetic transaminase with return of the liver function tests to normal over a 3-month period.

The mechanism whereby this patient developed liver disease is not clear. Acetaminophen is normally oxidized by cytochrome P-450 oxidases to a reactive metabolite, which is then conjugated with glutathione. If there were deficient stores of glutathione present, the active metabolite of acetaminophen could bind with nuclear proteins in the liver and directly cause *de novo* liver disease. If subclinical liver disease was already present in the above-mentioned patient, it was markedly aggravated by therapeutic doses of acetaminophen not generally thought to be hepatotoxic.

ALLOPURINOL

Allopurinol and its major metabolic product, oxypurinol, are analogues of hypoxanthine and xanthine, respectively, and are both inhibitors of xanthine oxidase, the enzyme that converts hypoxanthine to xanthine and xanthine to uric acid. As such, they are very effective in lowering serum uric acid levels. In general, allopurinol is well tolerated; only 5 per cent or less of patients who receive it develop side effects serious enough to require discontinuation of the drug. Among the side effects reported, however, are jaundice and a granulomatous hepatitis. In a group of seven patients with decreased creatinine clearances (32 to 64 ml/min), five developed elevations of alkaline phosphatase and two developed clinical jaundice. Biopsy in those two patients revealed an intrahepatic cholestasis.[35] In another case with acute renal failure secondary to rhabdomyolysis and myoglobinuria, the patient developed fever, eosinophilia, and abnormal liver function studies (primarily an increase in alkaline phosphatase levels) after 3 weeks of taking 300 mg of allopurinol daily.[36] Liver biopsy demonstrated focal necrosis and noncaseating granulomas. One month following discontinuation of the drug, liver function studies were normal, as was a repeat liver biopsy. It would thus appear that allopurinol must be used with caution and in lower dosage (200 mg daily) in anyone with even mild to moderate renal failure. In addition, allopurinol has also been reported to cause interstitial nephritis (see Chap. 7).

THE SPECIFIC USE OF ANTIRHEUMATIC DRUGS IN RENAL AND HEPATIC DISEASE

ASPIRIN AND THE SALICYLATES

More than 50 aspirin and salicylate preparations are listed in the 1979 *Physicians' Desk Reference*.[37] Thus, their use, either for acute conditions (such as headaches), or on a chronic basis (for diseases such as degenerative disc disease), is encountered in almost all individuals, including those with renal or liver disease. Because of this and their potential toxicity when used under these circumstances, a brief review of the pharmacology and chemistry of salicylates follows.

All salicylates are absorbed readily, primarily from the stomach and to a lesser extent, from the small intestine. Aspirin (acetylsalicylic acid) has a plasma half-life of only 15 minutes, therefore, its metabolite, salicylic acid, is the substance that is distributed to tissues, and it is also what is predominantly measured when a salicylate level is obtained. In plasma, salicylates are bound to albumin at two sites, with binding decreasing with increasing concentrations of the drug. Thus, at serum concentrations below 10 mg/dl, it is over 90 per cent bound, while at concentrations of 30 mg/dl, it is only 80 per cent bound. Consequently, at higher concentrations of the drug or in conditions in which serum albumin is decreased (cirrhosis), more salicylate is free and able to distribute into tissues. Changes in body pH also affect the distribution of salicylates, since non-ionized drug diffuses through cell membranes more easily than ionized drug. A decrease in arterial pH, as may occur in chronic renal disease, increases the proportion of nonionized drug and thus makes more salicylate available for distribution into tissue.

The liver is the principal site for salicylate metabolism. Four salicylate metabolites and also salicylic acid are formed in the liver and then excreted by the kidney. Thus, renal failure or severe liver disease will prolong the action of the salicylates.

Salicylates, particularly the acetylated compounds, also have a significant effect on platelet function. Platelet aggregation and adhessiveness along with adenosine diphosphate (ADP) release and platelet factors 3 and 4 are all inhibited for up to 72 hours after aspirin therapy. In addition, aspirin can also cause prolongation in bleeding time and prothrombin time. Because of these potentially serious toxicity problems, chronic therapy with high doses of aspirin and any salicylate derivative are not recommended for use in patients with either chronic renal or chronic liver disease.

PHENACETIN AND ACETAMINOPHEN

Both phenacetin and acetaminophen are in common use as analgesics, being available alone or in combinations with other drugs, especially aspirin, codeine, and caffeine. Both compounds are rapidly absorbed from the gastrointestinal tract, reaching peak plasma levels in about 1 hour for acetaminophen and 2 hours for phenacetin. Phenacetin is converted to acetaminophen, and acetaminophen is then metabolized by the microsomal enzyme system of the liver. Measurement of renal tissue concentrations of these metabolites indicates that they are found in the renal papilla. Since analgesic nephropathy appears related to overuse of these compounds, with the development of interstitial nephritis and papillary necrosis, they should not be used chronically in any patients with renal insufficiency. Similarly, since they are metabolized by the liver, chronic ingestion is not recommended. Occasional use of these compounds for mild pain relief, however, is acceptable.

NONSTEROIDAL ANTI-INFLAMMATORY DRUGS

The NSAIDs are organic acid derivatives capable of reducing the signs and symptoms of inflammation within a few days of administration. These drugs share many of the same pharmacologic properties in that they are all well absorbed orally, are greater than 90 per cent bound to protein in plasma, and are metabolized by the liver. Their mechanisms of action have still not been completely defined, although it is known that prostaglandin synthetase is inhibited by the NSAIDs, resulting in decreased levels of prostaglandins. Since prostaglandins can cause edema, erythema, and some of the histologic changes of inflammation, a reduction in prostaglandins may partially explain why the NSAIDs are effective in suppressing inflammation.

Besides sharing some common pharmacologic properties, these compounds are all capable of causing similar side effects with regard to gastrointestinal toxicity, a major limiting feature in their use. Each of the compounds, however, does possess certain distinctive features that may make them more or less useful in renal or liver failure. These are discussed in the following paragraphs.

PHENYLBUTAZONE

In adults, phenylbutazone has a very long half-life of approximately 80 hours. Because of this and the fact that 23 per cent of its active metabolites are excreted unchanged by the kidney, the daily dosage should be reduced approximately 50 per cent (to 100 to 200 mg/day) in patients with a glomerular filtration rate (GFR) of less than 20 ml/min and probably should not be used at all if the GFR falls below 10 ml/min.[38] Phenylbutazone can also cause increased renal tubular reabsorption of sodium with resultant formation or worsening of edema and hypertension. Thus, it should not be used in anyone with overt or borderline cardiac function or elevated blood pressure.

Significant drug interactions can also occur with the use of phenylbutazone, especially with drugs it is able to displace from their protein-binding sites. For example, a marked increase in prothrombin time will usually occur if phenylbutazone is given to a patient using warfarin. Finally, in chronic liver disease, even though it is metabolized by the liver, full doses of phenylbutazone are generally well tolerated if given for short periods of up to 7 to 10 days.

INDOMETHACIN

In contrast to phenylbutazone, indomethacin has a relatively short half-life of between 2 and 11 hours, requiring three or four times a day dosing. Indomethacin is converted in the liver to inactive metabolites; therefore, even in severe renal failure (GFR < 10 ml/min), it is not necessary to modify its dosage.[39] It has been shown in elderly patients, however, that renal elimination is decreased; thus, gastrointestinal elimination is increased. One would thus expect more gastrointestinal toxicity in the elderly. Similarly, because of their decreased renal excretion, patients with renal disease may be more at risk for dyspepsia and gastrointestinal bleeding.

Central nervous system side effects are more common with indomethacin than with the other NSAIDs. Headaches may be quite severe and vertigo, dizziness, and a feeling of unreality are found, especially in the elderly patient. The use of indomethacin in chronic liver disease has not been well studied. If a patient does not have a bleeding tendency, however, a short course of indomethacin may be employed.

IBUPROFEN

Like indomethacin, ibuprofen has a short half-life (2 hours) and is metabolized primarily in the liver. When first introduced, it was used in dosages up to 1200 mg/day and demonstrated good analgesic but no significant anti-inflammatory activity. At these doses, side effects, including gastrointestinal toxicity, were less than with salicylates. At higher dosage schedules, ibuprofen becomes more of an anti-inflammatory drug but correspondingly shows more side effects. Because of these findings and because so little of ibuprofen is cleared unchanged by the kidney, it makes an excellent choice when one is looking solely for an analgesic effect. Ibuprofen can, however, be used in full anti-inflammatory doses even in severe renal failure.[40] Although ibuprofen is metabolized by the liver, it has not been found necessary to reduce its dosage even in severe liver disease.

NAPROXEN

Under conditions of normal renal and liver function, naproxen offers the advantage of a longer half-life (12 to 15 hours), requiring only twice-a-day dosing. Since naproxen is almost entirely metabolized by the liver, it can be used in full dosages (500 to 750 mg/day) in patients with chronic renal disease, especially for short-term therapy. As with any of the NSAIDs, the consequences of long-term therapy with naproxen in patients with severe renal disease are not known. Since, however, a small part of the drug is excreted unchanged (10 per cent for naproxen), there is a theoretical danger of drug accumulation with an increased incidence of side effects.[41] The use of naproxen in chronic liver disease has not been well studied in humans; therefore, its use cannot be recommended until such studies are available.

TOLMETIN SODIUM

Tolmetin sodium is a pyrroleacetic acid derivative, similar to indomethacin except for the substitution of the pyrrole nucleus for the indole structure. It is rapidly absorbed after oral administration with a half-life of 4.5 to 6.0 hours. It is excreted by the kidney in largely an inactive form, although some unchanged drug remains. It has not been well studied in either chronic renal or liver disease; therefore, it should be used with caution in patients with moderate or severe disease of these organs. Its major advantage over indomethacin is a decrease in central nervous system and gastrointestinal toxicity. The usual dosage is 1200 mg/day in three divided dosages with a maximum recommended dose of 1800 to 2000 mg/day.[42]

FENOPROFEN

Fenoprofen is a propionic acid derivative similar in its actions and metabolism to those of ibuprofen. As such, it can be used in end-stage renal disease in full dosage (up to 3200 mg/day given in four divided doses). Like others of the NSAIDs, its use in liver disease has not been well studied and should be used cautiously in severe liver disease, especially if bleeding problems are present.[43]

SULINDAC

Sulindac, a sulfoxide, is metabolized to its active sulfide form in the intestine as well as in the liver. The active sulfide has a half-life of 18 hours; therefore the drug has to be given only twice daily. Its metabolism and elimination are more complicated than those of most of the other NSAIDs because all forms of the drug undergo enterohepatic recirculation, with a large proportion of the inactive form, the sulfone, excreted in the gastrointestinal tract. Nevertheless, there is still some renal excretion of the parent compound, sulindac; thus, in severe renal failure it should be used only in one half the usual dosage. Its usual dose is 100 to 200 mg twice daily.[44]

In summary, the NSAIDs can all be used in mild renal disease and certain of them, including indomethacin, naproxen, ibuprofen, and fenoprofen, can be used in full dosages in end-stage renal disease. It is important to realize, however, that almost all the studies demonstrating the safety of these drugs have been short-term studies, and the effect of chronic administration for diseases such as osteoarthritis or rheumatoid arthritis is not really known.

In patients with chronic liver disease, the only drug that has been studied and found to be safe in full dosages is phenylbutazone. Further studies are necessary to define the role of the other NSAIDs. If, however, bleeding is a part of the clinical picture of the patient with chronic liver disease, none of these medications should be used, since they all decrease platelet adhesiveness and the majority of them may also prolong the prothrombin time.

GOLD SALTS

Intramuscular injection of gold salts (aurothiomalate or aurothioglucose) has been a generally accepted part of the treatment program for rheumatoid arthritis since the 1920's. Approximately one half to two thirds of the patients treated will derive some benefit from gold therapy. Although there are a few reports that gold therapy is useful in psoriatic arthritis, systemic lupus erythematosus, and chronic pemphigus, most physicians still employ it exclusively for the treatment of rheumatoid arthritis. As previously discussed, a small number of patients will develop a membranous glomerulonephritis while taking gold. If the gold is discontinued there is eventual clearing of the renal lesion.

Since the gold salts are deposited in tissues, especially the reticuloendothelial system, it is not advisable to continue this form of treatment in patients with significant liver disease. Likewise, since gold is not only deposited in, but is excreted via, the kidney, it should not be used in anyone with a creatinine clearance of 50 ml/min or less.

PENICILLAMINE

Among the rheumatic diseases, penicillamine has been definitely proven useful only for the treatment of rheumatoid arthritis, with approximately 80 per cent of patients noting clinical improvement after a few months of penicillamine therapy. Like gold, a small percentage of patients do develop signs of renal toxicity, generally a membranous glomerulopathy. Also, similar to gold, it is almost exclusively excreted through the kidney. Because of this, it should be avoided in anyone with a creatinine clearance of less than 50 ml/min.

Its use in liver disease has not been well studied except in Wilson's disease. In this disease, improvement in liver function is noted after penicillamine therapy. From these findings, however, it would appear that penicillamine could be used if needed even in the case of markedly impaired liver function.[25]

ANTIMALARIALS

The antimalarial drugs chloroquine and hydroxychloroquine can be used to treat rheumatoid arthritis and the arthritis and skin manifestations of systemic lupus erythematosus. The usual dose of hydroxychloroquine is 200 to 400 mg/day, and the usual dose of chloroquine is 125 to 250 mg/day. These drugs are only slowly excreted, with significant concentrations deposited in the liver and spleen, and smaller amounts found in the kidney and lung. They are largely broken down in the body with little excretion of active compound. They can be used in patients with the renal disease of systemic lupus erythematosus, but because of the large amounts deposited in the liver, they should not be used in the presence of chronic liver disease.

DRUGS USED SPECIFICALLY FOR THE TREATMENT OF GOUT

COLCHICINE

Colchicine has been used for centuries in the treatment of acute gouty arthritis. When used early in the course of an attack, it is very successful; however, when it is given by mouth, almost all patients develop gastrointestinal toxicity, especially diarrhea. If it is given intravenously, however, the gastrointestinal side effects are completely avoided. In both chronic liver and renal disease, it is well tolerated in short courses except for the gastrointestinal side effects after oral administration.

URICOSURIC DRUGS

Both probenecid (1.0 to 3.0 gm/day) and sulfinpyrazone (200 to 800 mg/day) are useful uricosuric agents in hyperuricemia and gout. Since their mechanism of action is to increase renal excretion of uric acid, they should not be used in anyone with a GFR less than 50 ml/min. They may, however, be used in full dosages in patients with chronic liver disease.

Probenecid has a number of drug interactions that must be kept in mind if it is used concurrently with other medications. Probenecid interferes with the excretion of indomethacin; therefore, if the drugs are being used together the dosage of indomethacin should be reduced about 50 per cent. Likewise, probenecid enhances the blood levels of ampicillin and penicillin and prolongs the half-life of rifampicin and cephradine. Lastly, the uricosuric effect of probenecid is completely blocked by the concomitant use of aspirin. This effect of aspirin is also noted on sulfinpyrazone.

ALLOPURINOL

Allopurinol and its major metabolic product, oxypurinol, are both potent inhibitors of xanthine oxidase and are thus very effective in controlling hyperuricemia. Since their major route of excretion is through the kidney, in patients with decreased GFR of 40 ml/min or less the total daily dosage should be reduced to 200 mg or 100 mg/day. With severe liver disease, most patients will demonstrate hypouricemia; therefore, there is no need to use allopurinol.

MISCELLANEOUS

Prednisone or its active metabolite, prednisolone, is used in the treatment of many chronic liver and renal diseases. There is no indication of any increased drug toxicity or renal or liver toxicity when these drugs are used, even if they are used in high doses.[45]

REFERENCES

1. Arthritis Foundation, Annual Report, New York, 1976.
2. Wands JR, Mann E, Alpert E, et al.: The pathogenesis of arthritis associated wtih acute hepatitis B surface antigen-positive hepatitis. J. Clin. Invest. *55*:930–936, 1975.
3. Steele TH, Rieselbach RE: The contribution of residual nephrons within the chronically diseased kidney to urate homeostasis in man. Am. J. Med. *43*:876–886, 1967.
4. Sarre H: Congres Internationale de la Goutte et de la Lithiase Urique. Evian, France, 1964.
5. Buchanan WW, Klinenberg JR, Seegmiller JR: The inflammatory response to injected microcrystalline monosodium urate in normal, hyperuricemic, gouty and uremic subjects. Arthritis Rheum. *8*:361–367, 1965.
6. Ellman MH, Brown, NL, Katzenberg CA: Acute pseudogout in chronic renal failure. Arch. Intern. Med. *139*:795–796, 1979.
7. Caner JEZ, Decker JL: Recurrent acute (? gouty) arthritis in chronic renal failure treated with periodic hemodialysis. Am. J. Med. *36*:571–582, 1964.
8. Moskowitz RW, Vertes V, Schwartz A, et al.: Crystal-induced inflammation associated with chronic renal failure treated with periodic hemodialysis. Am. J. Med. *47*:450–460, 1969.
9. Dieppe PA, Crocker P, Huskisson EC, et al.: Apatite deposition disease: a new arthropathy. Lancet *1*:266–269, 1976.
10. Schumacher HR, Smolyo AP, Tse RL, et al.: Arthritis associated with apatite crystals. Ann. Intern. Med. *87*:411–416, 1977.
11. Lain DL, Thorne G, Steigerwald JC: Apatite arthritis in patients on hemodialysis. Personal unpublished observations.
12. Mackay IR: Lupoid hepatitis and primary biliary cirrhosis: autoimmune disease of the liver? Bull. Rheum. Dis. *18*:487–494, 1968.
13. Golding PL, Smith M, Williams R: Multisystem involvement in chronic liver disease — studies on the incidence of pathogenesis. Am. J. Med. *55*:772–782, 1973.
14. Pietrograndi V, Mastromario R: Osteopatia da prolungata trattamento cortisonico. Ortop. Traumatol. appar. Motore. *25*:791, 1957.
15. Bravo JF, Herman JH, Smyth CJ: Musculoskeletal disorders after renal homotransplantation — a clinical and laboratory analysis of 60 cases. Ann. Intern. Med. *66*:87–104, 1967.
16. Jones JP, Jr.: Alcoholism, hypercortisonism, fat embolism and osseous avascular necrosis. *In* Idiopathic Ischemic Necrosis of the Femoral Head in Adults. (WM Zinn, ed.) Stuttgart: Thieme, 1971, p. 130.
17. Coburn JW: Renal osteodystrophy. Kidney Int. *17*:677–693, 1980.
18. Kumar R: Renal osteodystrophy: a complex disorder. J. Lab. Clin. Med. *93*:895–898, 1979.
19. Coburn JW, Wong ECG, Sherrard DJ, et al.: Use of 24,25-dihydroxyvitamin D3 in dialysis osteomalacia: preliminary results. Clin. Res. *28*:532A, 1980.
20. Recker R, Schoenfeld, P, Letteri J, et al.: The efficacy of calcifediol in renal osteodystrophy. Arch. Intern. Med. *138*:857–863, 1978.
21. Massry SG, Ritz E: The pathogenesis of secondary hyperparathyroidism of renal failure. Arch. Intern. Med. *138*:853–856, 1978.
22. Kimberly RP, Plotz PH: Aspirin-induced depression of renal function. N. Engl. J. Med. *296*:418–424, 1977.
23. Kimberly RP: Renal prostaglandins in systemic lupus erythematosus. Lancet *2*:553–555, 1978.
24. Seaman WE, Plotz PH: Effect of aspirin on liver tests in patients with RA or SLE and in normal volunteers. Arthritis Rheum. *19*:155–160, 1976.
25. Kimberly RP, Bowden RE, Keiser HR, et al.: Reduction of renal function by newer nonsteroidal anti-inflammatory drugs. Am. J. Med. *64*:804–807, 1978.
26. Brandstetter RD, Mar DD: Reversible oliguric renal failure associated with ibuprofen treatment. Br. Med. J. *1*:1194–1195, 1978.
27. Brezen JH, Katz SM, Schwartz AB, et al.: Reversible renal failure and nephrotic syndrome associated with nonsteroidal anti-inflammatory drugs. N. Engl. J. Med. *301*:1271–1273, 1979.
28. Kimberly RP, Brandstetter RD: Exacerbation of phenylbutazone-related renal failure by indomethacin. Arch. Intern. Med. *138*:1711–1712, 1978.

29. Jaffe IA: Penicillamine treatment in rheumatoid arthritis. *In* Arthritis and Allied Conditions (DJ McCarty ed.). Phiadelphia: Lea & Febiger, 1979, pp. 368–374.
30. Spuhler O, Zollinger H: Die chronisch-interstitielle Nephritis. Z. Klin. Med. *151*:1–50, 1953.
31. New Zealand Rheumatism Association: Aspirin and the kidney. Br. Med. J. *1*:593–596, 1974.
32. Mitchell JR, McMurtry RJ, Statham CN, et al.: Molecular basis for several drug induced nephropathies. Am. J. Med. *62*:518–526, 1977.
33. Molland EA: Experimental renal papillary necrosis. Kidney Int. *13*:5–14, 1978.
34. Johnson GK, Tolman KG: Chronic liver disease and acetaminophen. Ann. Intern. Med. *87*:302–304, 1977.
35. Lidsky MD, Sharp JT: Jaundice with the use of 4-hydroxypyrazole (3,4-D) pyrimidine (4-HPP). Arthritis Rheum. *10*:294, 1967.
36. Simmons F, Fedlman, B, Geretz D: Granulomatous hepatitis in a patient receiving allopurinol. Gastroenterology *62*:101–104, 1972.
37. Physicians' Desk Reference: Publisher, Charles E. Baker, Jr., Oradell, N.J.: Medical Economics Co., 1979, p. 206.
38. Held H, Enderle C: Elimination and serum protein binding of phenylbutazone in patients with renal insufficiency. Clin. Nephrol. *6*:388–393, 1976.
39. Paulus HE, Furst DE: Aspirin and Nonsteroidal Anti-Inflammatory Drugs. *In* Arthritis and Allied Conditions (DJ McCarty, ed.). Philadelphia: Lea & Febiger, 1976, pp. 331–354.
40. Kantor TG: Ibuprofen. Ann. Intern. Med. *91*:877–882, 1979.
41. Brogden RN, Heel RC, Speight TM, et al.: Naproxen up to date: a review of its pharmacologic properties and therapeutic efficacy and use in rheumatic diseases and pain states. Drugs *18*:241–277, 1979.
42. Ehrlich GE: Tolmetin sodium: meeting the clinical challenge. Clin. Rheum. Dis. *5*:481–497, 1979.
43. Brogden RN, Pinder RM, Speight TM, et al.: Fenoprofen: a review of its pharmacological properties and therapeutic efficacy in rheumatic diseases. Drugs *13*:241–265, 1977.
44. Rhymer AR: Sulindac. Clin. Rheum. Dis. *5*:553–568, 1979.
45. Gambertoglio JG, Amend WJC, Benet LZ: Pharmacokinetics and bioavailability of prednisone and prednisolone in healthy volunteers and patients: a review. J. Pharmacokinet. Biopharm. *8*:1–52, 1980.

Chapter 18

Cytotoxic and Immunosuppressive Drugs

by

L. Michael Glode

Immunologically mediated renal glomerular and interstitial diseases are often treated with corticosteroid and immunosuppressive agents. Other indications for the use of these agents in kidney disease include therapy of acute and chronic rejection following renal transplantation and as antineoplastic therapy. Regarding the latter possibility, there are some suggestions that the incidence of *de novo* neoplasia is increased in patients on chronic maintenance dialysis programs.[1, 2] Moreover, hemodialysis supportive care in patients with concomitant neoplastic disease and renal failure, such as occurs during the course of multiple myeloma, is being utilized with greater frequency.[3]

Corticosteroid and immunosuppressive agents have been utilized in the therapy of chronic active hepatitis and following hepatic transplantation.[4] Moreover, patients with advanced neoplastic disease treated with cytotoxic agents often have impaired hepatic function due to tumor metastases.

This chapter will briefly review the indications for cytotoxic chemotherapy in the setting of presumed immunologically mediated renal and hepatic disease. The causes and effects of renal and hepatic dysfunction on drug metabolism in the setting of neoplastic disease will also be reviewed. Finally, the clinical pharmacology of each cytotoxic and immunosuppressive agent will be discussed with particular reference to dosage modifications required for patients with kidney and liver disease.

USE OF CYTOTOXIC AND IMMUNOSUPPRESSIVE THERAPY IN RENAL AND HEPATIC DISEASE

CYTOTOXIC AND IMMUNOSUPPRESSIVE AGENTS IN KIDNEY DISEASES

Current evidence indicates that the majority of glomerulonephritides are mediated by immunologic processes in which circulating antigen-antibody complexes are deposited in the glomerulus. In some cases (e.g., Goodpasture's syndrome and some cases of idiopathic rapidly progressive glomerulonephritis), circulating antibodies are directed against the glomerulus and induce glomerulonephritis.[5] Regardless of the mechanism involved, the potential of cytotoxic drugs to inhibit both humoral and cellular immune responses makes them useful in the therapy of glomerulonephritis. However, there are few well-controlled trials in which either corticosteroid or cytotoxic drug therapy has been proven to be of benefit.

POSTINFECTIOUS GLOMERULONEPHRITIS

Postinfectious glomerulonephritis occurs when an infectious agent serves as an antigen. If the host forms antibody and the resultant antigen-antibody complexes are of the right size and have certain physicochemical properties, immune complexes may be deposited in the glomerulus with resultant glomerulonephritis. The best-studied example of this form of glomerulopathy is poststreptococcal glomerulonephritis, which occurs a week or more after cutaneous or pharyngeal infection with certain serotypes of the group A, β-hemolytic streptococci. Other acute infectious illnesses of bacterial, viral, parasitic, or fungal origin can also result in postinfectious glomerulonephritis. In addition, chronic, indolent infections, such as visceral abscesses and subacute bacterial endocarditis, can result in this form of glomerulonephritis. This form of glomerulonephritic disease is usually self-limited, and therapy should be directed toward finding and eradicating the responsible antigen. There is no convincing evidence that therapy with either steroids or cytotoxic drugs is of any benefit in shortening the course of the disease or in preventing the occasional development of progressive glomerulosclerosis.

"NIL DISEASE" OR MINIMAL CHANGE NEPHROPATHY

Among the idiopathic (primary) glomerulopathies, corticosteroids and cytotoxic drugs have been shown to be of definite benefit in the therapy of minimal change (nil) disease. This disorder, which accounts for over three fourths of nephrotic syndromes in children, is characterized by the development of heavy proteinuria, edema, hypoalbuminemia, and hypercholesterolemia. Renal biopsy reveals no visible changes at the light microscopic level, but fusion of the epithelial foot processes is observed at the electron microscopic level. While most patients with this disorder respond to short-term corticosteroids, up to 50 to 85 per cent relapse. The use of cyclophosphamide (2.5 to 3.0 mg/kg/day for 8 weeks) during steroid-induced remission has produced a highly significant reduction in the number of relapses.[6] Similarly, chlorambucil, another alkylating agent, has prolonged the duration of relapse-free periods in children with nil disease on maintenance corticosteroid therapy.[7] On the other hand, azathioprine, an antimetabolite, is of no benefit.[8] In view of the essentially benign course of nil disease, alkylating agents that can produce late myeloproliferative disorders and permanent sterility in males, should be reserved for patients in whom steroid toxicity or the psychologic burden of excessively prolonged therapy becomes problematic.

FOCAL GLOMERULOSCLEROSIS

Focal glomerulosclerosis is another less common major cause of idiopathic nephrotic syndrome of children and some adults. Some observers feel this process may represent the advanced stage of nil disease. This lesion is characterized by segmental focal sclerosis of glomeruli, starting in the juxtaglomerular area and then spreading to involve the remaining cortical areas of the kidney. There have been no controlled trials on therapy in this disorder. In general, progressive renal insufficiency and persistent nephrotic syndrome are observed. There are no data at present to suggest that either corticosteroid or cytotoxic therapy provides any benefit.[9-13] Focal glomerulosclerosis related to parenteral heroin abuse is discussed in Chapter 7.

MEMBRANOUS GLOMERULOPATHY

Membranous glomerulopathy is characterized by thickening of the glomerular basement membrane with deposition of electron-dense deposits containing immunoglobulin on the subepithelial side of the basement membrane. A number of chronic immunologic diseases, such as systemic lupus erythematosus, chronic hepatitis B antigen–positive hepatitis, carcinomas, and thyroiditis may be associated with this disorder. In addition, a number of pharmacologic agents may produce this type of lesion[5] (see Chap. 7). Membranous glomerulopathy usually presents as asymptomatic proteinuria or as the nephrotic syndrome.[5] In a multicenter prospective controlled trial, alternate-day corticosteroids (2 mg/kg on an every-other-day basis for 2 months) were of benefit in terms of slowing progression of renal failure and in causing a number of clinical remissions.[14] On the other hand, a small (20 patients) randomized prospective study on the effects of the cytotoxic agent cyclophosphamide on idiopathic membranous nephropathy revealed no difference in clinical outcome.[15] At the present time, corticosteroid, but not cytotoxic, therapy appears to be of value in some cases of membranous nephropathy.

In contrast to pure membranous nephropathy, the renal biopsy in *membranoproliferative glomerulonephritis* reveals dense deposits in the glomerular basement membrane and mesangium, as well as mesangial cell proliferation into the periphery of the glomerular capillary loops. Clinically, this entity presents as acute nephritis, including an active urinary sediment and often heavy proteinuria. Complement components are often reduced and component C3 can frequently be found in association with the dense deposits. To date, no prospective trial exists to suggest that steroid or cytotoxic drugs alter the relentless progression of this lesion. Therefore, most investigators have concluded that an effective therapeutic regimen has yet to be devised,[5] although retrospective studies suggest benefit from alternate-day corticosteroids.[16]

RAPIDLY PROGRESSIVE GLOMERULONEPHRITIS

Rapidly progressive glomerulonephritis may occur in association with a host of systemic diseases, including infective bacterial endocarditis, occult visceral sepsis, systemic lupus erythematosus, Henoch-Schönlein purpura, Berger's disease, antiglomerular basement membrane–mediated nephritis (Goodpasture's syndrome), polyarteritis nodosa, and mixed cryoglobulinemia.[5] However, in most cases, a clear-cut underlying cause cannot be found. The major distinguishing features of this form of nephropathy are the rapid progression of renal failure and an extensive extracapillary proliferation (crescents) in glomeruli on renal biopsy. While no controlled trial has been carried out with steroids or cytotoxic drugs, two reports suggest that cyclophosphamide and azathioprine can be used in conjunction with plasmapheresis to lower rapidly the anti–basement membrane antibody titers in patients with Goodpasture's syndrome.[17, 18] Moreover, preliminary reports also suggest that intermittent large doses of corticosteroid administered as "pulses" may benefit this disorder.[19] As will be discussed later, glomerular nephritis occurs in association with collagen vascular diseases. When rapidly progressive glomerulonephritis occurs in this setting, a response to corticosteroid and cytotoxic therapy may be observed.

RENAL INVOLVEMENT IN ASSOCIATION WITH CONNECTIVE TISSUE DISORDERS

Systemic lupus erythematosus (SLE) serves as the best example of the connective tissue disorders, since virtually any of the glomerulonephritis lesions discussed previously may be seen with SLE. Because renal involvement usually occurs in the setting of other systemic manifestations of SLE, the isolated effect of steroid and cytotoxic therapy on renal lesions has not been easily defined. No controlled trials comparing steroid-cytotoxic therapy with placebo are available. The controlled trials that have examined the efficacy of corticosteroid alone versus cytotoxic drugs plus corticosteroids in slowing the advance of SLE are inconclusive as to which regimen or combination is superior. Some studies suggest that cyclophosphamide plus corticosteroids is more efficacious in slowing progression of renal pathology than steroids alone. However, it remains controversial as to whether long-term benefits observed in patients treated with both drugs outweigh potential complications.[20, 21] The only other drug that has received extensive clinical evaluation is azathioprine, which again is probably best used in combination with corticosteroids. The ability of azathioprine to produce a salutory effect remains unproven.[20] Often, cytotoxic agents are utilized as "steroid-sparing" drugs in patients with active SLE who have significant adverse effects from corticosteroids.

In summary, lupus nephritis as well as the systemic manifestations of SLE continue to be treated empirically, with cytotoxic drugs held in reserve for those patients who progress or fail to respond to the usual doses of corticosteroids and other anti-inflammatory agents. In consideration of the potential long-term complications of cytotoxic immunosuppressive therapy, especially with alkylating agents, their routine use in the *initial* management of patients with SLE should be restricted to controlled clinical trials.

Among the remaining connective tissue disorders, special note should be made of the efficacy of cyclophosphamide in the therapy of Wegener's granulomatosis. Renal involvement, characterized by focal glomerulonephritis, occurs in up to 85 per cent of cases, and renal failure is the most common cause of death. Dramatic reversal of this lesion, along with amelioration of the other systemic manifestations (primarily necrotizing angiitis of the upper and lower respiratory tract), has been achieved using intensive cyclophosphamide therapy.[22] Interestingly, corticosteroid therapy has been far less successful.[22, 23]

Systemic necrotizing vasculitis, a term used for the vasculitides that include classic polyarteritis nodosa, frequently involves both the kidney and the liver. Recent evidence suggests that cyclophosphamide can produce complete remissions in a high percentage of patients (14 of 16 treated) in whom side effects or lack of response precludes further corticosteroid therapy.[24]

Mixed connective tissue disease, an entity recently separated from SLE and scleroderma on the basis of serologic studies, involves the kidney in about 10 per cent of cases. While steroids are thought to be beneficial, too few patients have been treated with either steroids or cytotoxic therapy to draw firm conclusions.[25] Similarly, the renal involvement seen with scleroderma, though often life threatening, has not been demonstrated to respond to corticosteroid and/or cytotoxic chemotherapy.[26]

CYTOTOXIC AND IMMUNOSUPPRESSIVE AGENTS IN INFLAMMATORY DISEASES OF THE LIVER

VIRAL HEPATITIS AND ACUTE FULMINANT HEPATITIS

The use of corticosteroids in viral hepatitis has had a long history. In general, it can be safely stated, on the basis of recent prospective randomized trials, that corticosteroids are of no benefit in the setting of acute viral hepatitis regardless of the severity. Indeed, the results of several trials suggest that patients treated with steroids fare worse than placebo-treated controls.[27]

CHRONIC ACTIVE HEPATITIS

Multiple trials with prednisone have been undertaken in patients with non–hepatitis B–related chronic active hepatitis. The results of the most recent trials all indicate that corticosteroid therapy is significantly effective in reducing mortality.[4, 28] One trial that included evaluation of azathioprine therapy concluded that the combination of azathioprine and prednisone was the initial treatment of choice, since fewer side effects were observed on the lower dose of prednisone that the combination allowed.[29]

OTHER LIVER DISEASES

Steroid and cytotoxic therapy has no proven role in the treatment of chronic persistent hepatitis or alcoholic liver disease.[27] In the first instance, the mild nature of the disease and good prognosis make the potential side effects of therapy outweigh any hoped-for benefit. In the second, there has been some evidence that patients with severe alcoholic hepatitis may derive short-term benefit from corticosteroids but studies have not allowed for characterization of patients most likely to respond to corticosteroids. Finally, uncontrolled series suggest corticosteroids are of benefit in the rare condition of granulomatous hepatitis.[30]

IMMUNOSUPPRESSIVE THERAPY IN KIDNEY AND LIVER TRANSPLANTATION

The use of cytotoxic agents, especially cyclophosphamide and azathioprine in conjunction with corticosteroids, has become standard therapy in both kidney and liver transplantation programs. Recipients commonly receive high-dose corticosteroids (100 mg prednisone/day) tapering gradually over the first few months after transplantation. Azathioprine is usually the drug utilized with corticosteroids. Cyclophosphamide may be substituted for azathioprine when the latter drug is suspected of contributing to hepatic toxicity. Additionally, cyclophosphamide has been used during episodes of acute rejection, especially with renal allografts.[31]

Two related issues are worthy of comment. First, in liver transplantation, the degree of immunosuppression necessary may be much less than for successful kidney transplantation.[32] The lower doses of immunosuppressive agents may explain why the anticipated hepatotoxicity of azathioprine (discussed later) and lack of metabolism of cyclophosphamide to active metabolites has not been observed with liver transplantation. Secondly, recent evidence suggests that important immunostimulation of the recipient may be induced by donor organ passenger lymphocytes. Thus, some observers feel these data support the use of cyclophosphamide and steroid pretreatment of the donor where feasible.[31]

RENAL AND HEPATIC DYSFUNCTION IN PATIENTS WITH NEOPLASTIC DISEASE

RENAL INSUFFICIENCY

Renal function may be compromised in the tumor-bearing patient by any of a number of mechanisms. In planning a therapeutic approach, the chemotherapist must have a thorough knowledge of both the metabolism and the excretion of the cytotoxic drugs to be employed as well as their activity against specific tumors.

The causes of renal insufficiency in patients receiving cytotoxic drugs for malignancy may be broadly categorized as the result of direct tumor invasion, the result of tumor-derived nephrotoxic metabolites, and as a direct complication of tumor chemotherapy (Table 18–1).[33] Secondary tumor involvement may occur when the kidney or ureters are invaded by metastatic or direct tumor invasion. In practice, only the leukemias and lymphomas frequently involve the kidneys secondarily, often producing bilateral renal enlargement on radiograms or presenting clinically as flank masses. As will be discussed later, two of the effective drugs used in the therapy of the lymphomas-leukemias, cyclophosphamide and methotrexate, are excreted primarily in the urine; thus, reduced dosages of these drugs may be necessary in the setting of renal failure due to tumor invasion. Obstructive uropathy may also be seen when the ureters or bladder are invaded by any of a number of solid tumors, including cervical, gastric, pancreatic, colonic, breast, ovarian, bladder, and prostatic carcinomas.[33] Again, the importance of recognizing the cause of renal insufficiency prior to administering cytotoxic drugs cannot be overstated. In many cases, the use of radiation therapy and diverting ureteral surgery may allow chemotherapy of the patient's malignancy.[34]

Toxic tumor metabolites are the second main cause of renal insufficiency in patients receiving chemotherapy. Patients with multiple myeloma often develop insidious renal failure on the basis of inadequate hydration and tubular precipitation of myeloma-related proteins as well as the direct toxic effects of paraproteins on the glomeruli and tubules.[35] Anecdotal evidence has been presented that suggests that reduction in the myeloma-related proteins with effective drugs, such as melphalan, vincristine, and prednisone, may lead to partial reversal of the renal damage.[36] Thus, while ominous, advanced renal insufficiency does not constitute a valid reason in itself to withhold cytotoxic drugs in the treatment of myeloma.

TABLE 18–1. CAUSES OF RENAL INSUFFICIENCY IN NEOPLASTIC DISORDERS

Direct tumor invasion
Parenchymal involvement (leukemias, lymphomas)
Ureteral obstruction
Toxic tumor metabolites
Paraproteins
Uric acid
Calcium
Toxic drug therapy
Methotrexate
Nitrosoureas
cis-Platinum
Streptozotocin
Mithramycin
Tumor-associated glomerulonephritis

Another tumor metabolite that exerts potential nephrotoxicity is uric acid. Uric acid formation occurs by the catabolism of purines and is increased in patients with lymphoma, leukemia, and, occasionally, solid tumors. While the kidney can compensate for the increased uric acid load, primarily by increasing tubular secretion of urate,[37] with the rapid cytoreduction seen following effective chemotherapy (especially in leukemias and lymphomas), this mechanism is often insufficient and the resultant increase in filtered uric acid load results in the precipitation of urate in the vasa recta, distal tubules, and collecting ducts. Prevention of urate nephropathy can generally be achieved by allopurinol treatment that inhibits xanthine oxidase, thus preventing uric acid formation.[33, 38] An infusion of mannitol to induce solute diuresis and sufficient bicarbonate to maintain the urinary pH at 7.0 or greater may also be utilized. Since uric acid nephropathy is usually seen as an acute complication of effective therapy of malignant disease, the administration of cytotoxic drugs should be delayed whenever possible to allow the utilization of the protective measures outlined previously before cytoreductive therapy is instituted. Moreover, since uric acid nephropathy is often temporary and since the patient may be in a group for whom long-term survival from the neoplastic disease is a realistic expectation, aggressive hemodialysis is indicated in management of acute renal failure secondary to hyperuricemia.

Hypercalcemia is another cause of renal failure in cancer patients who receive cytotoxic drugs. The potential causes of hypercalcemia include direct bone involvement by tumors or the elaboration of humoral substances such as parathormone-like substances, osteoclast-activating factor, and prostaglandins. In addition, dehydration and immobilization may contribute to hypercalcemia. As with uric acid, mannitol diuresis, often combined with a potent loop diuretic such as furosemide, may be the most effective means of therapy of hypercalcemia. Such therapy should be used in conjunction with specific antitumor therapy. The toxicity of hypercalcemia on the kidney is poorly understood but may relate to a direct effect on tubular function and decreased glomerular filtration from volume depletion, calcium-induced vasoconstriction, and nephrotoxicity. Two drugs, mithramycin and prednisone, have been found to be of benefit in the management of some patients with hypercalcemia associated with malignancy.[39]

Renal insufficiency may occur as a direct result of therapy with cytotoxic drugs or radiation. As will be discussed later, meCCNU, (methyl-1-[2-chloroethyl]-3-cyclohexyl-1-nitrosourea) streptozotocin, methotrexate, and *cis*-DDP (*cis*-platinum, *cis*-dichlorodiammineplatinum) have all been found to produce direct toxic effects on the kidney and may require major dose modification in the presence of renal failure. In addition, the use of radiation alone or in conjunction with cytotoxic drugs may produce irreversible renal damage, which is especially ominous if it is associated with malignant hypertension (Table 18–2).[40]

Finally, it should be noted that tumors may serve as antigens and induce an antigen-antibody form of glomerulonephritis. Although rare, renal insufficiency may result from this complication.

In the past two decades, in spite of extensive trials with more than 20 different cytotoxic agents, none has been found to produce objective responses in more than 20 to 30 per cent of patients with primary renal cancer. The most extensive trials have utilized vinblastine, a vinca alkaloid with notable activity in lymphomas, myeloma, and testicular cancer. Some 33 of 135 patients treated with vinblastine have had objective responses and it remains the single most effective drug available for use in therapy.[41]

HEPATIC INSUFFICIENCY

Hepatic insufficiency can arise in a number of clinical settings requiring the use of cytotoxic drugs. We have previously discussed the use of cyclophosphamide, azathioprine, and corticosteroids in primary inflammatory diseases such as fulminant viral hepatitis and chronic active hepatitis. The liver is also frequently involved in systemic lupus erythematosus, polyarteritis, and other collagen vascular diseases that may require cytotoxic therapy. Primary carcinoma of the liver or biliary tree, metastatic tumors arising from other primary sites, such as the colon, pancreas, stomach, or breast, and the leukemias and lymphomas all have been reported to produce hepatic disease due either to obstruction of bile ducts or to direct infiltration of the hepatic parenchyma. The median survival of patients with untreated metastases to the liver ranges from 2 to 12 months, an indication of the gravity of this condition and an explanation of the impetus for the use of cytotoxic therapy for metastatic and primary liver disease.[42] Finally, patients with alcoholic, cholestatic, postinflammatory, or drug-induced liver dysfunction may require cytotoxic therapy for malignancy arising independently or as a result of the primary liver disease.

In any of the settings listed previously, the pharmacokinetics of cytotoxic drugs may be radically altered. Since we will discuss the individual pharmacokinetics of each of the drugs later, it will suffice here simply to list those cytotoxic drugs that are extensively metabolized or excreted by the liver (Table 18–2). Caution should be observed in the

TABLE 18–2. CYTOTOXIC DRUGS REQUIRING CAREFUL OBSERVATION WHEN ADMINISTERED TO PATIENTS WITH KIDNEY AND LIVER DISEASE

Drugs primarily excreted by the kidney or exhibiting nephrotoxicity
Bleomycin
Busulfan
Cyclophosphamide
Cytosine arabinoside
Methotrexate
Mithramycin
Mitomycin C
Nitrosoureas
cis-Platinum
Streptozoticin
Drugs metabolized or excreted primarily by the liver or exhibiting hepatotoxicity
Adriamycin
Azathioprine
Cyclophosphamide
6-Mercaptopurine
5-Fluorouracil
Vincristine

administration of any of these drugs to a patient with hepatic insufficiency.

In contrast to the above-mentioned settings with abnormal liver function, the normally functioning liver that contains metastases provides the chemotherapist with the unique opportunity to use regional therapy at a higher dose rate than is usually possible with systemic therapy. An excellent example of this approach is the use of 5-fluorouracil (5-FU) or 5-fluorouracil deoxyriboside (FUdR). Since 19 to 51 per cent of 5-FU and 94 to 99 per cent of FUdR is extracted in a single pass through the liver, it is possible to infuse either of these agents at a higher dose rate in the hepatic artery than peripherally with no increase in toxicity.[43] The technique is even more attractive theoretically, since it is known that metastatic tumors derive their blood supply primarily from the hepatic artery rather than from the portal system. Use of this technique appears to be of benefit in patients with metastatic tumors from several different sites and may be safely combined with radiation therapy.[42] Other drugs that may be useful for hepatic artery infusion because of primary extraction by the liver include BCNU (1,3-bis[2-chloroethyl]-1-nitrosourea), adriamycin, and dichloromethotrexate.

Similar to the disappointing results in therapy of renal adenocarcinoma, treatment of primary liver neoplasms is far from ideal. Both 5-FU and adriamycin have some activity in this disease, but complete responses are rare and most patients succumb to advancing local and metastatic disease.[44] Nevertheless, most studies document improved survival of responding patients over the nonresponders and when measurable disease is present, a trial of chemotherapy is warranted.

PHARMACOLOGY OF INDIVIDUAL DRUGS

DRUGS PRIMARILY EXCRETED BY THE KIDNEY OR EXHIBITING NEPHROTOXICITY

METHOTREXATE

Methotrexate (MTX) and amethopterin were developed in the late 1940's and became the first antimetabolites to receive clinical trials. MTX remains a prominent drug in chemotherapy today. It acts by the nearly irreversible binding and inactivation of dihydrofolate reductase within cells, thus preventing the regeneration of tetrahydrofolate necessary for one-carbon synthetic steps in the synthesis of purines and deoxythymidine. The toxicity of MTX is critically dependent on both the level of free drug and duration of exposure. MTX is 50 per cent protein bound and its binding can be diminished by other organic acids such as salicylates, sulfonamides, phenytoin, and chloramphenicol.

Renewed interest in MTX pharmacology has been generated in recent years because of studies suggesting the increased efficacy of high-dose MTX in combination with leucovorin (folinic acid).[45, 46] Combining high-dose MTX therapy with appropriately timed "rescue" using leucovorin or thymidine is theoretically attractive for several reasons. First, it is known that some tumors become resistant to the usually achievable plasma MTX concentration by virtue of decreased transport. Since MTX and folinic acid share the same transport pathways, the achievement of high plasma levels with pharmacologic doses of MTX (1 to 15 gm/M^2) may allow passive diffusion of MTX into resistant cells. "Standard" doses of leucovorin given at later time points then effectively rescues the normal host target organs (bone marrow, gut epithelium), while the resistant tumor cells fail to take up the rescue agent. Secondly, using these doses of MTX, it has been shown that effective cytotoxic drug levels are achieved in the central nervous system, a common sanctuary for tumors, especially lymphomas and leukemias.[46] Finally, high-dose MTX in combination with thymidine rescue may induce "purineless death" in tumor cells that appear to be more dependent on endogenous purine synthesis than are normal host tissues.

MTX is well absorbed orally in doses less than 30 mg/M^2, but absorption falls with doses greater than 80 mg/M^2. Peak plasma levels after conventional doses (25 to 75 mg/M^2) are in the 10^{-5} to 10^{-6} M range, while high-dose regimens may achieve plasma levels in excess of 10^{-3} M. Following an initial rapid distribution phase, MTX is eliminated from the blood in a two-component pattern with half-time for plasma disappearance of 2 to 4 hours and 8 to 12 hours, respectively.[47] The major route of excretion is via the kidney with greater than 85 per cent of administered drug appearing in the urine within 24 hours. In humans, approximately 10 to 15 per cent of MTX is metabolized by the liver.

Since MTX is a soluble weak organic acid

with a pKA of 4.7, it comes as no surprise that the drug has been found to cause tubular crystal deposition when given at high doses.[46, 48] Delay in renal clearance leads to a prolonged plasma level that can result in lethal toxicity if unrecognized. Successful protection from such toxicity can be achieved by (1) urinary alkalinization that increases MTX and metabolite solubilities, (2) increasing urinary flow, and (3) prolonged administration of high doses of leucovorin.[46] While the pathophysiology of MTX nephrotoxicity has been thought to be due to crystalluric damage to the renal tubules and collecting ducts, its occurrence at much lower doses and the occurrence of the same toxicity syndrome using tenfold less aminopterin, a much more potent antifolate compound with similar solubility, raises the possibility that renal damage may also result in part from antifolate activity of the drug.[49]

Although relatively small (MW 454), the protein binding and wide tissue distribution of MTX limit its availability for removal by dialysis. Peritoneal clearance is negligible and clearance rates of various hemodialyzers range from 30 to 74 ml/min. Use of charcoal or exchange resins can raise the clearance rate to 40 to 137 ml/min; however, the relatively large volume of distribution makes it unlikely that extracorporeal removal of the drug will be of significant utility.[51] Enzymatic degradation of MTX using carboxypeptidase G1 has promise as a technique for the *in vivo* catabolism of the drug.[51]

Hepatic toxicity of MTX has been frequently reported following the administration of high doses and is associated with a chronic portal inflammatory reaction.[52] This reaction is usually transient and there is little evidence that the toxicity has any clinical implications such as dose or therapy limitation. On the other hand, the chronic use of low doses of MTX in patients with psoriasis has been reported to produce permanent liver damage in some patients.[53]

cis-PLATINUM

Cis-Platinum (*cis*-dichlorodiammineplatinum, *cis*-DDP) is a coordination complex with a broad range of antitumor activity, including the testicular and ovarian carcinomas, squamous cell carcinoma of the head and neck, lymphomas, and some lung cancers. Following intravenous administration, approximately 90 per cent of the drug is protein bound and highest tissue concentrations are found in the kidney, liver, spleen, and lungs. Thirty to 70 per cent of administered drug is recovered from the urine within 4 to 6 hours of administration.[54] The mechanism of action of *cis*-DDP, while incompletely understood, is markedly dependent on the *cis* configuration and appears to involve interaction with cellular DNA, especially guanine, with resultant strand breaks and cross links.[55]

Early clinical trials with *cis*-DDP quickly uncovered substantial dose-limiting nephrotoxicity in the form of acute tubular damage with resultant azotemia.[56] While the lesion is usually mild and not associated with oliguric renal failure, prolonged oliguria, and lack of recovery of renal function are occasionally observed.[57] Subsequent studies have reported a marked diminution in the incidence of nephrotoxicity using a number of different techniques to increase urine flow or decrease the urinary concentration of *cis*-DDP and its metabolites. These have included the use of forced saline diuresis with or without furosemide, mannitol diuresis, fractionation of the dose, and prolonging the infusion of a given dose. With these techniques, administration of doses in the 3 mg/kg (120 mg/M^2) range can be safely performed.[56] In addition to renal failure, *cis*-DDP may also induce selective renal tubular damage. Recent reports suggest that renal magnesium wasting may frequently accompany *cis*-DDP therapy and cases of renal tubular acidosis have been observed.[58]

There have been few reports on the use of *cis*-DDP in patients with renal failure, although impaired renal function is known to lead to higher plasma levels of filterable platinum with little change in the terminal half-life.[54] Anecdotal experience in patients with testicular carcinoma and severe obstructive uropathy suggests that *cis*-DDP should be used at full dosage and that no unusual toxicities are encountered.[59] There is no evidence of hepatic toxicity in patients receiving *cis*-DDP.

STREPTOZOTOCIN

Streptozotocin is a cytotoxic antibiotic with a glucosamine and nitrosourea moiety. It has clinical utility in therapy of islet cell carcinoma of the pancreas, although its mechanism of action is incompletely understood.[60] Following parenteral administration, it is rapidly taken up by the kidney, liver, and pancreatic islet cells, then disappears with a triphasic elimination curve having half-lives of 17, 16, and 13 minutes. Ten to 20 per cent of the drug is excreted unchanged in the urine within 24 hours of administration.[61]

Streptozotocin is a potent nephrotoxin, and renal damage is the principal treatment-limiting drug effect. Early manifestations of tubular damage include proteinuria, hypophosphatemia, and renal tubular acidosis. When nephrotoxicity is unrecognized or when therapy is continued out of necessity, reduction in creatinine clearance and azotemia may occur.[62] Pathologically, the kidneys show degeneration and necrosis of tubular epithelium. Patients with preexisting renal insufficiency appear to be at increased risk.

While no clinically significant hepatotoxicity has been reported with streptozotocin, transient elevation in serum transaminases has been noted in 15 to 65 per cent of patients receiving the drug. Therefore, prudence would dictate that great caution be used when administering streptozotocin to patients with either renal or hepatic disease.

NITROSOUREAS

The nitrosoureas in clinical use are 1,3-Bis(2-chloroethyl)-1-nitrosourea (BCNU), 1-(2-chloroethyl)-3-cyclohexyl-1-nitrosourea (CCNU), and 1-(2-chloroethyl)-3-(4-methyl cyclohexyl)-1-nitrosourea (Me CCNU). These drugs act both as alkylating agents and independently as inhibitors of DNA synthesis. The drugs are rapidly metabolized, with a majority of metabolites appearing in the urine after oral or intravenous administration. There is apparently a wide disparity in the half-lives of individual metabolites that may depend on variable protein binding.[63]

There is mounting evidence that in patients who survive long enough and in whom marrow tolerance to continued nitrosourea therapy exists, severe nephrotoxicity may occcur. In one study in children, all of whom had normal renal function at the start of therapy, five of six who received greater than 1500 mg/M^2 developed progressive azotemia at varying times after therapy had ceased. Histologic examination of damaged kidneys showed severe tubular loss and varying degrees of glomerular sclerosis.[64] Reversible minor hepatic abnormalities also have been noted in patients receiving nitrosoureas. Cirrhosis has been observed in animals administered high doses of nitrosoureas. At present, therapy with meCCNU in children should be limited in time and total dose until its toxicity is further clarified. There is no convincing evidence that dosage alteration should be made in patients with hepatic or renal insufficiency, and the dialyzability of these drugs is doubtful in view of their strongly lipophilic nature.

BLEOMYCIN

Bleomycin is an antibiotic with antiviral, antibacterial, and antitumor activity. Its mechanism of action is probably due to interaction with DNA, causing strand scission, especially in cells in the M (mitotic) or G2 (post-DNA synthetic) phase of the cell cycle.[65] In cancer therapy, it has activity against lymphoma and testicular and squamous cell carcinomas.

Following parenteral administration by subcutaneous, intramuscular, or intravenous injection, bleomycin achieves high plasma levels. Highest tissue levels may be found in the kidneys, liver, or lungs. It is rapidly excreted as immunoreactive or biologically active drug with about 80 per cent appearing in the urine. While renal failure results in prolongation of the normal 2-hour half-life, even patients with severe renal impairment (creatinine clearance 25 to 30 ml/min) show no detectable drug at 72 hours. Thus, twice-weekly bolus therapy with bleomycin would probably be safe in the setting of renal failure. Extrarenal metabolism may be due to the action of an enzyme, tentatively designated as bleomycin hydrolase.[66] Limited information suggests that the drug is not dialyzable.

The major dose-limiting toxicity of bleomycin is pulmonary fibrosis. It is not thought to be significantly toxic to liver or kidney. However, high doses or continuous infusion may result in hypertension, urinary burning, and hyperbilirubinemia in more than 17 per cent of cases.[67]

MITHRAMYCIN

Mithramycin is another antitumor antibiotic that has been used in the therapy of testicular carcinoma and to treat hypercalcemia associated with a variety of tumors and nonmalignant disorders. While it inhibits RNA synthesis, the actual mechanism of its hypocalcemic effect remains uncertain. Recent evidence suggests that it inhibits bone resorption with little effect on renal calcium clearance.[68]

Mithramycin is weakly acidic and has low lipid solubility. A two-phase plasma disappearance has been described with 10 to 30 per cent of intravenously administered drug appearing in the urine after a short time. Later, the drug appears in the stool. There is no information on the pharmacokinetics of mithramycin in the presence of kidney or liver disease.

Mithramycin has produced both hepatotoxicity in the form of elevated liver enzymes and nephrotoxicity with azotemia. Decreased synthesis of hepatic vitamin K–dependent clotting factors has been reported and may be severe enough to result in a hemorrhagic diathesis. Renal toxicity is cumulative with a slow loss of renal function apparently due to tubular necrosis. It is not known whether preexisting kidney or liver disease is an indication for a reduction in dosage.[69]

CYCLOPHOSPHAMIDE

Cyclophosphamide, a potent alkylating agent, has found widespread use as both an immunosuppressive and an antineoplastic agent. Following oral or intravenous administration, the drug, which is not active before biotransformation, is rapidly converted by the liver microsomal P-450 system to 4-hydroxycyclophosphamide, which is in equilibrium with the active alkylating moiety aldophosphamide. Aldophosphamide may be converted nonenzymatically to phosphoramide mustard and acrolein or may be oxidized by the liver to inactive carboxyphosphamide. Ultimately, 75 to 90 per cent of the drug is converted to these metabolites and less than 20 per cent is excreted unchanged in the urine. The alkylating metabolites are 50 to 60 per cent protein bound, while only 17 per cent of native cyclophosphamide is bound.[70, 71]

Renal failure results in a marked prolongation in the serum of protein-bound cyclophosphamide metabolites, while the disappearance of the parent drug is essentially normal owing to hepatic transformation. It is uncertain whether or not major modifications in cyclophosphamide dosage should be used in renal failure. In one study, a patient with a creatinine clearance of 18 ml/min had severe and prolonged myelosuppression after receiving 50 mg/kg over 5 days,[71] while another study reported no increase in toxicity in a group of 11 patients treated with a similar dose and comparable renal insufficiency.[72] Similarly, the influence of altered hepatic metabolism does not result in consistent changes in either the rate of cyclophosphamide metabolism or the development of toxicity.[71] Cyclophosphamide is readily dialyzable, with a clearance of 78 ml/min reported in one study. Dialysis has been effective in protecting dogs from hematopoietic toxicity.[73]

While cyclophosphamide has not been reported to be nephrotoxic (excepting one case report) or hepatotoxic, two other well-recognized toxicities are worthy of comment. First, the excretion of alkylating metabolites in the urine can lead to acute and chronic hemorrhagic cystitis, bladder fibrosis, and even bladder carcinoma.[74] Since this toxicity can be reduced by the simple measures of increased fluid ingestion, frequent bladder emptying, and avoidance of evening therapy, these maneuvers must be kept in mind. Second, cyclophosphamide may produce hyponatremia owing either to increased ADH (antidiuretic hormone) secretion or an increase in the renal tubular effect of ADH, or both. These side effects may be treated by water restriction.

MELPHALAN (L-PHENYLALANINE MUSTARD)

Melphalan, an alkylating agent with broad antitumor activity, has been most extensively used in the therapy of ovarian carcinoma, myeloma, and breast carcinoma. As with other alkylating agents, its mechanism of action is inhibition of DNA and RNA synthesis through covalent attachment to DNA. Although traditionally given as an oral tablet, the use of intravenous (IV) melphalan is gaining favor in some settings because higher and more reproducible peak levels are achieved. After oral administration, peak plasma levels are not achieved until 2 hours. Substantial drug appears in the feces. Following IV administration, a rapid clearance ($t1/2 = 67$ min) occurs followed by a prolonged terminal phase of clearance that is identical to that observed after oral administration ($t1/2 = 160$ hr).

Usually 60 to 90 per cent of melphalan is protein bound; preliminary data suggest less binding in the presence of jaundice.[75-77] Melphalan is not thought to be hepato- or nephrotoxic; therefore, there is no proven reason to alter the dose when treating patients with hepatic or renal insufficiency.

BUSULFAN

Busulfan is an alkylating agent used exclusively in the treatment of chronic myelogenous leukemia. It is well absorbed orally and 25 to 35 per cent appears in the urine as inactive metabolites. Since measurable amounts of busulfan persist in the urine up to 30 days, it is thought that tissue storage may occur. Based on limited information, busulfan dosage may not need to be altered in the presence of renal or hepatic insufficiency, and the dialyzability of the drug has not been characterized.[78, 79] A single report indicates that busulfan may, like cyclophosphamide, produce hemorrhagic cystitis.[80]

CYTOSINE ARABINOSIDE

Cytosine arabinoside (Ara-C) is an antimetabolite that, after intracellular conversion to cytosine arabinoside triphosphate, inhibits cell proliferation by interfering with DNA polymerase during the S phase of the cell cycle. Its major use is in the therapy of acute myelogenous leukemia, though it has activity against acute lymphocytic leukemia as well. Following intravenous administration, the drug is rapidly and ubiquitously deaminated to uracil arabinoside (Ara-U) by the enzyme cytidine deaminase. The drug and inactive metabolite are rapidly cleared by the kidney (clearance rate 78 ml/min) and disappear from the plasma in a biphasic manner with a short initial half-life of 8 to 11 minutes and longer terminal half-life of 111 to 157 minutes. Approximately 70 per cent of Ara-C and Ara-U appear in the urine in a ratio of 1:4 to 1:6, respectively.[81] Because of the short biologic and chemical half-life, Ara-C should be administered whenever possible by continuous infusion. The dosage need not be altered in hepatic or renal insufficiency because the drug is not toxic to either the liver or the kidney. The dialyzability of Ara-C is unknown.

MITOMYCIN C

Mitomycin C is an antitumor antibiotic that produces cell death by cross linking DNA, thus preventing replication. The major use of the drug has been as an important component of effective combinations for gastrointestinal malignancy.[82] Following IV administration, the drug is cleared from the plasma both by metabolism and by renal excretion. At higher doses (e.g., 30 mg/M^2) in humans, more and more of the drug is excreted in the urine and the terminal half-life is delayed. Thus, in the presence of renal failure, a reduction in mitomycin C may be indicated in patients receiving high doses.[83] Nephrotoxicity has been reported with mitomycin C; however, its true incidence and histopathologic appearance have not been determined. Thus, while remaining aware of this potential, physicians should not alter their use of the drug based on an attempt to prevent nephrotoxicity.[84] Mitomycin is not known to produce hepatotoxicity.

DRUGS EXCRETED PRIMARILY BY THE LIVER OR EXHIBITING HEPATOTOXICITY

ADRIAMYCIN AND DAUNOMYCIN

Adriamycin and daunomycin are anthracycline antibiotics with a wide spectrum of antitumor activity. They differ in structure only by the substitution in adriamycin of a hydroxyl group for a hydrogen atom in the acetyl radical of the aglycone of daunomycin. Their mechanism of action is inhibition of DNA synthesis by intercalation into the α helix. In addition, they produce a unique form of cardiac toxicity by facilitating the oxidation of lipids, and, perhaps, proteins in the myofibrils.[85] Following intravenous administration, the drugs are widely distributed in all tissues, except the central nervous system, and then are cleared from the plasma with a short initial half-life and prolonged and variable secondary half-lives.[86] Both drugs are enzymatically metabolized in liver, kidneys, and muscles by carbonyl reduction (via aldoketoreductases) to adriamycinol and daunomycin and by reductive glycosidic cleavage (via microsomal glycosidases) to aglycones. The parent drugs and metabolites then appear in the urine and the bile.[87] Approximately 10 to 30 per cent of adriamycin and its metabolites appear in the urine in 72 hours, accounting for the red urine seen in patients receiving the drug; the remainder appears primarily in the bile.

The presence of either renal or hepatic impairment may alter the excretion of anthracyclines, resulting in prolongation of the terminal plasma clearance. Although an increase in toxicity has not been reported in patients

TABLE 18–3. EFFECTS OF CYTOTOXIC AND IMMUNOSUPPRESSIVE DRUGS ON THE KIDNEY AND LIVER

	Renal Effects							Hepatic Effects	
	Renal Failure		*Defect in Water Balance*	*Proximal Tubular Defects*	*Nephrotic Syndrome*	*Dose Reduction**	*Miscellaneous*	*Hepato-toxicity*	*Dose Reduction**
Drug	*Acute*	*Chronic*							
Adriamycin	±	–	–	–	+	–	–	±	+
Azathioprine/6-mercaptopurine	+	–	–	±	–	±	6-MP crystalluria	+	±
Bleomycin	–	–	–	–	–	+	–	±	–
cis-Platinum	+	±	–	+	–	±	Renal Mg^{++} wasting	–	–
Cyclophosphamide	–	–	+	–	–	±	Hemorrhagic cystitis	–	–
Cytosine arabinoside	–	–	–	–	–	–	–	–	–
5-Fluorouracil	–	–	–	–	–	–	–	–	–
Melphalan	–	–	–	–	–	–	–	–	–
Methotrexate	+	–	–	–	–	+	–	+	–
Mithramycin	+	+	–	–	–	±	↓ serum Ca^{++}, ↓ phos, ↓ K^{+}	+	±
Mitomycin C	–	±	–	–	–	–	–	–	–
Nitrosoureas	–	+	–	–	–	–	–	+	–
Streptozotocin	+	+	–	+	±	+	↓ serum phos	±	–
Vinca alkaloids	–	–	+	–	–	–	–	–	±

*Reduced dosage may be indicated in the presence of renal or hepatic insufficiency.
↑ = Increase.
↓ = Decrease.

with renal failure, hepatic insufficiency is well known to lead to delays in clearance, resulting in severe adriamycin toxicity, with myelosuppression and mucositis being the primary clinical manifestations.[88] The recommended dosage reductions with hepatic impairment are as follows: for bilirubin greater than 3 mg/dl, 75 per cent reduction; for bilirubin levels between 1.2 and 3.0 mg/dl, 50 per cent reduction.

Neither adriamycin nor daunomycin has been reported to produce hepatotoxicity in humans. In animals and in one suggestive case in a patient, adriamycin has produced a toxic glomerular injury characterized by nephrotic syndrome, azotemia, and histologically, fusion of the epithelial foot processes with mild glomerular epithelial proliferation and tubular atrophy.[89]

AZATHIOPRINE AND 6-MERCAPTOPURINE

Azathioprine and 6-mercaptopurine (6-MP) are purine analogues that inhibit DNA synthesis by activity as antagonists of hypoxanthine. Azathioprine (Imuran) is rapidly converted ($t1/2 = 47$ min) to 6-MP *in vivo* but may also be directly metabolized to thiouric acid, the major metabolite of 6-MP. Since allopurinol inhibits the conversion of either drug to the inactive 6-thiouric acid by xanthine oxidase, the dose of either drug must be reduced 50 to 70 per cent when allopurinol is given concomitantly. In addition to direct oxidation, 6-MP may also be methylated at its sulfur atom prior to oxidation to 6-methyl-thiouric acid.[90] The drugs are 30 per cent protein bound. Following oral administration, 50 to 70 per cent of the drug is found in the urine, mostly as metabolites.[91] These two drugs are widely used in immunosuppressive therapy (discussed previously) as well as in the therapy of acute leukemia.

The nephrotoxicity of the mercaptopurine analogues is an interesting and controversial topic. There is little doubt that 6-MP can produce direct nephrotoxicity in high doses by the direct precipitation of drug, causing crystalluria and hematuria.[92] In addition, the use of azathioprine has resulted in oliguric renal failure due to allergic interstitial nephritis.[93] Early studies suggested that renal failure enhanced 6-MP–induced neutropenia while later studies have not. *In vitro* dialysis of azathioprine and metabolites has been observed.[94]

Both 6-MP and azathioprine can produce hepatic damage, especially after long-term administration.[95] In prolonged immunosuppressive therapy following renal transplantation, cholestatic jaundice is commonly observed, but chronic liver disease is unusual.[96] The combination of adriamycin and 6-MP has been reported to produce severe hepatotoxicity in some patients with leukemia.[97] Liver disease probably does not affect the plasma decay of azathioprine but may diminish the conversion of azathioprine to 6-MP.

5-FLUOROURACIL

5-Fluorouracil (5-FU) is an antimetabolite with antitumor activity in gastrointestinal and breast neoplasia. Its mechanism of action is in the inhibition of DNA synthesis by preventing thymidylate synthesis, although it may interfere with RNA metabolism as well. The active metabolite of the drug, 5-fluorouracil deoxyribose monophosphate, can be found in many tissues, while inactivation of the drug occurs primarily in the liver.[98] This degradative process in the liver is saturable but efficient, with up to 51 per cent of 5-FU extracted in a single pass.[33] The renal clearance of 5-FU is 170 ml/min; however, the drug, which is readily dialyzable, need not be given at a reduced rate in renal failure.[99] 5-FU does not produce known hepatic or renal toxicity.

VINCA ALKALOIDS

Vincristine and vinblastine are both derivatives of the periwinkle plant, *Vinca rosea* Linn., and have a broad spectrum of antitumor activity. Their mechanism of action is by interfering with microtubule formation. Following IV administration, the drugs are eliminated in a multiphasic fashion with half-lives of 3 to 4 minutes, 1.0 to 1.5 hours, and 20 hours.[100, 101] Ten to 20 per cent of administered drug can be recovered unchanged from the urine; 60 to 70 per cent of vincristine metabolites are excreted in the bile, but much less is present after vinblastine administration.[101] What happens to the unexcreted drug is uncertain; however, there is extensive binding to tubulin in leukocytes, platelets, and neural tissue. There is no information on the effects of hepatic or renal disease on vinca metabolism, nor are there data on the dialyzability of the drugs. Based on the available pharmacokinetic measurements that show wide distribution and attachment to cellular proteins, it seems unlikely that major dose modification would be required in the setting of hepatic or renal insufficiency.

While neither vincristine nor vinblastine produces hepatotoxicity or nephrotoxicity, both can produce hyponatremia with abnormal water retention due (probably) to the nonosmotic release of ADH. Typically, hyponatremia develops 3 to 14 days following the last dose and lasts for 5 to 10 days. Peripheral autonomic neuropathy is usually evident and may play a role in stimulating ADH release.[102, 103]

REFERENCES

1. Matas AJ, Simmons RL, Kjellstrand CM, et al.: Increased incidence of malignancy during chronic renal failure. Lancet *1*:883–885, 1975.
2. Herr HW, Engen DE, Hostetler J: Malignancy in uremia: Dialysis versus transplantation. J. Urol. *121*:584–586, 1979.
3. Jolison WJ, Kyle RA, Dahlberg PJ: Dialysis in the treatment of multiple myeloma. Mayo Clin. Proc. *55*:65–72, 1980.
4. Czaja AJ, Ammon HV, Summerskill WHJ: Clinical features and prognosis of severe chronic active liver disease (CALD) after corticosteroid-induced remission. Gastroenterology *78*:518–523, 1980.
5. Glassock RJ: Clinical features of immunologic glomerular disease. *In* Immunologic Mechanisms of Renal Disease. CB Wilson, BM Brenner, and JH Stein, eds. New York: Churchill Livingstone, 1979, pp. 255–322.
6. Barratt JM, Soothill JF: Controlled trial of cyclophosphamide in steroid sensitive relapsing nephrotic syndrome of childhood. Lancet *2*:479–482, 1970.
7. Grupe WE, Makker SP, Inglefinger JR: Chlorambucil treatment of frequently relapsing nephrotic syndrome. N. Engl. J. Med. *295*:746–749, 1976.
8. Barratt JM, Cameron JS, Chantler C, et al.: Controlled trial of azathioprine in treatment of steroid-responsive nephrotic syndrome of childhood. Arch. Dis. Child. *52*:462–463, 1977.
9. Matalon R: Glomerular sclerosis in adults with nephrotic syndrome. Ann. Intern. Med. *80*:488–495, 1974.
10. Lim VS: Adult lipoid nephrosis: clinicopathological correlations. Ann. Intern. Med. *81*:314–320, 1974.
11. Cameron JS, et al.: The long-term prognosis of patients with focal segmental glomerulosclerosis. Clin. Nephrol. *10*:213–218, 1978.
12. Beaufils H: FGS: Natural history and treatment. Nephron *21*:75–85, 1978.
13. Velosa JA, et al.: Focal sclerosing glomerulopathy. A clinicopathologic study. Mayo Clin. Proc. *50*:121–133, 1975.
14. Coggins CH, Pinn V, Glassock RR: Collaborative study of the adult idiopathic nephrotic syndrome. A controlled study of short term prednisone treatment in adults with membranous nephropathy. N. Engl. J. Med. *301*:1301–1306, 1979.
15. Donadio JV, Holley KE, Anderson CF, et al.: Controlled trial of cyclophosphamide in idiopathic membranous nephropathy. Kidney Int. *6*:431–439, 1974.
16. McEnery PT, McAdams AJ, West CD: Membranoproliferative glomerulonephritis: improved survival with alternate day prednisone therapy. Clin. Nephrol. *13*:117–124, 1980.
17. Lockwood CM, Pearson TA, Rees AJ, et al.: Immunosuppression and plasma exchange in the treatment of Goodpasture's syndrome. Lancet *1*:711–715, 1976.
18. Rossen RD, Hersh EM, Sharp JF, et al.: Effect of plasma exchange on circulating immune complexes and antibody formation in patients treated with cyclophosphamide and prednisone. Am. J. Med. *63*:674–682, 1977.
19. Bolton WK, Couser WG: Intravenous pulse methylprednisolone therapy of acute cresentic rapidly progressive glomerulonephritis. Am. J. Med. *66*:495–502, 1979.
20. Wagnen L: Immunosuppressive agents in lupus nephritis. A critical analysis. Medicine *55*:239–250, 1976.
21. Donadio JV, Holley KE, Ferguson RH, et al.: Treatment of diffuse proliferative lupus nephritis with prednisone and combined prednisone and cyclophosphamide. N. Engl. J. Med. *299*:1151–1155, 1978.
22. Fauci AS: The spectrum of vasculitis: clinical, pathologic, immunologic and therapeutic considerations. Ann. Intern. Med. *89*:660–680, 1978.
23. Hensley MJ, Feldman NT, Lazarus JM, et al.: Diffuse pulmonary hemorrhage and rapidly progressive renal failure. An uncommon presentation of Wegener's granulomatosis. Am. J. Med. *66*:894–898, 1979.
24. Fauci AS, Katz P, Haynes BF et al: Cyclophosphamide therapy of severe systemic necrotizing vasculitis. N. Engl. J. Med. *301*:235–238, 1979.
25. Brook AS: Mixed connective tissue diseases. Aust. N. Z. J. Med. *8*:130–133, 1978.
26. Cheigh JS, Kim SJ: Scleroderma kidney disease: a therapeutic approach with nephrectomy and hemodialysis. J. Dial. *1*:349–356, 1977.
27. Tanner AR, Powell LW: Progress Report. Corticosteroids in liver disease: Possible mechanisms of action, pharmacology and rational use. Gut *20*:1109–1124, 1979.
28. Wright EC, Seeff LB, Berk LB, et al.: Treatment of chronic active hepatitis. An analysis of three controlled trials. Gastroenterology *73*:1422–1430, 1977.
29. Summerskill WHJ, Korman MG, Ammon HV, et al.: Prednisone for chronic active liver disease: dose titration, standard dose, and combination with azathioprine compared. Gut *16*:876–883, 1975.
30. Simon HB, Wolff SM: Granulomatous hepatitis and prolonged fever of unknown origin: A study of 13 patients. Medicine *52*:1–21, 1973.
31. Guttman RD: Renal transplantation. N. Engl. J. Med. *301*:975–982, 1038–1048, 1979.

32. Terblanche J, Koep LJ, Starzl TE: Liver transplantation. Med. Clin. North Am. *63*:507–521, 1979.
33. Garnick MB, Meyer RJ: Acute renal failure associated with neoplastic diseases and its treatment. Seminars Oncol. *5*:155–165, 1978.
34. Washington JH, Holland JM, Ketcham AS: Return of renal function following diversion of the obstructed ureter. Cancer *18*:1457–1461, 1965.
35. Rees ED, Waugh WH: Factors in the renal failure of multiple myeloma. Arch. Intern. Med. *116*:400–405, 1965.
36. Brown WW, Herbert LA, Piering WF, et al.: Reversal of chronic and end-stage renal failure due to myeloma kidney. Ann. Intern Med. *90*:793–794, 1979.
37. Mir MA: Renal excretion of uric acid and its relationship to relapse and remission in acute myeloid leukemia. Nephron *19*:69–80, 1977.
38. Conger JD, Falk SA: Intrarenal dynamics in the pathogenesis and prevention of acute uric nephropathy. J. Clin. Invest. *59*:786–793, 1977.
39. Mazzaferri EL, O'Dorisio TM, LoBuglio AF: Treatment of hypercalcemia associated with malignancy. Seminars Oncol. *5*:141–153, 1978.
40. Luxton R: Radiation nephritis. A long term study of 54 patients. Lancet *2*:1221–1224, 1961.
41. Hrushesky WJ, Murphy GP: Current status of the therapy of advanced renal carcinoma. J. Surg. Oncol. *9*:277–288, 1977.
42. Webber BM, Soderberg CH, Leone LA, et al.: A combined approach to the management of hepatic metastases. Cancer *42*:1087–1095, 1978.
43. Ensminger WD, Rosowsky A, Raso V, et al.: A clinical-pharmacological evaluation of hepatic arterial infusions of 5-fluoro-2′-deoxyuridine and 5-fluorouracil. Cancer Res. *38*:3784–3792, 1978.
44. Olweny CLM, Toya T, Katongole-Mbbidde E, et al.: Treatment of hepatocellular carcinoma with adriamycin. Cancer *36*:1250–1257,1975.
45. Frei E, III, Jafee N, Tattersall MHN, et al.: New approaches to cancer chemotherapy with methotrexate. N. Engl. J. Med. *292*:846–851, 1975.
46. Pitman SW, Frei E: Weekly methotrexate-calcium leucovorin rescue: effect of alkalinization on nephrotoxicity: pharmacokinetics in the CNS and use in CNS non-Hodgkin's lymphoma. Cancer Treat. Rep. *61*:695–702, 1977.
47. Stoller RG, Hande KR, Jacobs SA, et al.: Use of plasma pharmacokinetics to predict methotrexate toxicity. N. Engl. J. Med. *287*:630–634, 1977.
48. Von Hoff DD, Penta JS, Helman LJ, et al.: The incidence of drug related deaths secondary to high-dose methotrexate and citrovorum factor administration. Cancer Treat. Rep. *61*:745–748, 1977.
49. Glode LM, Pitman SW, Ensminger WD, et al.: A Phase I study of high dose aminopterin with leucovorin rescue in patients with advanced metastatic tumors. Cancer Res. *39*:3707–3714, 1979.
50. Gibson TP, Reich SD, Krumlovsky FA, et al.: Hemoperfusion for methotrexate removal. Clin. Pharmacol. Ther. *23*:351–355, 1978.
51. Abelson HT, Ensminger W, Rosowsky A, et al.: Comparative effects of citrovorum factor and carboxypeptidase G1 on cerebrospinal fluid-methotrexate pharmacokinetics. Cancer Treat. Rep. *62*:1549–1552, 1978.
52. Hersh EM, Wong VD, Henderson ES, et al.: Hepatotoxic effects of methotrexate. Cancer *19*:600–606, 1966.
53. Podurgiel BJ, McGill DB, Ludwig J, et al.: Liver injury associated with methotrexate therapy for psoriasis. Mayo Clin. Proc. *48*:787–792, 1972.
54. Belt RJ, Himmelstein KJ, Patton TF, et al.: Pharmacokinetics of non-protein bound platinum species following administration of cis-dichlorodiammineplatinum (II). Cancer Treat. Rep. *63*:1515–1521, 1979.
55. Rosenberg B: Anticancer activity of cis-dichlorodiammineplatinum (II) and some relevant chemistry. Cancer Treat. Rep. *63*:1433–1438, 1979.
56. Krakoff IH: Nephrotoxicity of cis-dichlorodiammineplatinum (II). Cancer Treat. Rep. *63*: 1523–1525, 1979.
57. Madias NE, Harrington JT: Platinum nephrotoxicity. Am. J. Med. *65*:307–314, 1978.
58. Schilsky RL, Anderson T: Hypomagnesemia and renal magnesium wasting in patients receiving cisplatin. Ann. Intern. Med. *90*:929–931, 1979.
59. Einhorn LH, Wetlaufer J: Personal communication.
60. Schein PS, O'Connell MJ, Blom J, et al.: Clinical antitumor activity and toxicity of streptozotocin. Cancer *34*:993–1000, 1974.
61. Johansson EB, Tjalve H: Studies in the tissue distribution and fate of ^{14}C-streptozotocin with special reference to pancreatic islets. Acta Endocrinol. *89*:339–351, 1978.
62. Schein PS, O'Connell MJ, Blom J, et al.: Clinical antitumor activity and toxicity of streptozotocin. (NSC-85998). Cancer *34*:993–1000, 1974.
63. Oliverio VT: Toxicology and pharmacology of the nitrosoureas. Cancer Chemother. Rep. *4*(3):13–20, 1973.
64. Harmon WE, Cohen HS, Schneeberger EE, et al.: Chronic renal failure in children treated with methyl CCNU. N. Engl. J. Med. *21*:1200–1209, 1979.
65. Bennett JM, Reich SD: Bleomycin. Ann. Intern. Med. *90*:945–948, 1979.
66. Crooke ST, Comis RL, Einhorn LH, et al.: Effects of variation in renal function on the clinical pharmacology of bleomycin administered as an IV bolus. Cancer Treat. Rep. *61*:1631–1636, 1977.
67. Samuels MC, Johnson DE, Haloye PY: Continuous infusion bleomycin therapy with vinblastine in stage III testicular neoplasia. Cancer Chemother. Rep. *59*:563–571, 1975.
68. Kiang DT, Loken MK, Kennedy BJ: Mechanism of the hypercalcemic effect of mithramycin. J. Clin. Endocrinol. Metab. *48*:341–344, 1979.
69. Kennedy BJ: Metabolic and toxic effects of mithramycin during tumor therapy. Am. J. Med. *49*:494–503, 1970.
70. Grochow LB, Calvin M: Clinical pharmacokinetics of cyclophosphamide. Clin. Pharmacokinet. *4*:380–394, 1979.
71. Bagley CM, Bostick FW, et al.: Clinical pharmacology of cyclophosphamide. Cancer Res. *33*:226–233, 1973.
72. Humphrey RL, Dvols LK: The influence of renal insufficiency on cyclophosphamide induced he-

matopoietic depression and recovery. Proc. Am. Assoc. Cancer Res. *15*:84, 1974.
73. Bending MR, Finch RE: Haemodialysis during cyclophosphamide treatment. Br. Med. J. *1*:1145–1146,1978.
74. Plotz PH, Klippel JH, Decker JL, et al.: Bladder complications in patients receiving cyclophosphamide for systemic lupus erythematosus or rheumatoid arthritis. Ann. Intern. Med. *91*: 221–223, 1979.
75. Tattersall MH, Jarman M, Newlands ES, et al.: Pharmacokinetics of melphalan following oral or intravenous administration. Eur. J. Cancer *14*:507–513, 1978.
76. Alberts DS, Chang SY, Chen HS, et al.: Kinetics of intravenous melphalan. Clin. Pharmacol. Ther. *26*:73–80, 1979.
77. Alberts DS, Chang SY, Chen HG, et al.: Oral melphalan kinetics. Clin. Pharmacol. Ther. *26*:737–745, 1979.
78. Vodopick H, Hamilton HE, Jackson HL: Metabolic fate of tritiated busulfan in man. J. Lab. Clin. Med. *73*:266, 1969.
79. Nadkarni MB, Trans EG, Smith PK: Preliminary studies on the distribution and fate of TEM, TEPA, and Myleran in the human. Cancer Res. *19*:713, 1959.
80. Millard RJ: Busulfan hemorrhagic cystitis. Br. J. Urol. *50*(3):210, 1978.
81. Wan SH, Huffman DH, Azarnoff DL, et al.: Pharmacokinetics of 1-beta-D-arabinofuranosylcytosin in humans. Cancer Res. *34*:392–397, 1974.
82. Schein PS, McDonald JS, Hoth DF, et al.: The FAM (5-fluorouracil, adriamycin, mitomycin C) and SMF (streptozotocin, mitomycin C, 5-fluorouracil) chemotherapy regimens. *In* Mitomycin C. Current Status and New Developments. SK Carter and ST Crooke, eds.). New York: Academic Press, 1979, pp. 133–143.
83. Reich SD: Clinical pharmacology of mitomycin C. *In* Mitomycin C. Current Status and New Developments. (SK Carter and ST Crooke, eds.). New York: Academic Press, 1979, pp. 243–250.
84. Ratanatharathorn V, Baker CH, Cadnapaphornchai P, et al.: Clinical and pathologic study of mitomycin C nephrotoxicity. *In* Mitomycin C. Current Status and New Developments. (SK Carter and ST Crooke, eds.). New York: Academic Press, 1979, pp. 219–229.
85. Myers C, McGuire W, Liss R, et al.: Adriamycin: The role of lipid peroxidation in cardiac toxicity and tumor response. Science *197*:165–167, 1977.
86. Chann KK, Cohen JL, Gross JF, et al.: Prediction of adriamycin deposition in cancer patients using a physiologic, pharmacokinetic model. Cancer Treat. Rep. *62*:1161–1170, 1978.
87. Loveless H, Arena E, Felsted RL, et al.: Comparative mammalian metabolism of adriamycin and daunorubicin. Cancer Res. *38*:593–598, 1978.
88. Benjamin RS, Wiernik PH, Bachur NR: Adriamycin chemotherapy — efficacy, safety and pharmacologic basis of an intermittent high dosage schedule. Cancer *33*:19–27, 1974.
89. Burke JF, Laucius JF, Biodovsky HS, et al.: Doxorubicin hydrochloride-associated renal failure. Arch. Intern. Med. *137*:385–388, 1977.
90. Chalmers AH, Knight PR, Atkins MR: 6-Thiopurines as substrates and inhibitors of purine oxidases: a pathway for conversion of azathioprine into 6-thiouric acid without release of 6-mercaptopurine. Aust. J. Exp. Biol. Med. Sci. *47*:263, 1969.
91. Elion GB: Biochemistry and pharmacology of purine analogues. Fed. Proc. *26*:898, 1967.
92. Duttera MJ, Carolla RL, Gallelli, Jr, et al.: Hematuria and crystalluria after high dose 6-mercaptopurine administration. N. Engl. J. Med. *287*:292, 1972.
93. Sloth K, Thomsen AC: Acute renal insufficiency during treatment with azathioprine. Acta Med. Scand. *189*:145, 1971.
94. Bach J, Dardenne M: The metabolism of azathioprine in renal failure. Transplantation *12*:253, 1971.
95. Einhorn M, Davidsohn I: Hepatotoxicity of mercaptopurine. J.A.M.A. *802*:102–106, 1964.
96. Ware AJ, Luby JP, Hallinger B, et al.: Etiology of liver disease in renal-transplant patients. Ann. Intern. Med. *91*:364–371, 1979.
97. Rodriquez V, Bodey GP, McCredie KB, et al.: Combination 6-mercaptopurine-adriamycin in refractory adult acute leukemia. Clin. Pharmacol. Ther. *18*:462–466, 1975.
98. Christophidis N, Vajda FJ, Lucas I, et al.: Fluorouracil therapy in patients with carcinoma of the large bowel: a pharmacokinetic comparison of various rates and routes of administration. Clin. Pharmacokinet. *3*:330–336, 1978.
99. Galletti PM, Pasqualino A, Geering RC: Hemodialysis in cancer chemotherapy. Trans. Am. Soc. Artif. Intern. Organs *12*:20, 1966.
100. Owellen RJ, Roat MA, Hains FO: Pharmacokinetics of vindesine and vincristine in humans. Cancer Res. *37*:2603–2607, 1977.
101. Owellen RJ, Hartke CA, Hains, FO: Pharmacokinetics and metabolism of vinblastine in humans. Cancer Res. *37*:2597–2602, 1977.
102. Waken C: Inappropriate ADH secretion associated with massive vincristine overdose. Aust. N. Z. J. Med. *5*:266, 1975.
103. Winter S: SIADH secondary to vinblastine overdose. Can. Med. Assoc. J. 1117:1134, 1977.

Chapter 19

Use of Neuropsychiatric Drugs

by

John G. Gambertoglio and Roger M. Lauer

This chapter discusses the clinical use of neuropsychiatric drugs for patients with renal or hepatic disease. The two major areas covered are the psychiatric drugs (antipsychotics, tricyclic antidepressants, monoamine oxidase inhibitors, and lithium) and anticonvulsants (phenytoin, phenobarbital, carbamazepine, valproic acid, ethosuximide, and trimethadione). Brief attention is given to drugs used in Parkinson's disease (levodopa, carbidopa, and amantadine) and myasthenia gravis (pyridostigmine and neostigmine).

For each drug we discuss its rational use in the presence of kidney or liver dysfunction. We describe the pharmacokinetics of each drug, the effect of kidney and hepatic disease on its disposition, and the effect of dialysis on drug removal. Common side effects and adverse reactions are mentioned, especially those with special relevance to patients with kidney or liver disease. Finally, dosage recommendations are provided, although in many cases adequate information is unavailable and the clinician must carefully titrate the dose between therapeutic response and toxic effects. Overall, the neuropsychiatric drugs must be used with caution in patients with kidney or liver disease because of their central nervous system effects as well as for other reasons.

PSYCHIATRIC DRUGS

This section surveys the use of antipsychotic medications, tricyclic antidepressants, and lithium in patients with renal or hepatic disease. We will minimize purely theoretic or esoteric issues, and instead emphasize practical points. We will draw on our clinical experience as well as on the literature concerning the appropriate use of these drugs. Further relevant information on psychopharmacology is available from many sources.[1-7]

First, the physician must keep in mind that psychotropic drugs are superfluous for many psychiatric problems, and particularly for the psychiatric problems of patients with renal or hepatic disease. The mental turmoil of such patients is often produced by the enormous stress of their illness, and is best treated by allowing them to ventilate their feelings, and with encouragement, reassurance, and other psychologic approaches. Some mental disturbances can be precipitated by drugs or medical illness and can be treated through medical rather than psychiatric means.

Short-term situational stresses occasionally may warrant brief use of diazepam or other minor tranquilizers (discussed further in Chap. 14). Severe psychiatric conditions (particularly when there is a serious risk that the patient may harm himself or herself or others) may warrant the use of antipsychotics, tricyclics, or lithium.

For those severe conditions in which antipsychotics, tricyclics, or lithium might be appropriate, other considerations arise. Generally, these psychotropic medications seem less effective in patients with renal or hepatic disease than in people in better health. In part, this is due to the heavy overlay of long-term situational stress on their mental state. It is also due to the patients' low tolerance of psychotropics—their susceptibility to side effects and inability to take therapeutic dosages of medication. In summary, psychotropic drugs tend to have high risks and low therapeutic yields in this patient population and thus have limited usefulness.

A general principle in administering psychotropic drugs is that the dosage should be started lower than one would ordinarily give to patients without renal or hepatic disease. After establishing the patient on medication, the dose should be increased slowly and cautiously, watching for both side effects and therapeutic effects. The level at which either can occur is highly variable. Toxic effects tend to occur at lower doses than would be the case with physically healthy patients. Toxic effects are particularly likely in patients with severe renal or hepatic disease. Injudicious use of these drugs might compromise an already depressed central nervous system and might even precipitate coma.

Modern drug treatment of psychiatric problems is based on target symptoms; it is empiric rather than etiologic. In order to use these psychotropic medications effectively, careful diagnoses and evaluation are important.

Each group of psychotropic drugs will be discussed in terms of pharmacology, indications, dosage, side effects, and interaction with other medications.

ANTIPSYCHOTICS

Chlorpromazine. Chlorpromazine, the prototypic drug of the phenothiazines, was synthesized in 1952. That same year, it was noted to produce a "calm" without sedation by Laboret, a French anesthesiologist; later psychiatric use sprang from his observation. The antipsychotics fall into several classes (Table 19–1). Although their mechanism of action is unclear, a number of hypotheses have been presented, including blockade of norepinephrine receptors.

TABLE 19–1. COMMON ANTIPSYCHOTIC DRUGS AND THEIR USAGE IN PATIENTS WITH RENAL OR HEPATIC DISEASE

Group	Generic Name	Brand Name	Starting Dosage (mg/day)	High Dosage (mg/day)	Comments
Phenothiazines					
Aliphatic	Chlorpromazine	Thorazine	25–50	1000	Inexpensive.
Piperidine	Thioridazine	Mellaril	25–50	300	Retinitis risk with dose above 800 mg daily in patients without renal and hepatic disease.
	Mesoridazine	Serentil	25–50	400	Similar to Mellaril, but retinitis not yet reported.
Piperazine	Trifluoperazine	Stelazine	2–4	60	–
	Perphenazine	Trilafon	2–4	64	Available as a fixed dose combination with amitriptyline.
	Fluphenazine	Prolixin, Permitil	1–5	60	Depot form available.
Thioxanthenes	Chlorprothixene	Taractan	10–25	600	Actions similar to aliphatic phenothiazines.
	Thiothixene	Navane	1–5	60	Actions similar to piperazine phenothiazines.
Dibenzoxazepine	Loxapine	Loxitane	10–20	100	Actions intermediate between aliphatic and piperazine phenothiazines.
Indole	Molindone	Moban	5–10	200	Less likely to increase appetite.
Butyrophenone	Haloperidol	Haldol	2	20	Popular choice for psychiatric problems in many medically ill patients.

In terms of pharmacology and metabolism, chlorpromazine will be discussed as the prototypic phenothiazine, since it has been more extensively studied than other antipsychotic drugs.[8] Following administration of equal doses of chlorpromazine, patients exhibit quite variable steady-state plasma concentrations of unchanged drug and metabolites. This is mostly due to interindividual variability in metabolism and bioavailability. The latter is secondary to a substantial first-pass effect during absorption. Chlorpromazine is extensively metabolized by the liver to a large number of metabolites, some of which are active. Less than 1 per cent of an administered dose is excreted in the urine as unchanged chlorpromazine, the remainder being recovered as metabolites.

Haloperidol. Haloperidol, another commonly prescribed antipsychotic, is not a phenothiazine, but a butyrophenone.[8] Like chlorpromazine, it displays variable bioavailability and is extensively metabolized by the liver. The metabolites of haloperidol are inactive, except one is considered markedly less active than the parent drug. Of an administered dose, approximately 1 per cent is excreted as unchanged drug in the urine; the rest is excreted as metabolites.

Insufficient data are available on the disposition of chlorpromazine or haloperidol in patients with renal failure. Since very little unchanged drug is excreted in the urine, accumulation is unlikely; however, the pharmacologic activity of some of the metabolites, especially those of chlorpromazine, must be considered. Limited studies in patients with hepatic disease, such as compensated cirrhosis, suggest no significant alteration in plasma disappearance of chlorpromazine compared to that in control patients.[9] However, these patients were more sensitive to the central nervous system effects of these drugs.

Few data are available on the dialyzability of the antipsychotics. Clinically, hemodialysis or peritoneal dialysis does not seem effective in treating overdoses.[10] The very large volume of distribution, which limits the effect of hemoperfusion, and high degree of plasma protein binding would limit significant dialyzability. However, these drugs have multiple metabolites whose removal by dialysis is unknown.

A major indication for giving antipsychotic medications to anyone, including patients with renal or hepatic disease, is to reduce delusions, hallucinations, ideas of reference, loose associations, or other manifestations of psychotic thinking. A second indication would be to correct severe disturbances in social and motor behavior. The antipsychotics can correct some pathologically low activity levels (e.g., catatonia), as well as some pathologically high ones (e.g., mania).

Severe disturbances in thinking and social and motor behavior can occur in many psychiatric conditions — the common ones being schizophrenic disorders, major affective disorders, and organic brain syndromes. The accepted guidelines[11] for diagnosing such conditions are complicated and thus beyond the scope of this chapter.

The likely effectiveness of antipsychotic medications varies depending on diagnostic and other factors. Acute psychoses often improve, especially if there are components of affective disturbance, anxiety, or disorganization, while chronic psychosis states are much less responsive. Mania often remits. Psychotic manifestations of depression, particularly paranoid delusions, tend to be decreased. Symptoms of organic brain syndromes may decrease, but many patients with brain syndromes have extremely low tolerance to antipsychotic medications and become more confused. In general, the antipsychotic drugs are not indicated for anxious, nonpsychotic patients and may, in fact, make them worse.

Dosage of antipsychotic medication should be started low and the patient's response closely observed. Suggested starting doses in Table 19–1 are guidelines only; specific situations might indicate lower or higher doses. Medication should be increased slowly until a therapeutic or toxic response occurs. This titration likely would stop at a level below what is labeled as "high" in Table 19–1, and only rarely would it go above this level. There is no absolute maximum dose (other than for thioridazine) and in some extraordinary situations, very large doses may be necessary. Depending on the particular clinical situation, the antipsychotics could be given in a single daily dose (usually at bedtime) or in divided doses two or three times a day. It should seldom be necessary to give two different types of antipsychotic drugs simultaneously. To the extent possible, antipsychotic drugs should be given in small doses for short periods of time because of the serious risk of side effects. Long-term maintenance therapy usually can be avoided.

A great deal of research is being done on measuring antipsychotics in plasma in order to guide dosage regimens.[12] Unfortunately, at this time, there is no agreement on a therapeutic range, and the analytic capabilities for measurement of these drugs are not always available. Thus, the routine monitoring of plasma levels is not practical and one must rely on close clinical observation of the patient to adjust dose.

To illustrate antipsychotic dosage and clinical response, a case example will be provided.

E. M., a 26-year-old single white woman on chronic hemodialysis, developed an exacerbation of her chronic schizophrenia. No organic cause of this exacerbation was noted. She became overwhelmed by paranoid delusions and felt that she might have to strike out at her enemies before they could hurt her. Several years earlier, in another psychotic decompensation, E. M. had attacked her mother with a knife and was treated for 6 months in a state mental hospital. During that time, she was given haloperidol and seemed to respond satisfactorily. E. M. was agreeable to taking haloperidol again, and there was no reason to try a different antipsychotic. She was started on haloperidol 2 mg orally at bedtime and followed closely as an outpatient. After 3 days, there was modest improvement and no significant side effects, so the dose was increased to 4 mg at bedtime. Gradually, over the next 2 weeks, her symptoms cleared until she had regained her premorbid state. Then, because of her complaints of akathesia, haloperidol was discontinued. She continued to be followed closely for several years. Despite no antipsychotic medications, her thinking and behavior were satisfactory.

Different antipsychotic medications have varying tendencies to cause particular side effects (Table 19–2). At times, the choice of drug is on the basis of the relative incidence of what would be an especially undesired side effect for a given patient. The range of possible side effects is summarized in Table 19–3.

Orthostatic hypotension and confusion are side effects that seem to occur more frequently in patients with renal or hepatic disease than in normal subjects. The vulnerability to hypotension in patients with renal dysfunction may relate to antihypertensive medication, dialysis, and fluid volume deficits. The vulnerability to confusion for patients with either renal or hepatic disease may relate to metabolic cortical impairment. Hypotension tends to occur more with chlorpromazine and thioridazine (Table 19–2) and less with trifluoperazine, fluphenazine, and haloperidol. Confusion occurs about as often with any of the antipsychotics. Cholestatic jaundice, due to hypersensitivity, occurs most often with alipha-

TABLE 19–2. COMMON ANTIPSYCHOTIC DRUGS AND THEIR RELATIVE INCIDENCE OF SIDE EFFECTS

			Side Effects		
Group	Generic Name	Brand Name	*Sedation-Hypotension*	*Extra-pyrimidal*	*Anti-cholinergic*
Phenothiazines					
Aliphatic	Chlorpromazine	Thorazine	↑	moderate	moderate
Piperidine	Thioridazine	Mellaril	↑	↓	↑
	Mesoridazine	Serentil	↑	↓	moderate
Piperazine	Trifluoperazine	Stelazine	moderate	↑	↓
	Perphenazine	Trilafon	↓	↑	↓
	Fluphenazine	Prolixin, Permitil	↓	↑	↓
Thioxanthenes	Chlorprothixene	Taractan	↑	↓	↑
	Thiothixene	Navane	↓	↑	↓
Dibenzoxazepine	Loxapine	Loxitane	moderate	↑	↓
Indole	Molindone	Moban	moderate	↑	moderate
Butyrophenone	Haloperidol	Haldol	↓	↑	↓

↑ = Increased. ↓ = Decreased.

tic phenothiazines, such as chlorpromazine, and typically after 2 to 4 weeks of treatment. This side effect was more frequent in the 1960's than it is at present — possibly because the drugs are manufactured with greater purity now. Although the risk of jaundice is low, this possible side effect may need to be weighed for patients who already have hepatic disease.

Owing to their anticholinergic effects, the antipsychotics commonly cause dry mouth, constipation, and blurred vision, but less commonly urinary retention. The latter risk may be particularly significant in clinical situations in which patients already have impaired bladder function, in which precise measurements of urine volume are necessary, and in which patients are already taking other anticholinergic agents. Urecholine has commonly been used to alleviate antipsychotic-induced urinary retention.

A common side effect for all users of antipsychotics, including patients with hepatic or renal disease, is extrapyramidal symptoms. Patients may develop parkinsonism with tremor, rigidity, akinesia, shuffling gait, masklike facies, and hypersalivation. They may develop akathesia in which they fidget and feel restless; this tends to occur early in treatment and may be misdiagnosed as anxiety or psychotic agitations. They may develop acute dystonia — bizarre muscular spasms of sudden onset, mainly in the muscles of the head and neck; this tends to occur mainly in young males, 1 to 2 days after treatment starts, and may be misdiagnosed as hysteria or tetany. In

TABLE 19–3. SIDE EFFECTS OF ANTIPSYCHOTICS

Central Nervous System	Cardiovascular
Extrapyramidal reaction: Parkinsonism: tremor, rigidity, bradykinesia, shuffling gait, masklike facies, hypersalivation Dystonia: torticollis, opisthotonos, dysphagia, laryngospasm, oculogyric crisis Akathesia Tardive dyskinesia Sedation Confusional state (toxic psychosis)* Seizure EEG changes Autonomic effects: α-antiadrenergic: orthostatic hypotension*; inhibited ejaculation (especially Mellaril) Anticholinergic: dry mouth and skin, tachycardia, blurred vision, urinary retention,* constipation–fecal impaction–adynamic ileus	See CNS–autonomic effects Hypertension EKG changes (nonspecific) Cardiac arrhythmia (ventricular tachycardia)

Gastrointestinal	Skin	Eye
See CNS Heartburn Abdominal cramps Diarrhea Cholestatic jaundice* Weight gain (may be due to increased appetite and/or decreased activity)	Seborrhea Allergic dermatitis: urticaria, maculopapular eruptions, petechiae Photosensitivity (especially with Thorazine)	See CNS–autonomic effects Oculocutaneous syndrome (skin pigmentation, eye opacities) Pigmentary retinopathy (Mellaril)

Endocrine	Blood	Other
Hyperglycemia Lactation Gynecomastia Menstrual dysfunction Decreased libido Hyperprolactinemia (with possible stimulation of breast tumors)	Anemia Leukopenia Antinuclear antibodies Thromboembolic disease Agranulocytosis Transient eosinophilia Purpura Pancytopenia	Neuroleptic malignant syndrome: muscular rigidity, hyperthermia, altered consciousness, autonomic dysfunction Peripheral edema Water intoxication

*Of particular concern for patients with renal or hepatic disease.

general, extrapyramidal side effects can be treated with benztropine (Cogentin, 1 to 2 mg b.i.d.) or trihexyphenidyl (Artane, 2 to 4 mg b.i.d.). Small doses should be used for as short a time as possible, since these drugs, like antipsychotics, have anticholinergic effects. It is seldom necessary to give antiparkinson treatment on a prophylactic basis.

Tardive dyskinesia is a disfiguring side effect (most commonly manifested as buccolinguomasticatory movement) that generally occurs after long-term high dosage of antipsychotics, especially in the elderly, women, and in patients with a prior history of brain damage. It may worsen under emotional distress and disappear during sleep. At present, there is no accepted treatment.

Blood dyscrasias, such as leukopenia, agranulocytosis, purpura, and pancytopenia, sometimes are caused by antipsychotic medication, and may be associated with sore throat, cellulitis, fever, or asthenia. Elderly white women in poor general health may be at increased risk. Sedation may result from antipsychotic medication, although this is usually temporary and patients adapt. In terms of the eye, corneal and lens opacities have been recorded. Thioridazine in doses above 800 mg a day has caused a retinitis in patients without renal or hepatic disease. For patients with renal or hepatic disease, it might be wise to set a limit lower than 800 mg a day.

Since patients with renal and hepatic disease commonly take a multiplicity of drugs, several drug interactions with the antipsychotics are worth emphasizing.[13] The central nervous system depressant and hypotensive effects of the antipsychotics are additive to those of the narcotics, sedative hypnotics, antihistamines, alcohol, and antihypertensives such as methyldopa. Antacids such as aluminum or magnesium gels may decrease the gastrointestinal absorption of oral antipsychotics; thus, the two should be ingested separately. Phenothiazines may decrease the hypoglycemic effect of insulin and oral hypoglycemic agents. The potassium loss induced by diuretics or glucocorticoids may enhance cardiac toxicity of psychoactive drugs.

Finally, it is worth pointing out that there has been some interest in using dialysis to treat schizophrenia. A number of studies have been reported, but the results are conflicting.[14] At present, we believe that there is insufficient evidence to justify using dialysis for schizophrenia.

TRICYCLIC ANTIDEPRESSANTS

After the introduction of chlorpromazine in the early 1950's, the effort to develop improved antipsychotics led to the discovery by Kuhn, in Switzerland (1957), that a phenothiazine-like compound (imipramine) had antidepressant effects. Other tricyclic antidepressants were then developed (Table 19–4). The tricyclics produce several effects on brain chemistry, including blocking of reuptake of norepinephrine at synapses, but precisely what chemical events are associated with the antidepressant effect is unknown. The tricyclics are not stimulants; in fact, they enervate people who are of normal mood or are merely tired.

The tricyclic compounds are structurally and pharmacologically similar to the phenothiazines.[15, 16] They are readily absorbed after oral administration and then undergo pronounced and variable first-pass metabolism. Some bioequivalence problems have arisen with generic tricyclics; consequently, many clinicians prefer to use brand name products. Different patients treated with equal doses of tricyclics exhibit quite variable steady-state plasma levels. These drugs are almost entirely metabolized by the liver, resulting in the formation of a number of metabolites. Five per cent or less of the dose is excreted as unchanged drug in the urine. Imipramine and amitriptyline are demethylated to desmethylimipramine and nortriptyline, respectively, which are then further degraded. Most of the metabolites formed are excreted by the kidney and some are believed to possess weak pharmacologic activity.

Data are unavailable on the pharmacokinetic disposition of these drugs in patients with renal or hepatic disease. In one study, the plasma protein binding of desmethylimipramine in uremic patients was not significantly different from that of normal subjects.[17] The high degree of protein binding and the extremely large volume of distribution of these compounds prohibits adequate removal by dialysis. Despite reports of rapid clinical improvement after dialysis is begun in patients who have overdosed on tricyclics, only minute quantities of drug (less than 1 per cent when compared to the amount ingested) seem to be removed. The toxicity and dialyzability of the tricyclic metabolites are unknown.

The major indication for tricyclics is a severe depression of the type that has been labeled endogenous or psychotic. Present no-

TABLE 19–4. COMMON TRICYCLIC ANTIDEPRESSANTS AND THEIR USAGE IN PATIENTS WITH RENAL AND HEPATIC DISEASE

Group	Generic Name	Brand Name	Starting Dose (mg/day)	High Dose (mg/day)	Comments
Dibenzazepines	Desipramine	Norpramin Pertofrane	25–50	200	
	Imipramine	Tofranil, Imavate, SK-Pramine	25–50	200	
Dibenzocycloheptadenes	Protriptyline	Vivactil	5–10	50	
	Nortriptyline	Aventyl Pamelor	10–20	150	
	Amitriptyline	Elavil, Endep, Amitid, Amitril, SK-Amitriptyline	25–50	200	Available as a fixed dosage combination with phenothiazine
Dibenzoxepin	Doxepin	Sinequan Adapin	25–50	200	May have lower cardiac toxicity

menclature would call this a "major depression," and it may be associated with "melancholia" or "psychotic features."[11] *Melancholia* refers to a loss of pleasure in almost all activities and at least three of the following: (1) mood that is perceived as distinctively different from other kinds of lows, (2) depression that is regularly worse in the morning, (3) early morning awakening, (4) marked psychomotor retardation or agitation, (5) anorexia and weight loss, and (6) excessive guilt. *Psychotic features* refers to delusions, hallucinations, depressive stupor (mute and unresponsive), and other gross impairments in reality testing. Tricyclics generally are not indicated for what has been called a mild, reactive or exogenous depression.

In studies of patients with major depressions, tricyclics have been highly successful, producing marked clinical improvement 70 per cent of the time. However, there are no statistics available as to their effectiveness in patients with renal or hepatic disease. Our clinical impression is that their effectiveness is much lower in this patient population.

Tricyclic dosage should be started lower than for patients without renal or hepatic disease. Then it should be increased slowly until a therapeutic or toxic response occurs. Medication may be given in divided daily doses or at bedtime only. Guidelines for starting doses and the high doses that may be needed for a full therapeutic response are shown in Table 19–4. In many patients with renal or hepatic disease, side effects prevent the administration of high doses. Fortunately, some patients are sensitive at low doses to the antidepressant effects of tricyclics. However, others are not and they may need 3 to 4 weeks of the high dose before showing a response. Occasionally, even higher doses than listed in Table 19–4 may be needed.

The concept of a "therapeutic window" has been used regarding tricyclics. This refers to an optimum range of medication in the blood. Tricyclic levels above or below this range may not be effective. At this time, measurement of blood tricyclics need not be done routinely, but may be useful if dosage questions arise.

Although the tricyclics developed as an outgrowth of phenothiazine research, there are biologic differences between the two groups of compounds. Tricyclics often aggravate schizophrenia, while phenothiazines tend to improve it. Tricyclics rarely cause parkinsonian symptoms or tardive dyskinesia, while phenothiazines are more likely to do so.

With the previously mentioned exception of parkinsonism and tardive dyskinesia, the tricyclics have most of the side effects of the antipsychotic agents. The most important side effects in patients with renal or hepatic disease are confusion, orthostatic hypotension, and jaundice. Other potentially important side effects are cardiac arrhythmias, sedation, and anticholinergic effects. Different tricyclics have varying tendencies to cause the latter two effects (Table 19–5). Depending on the

TABLE 19–5. COMMON TRICYCLIC ANTIDEPRESSANTS AND THEIR INCIDENCE OF SIDE EFFECTS

Group	Generic Name	Brand Name	Side Effects	
			Sedation	*Anticholinergic*
Dibenzazepines	Desipramine	Norpramin Pertofrane	↓	↓
	Imipramine	Tofranil Imavate SK-Pramine	moderate	moderate
Dibenzocycloheptadenes	Protriptyline	Vivactil	↓	moderate
	Nortriptyline	Aventyl Pamelor	moderate	↓
	Amitriptyline	Elavil, Endep, Amitid, Amitril, SK-Amitriptyline	↑	↑
Dibenzoxepin	Doxepin	Sinequan Adapin	↑	↑

↑ = Increased. ↓ = Decreased.

TABLE 19–6. SIDE EFFECTS OF TRICYCLIC ANTIDEPRESSANTS

Central Nervous System	
Parkinsonism (rare) Tardive dyskinesia (rare) Sedation Confusional state (toxic psychosis)* Seizures Tremor Anxiety Insomnia Headache Fatigue	Autonomic effects: α-antiadrenergic: orthostatic hypotension* Anticholinergic: dry mouth and skin, tachycardia, blurred vision, urinary retention,* constipation–fecal impaction–adynamic ileus

Cardiovascular	Gastrointestinal	Skin
See CNS–autonomic effects Hypertension EKG changes Cardiac arrhythmia	See CNS Cholestastic jaundice* Weight gain (may be due to increased appetite or decreased activity) Anorexia Nausea and vomiting	Allergic dermatitis (rare) Photosensitivity (rare) Diaphoresis

Eye	Endocrine	Blood
See CNS – autonomic Aggravation of angle closure glaucoma	Inappropriate ADH secretion Impotence	Leukopenia Agranulocytosis Eosinophilia Leukocytosis Thrombocytopenia

*Of particular concern for patients with renal or hepatic disease.

clinical situation, this may influence the choice of medication. A summary of all tricyclic side effects is presented in Table 19–6.

Tricyclics may interact with other drugs commonly given to patients with renal or hepatic disease. The sedative and hypotensive effects of the tricyclics are additive to sedative-hypnotics and alcohol. Anticonvulsants may increase the metabolism of tricyclics and thus decrease plasma levels. Additionally, tricyclics can lower the seizure threshold. The tricyclics can reverse the antihypertensive action of guanethidine, methyldopa, and clonidine. They may also potentiate the effects of anticholinergics or adrenergics.

Tricyclics may be used with other somatic psychiatric treatments. They are compatible with the antipsychotic agents and may be given together in special circumstances. For example, psychotic depression occurs with marked paranoia. Fixed dosage combinations of antipsychotics and tricyclics (Tables 19–1 and 19–4) are available, but single drug preparations are preferred, since dosages can be controlled separately. Tricyclics may be combined with electroconvulsive treatment or may be potentiated by small doses of thyroid.

To illustrate the limited usefulness of tricyclics, a case example will be provided.

B. M., a 32-year-old black divorced woman with a 4-year-old son, had end-stage renal disease secondary to diabetes. After a year of chronic hemodialysis in a local center, she received a cadaver renal transplant at a university medical center 400 miles from her home. Her transplant was rejected, and numerous medical and surgical complications prolonged her hospital stay. Under the stress of prolonged hospitalizations far from her son, she became severely depressed — withdrawing from human contact, sleeping poorly, crying incessantly, eating minimal food because of "no appetite," and ruminating about suicide. Verbal counseling was ineffective and the risk of death from inanition or suicide seemed great. In the face of a life-threatening mental disorder, she was started on amitriptyline, 25 mg at bedtime. There was little reason in this clinical situation to choose one tricyclic over another, although amitriptyline had the advantage of being highly sedating. During 3 days of close follow-up, there were neither therapeutic nor toxic effects — then B. M. developed severe orthostatic hypotension and amitriptyline had to be discontinued. Fortunately, at this time, new developments permitted her to make plans to leave the hospital and receive care locally. With the news of impending discharge her mood began to improve.

MONOAMINE OXIDASE INHIBITORS

At times, monoamine oxidase (MAO) inhibitors might be considered for some patients with renal or hepatic disease, particularly those with an "atypical depression" or with a depression unresponsive to tricyclics. Strict avoidance of certain foods is necessary in order to safely take MAO inhibitors; dietary indiscretions (e.g., cheddar cheese, chianti wine) have caused severe cardiovascular side effects and even death because tyramine in these foods releases catecholamines. It is suggested that these agents be given only when supervised by a physician thoroughly experienced in their use and probably only for a hospitalized patient. Generally, MAO inhibitors and tricyclics have been considered to be incompatible, but in the past few years, some practitioners have given the two agents together without significant problem. How effective the combination might be in patients with renal or hepatic disease is not known.

LITHIUM

In the late nineteenth century, lithium bromide was used as a sedative; bromine, not lithium, was thought to be the effective ingredient. In the 1940's, lithium was used as a salt substitute, but fell into disrepute after causing deaths. The modern use of lithium in affective illness dates from Cade's observation (in Australia in 1949) of its calming effect. By the early 1970's, lithium had come into wide psychiatric use. Currently, several lithium preparations (Table 19–7) are available.

Lithium is a simple salt whose mechanism of action in mental illness is unknown. It is rapidly and almost completely absorbed when taken orally.[18-20] Complete plasma-tissue equilibration and steady-state plasma levels re-

TABLE 19–7. LITHIUM PREPARATIONS

Generic Name	Brand Name	Type of Preparation
Lithium carbonate	Eskalith	Capsule, tablet
	Lithane	Tablet
	Lithobid	Tablet
	Lithonate	Capsule
	Lithotabs	Tablet
	Pfi-Lith	Tablet
Lithium citrate	Lithonate-S	Liquid

quire 5 to 6 days because of slow tissue distribution. Lithium is not metabolized in the body, and essentially all of an administered dose is excreted in the urine. Of a given dose, one-third to two-thirds is excreted within 6 to 8 hours of administration; the remainder is slowly excreted over 10 to 14 days because of extensive tissue localization.

Lithium is freely filtered at the glomerulus, and 60 to 80 per cent is reabsorbed in the proximal tubule.[21] Sodium depletion and consequent extracellular fluid contraction result in enhanced proximal tubular reabsorption of lithium and, subsequently, increased serum levels. Increasing water intake or urinary acidification does not increase renal lithium excretion.

In patients with decreased renal function, the renal clearance of lithium is decreased, and the plasma half-life is increased. Lithium is dialyzable owing to its lack of plasma protein binding and relatively limited volume of distribution. Substantial lowering of serum lithium levels occurs with either peritoneal dialysis or hemodialysis; clinical improvement in toxic patients is reported during or immediately following dialysis. However, rebound increases in serum lithium levels frequently occur a few hours following dialysis because of slow equilibration between the intra- and extracellular fluid.

Patients with liver impairment would not be expected to have altered kinetics of lithium; however, data on these patients are unavailable.

In physically healthy patients, the major indication for lithium therapy is to treat or prevent the manic phases of bipolar disease (manic-depressive psychosis). Secondary, less compelling indications are to treat or prevent recurrent major depressions. (Further discussion of the indications for the use of lithium is available in reference 22.)

For patients with renal impairment, lithium has been used only on rare occasions; consequently, little clinical experience has accumulated. There are many potential hazards in administering lithium to such patients. Lithium has formidable side effects (Table 19–8). Many are dose related, tending to occur at elevated serum levels. In the face of decreased or fluctuating renal clearances, maintaining the proper serum level can be difficult. In addition, further renal damage could occur,

TABLET 19–8. LITHIUM SIDE EFFECTS

Central Nervous System	
Abnormal movements: tremor, ataxia, fasciculations, clonic movements, choreoathetosis, seizures, nystagmus	Fatigue–weakness–myasthenia-like syndrome
Dysarthria	Hyperreflexia
Sedation-stupor-coma-death*	Headache
Dizziness	Extrapyramidal syndrome
	Tinnitus
Confusion (toxic psychosis)	Aphasia

Cardiovascular	Gastrointestinal	Skin
EKG changes	Nausea-vomiting	Acne
Arrhythmia	Diarrhea-constipation	Maculopapular rash
Syncope	Cramps	Cutaneous ulcers
	Anorexia	Psoriasis
	Dry mouth	

Eye	Endocrine	Blood	Other
Blurred vision	Changes in carbohydrate metabolism	Leukocytosis	Renal tubular acidosis
	Goiter-hypothyroidism-hyperthyroidism		Polydipsia–polyuria–nephrogenic diabetes insipidus*
			Oliguria*
			Malaise
			Peripheral edema
			Metallic taste
			Teratogenic effects (especially congenital heart disease)
			Weight gain

*Of particular concern for patients with renal or hepatic disease.

since several studies indicate that lithium is nephrotoxic.

For patients with either renal or hepatic disease, metabolically induced confusion might interfere with patients taking medication properly, reporting side effects promptly, or cooperating in other ways. Furthermore, lithium alone might precipitate or aggravate confusion.

Because of the risks, some experts argue that lithium should never be used in patients with significant renal disease. Our view is that lithium should be avoided whenever possible — and used only in extraordinary circumstances. Other treatments may be effective, safer, and less problematic; they should be considered first. For acute affective illness, this would mean the use of antipsychotics, tricyclics, or electroconvulsive treatment, depending on the clinical situation. For recurrent illness, patients should be monitored closely and given antipsychotics or tricyclics at the first sign of deterioration. If this fails, then maintenance use of the same medication could be tried. Regarding patients with hepatic disease, there is less reason to avoid lithium, but here, too, other treatment options should be considered. In summary, renal disease is a strong contraindication to the use of lithium; hepatic disease is less of a contraindication.

Before starting lithium, a complete physical examination should be performed as well as an assessment of renal, thyroid, and hematologic function. Lithium is available in tablet, capsule, or liquid form (Table 19–7). Some patients dislike the tablets because of the metallic taste or the capsules because of the large size. Lithium dosage should be adjusted in order to maintain a serum level in the range of 0.6 to 1.2 mEq/L. Serum levels are ordinarily measured with a 12-hour sampling interval from the last oral dose. No specific methods have been proposed for dosing lithium in the setting of hepatic or renal disease. However, two general methods are available for determining the proper dosage of lithium that could be applied to such patients. These methods involve measuring renal lithium clearance and assessing single plasma concentrations after a test dose.[23, 24] For patients with renal disease who are on hemodialysis, case reports have described the successful use of a single dose (300 to 600 mg lithium carbonate) after each dialysis.[25, 26] In all cases, close attention to serum lithium levels is essential.

With our present state of knowledge, lithium seems to have few problem interactions with other drugs. A major interaction to remember is that most diuretics (loop, mercurial, thiazide, spironolactone) cause lithium retention, not excretion. Consequently, lithium may be contraindicated in patients taking diuretics. On the other hand, lithium excretion can be increased by aminophylline, osmotic diuretics, acetazolamide, and sodium bicarbonate. There have been some data to suggest adverse interactions of lithium with iodine, methyldopa, succinylcholine, baclofen, and digitalis.

NEUROLOGIC DRUGS

Patients with renal or hepatic disease can develop a variety of neurologic disturbances. Convulsions occur commonly in the setting of severe acute and chronic renal failure and are usually generalized major seizures, but may be focal motor. Treatment may be limited to measures to improve the uremic state. However, anticonvulsants are often necessary because of recurrent seizures. Convulsions may also occur in the setting of hemodialysis-related dysequilibrium syndrome and are usually self-limited. Seizures are a particular problem for hypertensive children with kidney transplants. Additionally, relatively excessive doses of penicillin may induce seizures, especially in patients with renal failure. On the other hand, seizures are less commonly a primary manifestation of liver failure. Rather, the frequent occurrence of seizures in this setting represents manifestations of associated previous head trauma and, perhaps, alcohol abuse.

Several commonly used anticonvulsant drugs will be discussed in relation to their pharmacokinetic disposition, side effects, and dosage in patients with renal and hepatic dysfunction. Most anticonvulsants are eliminated mainly by hepatic metabolism, and it is generally believed that hepatic function must be severely impaired to alter significantly plasma drug levels. The effect of renal failure on phenytoin disposition has been well studied and will be discussed in detail, since there is prominent clinical relevance.

Parkinson's disease and myasthenia gravis are less common problems in patients with renal or hepatic disease; nevertheless they may occur. A brief discussion of drugs used to treat these disorders will also be included.

ANTICONVULSANTS

PHENYTOIN

Phenytoin is one of the most commonly used anticonvulsant drugs. It is used for a variety of seizures, such as generalized tonic-clonic seizures and simple or complex partial seizures. It is not indicated in the setting of generalized absence seizures (formerly called petit mal), febrile convulsions, withdrawal convulsions, and a variety of particular generalized seizures of the pediatric age group. The absolute bioavailability of orally administered phenytoin is generally good with high-quality products.[27] However, the rate of absorption may be slow and erratic with peak plasma levels occurring from 4 to 12 hours after the dose. Phenytoin is extensively metabolized in the body with less than 5 per cent excreted in the urine unchanged.[28] It undergoes parahydroxylation in the liver to its major metabolite, 5-(*p*-hydroxyphenyl)-5-phenylhydantoin (*p*-HPPH), which is then mostly conjugated with glucuronic acid and excreted in the urine. Other metabolites of phenytoin have been identified in the urine, but are quantitatively less important. None of the metabolites, including *p*-HPPH, are considered to be significantly pharmacologically active or toxic.[28] The half-life of phenytoin is variable and ranges from 10 to 30 hours in normal subjects. Owing to the concentration-dependent, nonlinear kinetics of phenytoin (within the therapeutic concentration range), the elimination half-life of the drug is longer at higher plasma levels and with larger doses. The same dose given to different patients results in quite variable half-lives, dependent on the individual level of saturation of metabolism. Furthermore, small increases in the dose can result in a more than proportionate increase in plasma level.[28]

Several studies have discussed the pharmacokinetic disposition of phenytoin in patients with renal disease.[17, 29, 30] Renal failure decreases the plasma protein binding of phenytoin to 70 to 90 per cent (normal 85 to 95 per cent), the degree of decreased binding being related to the degree of renal failure.[17, 30] The plasma protein binding is also related to the albumin concentration. In patients with the nephrotic syndrome and a creatinine clearance > 50 ml/min, the protein binding of phenytoin is decreased from 90 to 81 per cent. Renal transplantation restores the protein binding to almost normal values. The apparent volume of distribution of phenytoin is increased in uremic patients to approximately 1.0 to 1.8 L/kg (normal 0.5 to 0.7 L/kg) owing to the decrease in plasma protein binding.[29]

Furthermore, in patients with impaired renal function, the half-life of phenytoin has been found to be shorter than that of a control group. Patients with decreased renal function have significantly lower total plasma phenytoin levels than subjects with normal renal function given the same dose owing to the changes in binding and distribution. However, since the unbound fraction of phenytoin in plasma is increased, the concentration of free phenytoin in plasma is similar to that of normal subjects. Thus, the therapeutic and toxic phenytoin levels in uremic subjects (i.e., total plasma concentrations) are lower in comparison to patients with normal renal function.[31] Figure 19–1 illustrates how the normal therapeutic range of 10 to 20 μg/ml is reduced in patients with varying degrees of renal failure.

The plasma protein binding of phenytoin may be decreased in liver disease, correlating with alterations in albumin and bilirubin levels. In patients with acute viral hepatitis, a significant decrease in protein binding has been shown during the acute illness phase compared to the control phase.[32] The mean increase in unbound phenytoin was close to one-third over that of the control values. However, these patients showed no significant change in average phenytoin half-life, volume of distribution, or plasma clearance compared to their control recovery phase values. On an individual basis, some patients showed a decreased plasma clearance and others an increased clearance during the hepatitis phase. In most patients with alcoholic liver disease with cirrhosis, the protein binding of phenytoin is not significantly altered.[33] However, a few of these patients and others with different types of liver disease may exhibit a substantial decrease in plasma protein binding. In an earlier study of patients with liver disease (mostly alcoholic cirrhosis), a few were observed to have a decreased tolerance to phenytoin, exhibiting nystagmus and ataxia at usual doses.[34] This was associated with an accumulation of unmetabolized drug and decreased urinary excretion of metabolites. Thus, in liver disease, the net effect on phenytoin disposition will be a balance between an increased clearance due to decreased protein

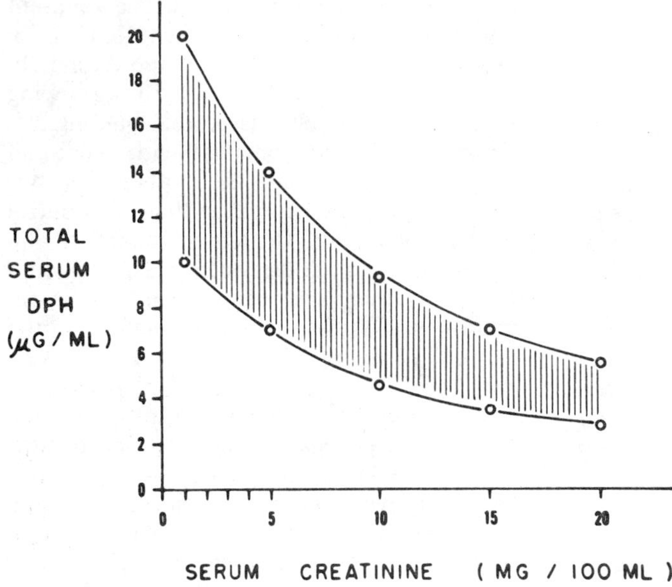

Figure 19–1. Total serum phenytoin (DPH) concentrations calculated for patients with varying degrees of renal failure that provide levels of free (unbound) drug comparable to those found in epileptic patients with normal renal function. (Reproduced with permission from Reidenberg, M. M., and Affrime, M.: Influence of disease on binding of drugs to plasma proteins. Ann. N.Y. Acad. Sci., *226*:115–26, 1973.)

binding and a reduced intrinsic ability of the liver to metabolize the drug.

The frequency of adverse reactions to phenytoin has been shown to be inversely proportional to the serum albumin level and, presumably, results from excess unbound drug. Neurologic manifestations of toxicity, such as ataxia, nystagmus, vertigo, and confusion, correlate well with specific concentrations and are used as clinical toxic end points in dosing. Peripheral neuropathies, hypersensitivity reactions, including acute renal failure, and a systemic lupus erythematosus–like illness can also occur, but are rare and not clearly related to dose or drug level. Hematologic side effects include bone marrow suppression, folic acid deficiency, and generalized lymphadenopathy.

Among the interesting metabolic effects are suppression of insulin release with resultant hyperglycemia and hypocalcemia, hypophosphatemia, and radiographic changes of rickets secondary to diminished vitamin D activity. Miscellaneous reactions include hirsutism, gingival hyperplasia, hepatitis, and pulmonary fibrosis.

Usual doses of phenytoin may be administered to patients with renal failure. However, owing to the altered kinetics of this drug in renal failure, the therapeutic plasma concentration range is lower, approximately 4 to 8 μg/ml in severe renal dysfunction. The usual therapeutic range (Table 19–9) would represent excessive levels of free drug in the plasma and toxicity for renal patients. Insignificant amounts of phenytoin are removed by dialysis, and no supplemental doses are needed postdialysis.[35] No dosage change for phenytoin appears necessary for patients with acute viral hepatitis. Furthermore, most patients with cirrhosis tolerate usual doses. However, some patients with severe liver dysfunction may have significant changes in phenytoin disposition, requiring some dose reduction. For any patient receiving phenytoin, it must be kept in mind that this drug exhibits concentration-dependent kinetics and that small increases in dose may lead to more than proportionate increases in plasma concentration. Specific approaches to dosing of phenytoin, taking these factors into consideration, are available.[28]

PHENOBARBITAL

Phenobarbital is commonly used in the treatment of generalized tonic-clonic seizures and in simple or complex partial seizures and some cases of febrile seizures. Although phenobarbital has been in use since 1912, relatively little is known about its pharmacokinetics. Data on the absolute bioavailability of phenobarbital are unavailable, although it is generally considered to be almost completely absorbed after oral doses.[36] Phenobarbital is metabolized in the liver and excreted unchanged through the kidneys. The major metabolite formed, parahydroxyphenobarbi-

TABLE 19–9. COMMON ANTICONVULSANTS AND USUAL DOSAGES AND THERAPEUTIC PLASMA LEVELS

GENERIC NAME	BRAND NAME	USUAL DOSAGE (MG/DAY)	THERAPEUTIC PLASMA LEVEL (μG/ML)
Phenytoin	Dilantin	300–400	10–20
Phenobarbital	Luminal	100–200	10–40
Carbamazepine	Tegretol	600–1200	4–10
Valproic acid	Depakene	750–2000	50–100
Ethosuximide	Zarontin	750–2000	40–80
Trimethadione	Tridione	600–1800	>700 (as dimethadione)

tal, is inactive, and other metabolites have been identified, but not quantitated. The amount of unchanged phenobarbital excreted in the urine ranges from 10 to 40 per cent of the dose depending on urine flow and pH.[36, 37] Forced alkaline diuresis has been commonly employed in the treatment of barbiturate overdose and can result in enhanced elimination of long-acting barbiturates like phenobarbital.

Since phenobarbital has a relatively long half-life, varying from 60 to 150 hours, accumulation with repeated doses occurs. The mean half-life of phenobarbital is significantly increased in patients with cirrhosis; 130 hours compared to 86 hours in normal controls.[38] In patients with acute viral hepatitis, the mean half-life of 104 hours was not significantly greater than that in the controls, although some individual half-life values were high. Information on the effect of renal disease on phenobarbital half-life is unknown, although some increase would be expected.

Side effects of phenobarbital that have been reported during therapeutic use include sedation, slowness, dizziness, ataxia, and confusion. In addition, various rashes, stomatitis, fever, blood dyscrasias, nonspecific hepatic changes, osteomalacia, and other non–dose-related side effects have been observed.

Barbiturates induce the microsomal enzyme system of the liver, causing numerous drug interactions. Of interest for patients with renal failure is the interaction between vitamin D and barbiturates. The administration of phenobarbital has been shown to accelerate the biotransformation of vitamin D_3 to 25-hydroxycholecalciferol. Furthermore, both of these may undergo accelerated conversion to more polar metabolites, some of which are inactive. However, the presence of phenobarbital does not appear to affect the conversion of 25-hydroxycholecalciferol to 1,25-dihydroxycholecalciferol.

Since phenobarbital has a long half-life, maximum effect from a given dose will not be achieved until days after therapy is initiated, unless a loading dose is administered. In patients with severe renal or liver dysfunction, accumulation of phenobarbital may occur, especially in those with liver failure. Furthermore, since these patients are probably more sensitive to the effects of barbiturates, lower doses should be used initially, with gradual increases until the desired effect and plasma levels or side effects (Table 19–9) are attained. A supplemental dose after dialysis may be needed depending on the type and duration of dialysis, the individual patient's plasma phenobarbital concentration, and the changes in concentration during dialysis.

CARBAMAZEPINE

Carbamazepine is useful in the chronic treatment of generalized tonic-clonic seizures and simple and particularly complex partial seizures (e.g., temporal lobe seizure). Uncomfortable side effects associated with the abrupt initiation of usual maintenance doses precludes its use in acute situations. It is also the drug of choice for treating trigeminal neuralgia.[39] Absorption of carbamazepine from the gastrointestinal tract is variable and slow, with peak plasma levels being reached several hours after the dose.[39] Carbamazepine is extensively metabolized by the liver to several metabolites.[39, 40] One metabolite, carbamazepine-10,11-epoxide, has similar anticonvulsant activity to that of carbamazepine in animal studies. It is believed that this metabolite may be responsible in part for therapeutic as well as toxic effects in patients. Only 1 to 2 per cent of a dose of carbamazepine is excreted unchanged in the urine along with a similar amount of the epoxide metabolite. Other metabolites are also excreted renally, and also through the biliary route. Carbamazepine exhibits large interindividual differences in metabolism, accounting for its wide range of half-life values. Furthermore, the half-life decreases with multiple oral doses and in epileptic patients treated with the drug chronically (9 to 21 hours) as compared to single doses (19 to 55 hours). The reason for this shorter half-life is the self-induction of carbamazepine metabolism, as well as enhanced metabolism secondary to other drugs (e.g., phenobarbital and phenytoin) given concomitantly with carbamazepine.

No data are available on the pharmacokinetic disposition of carbamazepine in patients with renal or hepatic disease. It has been shown that renal disease has no significant influence on the plasma protein binding of carbamazepine.[41] Although patients with various types of hepatic disease (hepatitis and cirrhosis) exhibited significantly lower protein binding compared to controls, the difference is slight and clinically unimportant.

Common dose-related side effects due to carbamazepine are diplopia, vertigo, dizziness, and drowsiness. Other toxic effects include anorexia, nausea, vomiting, and diarrhea. Blood dyscrasias, such as agranulocytosis, thrombocytopenia, and leukopenia, have been reported, but their incidence is low. Elevated levels of alkaline phosphatase may occur in the absence of other signs of liver abnormalities. Proteinuria can occur but disappears when the drug is discontinued. A single case report of nonoliguric renal failure with suspected tubular toxicity secondary to carbamazepine has been observed; on discontinuing the drug, the patient recovered. Carbamazepine has antidiuretic effects and may lead to serious water intoxication.[42]

No dosage guidelines are available for carbamazepine for patients with renal or hepatic disease. Normal doses in renal failure seem appropriate, since only small amounts of unchanged carbamazepine and its active epoxide metabolite are excreted in the urine. There is no information on the dialyzability of carbamazepine or its epoxide metabolite. The drug should be used cautiously in patients with liver failure. Owing to the variable half-life of carbamazepine and its enhanced metabolism with chronic dosing, causing plasma levels to decline, patients must be monitored closely and plasma carbamazepine levels (Table 19–9) measured periodically. The most useful parameter in dosing these patients remains clinical evidence of toxicity.

VALPROIC ACID

Valproic acid is a relatively new anticonvulsant. It is generally used as an adjunct in the treatment of generalized absence seizures (formerly called petit mal), although it may be used alone in this situation. It has also been used as an adjunct in the treatment of generalized tonic-clonic seizures, simple and complex partial seizures, and some refractory seizures of childhood.[43-45] As with carbamazepine, a valproic acid regimen is also initiated slowly and therefore is not used in the acute setting.

Valproic acid is completely and rapidly absorbed following its oral administration.[46, 47] It undergoes extensive hepatic metabolism with the formation of some metabolites shown to be active in animal studies. Very little valproic acid is excreted unchanged in the urine.[46, 47]

The pharmacokinetics of valproic acid have not been studied in renal failure patients. However, significant reductions in plasma protein binding have been demonstrated in renal failure.[48, 49] In therapeutic concentrations, the percentage of free valproic acid has been shown to double in patients with varying degrees of renal impairment. A good correlation was observed between the unbound fraction of valproic acid in plasma and serum creatinine and creatinine clearance.[49] Although the kidney is a minor route of elimination for unchanged valproic acid, active metabolites could accumulate in renal failure and contribute to the pharmacologic effect.

Patients with alcoholic cirrhosis and patients in the recovery phase of acute hepatitis have been shown to have a significant decrease in the plasma protein binding and increase in the volume of distribution of valproic acid.[50] Plasma half-life was also prolonged in both groups of patients compared to healthy controls; however, total plasma clearance was not impaired. In patients during the acute stage of viral hepatitis, the half-life of valproic acid was increased and total plasma clearance decreased.[46]

The most common side effects of valproic acid are gastrointestinal disturbances, such as anorexia, nausea, vomiting, diarrhea, and abdominal cramps.[43-45] Drowsiness and sedation are also common, usually occurring at the initiaton of therapy and especially when used in combination with barbiturates. Any associated phenobarbital dose should automatically be reduced by one third with initiation of valproic acid therapy. Hepatic toxicity may occur as a result of valproic acid, and ranges from temporary asymptomatic serum liver enzyme elevations to toxic hepatitis and even death.[51] Valproic acid can cause inhibition of the secondary phase of platelet aggregation, decreased platelet adhesiveness, thrombocytopenia, decreased serum fibrinogen, and prolonged partial thromboplastin and prothrombin times. This problem may be especially important when patients are given other drugs affecting coagulation or have an underlying coagulopathy, as can occur with renal or hepatic disease. Other reported side effects due to valproic acid include alopecia, tremor, ataxia, incoordination, diplopia, headache, depression, psychosis, paresthesias, asterixis, rash, and leukopenia. Urinary tests for ketones may show false-positive results in patients taking valproic acid.

No specific dosage recommendations are available for patients with renal or hepatic disease. In some cases of hepatic failure and during severe renal failure, some decrease in the usual dose seems warranted. No information is available on the dialyzability of valproic acid. Since this drug can cause significant gastrointestinal symptoms, sedation, hepatic, and coagulation-related side effects, it must be used very cautiously in patients with renal or hepatic disease.

SUCCINIMIDES

The succinimides (ethosuximide, methsuximide, and phensuximide) have been used in the treatment of generalized absence seizures (formerly called petit mal). Ethosuximide is the only currently used agent in this group.[36]

Ethosuximide. Ethosuximide is considered to be completely absorbed after oral dosing. Owing to its long half-life (50 to 60 hours in adults, 25 to 40 hours in children) steady-state plasma levels are reached after approximately 8 to 10 days of administration.[52, 53] Little information on the metabolism of ethosuximide is available, although the metabolites formed are believed to be inactive. Approximately 10 to 20 per cent of ethosuximide is excreted unchanged in the urine.[52-54] No pharmacokinetic information is known for ethosuximide in patients with renal or hepatic failure.

Dose-related side effects of ethosuximide include gastric distress, nausea, vomiting, anorexia, fatigue, headache, dizziness, euphoria, and hiccups. Parkinsonian symptoms and photophobia have also been reported with this drug. Toxic effects considered unrelated to dose are skin rashes, urticaria, Stevens-Johnson syndrome, systemic lupus erythematosus, eosinophilia, leukopenia, and pancytopenia.

Owing to the small amount of unchanged ethosuximide excreted in the urine, only a slight reduction in dose is suggested for patients with severely impaired kidney function. Furthermore, the dialyzability of ethosuximide is unknown, but owing to negligible protein binding and small distribution volume, some removal would be expected.[52, 54] Because of insufficient information, this drug should be used cautiously in patients with renal or hepatic disease. Close observation for dose-related side effects and measurement of plasma concentrations (Table 19–9) may help guide dosage.

TRIMETHADIONE

Trimethadione, although now rarely used, is indicated for treating generalized absence seizures (formerly called petit mal). Following absorption, it is rapidly and quantitatively demethylated, primarily in the liver, to dimethadione.[55] Both trimethadione and dimethadione have similar anticonvulsant activity. Since patients treated chronically with trimethadione have serum level ratios of 20:1 of dimethadione to trimethadione, it is felt that the majority of the anticonvulsant effect of trimethadione is due to dimethadione.[56] Very little trimethadione is excreted unchanged in the urine; the dimethadione formed is not further metabolized, but is virtually all excreted very slowly into the urine.[56] Dimethadione is a weak acid that is filtered at the glomerulus and then undergoes extensive tubular reabsorption with an acid urine. Thus, its renal excretion can be markedly enhanced by urinary alkalinization and increasing urine flow.[57] The half-life of dimethadione is extremely long and is estimated to range from 100 to 350 hours depending on urine flow and pH.[57]

Owing to this prolonged half-life, steady-state levels of dimethadione will not be achieved until weeks after initiating trimethadione therapy. No pharmacokinetic studies for trimethadione or dimethadione are available in patients with impaired renal or hepatic function.

Sedation, hemeralopia (glare effect), precipitation of grand mal seizures, rashes, erythema multiforme, exfoliative dermatitis, leukocyte shift, neutropenia, pancytopenia, and a myasthenia-like syndrome have all been reported as toxic effects of trimethadione.[58] The development of the nephrotic syndrome has been reported in a number of patients treated with trimethadione. This is usually reversible within 4 to 6 weeks following discontinuation of the drug.

Since dimethadione is principally excreted by the kidneys and has an extremely long half-life in patients with normal renal function, substantial accumulation would be anticipated in patients with renal failure. The dialyzability of trimethadione or dimethadione is unknown, although some removal is expected on account of their small molecular weight, small distribution volume, and lack of protein binding.

Owing to the lack of adequate information on the disposition of trimethadione in renal as well as hepatic disease, it should be used with extreme caution or avoided.

DRUGS USED IN PARKINSON'S DISEASE

LEVODOPA AND CARBIDOPA

Treatment strategy in Parkinson's disease has continued to evolve over the past 5 years. Over the past decade, it has become clear that chronic use of levodopa is associated with decreased efficacy and diminished tolerance. For this reason, anticholinergics, amantadine, and antihistamines have regained a prominence in the treatment of mild Parkinson's disease. Levodopa is reserved for more disabling symptoms and, moreover, is frequently used in association with anticholinergics, amantadine, and antihistamines late in the disease.[59] Levodopa is commonly administered with a peripheral decarboxylase inhibitor, such as carbidopa, in order to allow reduction in ingested dose and amelioration of many side effects.[60] Levodopa is extensively metabolized to a variety of metabolites, some of which are pharmacologically active. Of an administered dose, over 80 per cent is excreted in the urine, mostly as metabolites.[59-63] The primary route of metabolism of levodopa is decarboxylation to dopamine via enzymatic conversion by dopa decarboxylation present in the gut wall, liver, kidneys, pancreas, capillary walls, neurons, and brain. The basis for the action of carbidopa is inhibition of dopa decarboxylase in peripheral tissue, but not in the central nervous system, thus providing more levodopa within the brain for conversion to dopamine. Carbidopa is mostly metabolized.[60] The pharmacokinetic disposition of levodopa or carbidopa has not been studied in patients with impaired renal or hepatic function.

With chronic use, there is a predictable decrease in the threshold to side effects. These include gastrointestinal symptoms (anorexia, nausea, and vomiting) cardiovascular symptoms (postural hypotension, various cardiac arrhythmias), and mental disturbances (depression, psychotic disorders, anxiety, and chorea).[59, 60] The concomitant administration of carbidopa may decrease the incidence and severity of gastrointestinal and cardiovascular effects. Other side effects that have been reported include red-black urine and polyuria, increased blood urea nitrogen (BUN), and one case of interstitial nephritis. An interesting observation is that levodopa has been demonstrated to increase renal plasma flow, glomerular filtration rate, and sodium and potassium excretion. It has been shown not to suppress the renin-aldosterone system.

In terms of drug interactions, the efficacy of levodopa is decreased by pyridoxine or by multivitamins containing pyridoxine. However, the efficacy of the levodopa-carbidopa combination is not affected by pyridoxine.[59, 60] Methyldopa can potentiate the therapeutic effect of levodopa and decrease its daily dose requirements.

Levodopa and carbidopa should be administered cautiously to patients with renal or hepatic failure, especially those with concomitant cardiovascular disease. Low doses should be used initially and the patient slowly titrated between adequate clinical response and side effects.

AMANTADINE

In the late 1960's, the antiviral agent amantadine was observed to produce amelioration in the symptoms of Parkinson's disease. This drug is not metabolized and approximately 90 per cent of a dose is excreted unchanged in the urine. Thus, patients with renal impairment have a decreased ability to eliminate the drug and accumulation can occur.[64, 65] Patients with severe renal failure receiving amantadine have developed central nervous system toxicity, such as nightmares, confusion, depression, visual and auditory hallucinations, restlessness, and aggressive behavior, associated with elevated plasma drug concentrations. Additional adverse effects secondary to amantadine use are anorexia, nausea, vomiting, constipation, urinary retention, heart failure, edema, and livedo reticularis. Patients with renal failure require a reduced dosage of amantadine depending on the degree of renal dysfunction and should be monitored carefully for dose-related neuropsychiatric toxic effects. Very small amounts of amantadine are removed by hemodialysis or peritoneal dialysis.[66]

MISCELLANEOUS

Other drugs commonly used in the treatment of Parkinson's disease are the anticholinergics (e.g., trihexyphenidyl, benztropine) and antihistamines (e.g., diphenhydramine). These drugs are primarily metabolized and very little is excreted unchanged in the urine. There are no data available on the disposition of these drugs in patients with kidney or liver disease. Side effects associated with these drugs are mainly anticholinergic, such as dry mouth, blurred vision, dizziness, drowsiness, weakness, confusion, and urinary retention. In high doses, tachycardia, agitation, hallucinations, and increased body temperature can occur. Some of these side effects may aggravate already existent problems in patients with renal or hepatic disease. It is recommended to initiate therapy with low doses and closely titrate the patient to the desired response.

DRUGS USED IN MYASTHENIA GRAVIS

NEOSTIGMINE AND PYRIDOSTIGMINE

Neostigmine and pyridostigmine are reversible anticholinesterase agents and are commonly used in patients with myasthenia gravis. Structurally, they possess a charged quaternary ammonium group that allows high water solubility, but also makes it difficult to traverse cell membranes easily. Following oral administration, they are generally poorly and irregularly absorbed.[67] Pyridostigmine appears to be better absorbed and less metabolized than neostigmine when taken orally. Both drugs undergo rapid and extensive metabolism, primarily in the liver but also at other sites, to several metabolites, some of which are active. Unchanged drug and metabolites are excreted in the urine, with a substantially larger percentage of the dose being recovered unchanged following parenteral versus oral administration.[68] No data are available on the kinetics of these drugs in patients with liver disease. The pharmacokinetics of intravenous neostigmine was studied in patients undergoing anesthesia who were either anephric or had normal kidney function.[69] In anephric patients, the half-life was significantly increased (more than doubled) and total serum clearance was significantly decreased by approximately 50 per cent. Following kidney transplantation, neostigmine elimination was not different from that in patients with normal renal function.

Side effects associated with neostigmine and pyridostigmine include miosis, wheezing, increased bronchial secretions, abdominal cramps, diarrhea, diaphoresis, lacrimation, bradycardia, hypotension, weakness, muscle fasciculations, and paralysis.

Individual dosage requirements of anticholinesterase agents are quite variable depending on differences in drug disposition and severity of disease state. A greater percentage of unchanged drug is excreted in the urine after parenteral as compared to oral doses. Thus, empiric dose reductions would be required, especially with parenteral therapy in patients with impaired renal function. The exact dose for patients with renal and hepatic failure must be determined by clinical response and toxicity.

Acknowledgments

We would like to acknowledge the assistance of M.D. Goldfield, M.D., W.J.C. Amend, Jr., M.D., Howard Siu, M.D., and M. W. Marshall in reviewing this chapter.

REFERENCES

1. Shader, RI: Manual of Psychiatric Therapeutics. Boston: Little, Brown, 1975.
2. Denber, HCB: Textbook of Clinical Psychopharma-

cology. New York: Stratton Intercontinental, 1979.

3. Nicholi, AM: The Harvard Guide to Modern Psychiatry. Cambridge, Mass.: The Belknap Press of Harvard University Press, 1978.
4. AMA Drug Evaluation. American Medical Association, 1980.
5. Hollister, LE: Clinical Pharmacology of Psychotherapeutic Drugs. Boston: Churchill Livingstone, 1978.
6. Hackett, TP, Cassem, NH: Handbook of General Hospital Psychiatry. St. Louis, Mosby, 1978.
7. Viederman, M, Rusk, G: Psychotherapeutic agents in renal failure. Am. J. Med. *62*:529–532, 1977.
8. Hollister, LE: Antipsychotics. *In* Clinical Pharmacology of Psychotherapeutic Drugs. Boston: Churchill Livingstone, 1978, pp. 131–191.
9. Maxwell, MD, Carrella, M, Parkes, JD, et al.: Plasma disappearance and cerebral effects of chlorpromazine in cirrhosis. Clin. Sci. *43*:143–151, 1972.
10. Avram, MM, McGinn, JT: Extracorporeal hemodialysis in phenothiazine overdosage. J.A.M.A. *197*:142–143, 1966.
11. Diagnostic and Statistical Manual of Mental Disorders. 3rd ed. American Psychiatric Association, 1980.
12. Cooper, TB: Plasma level monitoring of antipsychotic drugs. Clin. Pharmacokinet. *3*:14–38, 1978.
13. Gaultieri, CT, Powell, SF: Psychoactive drug interactions. J. Clin. Psychiatry *39*:720–729, 1978.
14. Fogelson, DL, Marder, SR, Van Putten, T: Dialysis for schizophrenia: A review of clinical trials and implications for further research. Am. J. Psychiatry *137*:605–607, 1980.
15. Gram, LF: Plasma level monitoring of tricyclic antidepressant therapy. Clin. Pharmacokinet. *2*: 237–251, 1977.
16. Hollister, LE: Antidepressants. *In* Clinical Pharmacology of Psychotherapeutic Drugs. Boston: Churchill Livingstone, 1978, pp. 68–130.
17. Reidenberg, MM, Odar-Cederlöf, I, von Bahr, C, et al: Protein binding of diphenylhydantoin and desmethylimipramine in plasma from patients with poor renal function. N. Engl. J. Med. *285*:264–267, 1971.
18. Amdisen, A: Serum level monitoring and clinical pharmacokinetics of lithium. Clin. Pharmacokinet. *2*:73–92, 1977.
19. Hollister, LE: Lithium and manic-depressive disorder. *In* Clinical Pharmacology of Psychotherapeutic Drugs. Boston: Churchill Livingstone, 1978, pp. 192–226.
20. Baldessarini, RJ, Lipinski, JF: Lithium salts: 1970–75. Ann. Intern. Med. *83*:527–533, 1975.
21. Thomsen, K, Schou, M: Renal lithium excretion in man. Am. J. Physiol. *215*:823–827, 1968.
22. Jefferson, J, Greist, J: Primer of Lithium Therapy. Baltimore: Williams and Wilkins, 1977.
23. Schou, M, Baastrup, PC, Grof, P, et al.: Pharmacological and clinical problems of lithium prophylaxis. Br. J. Psychiat. *116*:615–619, 1970.
24. Cooper, TB, Simpson, GM: The 24-hour lithium level as a prognosticator of dosage requirements: a 2-year follow-up study. Am. J. Psychiatry *133*:440–443, 1976.
25. Port, FK, Kroll, PD, Rosenzweig, J: Lithium therapy during maintenance hemodialysis. Psychosomatics *20*:130–131, 1979.
26. Procci, WR: Mania during maintenance hemodialysis successfully treated with oral lithium carbonate. J. Nerv. Ment. Dis. *164*:355–358, 1977.
27. Neuvonen, PJ: Bioavailability of phenytoin: clinical pharmacokinetic and therapeutic implications. Clin. Pharmacokinet. *4*:91–103, 1979.
28. Richens, A: Clinical pharmacokinetics of phenytoin. Clin. Pharmacokinet. *4*:153–169, 1979.
29. Odar-Cederlöf, I, Bórga, O: Kinetics of diphenylhydantoin and uremic patients: consequences of decreased plasma protein binding. Eur. J. Clin. Pharmacol. *7*:31–37, 1974.
30. Olsen, GD, Bennett, WM, Porter, GA: Morphine and phenytoin binding to plasma proteins in renal and hepatic failure. Clin. Pharmacol. Ther. *17*:677–684, 1975.
31. Reidenberg, MM, Affrime, M: Influence of disease on binding of drugs to plasma proteins. Ann. N.Y. Acad. Sci. *226*:115–126, 1973.
32. Blaschke, TF, Meffin, PJ, Melmon, KL, et al.: Influence of acute viral hepatitis on phenytoin kinetics and protein binding. Clin. Pharmacol. Ther. *17*:685–691, 1975.
33. Affrime, M, Reidenberg, MM: The protein binding of some drugs in plasma from patients with alcoholic liver disease. Eur. J. Clin. Pharmacol. *8*:267–269, 1975.
34. Kutt, H, Winters, W, Scherman, R, et al.: Diphenylhydantoin and phenobarbital toxicity, the role of liver disease. Arch. Neurol. *11*:649–656, 1964.
35. Martin, E, Gambertoglio, JG, Adler, DS, et al.: Removal of phenytoin by hemodialysis in uremic patients. J.A.M.A. *238*:1750–1753, 1977.
36. Hvidberg, EF, Dam, M: Clinical pharmacokinetics of anticonvulsants. Clin. Pharmacokinet. *1*:161–188, 1976.
37. Whyte, MP, Dekaben, AS: Metabolic fate of phenobarbital. Drug Metab. Dispos. *5*:63–69, 1977.
38. Alvin, J, McHorse, T, Hoyumpa, A, et al.: The effect of liver disease in man on the disposition of phenobarbital. J. Pharmacol. Exp. Ther. *192*: 224–235, 1975.
39. Bertilsson, L: Clinical pharmacokinetics of carbamazepine. Clin. Pharmacokinet. *3*:128–143, 1978.
40. Morselli, PL, Frigerio, A: Metabolism and pharmacokinetics of carbamazepine. Drug Metab. Rev. *4*:97–113, 1975.
41. Hooper, WD, Dubetz, DK, Bocher, F, et al.: Plasma protein binding of carbamazepine. Clin. Pharmacol. Ther. *17*:433–440, 1975.
42. Sordillo, P, Sagransky, DM, Mercado, R, et al.: Carbamazepine-induced syndrome of inappropriate antidiuretic hormone secretion. Arch. Intern. Med. *138*:299–301, 1978.
43. Browne, TR: Valproic acid. N. Engl. J. Med. *302*:661–666, 1980.
44. Pinder, PM, Brogden, RN, Speight, TM, et al.: Sodium valproate: a review of its pharmacological properties and therapeutic efficacy in epilepsy. Drugs *13*:81–123, 1977.
45. Bruni, J, Wilder, BJ: Valproic acid, review of a new antiepileptic drug. Arch. Neurol. *36*:393–398, 1979.
46. Gugler, R, vonUnruh, GE: Clinical pharmacokinetics of valproic acid. Clin. Pharmacokinet. *5*:67–83, 1980.
47. Perucca, E, Gatti, G, Grigo, GM, et al.: Pharmaco-

kinetics of valproic acid after oral and intravenous administration. Br. J. Clin. Pharmacol. *5*:313–318, 1978.

48. Brewster, D, Muir, NC: Valproate plasma protein binding in the uremic condition. Clin. Pharmacol. Ther. *27*:76–82, 1980.
49. Gugler, R, Mueller, G: Plasma protein binding of valproic acid in healthy subjects and in patients with renal disease. Br. J. Clin. Pharmacol. *5*:441–446, 1978.
50. Klotz, U, Rapp, T, Müller, WA: Disposition of valproic acid in patients with liver disease. Eur. J. Clin. Pharmacol. *13*:55–60, 1978.
51. Suchy, FJ, Balistreri, WF, Buchino, JJ, et al.: Acute hepatic failure associated with the use of sodium valproate. N. Engl. J. Med. *300*:962–966, 1979.
52. Buchanan, RA, Kinke, AW, Smith, TC: The absorption and excretion of ethosuximide. Int. J. Clin. Pharmacol. *7*:213–218, 1973.
53. Goulet, JR, Kinkel, AW, Smith, TC: Metabolism of ethosuximide. Clin. Pharmacol. Ther. *20*:213–218, 1976.
54. Chang, T, Dill, WA, Glazko, AJ: Ethosuximide. Absorption, distribution and excretion. *In* Antiepileptic Drugs. (DM Woodbury, JK Penry, RP Schmidt, eds.). New York: Raven Press, 1972, pp. 417–423.
55. Withrow, CD, Woodbury, DM: Trimethadione and other oxazolidinediones. Absorption, distribution and excretion. *In* Antiepileptic drugs. (DM Woodbury, JK Penry, and RP Schmidt, eds.) New York: Raven Press, 1972, pp. 389–393.
56. Booker, HE: Trimethadione and other oxazolidinediones. Relation of plasma levels to clinical control. *In* Antiepileptic Drugs. (DM Woodbury, JK Penry, and RP Schmidt, eds.). New York: Raven Press, 1972, pp. 403–407.
57. Waddell, WJ, Butler, TC: Renal excretion of 5,5-dimethyl-2,4-oxazolidinedione (product of demethylation of trimethadione). Proc. Soc. Exp. Biol. Med. *96*:563–565, 1957.
58. Gallagher BB: Trimethadione and other oxazolidinediones. Toxicity. *In* Antiepileptic Drugs. (DM Woodbury, JK Penry, and RP Schmidt, eds.). New York: Raven Press, 1972, pp. 409–411.
59. Brogden, RN, Speight, TM, Avery, GS: Levodopa: a review of its pharmacological properties and therapeutic uses with particular reference to parkinsonism. Drugs *2*:262–400, 1971.
60. Pinder, RM, Brogden RN, Sawyer, PR, et al.: Levodopa and decarboxylase inhibitors: a review of their clinical pharmacology and use in the treatment of parkinsonism. Drugs *11*:329–377, 1976.
61. Calne, DB, Reid, JL: Antiparkinsonian drugs. Pharmacological and therapeutic aspects. Drugs *4*:49–74, 1972.
62. Bianchine, JR, Shaw, GM: Clinical pharmacokinetics of levodopa in Parkinson's disease. Clin. Pharmacokinet. *1*:313–338, 1976.
63. Dunner, DL, Brodie, HKH, Goodwin, FK: Plasma DOPA response to levodopa administration in man: effects of peripheral decarboxylase inhibitor. Clin. Pharmacol. Ther. *12*:212–217, 1971.
64. Armbruster, KFW, Rahn, AC, Ing, TS, et al.: Amantadine toxicity in a patient with renal insufficiency. Nephron *13*:183–186, 1974.
65. Ing, T, Daugirdas, JT, Soung, LS, et al.: Toxic effects of amantadine in patients with renal failure. Can. Med. Assoc. J. *120*:695–698, 1979.
66. Soung, LS, Ing, TS, Daugirdas, JT, et al.: Amantadine hydrochloride pharmacokinetics in hemodialysis patients. Ann. Intern. Med. *93*:46–49, 1980.
67. Chan, K, Calvey, TN: Plasma concentration of pyridostigmine and effects in myasthenia gravis. Clin. Pharmacol. Ther. *2*:596–601, 1977.
68. Nowell, PT, Scott, CA, Wilson A: Determination of neostigmine and pyridostigmine in the urine of patients with myasthenia gravis. Br. J. Pharmacol. *18*:617–624, 1962.
69. Cronnelly, R, Stanski, DR. Miller, RD, et al.: Renal function and the pharmacokinetics of neostigmine in anesthetized man. Anesthesiology *51*:222–226, 1979.

Chapter 20

Use of Dialysis and Hemoperfusion in Drug Overdose — An Overview

by

Serafino Garella
and *Jonathan A. Lorch*

The incidence of self-inflicted and accidental drug overdose has been increasing during the past several decades and can now be considered of epidemic proportion. In England and Wales, self-poisoning accounts for 6.8 per cent of all medical admissions to hospitals. Similar figures are available for other European countries and Australia.[1] It is unfortunate that no comprehensive system of poisoning reporting has been established in the United States. Data from the National Center for Health Statistics reveal 5339 deaths due to poisoning in 1977. Of these deaths 3125 were attributed to suicidal intent, making death due to self-poisoning the third most common mode of suicide, after firearms and hanging.[2] The frequency of all instances of drug overdose is extremely difficult to estimate, and many consultants feel that self-inflicted poisoning is underreported. Data from the National Clearinghouse for Poison Control Centers show that only 0.07 per cent of all cases of accidental and self-inflicted overdose end fatally, and that about 9 per cent require hospitalization.[3] If these figures are representative, then one can estimate that there are about 7.5 million instances of drug overdose per year in the United States, of which about 675,000 require hospitalization. Obviously, these figures are intended only to provide a coarse approximation of the magnitude of the problem. In any event, it is clear that many practicing physicians, especially those working in Emergency Departments or Intensive Care Units, must be well acquainted with drug overdose victims.

Of the thousands of patients presenting each year to hospitals for treatment of drug overdose, about 50 per cent are found to have mild intoxications, and are discharged. Of those who are admitted, about 28 per cent suffer from "serious" or "critical" intoxication, and require major treatment efforts to preserve life.[4] This latter pool of patients (estimated to be in the range of 11,000 patients per year) represents the group that has received most attention. It is now clear that all such patients should be approached and treated vigorously with the so-called "Scandinavian method," developed in the 1950's and described in 1961 by Clemmesen and Nilsson.[5]

IMPORTANCE OF SUPPORTIVE THERAPY FOR DRUG OVERDOSE

Before World War II, therapy for drug overdose consisted of massive gastric lavage and administration of analeptics; this resulted in an overall mortality of about 20 per cent of hospitalized patients.[6] Mortality began to decline in the 1940's and 1950's following introduction of more physiologic methods to combat hypotension and recognition of the importance of establishing a patent airway. Mortality further dropped to the present 1 to 2 per cent with the widespread use of the "Scandinavian method."[5, 7-9] This attentive, conservative means of management demands rapid establishment of a patent airway and support of ventilation if necessary. Monitoring and maintaining proper cardiac and hemodynamic function are important. Thus, intravenous lines for administration of necessary fluids and/or drugs are often required. In summary, supportive therapy to maintain vital functions until the drug is metabolized and/or excreted is the mainstay of this method. Removal of stomach contents and establishment of an adequate diuresis are important objectives, but remain secondary to the maintenance of basic vital functions.

More recent attempts at decreasing morbidity and mortality rates and shortening length of hospital stay have resulted in the employment of techniques directed at increasing the rate of clearance of the intoxicating agents. Initially, these techniques consisted of forced diuresis. More recently, peritoneal dialysis, hemodialysis, and hemoperfusion have been used to facilitate drug removal. These techniques are generally reserved for the most severely affected patients with overdose, a relatively small segment of the total population of overdose patients.[10, 11] In contrast, the supportive measures constituting the Scandinavian method are important in all cases of drug overdose. We therefore developed an algorithm (Fig. 20–1) to provide a guideline for the rapid and effective treatment of patients who present to a physician with a suspected diagnosis of drug intoxication.

In many such patients, metabolic or central nervous system (CNS) disturbances may eventually be found to have been the cause of the clinical syndrome. In addition, events such as narcotic overdose, hypoglycemia, and carbon monoxide poisoning must be suspected and treated promptly (note that "cherry red" cyanosis is a poor clue to carbon monoxide poisoning, as it tends to occur only in lethal exposures).[12] In proceeding down this algorithm, disagreement might arise regarding the proper place of gastric lavage versus emesis,[13] and which kind of emetic agent should be used. We feel that an attempt at emptying the stomach should be made, except in those patients who show evidence of having taken petroleum products or caustic agents. The best results, as far as recovery of nondigested drugs is concerned, are obtained by emesis. This can be used only in patients who are alert and capable of following directions. Syrup of ipecac is usually preferred over apomorphine, since it causes none of the CNS depression frequently seen with the latter[14]; however, syrup of ipecac has the disadvantages of being slower to act and of requiring completed emesis before activated charcoal is administered, otherwise it will be inactivated by the charcoal. In contrast, apomorphine and activated charcoal can be administered simultaneously, thereby effecting a prompter reduction of toxin absorption. If the patient cannot cooperate fully, or becomes stuporous after administration of the emetic, then gastric lavage performed through a 16 or 18 Fr. nasogastric tube and with repetitive, small (150 to 200 ml) volumes of water, should be carried out. Plain abdominal x-rays may be useful not only in confirming a drug ingestion, but also in determining whether or not lavage has been effective in removing the ingested material, in those cases in which the preparations result in radiologically detectable patterns.[15]

As a rule, before introducing the nasogastric tube, endotracheal intubation must be attempted in any uncooperative or comatose patient. If the patient resists endotracheal intubation, then the attempt must be stopped, since inappropriate forceful intubation can induce aspiration just as easily as inappropriate emesis. In this case, the patient should be placed in the left lateral decubitus position as the nasogastric tube is inserted. After the stomach is emptied, 30 to 60 gm of activated charcoal should be given as a slurry,[16] except when one is dealing with acetaminophen intoxication. Here, *N*-acetylcysteine appears to be a specific antidote,[17, 18] and it is inactivated by the charcoal. Following charcoal administration, it is common practice to give a cathartic, usually magnesium citrate, although some question has been raised about the effectiveness of this maneuver.

With the careful use of the Scandinavian method as the cornerstone of treatment of drug intoxication, the overall rate of mortality has been relatively low at 1 to 2 per cent of all patients admitted to the hospital with drug intoxication. However, some series show mortality as high as 35 per cent in selected patients who present in Stage IV coma. (For the purposes of this discussion, the staging of coma will be that of the criteria of Reed,

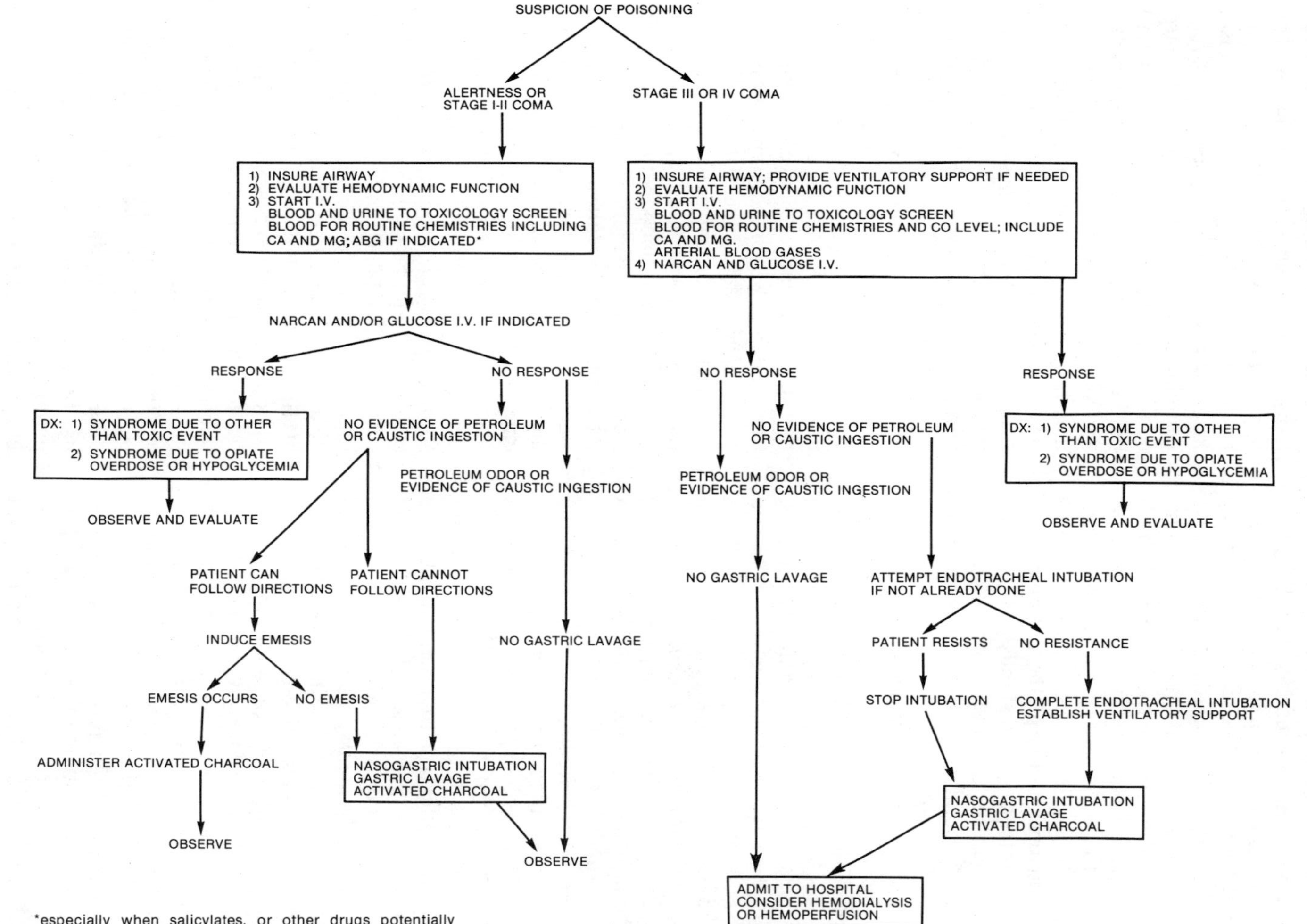

*especially when salicylates, or other drugs potentially resulting in acid-base disorders are suspected. ABG = arterial blood gases.

Figure 20–1. Initial approach to the diagnosis and treatment of suspected drug overdose.

Driggs, and Foote, as modified by Arieff and Friedman,[19] which is as follows:

Stage I — patient withdraws to painful stimuli and deep tendon reflexes are preserved.

Stage II — deep tendon reflexes are generally present and blood pressure and respiration are not depressed; however, patient does not withdraw from painful stimuli.

Stage III — respiration and blood pressure are not depressed, but most reflexes are diminished or absent.

Stage IV — in addition to absence of most reflexes and lack of withdrawal to painful stimuli, there is depression of respirations to less than 8 per min and/or hypotension with a systolic blood pressure lower than 85 mm Hg).[19]

In these selected patients, several maneuvers have been attempted to decrease the rate of complications and/or the length of hospitalization.

ADDITIONAL MODALITIES OF THERAPY FOR DRUG INTOXICATION

For the last two decades, the hope of accomplishing these goals has been focused on techniques originally designed to treat endogenous intoxications. Thus, peritoneal dialysis and hemodialysis and, more recently, adsorbent hemoperfusion were widely anticipated to result in dramatic improvements in the treatment of drug intoxication. The attraction of these techniques and their range of employment can be gauged by looking at the number of papers cited by the *Cumulated Index Medicus*. In 1968, 11 publications in the English language reporting of successes in the treatment of several types of intoxicants were listed under the heading "Hemodialysis." In 1968, the heading "Hemoperfusion" did not yet exist. In 1978, only four papers claiming success for dialysis in the treatment of overdose were listed. Also in 1978, 28 publications claimed that hemoperfusion could produce remarkable results in the treatment of a wide variety of intoxications.

Every physician who is involved in the medical care of severely intoxicated patients is forced either by the current literature or by the questions of his colleagues to decide whether to employ one or the other of these techniques in the severely intoxicated patient. It is therefore necessary to review the basic principles of operation of these techniques, the relationship of these techniques to the pharmacokinetics of poisons, and the experimental and clinical information currently available to arrive at a set of reasonable recommendations. We must caution that some of the conclusions that we will reach are as yet tentative, since this is a rapidly evolving field in which there is much need for additional research.

PERITONEAL DIALYSIS

Peritoneal dialysis is the simplest, easiest to perform, and most widely available form of dialytic therapy. It requires the placement of a catheter in the peritoneal cavity. Commercially available dialysis solutions are then instilled and withdrawn through this catheter at the usual rate of 2 L/hr. Peritoneal dialysis can be carried out for up to 48 hours or more. Complications include perforations of intra-abdominal organs or vessels, peritonitis, abnormalities in glucose and electrolyte concentration, and alterations in volume of body fluids. This form of dialysis has rates of clearance and removal of most intoxicants that are well below those of hemodialysis or hemoperfusion. Therefore, it should be chosen only under exceptional circumstances.

HEMODIALYSIS

Hemodialysis is the most complex of the three procedures under discussion. It requires special equipment, solutions not universally available, and a specially trained staff. An access to circulating blood capable of yielding 250 to 300 ml/min must be established, either by the surgical insertion of a Scribner arteriovenous shunt or by the percutaneous cannulation of large venous vessels (usually the femoral vein). The blood is pumped through a system of tubing and comes in contact with balanced electrolyte solutions through a semipermeable membrane. The rate of fluid removal or addition, and the rate of change in electrolyte or acid-base composition can be varied with appropriate maneuvers to change hydrostatic pressure, osmotic pressure, and chemical composition within the extracorporeal circulation. The patient must be heparinized to prevent clotting of the extracorporeal circuit. The patient must be hemodynamically stable to provide an adequate blood flow through the dialyzer, a condition sometimes difficult to achieve in Stage IV coma. Complications include infection of vascular access sites, septicemia, bleeding, sudden changes in the volume of body fluid compartments, rapid alterations in serum electrolyte composition, and aggravation of hypotension and hypoxemia.

Hemodialysis has been reported to achieve clearance rates of up to 150 ml/min for some intoxicants. As a rule of thumb, any poison dialyzable by the peritoneal route is more efficiently cleared by hemodialysis. An added advantage of hemodialysis is that it allows the treatment of eventual concurrent problems in acid-base or electrolyte composition and is, of course, indicated in cases of coexistent renal failure.

HEMOPERFUSION

Hemoperfusion is the most recent addition to the therapeutic armamentarium for the treatment of poisoning. It is the technique that has been felt by many to be widely applicable to a large variety of toxins. The principles of hemoperfusion were explored by Yatzidis in 1964 and resulted in the introduction of devices that began to be used clinically in the early 1970's. The technique requires the same type of access to the circulation, pumps, tubing, and staff support as hemodialysis. However, the dialyzer and dialysis solutions are replaced by the hemoperfusion cartridge. These cartridges are relatively compact plastic containers filled with adsorbent materials. Three basic models of cartridges are commercially available. These cartridges contain fixed-bed uncoated charcoal, charcoal granules coated with a semipermeable membrane, or polymer resins. Blood is perfused through the adsorbent materials at the rate of 200 to 300 ml/min. Relatively little is known about the factors that affect the interrelationship between charcoal or resins and the solutes present in plasma. In general, it appears that activated charcoal is more effective in adsorbing hydrophilic substances, whereas lipophilic substances are more readily adsorbed onto resins.

Although hemoperfusion as a technique cannot be employed to reverse alterations in acid-base parameters or electrolyte composition, its theoretic advantages in the treatment of poisonings are numerous. The surface area of the adsorbent material is several thousand times larger than the 1 to 2 square meters of a conventional hemodialyzer, thus allowing more interaction between toxin and adsorbent. This is further increased greatly by the fact that the thickness of the membrane coating the microcapsules is only about one-hundredth that of a standard hemodialysis membrane (0.05 versus 5μ). Finally, and most importantly, the adsorbents used for hemoperfusion bind virtually all common poisons, in contrast to the rather restricted list for hemodialysis and peritoneal dialysis. With few exceptions, these features allow hemoperfusion to achieve higher clearances for most intoxicants than previously possible and markedly decrease the limitations imposed by molecular size and/or protein binding that diminish the effectiveness of hemodialysis. Of course, the procedure is not without its potential complications and disadvantages. These include sepsis from vascular invasion, reduction in platelet and white cell counts, bleeding from heparinization, and decline in cartridge efficiency after 3 to 4 hours due to saturation of the column with toxins.

PHARMACOKINETIC PRINCIPLES IN DIALYSIS AND HEMOPERFUSION

The theoretic usefulness of dialysis and hemoperfusion in treating poisoning depends on the capacity of these techniques to transfer and hold a given toxin outside the blood stream. Several factors have an effect on this capacity; some depend on the procedure chosen and have been mentioned previously. Others depend on the intoxicating drug itself. The characteristics and metabolic behavior of the intoxicating drug that are most important in determining the potential effectiveness of dialysis and hemoperfusion are listed in Table 20–1.[20-24]

APPARENT VOLUME OF DISTRIBUTION

After absorption and equilibration, drugs will distribute differently in body fluid compartments, tissues, and even within different constituents of individual cells. However, drug concentrations are commonly measured only in blood or plasma. If a drug is preferentially distributed — to the intracellular compartment, for example — then its concentration in plasma will be lower than if it is distributed equally in all body constituents, or

TABLE 20–1. MOLECULAR WEIGHT, WATER SOLUBILITY, APPARENT VOLUME OF DISTRIBUTION, PROTEIN BINDING, AND CLEARANCE DATA FOR SOME COMMON INTOXICANTS*

Substance	Mol. Wt.	Water Solubility†	V_d‡	% Protein Binding	Plasma Clearance Rate (ml/min)§		
					P.D.	*H.D.*	*H.P.*
Analgesics							
Acetaminophen	151	S	1.02	10–20	< 10	120	200
Salicylates	138	S	9L/1.73 m^2		25	100	80
Sedative-Hypnotics							
Chlordiazepoxide	300		0.3	94			
Diazepam	285		0.9–1.1	98	0		0
Meprobamate	218						120
Ethchlorvynol	145	I	200L/1.73 m^2	45	20	60	120
Glutethimide	217	I	2.7	54		20	150
Methqualone	250		420L/1.73 m^2	80			90
Pentobarbital	248	S	1.0	50	10	15	40
Phenobarbital	232	S	0.75	50	10	40	100
Secobarbital	260	S	1.3	60	10	15	60
Tricyclic Antidepressants							
Amitriptyline	277	S	20	96			100
Imipramine	280	S	12	96		15	
Nortriptyline	263	S	20	94			
Antibiotics							
Aminoglycosides	460–590	S	0.2–0.3	0–5	6	20–40	100
Cephalosporins	350–450	S	10–20	20–80	< 10		100
Penicillin G	356	S	0.6	65			
Ampicillin	349	S	16L/1.73 m^2	20			
Carbenicillin	378	S	9L/1.73 m^2	20			
Methicillin	402	S	22L/1.73 m^2	35			
Nafcillin	436	S	1.06	90		10	
Oxacillin	441	S	13L/1.73 m^2	92			
Chloramphenicol	524	S	40L/1.73 m^2	70			
Vancomycin	1800	S	33L/1.73 m^2	10	6	0	
Isoniazid	137	S		10		70	140
5-Fluorocytosine	129	S	0.6	<5		80	
Amphotericin B	924	I		90		10	
Cardiac Drugs							
Digitoxin	765	S	0.6	90–97		<5	31
Digoxin	781	S	7–12	25		24	90
Disopyramide	339	S	0.7	20–40			100
Lidocaine	234	S	1.7	66			
Procainamide	219	S	1.9	3			
N-Acetylprocainamide	261	S	1.4	11		80	
Propranolol	259	S	3.6	90		80	
Quinidine	324	S	3.0	83		10	
Anticonvulsants							
Carbamazepine	236	I	1.0	70			
Primidone	218	I	0.6	0	see Phenobarbital		
Ethosuximide	141	S	0.7	0			
Phenytoin	252	I	0.6	90		10	
Miscellaneous							
Ethyl alcohol	46	S	0.6	<5	15	100	60
Methyl alcohol	32	S	0.6	<5	20	130	60
Ethylene glycol	62	S	0.6	<5		150	
Lithium carbonate	73	S	0.8	0	13	30	

*These data were derived primarily from recent reviews by Gibson[20] and Winchester et al.[23] It should be noted that large inconsistencies appear in published literature and that many values must be considered only approximate.

†S = Soluble. I = Insoluble.

‡V_d is reported in L/kg, or, when indicated, in L/1.73 m^2 of body surface area.

§These clearance data refer to exchange rates of 2 L/hr in peritoneal dialysis (P.D.), and to 200 ml/min of blood flow rates for hemodialysis (H.D.), and hemoperfusion (H.P.).

remains predominantly within the intravascular compartment. If the total amount of drug ingested is known, then its concentration in circulating blood or plasma will permit a calculation of the *apparent* volume of distribution (V_d). This is usually expressed in liters per kilogram of body weight, and it can be many times higher than the total volume of body fluids. For example, the tricyclic antidepressants have a V_d of approximately 20 L/kg. Thus, if a 70-kg patient ingests 1 gm of amitriptyline, at equilibrium the plasma concentration will be about 0.7 mg/L (V_d being 1400 L), or 0.0007 mg/ml. It is thus apparent that substances with high V_d's will have low plasma concentrations, and their removal will not be likely to be affected importantly by either dialysis or hemoperfusion.

EASE OF INTERCOMPARTMENTAL TRANSFER

Even in the presence of a high V_d, it is conceivable that a drug might be so loosely bound to its target compartment that a rapid clearing of the circulating drug would just as rapidly result in new drug being made available to the circulation. Thus, low binding could result in an effective rate of removal of drugs with large V_d's. Alternatively, tight binding would severely hinder the effectiveness of therapy to remove the drug. This is the case with the herbicide paraquat. Hemoperfusion can rapidly reduce the plasma concentration of this compound to zero. Tissue analysis, however, will continue to show toxic amounts. The drug is so tightly bound to tissues that its concentration in plasma will remain unmeasurably low even hours after hemoperfusion is stopped. Effectiveness of hemoperfusion in this circumstance would be minimal. Drugs that show a similar behavior, though not quite as extreme, are some lipid-soluble sedatives or hypnotics, such as glutethimide or thiopental, which are only slowly released by adipose tissue.

PHYSICAL CHARACTERISTICS

Molecular size, protein binding, and polarity of the drug are other factors that correlate with ease of dialyzability. In general, dialyzability diminishes with increasing size, protein binding, and drug polarity. It is particularly important to note that these factors represent serious limiting factors in the case of hemodialysis, less so in hemoperfusion. A high *water solubility* (in the presence of small molecular size and absence of significant protein binding) will allow more effective dialysis; this is the case with many alcohols, such as methyl and isopropyl alcohol, and ethylene glycol.

EFFECT OF DIALYSIS AND HEMOPERFUSION — THEORETIC CONSIDERATIONS

The criteria used to estimate the effectiveness of dialysis or hemoperfusion have been based on (1) clearance data; (2) total amount of drug removed; and (3) clinical results.

USE OF CLEARANCE DETERMINATIONS

Clearance data are the most easily obtained and readily available. The clearance rate of a toxin represents that amount of plasma that is completely cleared of the toxin per unit time. It is calculated from the known rate of plasma flow through either the dialyzer or the hemoperfusion cartridge, and the difference in drug concentration in the plasma before and after it has been through the device. There is no question that clearance rates can be very high for a large variety of intoxicants, especially when hemoperfusion is used.[23, 25, 26] Unfortunately, a high clearance rate tells us only that the procedure is capable of clearing a high volume of *plasma;* it gives no information whatsoever as to what may be occurring at the site of action of the drug. Moreover, clearance rates provide little information concerning the total amount of drug removed in relation to that ingested. To return to the previous example of amitriptyline, a clearance rate as high as 300 ml/min would remove only 0.21 mg of drug per minute, or about 50 mg during a 4-hour treatment if drug concentration remains stable in the plasma throughout the procedure and there is no saturation of the adsorbent in the hemoperfusion cartridge. Even more disturbing is what happens with paraquat,[27] in which clearance is high at the onset of the procedure. Then paraquat concentration in the plasma falls to zero, and clearance also falls to zero. Since there is no detectable movement of the toxin from its binding sites to the circulation, continuation of the procedure becomes futile. Thus, the widespread use of clearance data to justify the use of dialysis or hemoperfusion must be cautiously interpreted and is often misleading.

USE OF AMOUNT REMOVED

The total amount of drug removed can be estimated from clearance data. Alternatively, it can be derived from the amount either in the dialysate or adsorbed onto the granules of the hemoperfusion device at the end of the procedure. In either case, the available figures must be considered as relatively unreliable, since unpredictability of recovery rates and low drug concentrations in large volumes of fluid or over large adsorbent surfaces limit obtaining accurate data on total drug removal. Perhaps even more important, one does not know whether or not the active form of the drug or an inactive metabolite is being recovered. In any case, a review of the available data demonstrates that the total amount of drug removed is trivial and clinically unimportant in tricyclic antidepressant and digitalis compound intoxication.[8, 28] Both of these drugs have a high V_d. Most other common intoxicants, primarily the sedative and hypnotic agents, are removed at the rate of 1 gm or less per hemoperfusion treatment.[29-31] Even smaller amounts are removed with hemodialysis. Some exceptional instances have been reported. In one report, up to 13 gm of glutethimide were removed, but the patient had ingested the extreme amount of 75 gm.[26] Another report shows that multiple hemoperfusion treatments over a period of days were required to remove about one-third of the estimated amount of ingested ethchlorvynol;[32] it was felt that this represented an example of successful employment of hemoperfusion.

In view of the misleading nature of clearance data, and lack of reliable data on total drug removal, the issue as to whether or not dialysis or hemoperfusion should be used derives largely from clinical observations.

CLINICAL OBSERVATIONS

The recent literature is replete with reports of "miraculous awakenings" and low mortality rates in intoxicated patients treated with hemoperfusion. Favorable results have been claimed in the treatment of practically all known intoxicants, including hypnotics and sedatives, antidepressants, digitalis, theophylline, antibiotics, and such exotic intoxications as paraquat and *Amanita phalloides*. It is interesting to note, however, that a similar spectrum of favorable results had previously been attributed to treatment with hemodialysis.

The fundamental problem with this anecdotal reporting is that it is not known whether the patients might have survived without the treatment. Claims that treatment resulted in a faster resolution of the comatose state or in a lower rate of complications lack firm documentation. These claims can be substantiated only by carefully conducted controlled trials. Virtually no controlled studies are available. The few that have been attempted relate exclusively to those drugs that are usually ingested in suicidal attempts.

The types of drug ingestion requiring hospitalization in our experience (discussed later)[33] and in a British series are listed in Table 20–2. Important regional and temporal differences exist in the pattern of drug preference for sui-

TABLE 20–2. PERCENTAGE DISTRIBUTION OF DRUGS INGESTED IN THREE SERIES

Drug	R.I.H. Series[33] ("severe" intoxications) (1974–78)	Edinburgh Series[34] (all hospital admissions) *(1967)*	*(1976)*
Barbiturates	22.6	30	15
Benzodiazepines	22.2	9	42
Tricyclic antidepressants	20.0	5	11
Ethchlorvynol	6.5	not reported	–
Salicylates	6.1	16	10
Phenothiazines	6.1	not reported	–
Glutethimide	3.9	not reported	–
Acetaminophen	0.4	2	12
Multiple ingestions	57.5	not reported	–

cidal attempts.* It is obvious that the popularity of each class of drugs is not only subject to change from time to time in the same location, but also differs depending on the location of the population studied. The question of dialysis or hemoperfusion occasionally arises for the treatment of relatively unusual intoxications. In many of these cases, information on removal by dialysis or hemoperfusion is not available. In these cases, a decision is often based on the clinical condition of the patient and the previously discussed pharmacokinetic principles of the drug under question.

A brief examination of three noncontrolled studies that have compared patients treated with hemoperfusion with those not so treated yields contrasting observations. Volans et al.[35] reported on 57 patients with severe drug intoxication. These patients had a plasma level of the toxin generally considered lethal. In addition, these patients had advanced coma, or progressive deterioration, or prolonged coma with complications. This study concluded that the technique was "clinically safe and useful," despite the fact that mortality was 24 per cent in the treated patients and only 14 per cent in the untreated patients. Bismuth et al.[30] found that only 2.5 per cent of untreated patients in their series died, while mortality was 13 per cent in the hemoperfused patients. These authors concluded that hemoperfusion "does not seem to be a life saving procedure. . . and [is] not free from specific complications, especially infectious ones." Finally, Hampel et al.[40] reported on two groups of patients, 53 treated without hemoperfusion and 17 with hemoperfusion. Mortality was 21 per cent in the untreated versus only 6 per cent in the treated group. It is interesting to note, however, that of the 11 patients who died in the control group, one died at admission, no data were supplied for a second, and the remaining nine patients died several days after admission; only three of these patients had plasma drug levels that were high enough to require hemoperfusion.* This high mortality and its peculiar temporal pattern are inexplicable to us. Thus, of the three reports that made any attempt at comparing hemoperfusion with supportive treatment, only one seems to yield data favorable to hemoperfusion.

Thus, dialysis and hemoperfusion are procedures that should be reserved for the severely intoxicated patient. In order to determine more specific guidelines for the use of dialysis and hemoperfusion in the treatment of overdose, we examined our personal experience. Our purpose was to attempt to define a subset of patients that might require such procedures. Moreover, we wanted to determine if the addition of dialysis or hemoperfusion to the Scandinavian method would be likely to decrease hospital stay or rate of complications. Our series now covers all admissions to the Rhode Island Hospital over a consecutive 5-year period.[33] This hospital is the primary poison control center for a population base of approximately 1 million people; 600 admissions were analyzed. It should be noted that during this time, all patients admitted with this diagnosis were screened by gas chromatography — mass spectrometry.[41] Of these 600 patients, 24.3 per cent, or 146, were classified as "severe" according to the criteria of Winchester et al.[23] Hypotension was present in 42 patients and endotracheal intubation and ventilatory support were required in 99 patients. Aspiration and/or pneumonia was present in 33 patients, 19 were hypothermic or febrile, and eight had generalized seizures. Despite the obvious severity of intoxication in this group of patients, only seven died. Two patients died from cytoplasmic poisons (acetaminophen and thallium salts); one died from isopropyl alcohol within 2 hours of presentation with severe metabolic acidosis and cardi-

*Of particular concern is the great increase in acetaminophen intoxication in Great Britain, well evident by 1976 and still continuing. This intoxicant appears not to be amenable to hemoperfusion in view of its short half-life. Its treatment (especially with *N*-acetylcysteine) is being actively investigated and is likely to evolve markedly.[18] For up-to-date recommendations call the Rocky Mountain Poison Center, Tel. No. (303)534–0312.

*It should be noted that although plasma levels of drugs have been widely used as prognostic indicators, their interpretation is notoriously unreliable for this purpose. Unchanging, or even increasing, plasma concentrations can be seen at a time when the patient's clinical picture is clearly improving. This can be related to a number of factors, such as the presence of active metabolites,[36, 37] adaptation or development of tolerance to the depressant effects of the drug,[38] or changes in binding characteristics,[28] and internal redistribution.[39] Thus, drug levels may be most useful for purposes of identification of the intoxicating agents, and in some circumstances, to estimate total amounts of drug ingested, if the apparent volume of distribution is known.

ac arrhythmias. The remaining four patients (two of whom suffered from tricyclic antidepressant overdose, a type of intoxication not amenable to dialysis or hemoperfusion) died while being transported to the hospital or immediately on arrival. Thus, it is clear that neither dialysis nor hemoperfusion could have had a major impact on mortality in our series. The case of isopropyl alcohol intoxication may have responded to dialytic therapy; unfortunately, this patient expired before any procedure could be implemented.

If mortality rate cannot be decreased, can dialysis or hemoperfusion decrease morbidity or length of stay in intensive care units? Our data and a review of the literature indicate that even in severely intoxicated patients the length of stay in the intensive care unit is relatively short. For example, more than 80 per cent of all overdosed patients require less than 48 hours in an intensive care unit (Fig. 20–2). Moreover, the numerous complications resulting from overdose are usually present within 4 hours of admission and 76 per cent of all complications resolve within 24 hours (Fig. 20–3) of admission. These observations suggest that the morbidity of intoxications is generally not related to the length of coma, but rather to events occurring during the initial period of treatment,[42, 43] when vomiting and aspiration, traumatic intubation, hypoventilation, or arrhythmias are usually seen.

In view of these observations, it is untenable to suggest that all severely intoxicated patients should be dialyzed and/or hemoperfused. However, can a subset of this relatively

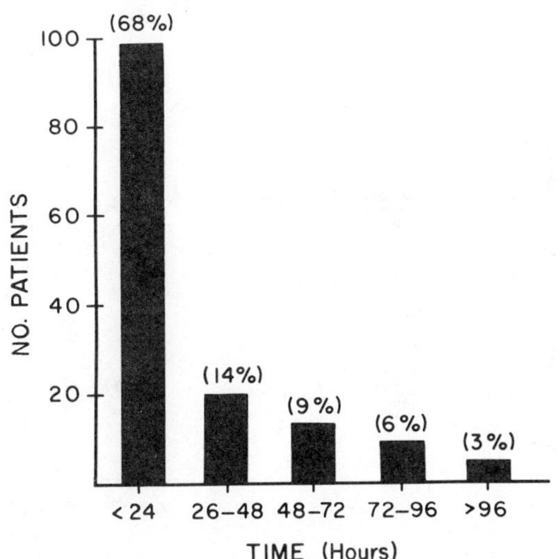

Figure 20–2. Total number (and percentage) of patients with "severe" intoxication, versus length of stay in Intensive Care Unit. Note that 82 per cent of patients required less than 48 hours of hospitalization. (Reproduced with permission from Garella, S., and Lorch, J. A.: Hemoperfusion for poisoning: who needs it? *In* Schreiner, G. E., et al. (eds.): Controversies in Nephrology. Washington, D. C.: Georgetown University Press, 1980.)

well-defined population be identified early after admission as a group of optimal candidates for treatment with dialysis or hemoperfusion? We attempted to do so by looking at the number of complications detected within 4 hours of admission in our patients (Fig. 20–4). We reasoned that an initial more severe clinical picture would identify the most severely ill patients at high risk for development of complications. Unfortunately, no clear correlation

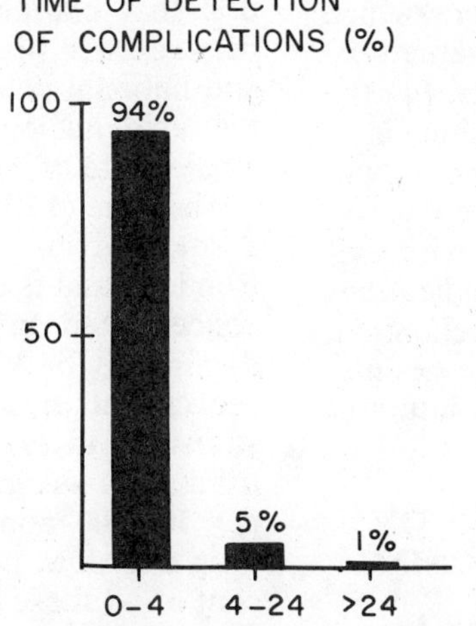

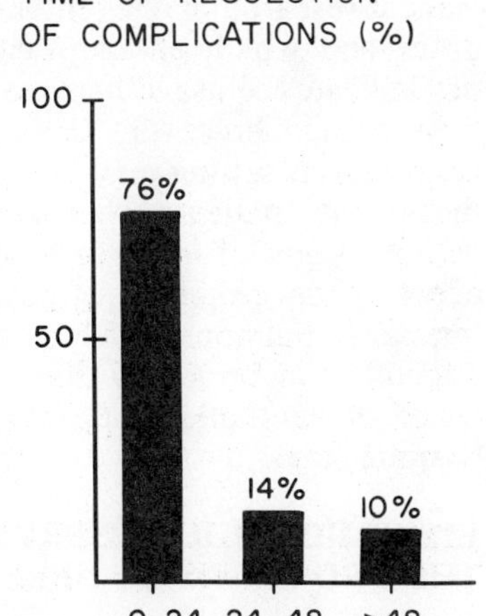

Figure 20–3. Time of detection and of resolution of all complications in 146 patients with "severe" drug overdose. Note that 94 per cent of all complications were detected within 4 hours of presentation to the hospital, and that 76 per cent resolved within 24 hours. (Reproduced with permission from Garella, S., and Lorch, J. A.: Hemoperfusion for poisoning: who needs it? *In* Schreiner, G. E., et al. (eds.): Controversies in Nephrology. Washington, D. C.: Georgetown University Press, 1980.)

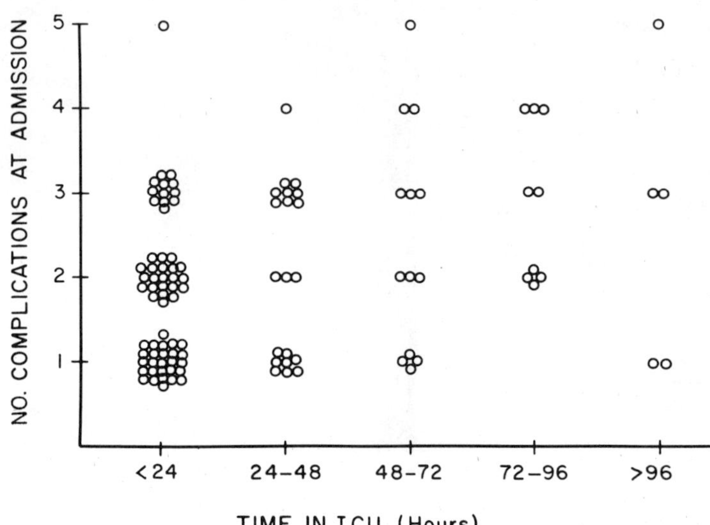

Figure 20–4. Number of complications detected within 4 hours of presentation to the hospital versus length of stay in the Intensive Care Unit. The patients who required the lengthiest treatment did not have at admission a clearly more severe clinical picture than those who were discharged within 24 hours. (Reproduced with permission from Garella, S., and Lorch, J. A.: Hemoperfusion for poisoning: who needs it? *In* Schreiner, G. E., et al. (eds.): Controversies in Nephrology. Washington, D. C.: Georgetown University Press, 1980.)

existed between severity of the clinical picture at admission and the length of stay in the intensive care unit.

Thus, despite the well-established evidence that hemoperfusion is extraordinarily effective in achieving high plasma clearance rates of most intoxicants, our data suggest that this form of therapy is not routinely indicated in the treatment of poisonings due to common intoxicants. The present inability to select a group of patients likely to benefit from the procedure results in the indiscriminate use of expensive technology with a number of potential side effects (both medical and socioeconomic) on a relatively large population whose prognosis is already by-and-large benign, with little likelihood of improving on hospital length of stay or complication rates. Ongoing clinical research may eventually define which drugs and which patient-related characteristics indicate the use of hemoperfusion. For the time being, however, hemoperfusion in a nonresearch setting may be justifiable only in those rare patients who remain comatose without signs of improvement and with evidence of development of new complications (primarily pulmonary: hypostatic pneumonia, difficulties in bronchial toilet, and/or maintenance of ventilation) after 24 to 48 hours of hospital stay.

EPIDEMIOLOGIC OBSERVATIONS ON THE PROGNOSIS OF SELF-POISONING

More than 3000 patients die yearly in the United States from the consequences of self-poisoning. Our series from the Rhode Island Hospital, which serves a population base of about 1,000,000, however, reveals an unexpectedly low mortality of seven patients during 5 years. Could this be due to the fact that our institution sees a segment of the population with a particularly benign prognosis, or to the fact that the state of Rhode Island has a peculiarly low incidence of death due to drug overdose? Neither of these two possibilities is tenable. The rate of hospital admissions is comparable to expected figures, and the degree of severity of intoxications is well documented by the frequency of complicating factors such as presence of hypotension, requirement for ventilatory support, and development of aspiration and/or pneumonia. However, the most pertinent piece of information that clarifies the apparent discrepancy between our hospital-generated observations and national data is provided by a review of the epidemiology of self-poisoning for the whole state of Rhode Island.[44]

The state of Rhode Island lends itself well to a study of the natural history of poisoning. Rhode Island is characterized by small size, a concentrated urban population served predominantly by Rhode Island Hospital, and by centralized agencies for tabulation of vital statistics. In 1978, there were 114 deaths attributed to suicide, representing a rate of 12.2 per 100,000 population per year. Voluntary drug overdose accounted for 21, or 18.4 per cent of all these deaths. Of these 21 suicides, 16 were found dead and never received medical attention. Of the remaining five, three have been reported previously as part of our hospital series; the final two represent a patient who died of imipramine intoxication (a tricyclic antidepressant that is not amenable to hemoperfusion) and one who expired of laryngospasm during extubation while she was awakening from barbiturate intoxication. It should be noted that the overall rate of death due to self-poisoning and the pattern of suicidal attempts in Rhode Island are comparable to national data.

Thus, we feel that although epidemiologic data show that death due to intoxication is a common problem, efforts such as hemoperfusion and dialysis directed at improving the prognosis of hospitalized patients are unlikely to result in significant changes in overall mortality statistics. The majority of patients who die of drug overdose expire without having obtained medical attention. Moreover, the prognosis of drug overdose appears determined at the time the patient is found. The majority of drug overdose suicides are found dead or expire during transportation to the hospital. The exceptional patient who expires despite reaching the hospital in relatively stable condition has ingested a toxin with generalized cytotoxic effects that cannot be reversed by any currently known therapy.

INDICATIONS FOR UNUSUALLY AGGRESSIVE THERAPY

We can find no firmly based evidence that hemoperfusion or dialysis significantly improves the prognosis of most patients who are intoxicated with the most common agents (Table 20–2) or with other less common or even exotic intoxicants (including digitalis compounds, theophylline, *Amanita phalloides,* or paraquat). There are, however, some situations in which dialysis may be indicated.

The clearest indication pertains to intoxications with alcohols,[45-47] primarily methanol, isopropyl alcohol, and ethylene glycol. These compounds are highly water soluble and have small molecular weights, properties that make them ideal candidates for removal with hemodialysis. In general, the majority of their toxic effects are not due to the ingested products themselves, but rather to some of their metabolites. Since they are all oxidized by alcohol dehydrogenase, it is recommended that patients be treated early during their clinical course with ethanol administration, to achieve a blood concentration between 100 and 200 mg/100 ml. At these levels, ethanol has a higher enzyme affinity, and it will be preferentially metabolized. The ingested toxin may be eliminated in large part intact through the kidneys and, more efficiently, by dialysis. The minimal blood concentration of intoxicant for which dialysis is recommended is about 50 mg/100 ml. The concurrent presence of metabolic acidosis and renal failure enhances the indications for urgency of dialysis. In the absence of availability of blood levels, a history of ingestion of more than 100 ml of these alcohols may be sufficient to initiate dialysis and ethanol administration.

In the presence of renal failure, intoxications due to salicylates or to lithium constitute another indication for dialysis. However, both of these compounds can be promptly excreted in the urine if renal function is normal. The induction of a large urine flow (with the use of diuretics and the administration of saline solutions) and, in the case of salicylates,[49] of an alkaline diuresis represent the treatment of choice. Because of the high mortality rate of some patients with blood salicylate levels greater than 100 mg/100 ml, some consultants recommend dialysis or hemoperfusion under these conditions.[50]

Despite a number of studies purporting to show the beneficial effects of hemoperfusion in a variety of intoxications, and the feeling expressed by some that this technique should be widely employed in patients with severe clinical pictures,[10, 11, 22-26] no specific indications exist at present for hemoperfusion. This topic is being extensively investigated at the present time, and the careful clinician could not be faulted for using the procedure in those patients who present with the most severe clinical picture, who do not improve with careful supportive management over a 24- to 48-hour period of time, and who may suffer concurrently from damage to liver and/or kidney function. In no instance, however, could one expect hemoperfusion to improve the prognosis of patients intoxicated with drugs with a high V_d and with tight cellular binding.

CONCLUSIONS

The treatment of drug intoxication must be based, in the majority of cases, on the Scandinavian method: careful, aggressive support of vital functions, supplemented by the evacuation of stomach contents and the administration of activated charcoal when possible. In the case of acetaminophen intoxication, the administration of *N*-acetylcysteine appears to have therapeutic efficacy.

Dialysis and hemoperfusion have not been shown to be capable of markedly improving prognosis in most severe intoxications. Although either method, especially hemoperfusion, can be shown to be able to achieve high plasma clearance rates for most common intoxicants, the reduction in total body burden of the intoxicant that they can achieve is trivial in many intoxications, and of questionable clinical validity in others.

Epidemiologic evaluation of the natural history of intoxications reveals that the prognosis in any given patient is usually fixed by the time the patient is discovered. Of the patients who reach the hospital and are admitted, very few will die; most of these deaths will be due to irreversible anoxic brain damage or to intoxications with cytotoxic drugs.

Hemodialysis is indicated in the treatment of intoxications with methanol, isopropyl alcohol, and ethylene glycol, especially if accompanied by metabolic acidosis and/or renal failure. It also is indicated for the treatment of salicylate intoxication if a large flow of alkaline urine cannot be induced, or, in the case of lithium intoxication, if a large diuresis cannot be established because of renal failure.

At the present time, there is no clear indication for the use of hemoperfusion in the treatment of intoxications. The usefulness of this form of therapy must be shown with carefully controlled studies of tightly defined populations of intoxicated patients. Until these data become available, it may be employed in patients who remain comatose and show a progressively deteriorating clinical picture beyond 24 to 48 hours after admission.

REFERENCES

1. Mills IH: Self-poisoning — a modern epidemic. Clin. Toxicol. *18*:11–20, 1977.
2. Vital Statistics of the United States, Vol. II, Mortality; 1977. Published by the U.S. Department of Health, Education, and Welfare, Public Health Service, Mortality Statistics Branch, Division of Vital Statistics, National Center for Health Statistics.
3. National Clearinghouse for Poison Control Centers — Bulletin. Tabulations of 1976 Case Reports; February 1978. Published by the U.S. Department of Health, Education, and Welfare. Public Health Service.
4. Brandwin MA: Drug overdose emergency room admissions. Am. J. Drug Alcohol Abuse *3*:605–619, 1976.
5. Clemmesen C, Nilsson E: Therapeutic trends in the treatment of barbiturate poisoning: the Scandinavian method. Clin. Pharmacol. Ther. *2*:220–229, 1961.
6. Eckenhoff JE, Dam W: The treatment of barbiturate poisoning with or without analeptics. Am. J. Med. *20*:912–918, 1956.
7. Piper KW, Griner PF: Suicide attempts with drug overdose. Arch. Intern. Med. *134*:703–706, 1974.
8. Lorch JA, Garella S: Hemoperfusion to treat intoxications. Ann. Intern. Med. *91*:301–304, 1979.
9. Dumont C, Rangno R: Argument against hemoperfusion in drug overdose. J.A.M.A., *242*:1611, 1979.
10. Gelfand MC: Hemoperfusion: present and future (editorial). J. Dial. *3*:1–9, 1979.
11. Better OS, Brunner G, Chang TMS, et al.: Controlled trials of hemoperfusion for intoxication. Ann. Intern. Med. *91*:925, 1979.
12. Done AK: Carbon monoxide: the silent summons. Emergency Med. *5*:269–276, 1973.
13. Goulding R, Volans GN: Emergency treatment of common poisons: emptying the stomach. Proc. R. Soc. Med. *70*:766–770, 1977.
14. Schofferman JA: A clinical comparison of syrup of ipecac and apomorphine use in adults. J.A.C.E.P. *5*:22–25, 1976.
15. Greensher J, Mofenson HC, Gavin WJ: The usefulness of abdominal x-rays in the diagnosis of poisoning. Vet. Hum. Toxicol. *21*:45–46, 1979.
16. Greensher J, Mofenson HC, Picchioni AL, et al.: Activated charcoal updated. J.A.C.E.P. *8*:261–263, 1979.
17. Ameer B, Greenblatt DJ: Acetaminophen. Ann. Intern. Med. *87*:202–209, 1977.
18. Peterson RG, Rumack BH: Toxicity of acetaminophen overdose. J.A.C.E.P. *7*:202–205, 1978.
19. Arieff AI, Friedman EA: Coma following nonnarcotic drug overdosage: management of 208 adult patients. Am. J. Med. Sci. *266*:405–426, 1973.
20. Gibson TP: Dialyzability of common therapeutic agents. Dialysis Transplant. *8*:24–40, 1979.
21. Golper TA: Drugs and peritoneal dialysis. Dialysis Transplant. *8*:41–43, 1979.
22. Rosenbaum JL: Haemoperfusion in the treatment of acute poisoning. Chapter 23 *in* Artificial Organs (RM Kenedi, et al., eds.) Baltimore: University Park Press, 1976, pp. 203–212.
23. Winchester JF, Gelfand MC, Knepshield JH, et al.: Dialysis and hemoperfusion of poisons and drugs — update. Trans. Am. Soc. Artif. Intern. Organs *23*:762–842, 1977.
24. Winchester JF, Gelfand MC, Tilstone WJ: Hemoperfusion in drug intoxications: clinical and laboratory aspects. Drug Metab. Rev. *8*:69–104, 1978.
25. Gelfand MC: Symposium on sorbents in uremia: Part 3. Charcoal hemoperfusion in treatment of drug overdosage. Dialysis Transplant. *6*:8–15, 1977.
26. Rosenbaum JL, Kramer MS, Raja R: Resin hemoperfusion for acute drug intoxication. Arch. Intern. Med. *136*:263–266, 1976.

27. Okonek S, Hoffman A, Henningsen B: Efficacy of gut lavage, hemodialysis, and hemoperfusion in the therapy of paraquat or diquat intoxication. Arch. Toxicol. *36*:43–51, 1976.
28. Callaham M: Tricyclic antidepressant overdose. J.A.C.E.P. *8*:413–425, 1979.
29. Crome P, Hampel G, Vale JA, et al.: Haemoperfusion in the treatment of drug intoxication. Br. Med. J. *1*:174, 1978.
30. Bismuth C, Conso F, Wattel F, et al.: Coated activated charcoal hemoperfusion: experience of French anti-poison centers in 60 cases. Vet. Hum. Toxicol. 21(Suppl):2–4, 1979.
31. Garella S, Lorch JA: Hemoperfusion for poisoning: who needs it? In Controversies in Nephrology (GE Schreiner, et al., eds.) Washington, D.C.: Georgetown University Press, 1980.
32. Lynn RI, Honig CL, Jatlow PI, et al.: Resin hemoperfusion for treatment of ethchlorvynol overdose. Ann. Intern. Med. *91*:549–553, 1979.
33. Garella S, Lorch JA: Hemoperfusion for acute intoxications: Con. Clin. Toxicol. *17*:515–527, 1980.
34. Proudfoot AT, Park J: Changing pattern of drugs used for self-poisoning. Br. Med. J. *1*:90–93, 1978.
35. Volans GN, Vale JA, Crome P, et al.: The role of charcoal haemoperfusion in the management of acute poisoning by drugs. *In* Artificial Organs (RM Kenedi, et al., eds.): Baltimore: University Park Press, 1976, pp. 178–187.
36. Hansen AR, Kennedy KA, Ambre JJ, et al.: Glutethimide poisoning. A metabolite contributes to morbidity and mortality. N. Engl. J. Med. *292*:250–252, 1975.
37. Chazan JA, Garella S: Glutethimide intoxication: a prospective study of 70 patients treated conservatively without hemodialysis. Arch. Intern. Med. *128*:215–219, 1971.
38. Greenblatt DJ, Woo E, Allen Divoll M, et al.: Rapid recovery from massive diazepam overdose. J.A.M.A. *240*:1872–1874, 1978.
39. Breimer DD: Clinical pharmacokinetics of hypnotics. Clin. Pharmacokinet. *2*:93–109, 1977.
40. Hampel G, Wiseman H, Widdop B: Acute poisoning due to hypnotics: the role of haemoperfusion in clinical prospective. Vet. Hum. Toxicol. 21(Suppl.):4–6, 1979.
41. Ullucci PA, Cadoret R, Stasiowski PD, et al.: A comprehensive GC/MS drug screening procedure. J. Anal. Toxicol. *2*:33–38, 1978.
42. Zwillich CW, Pierson DJ, Creagh CE, et al.: Complications of assisted ventilation: a prospective study of 354 consecutive episodes. Am. J. Med. *57*:161–170, 1974.
43. Jay SJ, Johanson WG, Pierce AK: Respiratory complications of overdose with sedative drugs. Am. Rev. Respir. Dis. *112*:591–598, 1975.
44. Annual Report from the Office of the Chief Medical Examiner, Rhode Island Department of Health, Providence, R.I., 1978.
45. Underwood F, Bennett WM: Ethylene glycol intoxication. J.A.M.A. *226*:1453–1454, 1973.
46. Parry MF, Wallach R: Ethylene glycol poisoning. Am. J. Med. *57*:143–150, 1974.
47. McCoy HG, Cipolle RJ, Ehlers SM, et al.: Severe methanol poisoning. Am. J. Med. *67*:804–807, 1979.
48. Rosenbaum AH, Maruta T, Richelson E: Clinical pharmacology. Series on pharmacology in practice. I. Drugs that alter mood. II. Lithium. Mayo Clin. Proc. *54*:401–407, 1979.
49. Done AK, Temple AP: Treatment of salicylate poisoning. Mod. Treatment *8*:528–551, 1971.
50. Anderson RJ, Potts DA, Gabow PA, et al.: Unrecognized adult salicylate intoxication. Ann. Intern. Med. *85*:745–748, 1976.

Appendix

These *Drug Reference Tables* are a compilation of data on the pharmacokinetic parameters of 160 drugs commonly used in medical practice. Included also in these tables is a summary of dosing recommendations for patients with renal or hepatic dysfunction. The contributors of the information contained in these tables are the authors of the individual chapters of this book.

The drugs are listed by their generic names and in alphabetical order. Eleven separate tables are included, with titles corresponding to the various chapters in the book. For each drug listed, various pharmacokinetic parameters are detailed. Oral availability is the percentage of an orally administered dose that is presented to the systemic circulation after passage through the gastrointestinal tract and liver, and available for pharmacologic effect. The per cent binding of the drug to plasma proteins and volume of distribution are also tabulated. A brief summary of the route of elimination—i.e. renal excretion, hepatic metabolism—for each drug is provided. The half-life of drug elimination from the body is given for individuals with normal renal and hepatic function, for patients with end-stage renal disease, termed "anephric" (i.e., creatinine clearance <10 ml/min), and for patients with liver disease (e.g., hepatitis, cirrhosis). Dosage guidelines for three categories of renal failure are given, based upon adjustments of either the normal dose (maintaining the usual dosage interval) or adjustments of the dosage interval (maintaining the usual dose). Dosage recommendations for liver dysfunction are generally given in more qualitative terms, since specific quantitative information is usually not available. Lastly, the effect of dialysis on drug removal is described. These data usually pertain to hemodialysis unless otherwise specified (numbers in parentheses refer to dialysis clearance values).

It should be emphasized that the tabular listing of this information has certain limitations. Drugs with complex pharmacokinetic characteristics or unusual dosing requirements in renal or hepatic disease cannot be sufficiently described. The purpose of these tables is to provide the clinician with some general guidelines regarding drug handling and the dosing of drugs in patients with renal or liver dysfunction. For additional details, reference should be made to specific chapters in this book.

JOHN G. GAMBERTOGLIO, PHARM.D.

TABLE 1. ANTIMICROBIAL AGENTS

Drug	Oral Availability (%)	Protein Binding (%)	Volume of Distribution (L/kg)	Metabolism & Elimination	T 1/2 (hours)	
					Normal	*Anephric*
Aminoglycosides						
Amikacin	Not available orally	<5.0	0.22–0.29	Similar to kanamycin	2–3	86
Gentamicin	0.5	<5.0	0.23–0.26	Renal excretion of unchanged drug is 97–99%.	2	60
Kanamycin	0.5	<10	0.19–0.23	Renal excretion of unchanged drug is 96–99%.	3	84
Neomycin	<1–5	<10	–	Excreted 95–97% as unchanged drug in urine.	2	12–24
Streptomycin	Not available orally	35	0.26	Renal elimination 95–97% as unchanged drug.	2.5	110
Tobramycin	0.5 (not available orally)	<5.0	0.22–0.25	Similar to gentamicin	2.5	70
Anthelmintics						
Mebendazole	5–10	–	–	90% metabolized by liver, 20% as inactive and 75% as unidentified metabolites; 2.5% excreted unchanged in the urine.	–	–
Pyrvinium pamoate	Not appreciable	–	–	Contribution of hepatic metabolism unknown; excreted mainly in feces; <1% eliminated renally as unchanged drug.	–	–
Quinacrine	Good	90	Very large	Metabolized peripherally by hydroxylase enzymes (88% to hydroxyacridine). Hepatic and renal elimination data not available.	120	–
Thiabendazole	Very good	–	–	90% hepatic metabolism, metabolites probably inactive; 1% excreted unchanged in urine; 9% eliminated unchanged in feces.	1–2	–
Antifungals						
Amphotericin B	Not available orally	90–95	4.0	95–97% metabolized in liver or inactivated in body tissues; elimination through bile or via gut metabolism may occur; 3.5–5.5% excreted unchanged in urine.	24 (Terminal, 360)	24–40
Flucytosine	85–90	3–49	0.6–0.7	<10% metabolized in liver; 85–90% excreted as unchanged drug in urine.	2.4–6	75–250
Griseofulvin	50	–	1.0–2.0	97–99% hepatic metabolism, activity of metabolites unknown; <1% excreted unchanged in urine.	10–22	–

TABLE 1. ANTIMICROBIAL AGENTS *(Continued)*

Liver Disease	Dose Change with Renal-Failure GFR (ml/min) >50	10–50	<10	Dose Change with Liver Failure	Effect of Dialysis
–	Dosage changes similar to kanamycin			None	Significant (22 ml/min)
Unchanged	75–100% normal dose	35–75% normal dose	25–35% normal dose	None	Significant (26–48 ml/min)
	[1 mg/kg administered every 8 × serum creatinine (every second to third half-life)]				
–	75% normal dose	35–50% normal dose	25% normal dose	None	Significant (30–40 ml/min)
–	None	q8–12h	q12–36h	None	Significant (30–50 ml/min)
May be increased in patients with concomitant renal and hepatic disease	q24h	q24–48h	q48–96h	None	Minimal (17 ml/min)
Unchanged	Same recommendations as for gentamicin			None	Significant (50–60 ml/min)
–	None	None	None	Decrease may be necessary in severe hepatic disease.	–
–	None	None	None	Close monitoring is warranted in significant liver disease.	–
–	–	–	–	–	–
–	None	None	None	Decrease may be necessary in severe hepatic failure.	–
–	None	None	q36–48h	Monitor closely for accumulation.	Insignificant
–	None	q12–24h	q24–48h	None	Significant (60–100 ml/min)
–	None	None	None	Decrease may be indicated with severe hepatic disease.	–

Table continues on following page.

TABLE 1. ANTIMICROBIAL AGENTS (*Continued*)

Drug	Oral Availability (%)	Protein Binding (%)	Volume of Distribution (L/kg)	Metabolism & Elimination	T 1/2 (hours)	
					Normal	*Anephric*
Miconazoie	Not available orally	90–93	21	50% metabolized to inactive metabolites; 1% eliminated renally as unchanged drug; 50% excreted unchanged in feces.	20–24	24
Antituberculous Drugs						
Ethambutol	75–80	20–30	1.6	8–15% hepatic metabolism; 65–80% excreted unchanged in urine.	3.3	>10
Isoniazid	Complete	<10	0.6	65–95% hepatic metabolism; 5–35% excreted as unchanged drug in the urine (depends on acetylator phenotype).	1.4 5.2 (slow acetylators)	2.3 10.7
Rifampin	Significant first-pass effect	60–90	0.93	85–95% hepatic metabolism; metabolites are active; 5–15% excreted unchanged in urine.	2.3	3.1–5
Antiviral Agents						
Amantadine	100	–	4.4–5.1	No evidence of hepatic metabolism; 90% excreted unchanged in the urine.	12–36	>24
Interferon	Not available orally	–	–	Normal body fluids (saliva, serum, bile, urine, and stool) can inactivate interferon. Little excreted unchanged in urine.	4–6	–
Vidarabine (Vira-A)	Not available orally	–	–	Rapidly deaminated peripherally to Ara-Hx (arabinosyl hypoxanthine), an active metabolite; 41–53% of Ara-Hx and 1–3% of Ara-A excreted unchanged in urine.	3.3 (active metabolite)	–
Cephalosporins						
Cefaclor	53	22–25	0.24–0.47	<90% excreted unchanged in urine.	0.6–1	1.5–3.5
Cefamandole	Not available orally	67–80	0.16	96% eliminated renally as unchanged drug.	0.5–1.8	15–24
Cefazolin	Not available orally	70–86	0.1–0.15	Renal elimination of unchanged drug 95–98%.	1.4–2	35–56
Cefoxitin	Not available orally	65–79	0.10–0.13	10–15% hepatically metabolized; >90% eliminated unchanged in urine.	0.6–1	8–33
Cephadroxil	89–93	20	0.31	88-93% excreted renally as unchanged drug.	1.0–1.4	10–25
Cephalexin	73–100	6–15	0.18–0.25	85–95% excreted renally as unchanged drug.	1–1.9	20–40
Cephaloglycin	25	5–30	–	75–90% excreted renally as unchanged drug.	0.7–1.5	–
Cephaloridine	Not available orally	10–30	0.19–0.26	70–85% unchanged drug excreted renally.	1.5	10–23
Cephalothin	Not available orally	62–79	0.15–0.31	Hepatic metabolism 33%; desacetyl metabolite weakly active; renally excreted 66% unchanged in urine.	0.5–0.9	3–18

TABLE 1. ANTIMICROBIAL AGENTS *(Continued)*

Liver Disease	Dose Change with Renal Failure GFR (ml/min) >50	10–50	<10	Dose Change with Liver Failure	Effect of Dialysis
–	None	None	None	Decrease may be necessary in severe hepatic insufficiency.	Insignificant
–	None	50% normal dose q24h or 100% q36h	25% normal dose q24h or 100% q48h	None	Significant
6.7	None	None	66–100% normal dose	Decrease may be necessary in moderate to severe hepatic disease.	Significant (20–49 ml/min)
Prolonged	None	None	None.	Patients with liver dysfunction or biliary obstruction may accumulate drug.	Insignificant
–	Accumulation in renal failure anticipated. Dosage changes with decreasing renal function may be necessary.			None	Slight (67 ml/min)
–	No dosage modification seems necessary.			Accumulation in liver failure would not be anticipated.	–
–	Accumulation of Ara-Hx in renal insufficiency warrants close monitoring and dosage adjustment.			Probably none	–
–	None	50–100% normal dose	25–33% normal dose	None	Insignificant
–	None	25–50% normal dose	10–25% normal dose	None	Significant
–	None	50% normal dose	25% normal dose	None	Significant
–	q8h	q8–12h	q24–48h	None	Significant
–	q8h	q12–24h	q24–48h	None	Significant
–	None	q6–12h	q12–24h	None	Significant
–	None	None	q6–12h	None	Peritoneal dialysis has been shown to remove small amounts.
–	Avoid [←——	Avoid Nephrotoxic	Avoid ——→]	None	Significant
–	None	None	q8–12h	Decrease may be warranted in moderate to severe hepatic disease.	Significant

Table continues on following page.

TABLE 1. ANTIMICROBIAL AGENTS *(Continued)*

Drug	Oral Availability (%)	Protein Binding (%)	Volume of Distribution (L/kg)	Metabolism & Elimination	T 1/2 (hours) Normal	T 1/2 (hours) Anephric
Cephapirin	Not available orally	44–54	0.15–0.50	40–59% hepatic metabolism, active desacetyl metabolite; 40–60% excreted unchanged in urine.	0.5	2.5
Cephradine	90–100	6–20	0.25–0.33	80–95% excreted unchanged in urine.	0.7–1.9	8–15
Chloramphenicol	75–90	25–60	0.57–1.0	85–95% metabolized in liver, inactive glucuronide metabolites may accumulate in ESRD and potentiate bone marrow toxicity; 5–10% excreted unchanged in urine.	2–4	3.5–7
Chloroquine	90	55	Very large	18% hepatic metabolism, activity of metabolites unknown; 39% excreted unchanged in urine, 10% unchanged in feces.	48–53	–
Clindamycin	23–38	60–95	0.61–1.14	85% hepatic metabolism to active and inactive metabolites; 15% excreted unchanged in urine.	2–4	3.5–5
Colistimethate (polymyxin E)	Poor	>75	0.54	25–40% metabolized; renal excretion of unchanged drug, 60–75%.	1.6–8	10–20
Erythromycin	Variable poor to good	70–93	0.5–0.7	Metabolized in liver and inactivated systemically (85–95%) to inactive compounds; renal excretion of unchanged drug 5–15%.	1.5–3	4–6
Lincomycin	30	70–72	0.31–0.60	50–70% hepatic metabolism to inactive compounds; 10–30% excreted unchanged in urine.	4–6.4	10
Methenamine	Good	–	–	10–25% metabolized in liver; 75–90% excreted unchanged in urine.	3–6	–
Metronidazole	Good but variable	20	0.6–0.8	60–70% metabolized in liver; hydroxy metabolite has 30% parent activity and may accumulate in renal failure; 30–40% excreted unchanged in urine.	6–14	8–15
Nalidixic acid	95	90–97	0.26–0.45	80% metabolized in liver to inactive and active metabolites; 10–15% excreted unchanged in urine.	1–2.5	21 (inactive metabolite)
Nitrofurantoin	Good but variable	25–60	0.3–0.7	50–70% metabolized by hepatic mechanisms or body tissues; 30–50% excreted unchanged in urine.	0.3	1
Oxolinic acid	Poor	77–85	–	82% metabolized in liver to active and inactive metabolites; renal excretion of unchanged drug, 1.4%.	6–7	–
Penicillins						
Amoxicillin	50–80	17–25	0.25–0.49	72–88% excreted unchanged renally.	0.5–2.3	7–20

TABLE 1. ANTIMICROBIAL AGENTS *(Continued)*

Liver Disease	Dose Change with Renal Failure GFR (ml/min) >50	10–50	<10	Dose Change with Liver Failure	Effect of Dialysis
–	None	None	q6–12h	Possible decrease in severe hepatic disease.	Significant
–	None	50% normal dose	25% normal dose	None	Significant
12	None	None	None	Decrease	Significant
–	None	None	50% normal dose	–	Insignificant (57 ml/min)
7–14	None	None	None	Decrease necessary in moderate to severe hepatic disease.	Insignificant
–	75–100% normal dose	50–75% normal dose	25–30% normal dose	None	Minimal (10 ml/min)
–	None	None	None	Decrease necessary in patients with moderate to severe hepatic disease.	Insignificant
11.8	q6h	q6–12h	q12–24h	Decrease necessary with moderate to severe hepatic disease.	Slight
–	None	None	Avoid	–	–
		[May produce systemic acidosis in renal insufficiency]			
–	None	q8–12h	q12–24h	Decrease in severe hepatic failure.	Moderate
–	None	None	Avoid	Use with caution in hepatic disease.	Significant (40–80 ml/min)
		[Metabolites may accumulate in renal failure.]			
–	None	Avoid	Avoid	Use with caution in hepatic disease.	Moderate
		[Metabolites can accumulate in renal failure, causing peripheral neuropathy.]			
–	None	None	None	Monitor for accumulation and toxicity.	–
–	None	q6–12h	q12–24h	None	Significant (50%)

Table continues on following page.

TABLE 1. ANTIMICROBIAL AGENTS *(Continued)*

Drug	Oral Availability (%)	Protein Binding (%)	Volume of Distribution (L/kg)	Metabolism & Elimination	T 1/2 (hours) Normal	Anephric
Ampicillin	30–60	18–25	0.17–0.31	76–88% excreted in urine as unchanged drug; some hepatic metabolism.	0.8–1.5	6–20
Carbenicillin	30–40	50–60	0.12–0.20	80% excreted as unchanged drug in the urine; some hepatic metabolism.	1	10–20
Cloxacillin	50	88–96	0.14–0.21	Hepatic metabolism 22%; renal excretion of unchanged drug, 88%.	0.5	0.8
Cyclacillin	40–60	20–25	–	Hepatic metabolism 20–25%; excreted 75–80% as unchanged drug in the urine.	0.5	10
Dicloxacillin	37–74	96–98	0.10–0.20	Hepatic metabolism 10%; renal excretion of unchanged drug, 90%.	0.7	1
Methicillin	Not available orally	17–43	0.31–0.33	Hepatic metabolism 8–10%; excreted 85–88% as unchanged drug in urine.	0.5–1	4
Nafcillin	50	85–90	0.28–0.70	Significant hepatic metabolism, 50–69%; renal excretion of unchanged drug, 31–50%.	0.6	1.2
Oxacillin	33	85–94	0.19–0.41	Significant hepatic metabolism, 50%; renal excretion of both metabolites and unchanged drug, 50%; metabolites are active.	0.4	1
Penicillin G	15–30	45–65	0.47	Renal excretion of 75–90% unchanged drug; some hepatic metabolism.	0.5	6–20
Ticarcillin	Not available orally	45–50	0.14–0.21	Similar to carbenicillin	1	10–20
Polymyxin B	Not available orally	–	–	60% excreted unchanged in urine.	4.5–6	36
Sulfonamides						
Sulfamethoxazole	90–100	60–70	0.14–0.36	65–80% hepatic metabolism to inactive compounds; 20–35% excreted unchanged in urine.	9–11	10–50
Sulfasalazine	10–33	80–95	–	85–98% hepatic metabolism; <15% excreted unchanged in urine.	5.7–10.4	10–40
Sulfisoxazole	100	85	0.13–0.28	46% hepatic metabolism to inactive metabolites; 50% excreted unchanged in urine.	4.5–7	6–12
Tetracyclines						
Doxycycline	90–100	80–93	–	50% metabolized in liver; up to 30% eliminated by chelation in gut; 20–50% excreted unchanged in urine.	15–24	25
Minocycline	90–100	70–75	0.40	87–90% metabolized in liver; <10% excreted in urine as unchanged drug.	12–15	14–30
Tetracycline	77–80	65	1.3–1.6	>30% hepatic metabolism; 50% excreted unchanged in urine.	6–15	7–75

TABLE 1. ANTIMICROBIAL AGENTS *(Continued)*

Liver Disease	Dose Change with Renal Failure *GFR (ml/min)* >50	10–50	<10	Dose Change with Liver Failure	Effect of Dialysis
1.9	None	q6–12h	q12–24h	None	Significant (40–80%)
1.9	q8–12h	q12–24h	q24–48h	None	Significant (20–40%)
Unchanged	None	None	None	None	Insignificant
–	None	[same as ampicillin]		None	Significant (70–80%)
Unchanged	None	None	None	None	Insignificant
–	None	q4–8h	q8–12h	None	Insignificant
1.7	None	None	None	Decrease in severe liver disease.	Insignificant
Possibly prolonged	None	None	None	Possible decrease with severe liver dysfunction.	Insignificant
–	None	q8–12h	q12–18h	None	Significant
–	Same recommendations as for carbenicillin			None	Significant
–	75–100% normal dose	50–75% normal dose	25–30% normal dose	None	Insignificant
–	q12h	q18h	q18–24h	Decrease may be necessary in severe hepatic disease.	Significant (22 ml/min)
–	None	None	None	Decrease in moderate to severe hepatic disease.	–
–	None	q8–12h	q12–24h	Decrease may be necessary in severe hepatic failure.	Moderate
–	None	None	None	Decrease	Insignificant
–	None [May have some antianabolic effects which require dosage interval increases.]	None	None	Decrease	Slight
–	Avoid	Avoid	Avoid	None	Slight

Table continues on following page.

TABLE 1. ANTIMICROBIAL AGENTS (*Concluded*)

Drug	Oral Availability (%)	Protein Binding (%)	Volume of Distribution (L/kg)	Metabolism & Elimination	T 1/2 (hours) Normal	T 1/2 (hours) Anephric
Trimethoprim	85–90	40–70	1.0–2.0	20–35% hepatic metabolism; 65–80% excreted unchanged in urine.	8–16	24–46
Vancomycin	Poor	<10	0.47–0.84	Renal excretion >90% as unchanged drug.	4–8	200–240

TABLE 2. ANALGESICS

Drug	Oral Availability (%)	Protein Binding (%)	Volume of Distribution (L/kg)	Metabolism & Elimination	T 1/2 (hours) Normal	T 1/2 (hours) Anephric
Acetaminophen	60–90	≤21	1.0	Hepatic conjugation with glucuronic and sulfuric acids. The oxidated metabolites via the p-450 microsomes may play a role in hepatotoxicity.	2	Unchanged
Acetylsalicylic acid (salicylate)	90–100	90 (abnormal in hepatic and renal disease)	0.1–0.2	Complete hydrolysis to salicylic acid. Hepatic metabolism to salicyluric acid, gentisic acid, salicyl acyl, and phenolic glucuronide (saturable pathways).	2–19 dose dependent	Unchanged
Codeine	40–70	7	3–4	Primarily hepatic metabolism; 5–17% excreted unchanged.	3.4	–
Dextropropoxyphene	Extensive first-pass metabolism	78	16.0	30–70% first pass; 7% unchanged; hepatic mono *N*-demethylation.	9–15	–
Meperidine	47–71	65–75	3.8	Hepatic hydrolysis and subsequent conjugation and demethylation (normeperdine is active); up to 10% excreted unchanged.	3	–
Methadone	90	71–87	5.0	10–30% eliminated unchanged by the kidneys.	13–55	–
Morphine	20–30	35	3.4	Glucuronide conjugation in liver and GI tract; 10% excreted unchanged.	2.3	–
Pentazocine	Low, significant first-pass effect	60–70	5.0	Hepatic amino acid conjugation; 2–15% excreted unchanged.	2	–

TABLE 1. ANTIMICROBIAL AGENTS (*Concluded*)

Liver Disease	Dose Change with Renal Failure *GFR (ml/min)* >50	10–50	<10	Dose Change with Liver Failure	Effect of Dialysis
–	q12h	q18h	q18–24h	None	Significant
–	q24–72h	q72–240h	q240h	None	Insignificant

TABLE 2. ANALGESICS (*Continued*)

Liver Disease	Dose Change with Renal Failure *GFR (ml/min)* >50	10–50	<10	Dose Change with Liver Failure	Effect of Dialysis
Unchanged	q4h	q4h	q4h	Avoid	Significant
Unchanged	q4h	q4–6h	Avoid	Avoid	Significant
–	q3–4h	q3–4h	q3–4h	Decrease	–
–	q4h	q4h	Avoid	Decrease	Poor
7	q3–4h	q3–4h	q3–4h	Decrease	–
–	q6h	q8h	q8–12h	Decrease	Insignificant
–	q3–4h	q3–4h	q3–4h	Decrease	–
–	q4h	q4h	q4h	Decrease	Significant

TABLE 3. SEDATIVE-HYPNOTICS

Drug	Oral Availability (%)	Protein Binding (%)	Volume of Distribution (L/kg)	Metabolism & Elimination	T 1/2 (hours) Normal	Anephric
Chloral hydrate (trichloroethanol)	Complete	35–40	1.6	Hepatic oxidation and glucuronide conjugation.	7–14	–
Chlordiazepoxide	100	94–97	0.3–0.5	Extensive hepatic metabolism via *N*-desmethylation and hydroxylation to active compounds.	5–30	–
Diazepam	100	94–98	0.7–2.6	Hepatic *N*-demethylation and hydroxylation (active metabolites).	20–90	–
Ethchlorvynol	Good	35–50	3–4	Hepatic oxidation and glucuronide conjugation.	19–32	–
Flurazepam	Good	–	–	Hepatic hydroxylation and dealkylation (active metabolite).	47–100 (desalkyl metabolite)	–
Glutethimide	Variable	54	2.7	Extensive hepatic metabolism, active 4-hydroxy metabolite.	5–22	–
Hexobarbital	–	42–52	1.1	Complete hepatic biotransformation.	3.7	–
Lorazepam	Complete	90	1.3	Glucuronide conjugation in the liver.	9–16	Unchanged
Meprobamate	Good	0–20	0.75	8–19% excreted unchanged and hepatic biotransformation.	6–17	–
Methaqualone	Complete	80	5–8	Hepatic biotransformation; 2% excreted unchanged by kidney.	10–43	–
Oxazepam	Complete	90	1.6	Extensive glucuronide conjugation in the liver.	6–25	Unchanged
Pentobarbital	Complete	60–70	1.0	Hepatic oxidation (hydroxylation); <1% excreted unchanged.	18–48	Unchanged
Phenobarbital (see Table 9)						
Thiopental	Parenteral only	72–86	–	Hepatic biotransformation.	3.8	–

TABLE 4. ANTIHYPERTENSIVE AGENTS

Drug	Oral Availability (%)	Protein Binding (%)	Volume of Distribution (L/kg)	Metabolism & Elimination	T 1/2 (hours) Normal	Anephric
Clonidine	80	20	3	Renal 50%	7–12	24
Guanethidine	3–50	0	–	Renal 50%; hepatic 50%	120–140	–
Hydralazine	10–30	90	1.6	Active metabolites – renal and hepatic	2–3	Prolonged metabolites
Methyldopa	25	<20	0.3	Renal 50–70%; liver 30–50%	2–3	6
Minoxidil	100	Very little	2.8	Mainly hepatic; small fraction renal	4.2	4.2
Prazosin	80	97	1.1	Mainly hepatic	2.5–4	Unchanged
Reserpine	Incomplete	–	–	Mainly hepatic	46–168	Unchanged

TABLE 3. SEDATIVE-HYPNOTICS *(Continued)*

Liver Disease	Dose Change with Renal Failure GFR (ml/min) >50	10–50	<10	Dose Change with Liver Failure	Effect of Dialysis
–	q24h	Avoid	Avoid	Decrease	Significant
63	q6–8h	q6–8h	q6–8h	Decrease	Poor
105–164	q8h	q8h	q8h	Decrease	Poor
–	q24h	Avoid	Avoid	Decrease	Slight
–	q24h	q24h	q24h	Decrease	Probably poor
–	q24h	Avoid	Avoid	Decrease	Poor
5–13	q8h	q8h	q8h	Decrease	–
28–41	q8h	q8h	q8h	None	–
32	q6h	q9–12h	q12–18h	Decrease	Moderate
–	q24h	Avoid	Avoid	Decrease	Slight
Unchanged	q8h	q8h	q8h	None	–
–	q8–24h	q8–24h	q8–24h	Decrease	Slight
–	None	None	Slight decrease	Decrease	Probably poor

TABLE 4. ANTIHYPERTENSIVE AGENTS *(Continued)*

Liver Disease	Dose Change with Renal Failure GFR (ml/min) >50	10–50	<10	Dose Change with Liver Failure	Effect of Dialysis
–	Decrease	Decrease	Decrease	Probably decrease	None
–	None	Decrease	Decrease	Probably decrease	None
–	Decrease ←— Accumulation of active metabolites	Decrease	Decrease —→	Decrease	Unpredictable
–	None ←— Active metabolite in brain	None	None —→	Avoid	Significant
–	None	None	None	Probably decrease	None
–	None	None	None	Probably decrease	Probably none
–	None	None	None	Probably decrease	None

TABLE 5. DIURETICS

Drug	Oral Availability (%)	Protein Binding (%)	Volume of Distribution (L/kg)	Metabolism & Elimination	T 1/2 (hours)	
					Normal	*Anephric*
Chlorthalidone	~50	98 (bound to RBCs)	3–13	Renal 50%	51	100
Ethacrynic acid	~100	95	0.1	Renal and hepatic	1	Prolonged
Furosemide	50–100	91–99	0.07–0.18	Renal 60–70%; hepatic 30–40%	0.5–1	Prolonged
Hydrochlorothiazide	~50–80	95	1.5	Mainly renal	2.5	24
Mercurials	Poor	0	–	Renal	2–3	>16
Metolazone	~50–80	95	1.6	Mainly renal	8–15	Prolonged
Spironolactone	~90	98 (for active metabolite canrenone)	–	Renal and hepatic for canrenone	16 (metabolite)	Prolonged
Triamterene	40–70	50	2–3	Mainly hepatic; renal 5%	2	Probably unchanged

TABLE 6. ANTIARRHYTHMICS AND CARDIAC GLYCOSIDES

Drug	Oral Availability (%)	Protein Binding (%)	Volume of Distribution (L/kg)	Metabolism & Elimination	T 1/2 (hours)	
					Normal	*Anephric*
Bretylium	–	–	–	80% excreted unchanged in urine.	4–17	31.5
Digitoxin	Complete	90–97	0.4–0.7	Primarily hepatic metabolism.	168–192	200
Digoxin	55–90	20–40	5.1–7.4	70% unchanged in urine.	30–40	87–100
Disopyramide	80–85	30–70	1.29	52% excreted unchanged; 16% first pass hepatic *N*-dealkylation	4.5–8.2	43
Lidocaine	Poor; parenteral only	60–65	0.8–2	2–3% excreted unchanged in urine; hepatic metabolites (MEGX + GX) are active.	1.3–2.3	1.3–2.5
Phenytoin (See Table 9)						
Procainamide	75–90	15	2.2	50–60% excreted unchanged in urine; hepatic actetylation to NAPA, active metabolite.	2.2–4	9–16
Propranolol	Low; saturable first-pass metabolism	95	3.9	Extensive hepatic metabolism	4	2–3.2
Quinidine	40–90	80–90 (altered in hypoalbuminemic condition – cirrhosis)	3	10–27% excreted unchanged; hepatic hydroxylation; active metabolites.	3–16	3–16
Verapimil	Complete	90	6.5	Hepatic metabolism, possibly active metabolites; majority excreted unchanged in urine.	3–7	–

TABLE 5. DIURETICS *(Continued)*

Liver Disease	Dose Change with Renal Failure GFR (ml/min) >50	10–50	<10	Dose Change with Liver Failure	Effect of Dialysis
–	None	← Probably ineffective →		None	None
–	Avoid	Avoid	Avoid	Probably decrease	None
–	None	None	None	Probably decrease	None
	←Will require more drug to achieve diuresis→				
–	None	← Probably ineffective →		None	None
–	Avoid	Avoid	Avoid	None	None
–	None	None	None	None	None
		← May require more drug to achieve diuresis →			
–	Decrease	Avoid	Avoid	Probably none	None
–	None	Avoid	Avoid	Decrease	None

TABLE 6. ANTIARRHYTHMICS AND CARDIAC GLYCOSIDES *(Continued)*

Liver Disease	Dose Change with Renal Failure GFR (ml/min) >50	10–50	<10	Dose Change with Liver Failure	Effect of Dialysis
–	q8h	q24–48h	Avoid	–	Significant
Unchanged	None	None	None	None	Insignificant
Unchanged	Unchanged	50% decrease	50–75% decrease	None	Insignificant
–	q6h	q12–24h	q24–48h	–	Significant
5	None	None	None	Normal loading dose and 1/2 infusion rate	Probably minimal
–	q3–6h	q6–12h	q12–24h	–	Significant
Prolonged	None	None	None	Significant decrease	Insignificant
–	None	None	None	–	Probably poor
–	← Careful use in renal failure because of possibility of active metabolite accumulation. →			–	Probably poor

TABLE 7. DRUGS USED IN GOUT, ARTHRITIS, AND INFLAMMATORY DISEASES

Drug	Oral Availability (%)	Protein Binding (%)	Volume of Distribution (L/kg)	Metabolism & Elimination	T 1/2 (hours) Normal	Anephric
Allopurinol	Good	0 (Allopurinol and oxipurinol)	Similar to total body water	Renal excretion; mainly active metabolite, oxipurinol, and allopurinol (<10%).	Allopurinol 0.7 Oxipurinol 14	Prolonged
Aurothiomalate sodium	Poor	95	–	Renal (major) and fecal; per cent excreted increases with cumulative dose.	143 (Serum)	–
Colchicine	–	0	2.2	Partly eliminated by renal excretion; some hepatic deacetylation.	0.3	0.7
Fenoprofen	>80	99	0.13–0.16	Hepatic metabolism; renal excretion of inactive metabolites and <5% unchanged drug.	1.5–2.9	–
Ibuprofen	–	99	–	Hepatic metabolism; renal excretion of inactive metabolites and <2% unchanged drug.	2	–
Indomethacin	98	90–99	0.3–1.6	Hepatic metabolism to inactive metabolites; renal and biliary excretion, 15% unchanged in urine.	2–11	2 (unchanged)
Naproxen	Complete	99.5	0.09	Hepatic metabolism; renal excretion of inactive metabolites and 10% unchanged drug.	12–15	Unchanged
Penicillamine	–	–	–	Renal excretion of metabolites.	–	–
Phenylbutazone	Good	87–99 (decreased in renal and hepatic disease)	0.09–0.17	Hepatic metabolism; renal excretion, 1% unchanged and 23% active metabolites.	40–140	27–96
Prednisone, (prednisolone, active moiety)	80–90	50–60 (high levels); 80–90 (low levels)	0.4–1	Hepatic metabolism; renal excretion of metabolites and 12–26% unchanged prednisolone; concentration-dependent kinetics.	2.5–3.5	Unchanged
Probenecid	Good	83–94	–	Renal excretion: active metabolites and 4–13% unchanged drug.	3–17 (dose-dependent)	–
Sulindac	>88	93 (sulindac); 98 (sulfide)	–	Metabolized to active sulfide and inactive metabolites; renal excretion: sulfide–none; sulindac–20%.	1.5–3.0 (sulindac) 18 (sulfide)	–

TABLE 7. DRUGS USED IN GOUT, ARTHRITIS, AND INFLAMMATORY DISEASES *(Continued)*

Liver Disease	Dose Change with Renal Failure *GFR (ml/min)* >50	10–50	<10	Dose Change with Liver Failure	Effect of Dialysis
–	300 mg/d (Oxipurinol accumulates with GFR < 40 ml/min)	200 mg/d	100 mg/d	–	Oxipurinol dialyzed as well as creatinine and uric acid.
–	None	Avoid	Avoid	–	Probably minimal
0.2	None	← Avoid prolonged use →		None	Probably minimal
–	None	None	None	–	Probably insignificant
–	None	None	None	–	Probably insignificant
–	None	None	None	–	Probably minimal
–	None	None	None	–	Naproxen not dialyzed; desmethyl metabolite is dialyzed.
–	None	Avoid	Avoid	–	–
40–149	None	None	Avoid	None	Probably minimal
3.5	None	None	None	None	Minimal
–	None	Avoid	Avoid	None	–
–	None	None	Start at half normal dose.	–	Probably insignificant

TABLE 8. IMMUNOSUPPRESSIVE AND ANTINEOPLASTIC DRUGS

Drug	Oral Availability (%)	Protein Binding (%)	Volume of Distribution (L/kg)	Metabolism & Elimination	T 1/2 (hours) Normal	Anephric
Adriamycin	Poor	50	1–4	Extensive hepatic metabolism; 10–30% renal excretion: 1/2 as unchanged drug, 1/2 as metabolites.	α–1 β–16 to 24	Unchanged
Azathioprine (6-mercaptopurine)	23–100	30	0.8 (AZA)	Extensive hepatic metabolism; 50–70% renal excretion, 80% as inactive thiouric acid and 20% as unchanged drug.	0.16 (AZA) 1 (6-MP)	Slightly prolonged
Bleomycin	Poor	0	0.2–0.4	Some metabolism by liver, kidney, and tumor tissue; 50–80% renal excretion.	2	Prolonged
Busulfan	Good	–	Large	Extensive metabolism probably in liver; 25–35% renal excretion as metabolic products.	Long	–
cis-Platinum	Poor	70–95	0.5	Some metabolism; 30–50% renal excretion, 1/2 as unchanged drug, 1/2 as metabolites.	α–0.4–0.8 β–58–73	Prolonged
Cyclophosphamide	75	0–15 (40–70 metabolites)	0.5–1.0 (0.5 metabolites)	Extensive hepatic metabolism to active and inactive metabolites; renal excretion, 5–20% unchanged drug, 60% as metabolites.	3–10	Prolonged
Cytosine arabinoside	Poor	13	2–3	Extensive metabolism in many tissues to inactive uracil arabinoside; >70% renal excretion: 10% as unchanged drug, rest as uracil arabinoside.	α–0.1 β–2.3	Unchanged
5-Fluorouracil	Poor	–	0.5	Metabolism in liver and other tissues to active and inactive metabolites. Most eliminated as CO_2, some renal excretion.	0.1	Unchanged
Melphalan	Poor	30–80	0.7	Metabolized to mono- and dihydroxy metabolites; 70% renal excretion, primarily as metabolites.	2	–
Methotrexate	Good at <30 mg/m^2; incomplete at >80 mg/m^2.	50	0.3–0.8	Hepatic metabolism 5–15% to 7-OH metabolite; renal excretion >80% as unchanged drug.	α–0.1 β–2.3 γ–10–30	Prolonged
Mithramycin	Poor	–	–	Renal excretion 10–30%; remainder in stool.	α–0.1 β–several hours	–
Nitrosoureas	Good	–	–	Some hepatic metabolism, some metabolites active; 30–60% renal excretion as metabolic products.	Very short	–
Streptozotocin	Poor	–	0.5	Metabolism 30–50%; rapid renal excretion of 10–20% of unchanged drug; later, renal excretion of metabolites.	0.25	–
Vinblastine	Poor	80	1–15	Some hepatic metabolism with biliary excretion of metabolites; renal excretion 10–20% and 10–35% in stool.	α–0.1 β–2.4 γ–60	–
Vincristine	Poor	–	1	Substantial hepatic metabolism, 60–80% in stool via biliary excretion. Renal excretion 10–20%.	α–0.1 β–2.3	–

TABLE 8. IMMUNOSUPPRESSIVE AND ANTINEOPLASTIC DRUGS *(Continued)*

Liver Disease	Dose Change with Renal Failure *GFR (ml/min)* >50	10–50	<10	Dose Change with Liver Failure	Effect of Dialysis
Prolonged	None	None	Slight decrease	Bilirubin >3.0. 75% reduction. Bilirubin <2.0–3.0, 50% reduction.	–
Slightly prolonged	None	None	Slight decrease	Liver failure predisposes to azathioprine and 6-MP hepatotoxicity. Azathioprine less effective with liver disease.	Significant
–	None	Probably decrease	Decrease	None	Minimal
–	None	None	Probably none	Probably none	–
Unchanged	None	Decrease	Decrease	None	–
Prolonged	None	None	Probably decrease	Slight decrease	Dialysis clearance of 78 ml/min.
Unchanged	None	None	Probably decrease	None	–
? Slightly prolonged	None	None	None	Slight decrease	Significant
–	None	None	None or slight decrease	Unchanged	–
–	None ← Use with caution due to nephrotoxicity →	Decrease	Decrease	Unchanged; use with caution because of hepatotoxicity.	Peritoneal removal negligible. Hemodialysis clearances of 40–70 ml/min. Charcoal clearances of 40–140 ml/min.
–	None	← Unknown; use with caution due to nephrotoxicity →		Unknown; use with caution due to hepatotoxic potential.	–
–	None	← Unknown; will induce chronic renal failure →		Unknown; use with caution due to hepatotoxic potential.	–
–	None ← Use with caution due to nephrotoxic potential →	None	Decrease	Slight decrease. Use with caution due to hepatotoxic potential.	–
Probably prolonged	None	None	None or slight decrease	Slight decrease	–
Probably prolonged	None	None	None of slight decrease	Slight decrease	–

TABLE 9. DRUGS USED IN NEUROLOGY AND PSYCHIATRY

Drug	Oral Availability (%)	Protein Binding (%)	Volume of Distribution (L/kg)	Metabolism & Elimination	T 1/2 (hours) Normal	T 1/2 (hours) Anephric
Anticholinesterases Neostigmine–N Pyridostigmine–P	Poor	Negligible	N–1.1–1.4 P–1.1	Extensive metabolism; renal excretion: unchanged drug (greater % after parenteral than oral doses) and metabolites, some active.	N–0.9–1.3 P–1.5–4.3	N–3 P–5.1–10.3
Carbamazepine	70, variable	70–80	0.8–1.4	Extensive liver metabolism; renal excretion: 1–2% unchanged, 2% active epoxide metabolite and other metabolites.	19–55 (single dose); 9–21 (chronic doses in epileptics)	–
Ethosuximide	Complete	Negligible	0.6–0.7	Primarily metabolized; renal excretion: 12–22% unchanged and inactive metabolites.	53–66 (adults) 25–42 (children)	–
Haloperidol	44–74	90–92	14–21	Extensive hepatic metabolism; renal excretion: 1% unchanged and mostly inactive metabolites.	10–36	–
Levodopa	Good	5–8	0.65	Extensive metabolism; metabolites (active and inactive) excreted in urine.	0.8–1.6	–
Lithium	100	0	0.5–0.9	Not metabolized; >90% excreted unchanged in urine.	14–28	Prolonged
Phenobarbital	Good	40–56	0.7–1	Hepatic metabolism; renal excretion: 10–40% unchanged (depending on urine flow and pH) and inactive metabolites.	60–150	–
Phenothiazines (e.g., chlorpromazine)	Variable, first-pass metabolism	91–99	7–9	Extensive hepatic metabolism; renal excretion: active and inactive metabolites, <1% unchanged.	11–42	–
Phenytoin	80–95	85–95 (decreased in renal and hepatic disease)	0.5–0.7 (increased in uremia)	Extensive hepatic metabolism, renal excretion of unchanged drug (<5%) and inactive metabolites.	10–30 (concentration-dependent)	6–11
Tricyclic antidepressants (e.g., nortriptyline)	Variable, first-pass metabolism	93–95	17–27	Extensive hepatic metabolism; renal excretion: ≤ 5% unchanged and various metabolites, some active.	12–56	–
Trimethadione (TMO)	–	0 (TMO and DMO)	0.6 for TMO (similar for DMO)	Hepatic demethylation to dimethadione (DMO); renal excretion: ≤ 4% TMO, rest as DMO; both active.	16 (TMO) 100–350 (DMO)	–
Valproic acid	100	89–93	0.1–0.2	Extensive hepatic metabolism; renal excretion: metabolites (some active) and 2–3% unchanged drug.	10–15	–

TABLE 9. DRUGS USED IN NEUROLOGY AND PSYCHIATRY *(Continued)*

Liver Disease	DOSE CHANGE WITH RENAL FAILURE *GFR (ml/min)* >50	10–50	<10	DOSE CHANGE WITH LIVER FAILURE	EFFECT OF DIALYSIS
–	None	None	50% decrease with parenteral, less with oral.	–	–
–	None	None	None	–	–
–	None	None	Slight decrease	–	–
–	None	None	None	None or slight decrease; use with caution.	Probably insignificant
–	None ←Titrate to desired effect→	None	None	–	–
–	None or slight decrease	Avoid	Avoid	None	Significant; rebound rise in plasma levels post dialysis.
Prolonged (cirrhosis, 100–208); unchanged (acute viral hepatitis, 60–134)	None	None	Minimal decrease; titrate with clinical response.	Moderate decrease in severe liver dysfunction, use with caution.	Significant
24	None	None	None or slight decrease	Slight decrease; use with caution.	Not significant; no data on metabolites
Unchanged–acute viral hepatitis, 7–24	None	None	None	None in most cases; severe liver failure may need decrease.	Insignificant
–	None	None	None	Slight decrease; use with caution.	Not significant; no data on metabolites
–	None	Avoid	Avoid	–	–
13–28	None	None	Slight decrease	Slight to moderate decrease	–

TABLE 10. HYPOGLYCEMIC AGENTS

Drug	Oral Availability (%)	Protein Binding (%)	Volume of Distribution (L/kg)	Metabolism & Elimination	T 1/2 (hours) Normal	T 1/2 (hours) Anephric
Acetohexamide	Good	>84–89	Extracellular fluid space	Extensive hepatic metabolism; renal excretion: active metabolites (hydroxyhexamide) and some unchanged drug.	0.4–2.4 (2–8 hydroxyhexamide)	Prolonged
Chlorpropamide	Good	72–96	0.14–0.18	Hepatic metabolism; renal excretion: ~25% unchanged drug; active and inactive metabolites.	25–42	Prolonged
Insulin	Poor, parenteral only	Negligible	0.2–0.3	Primarily liver metabolism, some renal clearance.	0.08–0.25	Prolonged
Tolazamide	Good	94	–	Extensive metabolism; renal excretion: active and inactive metabolites, ~5% unchanged drug.	7	–
Tolbutamide	93	90–99	0.10–0.18	Extensive hepatic metabolism; renal excretion: <5% unchanged; inactive and less active metabolites.	4–8	3–9

TABLE 11. MISCELLANEOUS DRUGS

Drug	Oral Availability (%)	Protein Binding (%)	Volume of Distribution (L/kg)	Metabolism & Elimination	T 1/2 (hours) Normal	T 1/2 (hours) Anephric
Cimetidine	60–75	13–26	0.45–1.15	Renal excretion: 40–80% unchanged, and metabolites.	1.4–2.4	3–10
Clofibrate (data for chlorphenoxyisobutyric acid, the active metabolite)	95	92–98 (decreased in renal failure and cirrhosis)	0.11–0.17 (increased in uremia and cirrhosis)	Primarily metabolized; renal excretion: 10–20% unchanged, and conjugated metabolites.	12–25	50–175
Diphenhydramine	26–60	98	3.3	Extensively metabolized; renal excretion: <4% unchanged and metabolites.	3–8	–
Heparin	Poor, Parenteral only	Extensive	0.04–0.07	Liver metabolism and reticuloendothelial system uptake.	1–2	Unchanged or slightly prolonged
Propantheline	Poor	–	–	Primarily metabolized; renal excretion: 1–17% unchanged, and metabolites.	2.2–3.7	–
Propylthiouracil	50–90	80	0.3–0.4	Primarily metabolized, 1–3% excreted unchanged in urine.	1–2	–
Theophylline	96–99	53–72 (decreased in cirrhosis)	0.3–0.7	Extensive hepatic metabolism; renal excretion: 7–13% unchanged, and metabolites.	3–12	–
Warfarin	93	97–99 (decreased in uremia)	0.09–0.16	Extensive hepatic metabolism; renal excretion: <1% unchanged, and inactive and less active metabolites.	15–87	21–43

TABLE 10. HYPOGLYCEMIC AGENTS (Continued)

Liver Disease	Dose Change with Renal Failure GFR (ml/min) >50	10–50	<10	Dose Change with Liver Failure	Effect of Dialysis
–	Slight decrease	Avoid	Avoid	Caution (hepatic damage reported)	Peritoneal dialysis – insignificant; hemodialysis – no data.
	← Prolonged hypoglycemia →				
–	Slight decrease	Avoid	Avoid	Caution (jaundice reported)	Peritoneal dialysis – insignificant; hemodialysis – no data.
	← Prolonged hypoglycemia →				
–	← Decreases required as renal function declines →			Titrate with blood sugar	Probably insignificant
–	Slight decrease	Avoid	Avoid	–	–
	← Prolonged hypoglycemia →				
3–7	None	None	None	None	Insignificant
	← Drug of choice in renal failure →				

TABLE 11. MISCELLANEOUS DRUGS (Continued)

Liver Disease	Dose Change with Renal Failure GFR (ml/min) >50	10–50	<10	Dose Change with Liver Failure	Effect of Dialysis
–	300 mg/6hrs	300 mg/8hrs	300 mg/12hrs	None	Some hemodialysis clearance; coincide doses after dialysis.
15–31 (acute hepatitis); 11–30 (cirrhosis)	None or slight decrease	50–75% decrease	90% decrease (1–1.5 g/wk)	None, acute hepatitis; 50% decrease, cirrhosis	Insignificant
–	None	None	None or slight decrease	–	Probably negligible
1.3	None	None	None	None	Insignificant
–	None	None	None or slight decrease	–	–
–	None	None	None	–	–
10–59 (cirrhosis)	None	None	None	Decrease by 50% or more	Significant hemodialysis and hemoperfusion removal
17–29 (acute viral hepatitis)	None	None	None	None	Probably insignificant
	← Caution: pre-existing altered hemostasis →				

Index

Numbers in *italics* refer to illustrations; numbers followed by (t) refer to tables.